ACL Injury and Its Treatment

Mitsuo Ochi • Konsei Shino • Kazunori Yasuda •
Masahiro Kurosaka
Editors

ACL Injury and Its Treatment

Springer

Editors
Mitsuo Ochi
Hiroshima University
Hiroshima
Japan

Konsei Shino
Sports Orthopaedic Center
Yukioka Hospital
Osaka
Japan

Kazunori Yasuda
Graduate School of Medicine
Hokkaido University
Sapporo
Japan

Masahiro Kurosaka
Graduate School of Medicine
Kobe University
Kobe
Japan

ISBN 978-4-431-55856-9 ISBN 978-4-431-55858-3 (eBook)
DOI 10.1007/978-4-431-55858-3

Library of Congress Control Number: 2016941930

Printed on acid-free paper

This Springer imprint is published by Springer Nature
The registered company is Springer Japan KK

Foreword

Anterior cruciate ligament (ACL) rupture is one of the most frequent orthopaedic sports-related injuries. An ACL injury can be devastating, particularly for a young athlete where high-level participation in strenuous sports is usually not possible without surgical reconstruction of the ACL. Furthermore, the long-term development of knee osteoarthritis is common. It is therefore extremely important to continue to develop new approaches to reconstruct the ACL, striving to provide patients with the best potential for a successful outcome, aiming to maintain both long-term knee health and quality of life.

Historically, ACL reconstruction was performed via an arthrotomy, with the goal to reproduce the native anatomy of the ACL. However, as with all modern surgery, minimally invasive surgical techniques were introduced in knee surgery, which subsequently led to the development of arthroscopically assisted ACL reconstruction. Arthroscopic ACL reconstruction was first performed using a two-incision and later a one-incision technique. Both techniques were fast and efficient, but unfortunately neither was consistent with respect to reproducing the native ACL anatomy. Surgeons attempting to learn the new, minimally invasive arthroscopic techniques characterized the early 1990s. However, the major advancements made with the introduction of arthroscopic ACL surgery were partially offset by new problems. Most of these problems pertained to the failure to restore anatomy.

Although ACL anatomy was described in detail as early as 1836 by Weber and Weber, the initial arthroscopic ACL reconstruction techniques did not accurately reproduce this native anatomy. For example, the Weber brothers described two functional bundles of the ACL, but the proposed techniques to reconstruct the ACL restored only one bundle. It was not until the 1990s that an arthroscopic method for double-bundle ACL reconstruction was described and popularized in Japan, under the direction of great pioneers such as Prof. Muneta as well as Prof. Yasuda, Prof. Ochi, Prof. Shino and Prof. Kurosaka. The efforts of these leaders in the field allowed us to take a more critical look at ACL anatomy.

These great surgeons, together with an excellent panel of their peers, have put together this outstanding book which presents detailed information on surgically relevant anatomy and histology of the ACL, biomechanics, diagnostics, surgery and rehabilitation. The anatomy section describes in detail the location and shape of the ACL insertion site, the orientation of its fibres and the double-bundle principle. In addition, it presents a summary of macroscopic anatomy as well as histological observations and addresses the presence of mechanoreceptors within the ACL. In the biomechanical section, the authors address the function of the normal ACL as well as how knee biomechanics are altered after a partial or complete ACL injury. The importance of the ACL remnant is also discussed here, which forms the basis for an individualized approach to reconstruction including augmentation and remnant preserving techniques. The biomechanics and kinematics of single- and multi-bundle ACL reconstruction are also presented in a concise and clinically relevant fashion.

Furthermore, the authors discuss in detail the importance of the history, physical examination and various imaging modalities used in the diagnosis and treatment of ACL injuries including MRI and 3D CT scan. Various important surgical nuances are addressed including graft selection, portal placement, the use of navigation, tunnel placement, graft tensioning protocols and fixation methods.

Finally, and perhaps most importantly, this book offers future perspectives. With the recent increase in interest for biologics in orthopaedic surgery such as platelet rich plasma, the authors offer strategies to enhance biological tendon-bone healing. In addition they offer a tissue engineering approach to ACL healing. Innovation is great thing. Like these Japanese leaders, we must never be afraid to learn from our past and seek improvement through our prior mistakes. For the future, the focus of ACL surgery will be on encouraging such innovation as displayed in this book and improve outcome measures to assess these new techniques.

This book is a must-read for orthopaedic surgeons as well as physical therapists specializing in ACL reconstruction. As medical professionals we must strive to continuously improve in an attempt to restore nature, replicate native anatomy and provide our patients with the best potential for a successful outcome. Congratulations to the editors: Prof. Ochi, Prof. Shino, Prof. Yasuda and Prof. Kurosaka on this incredible accomplishment. I continue to be a humble, dedicated student of these great Japanese masters.

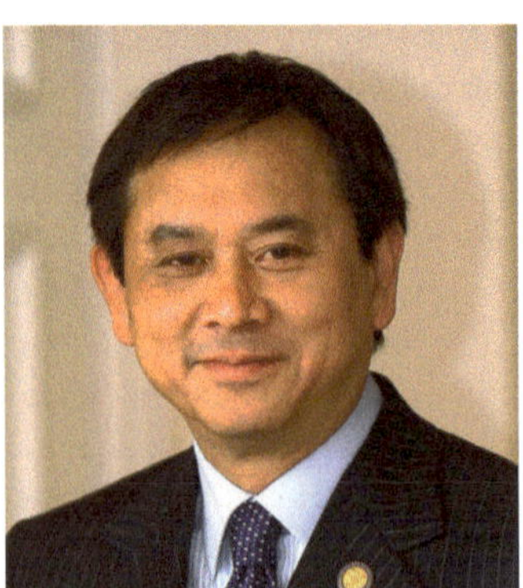

Distinguished Service Professor
University of Pittsburgh
David Silver Professor and Chairman
Department of Orthopaedic Surgery
University of Pittsburgh School of Medicine
Head Team Physician
University of Pittsburgh Department of Athletics

Freddie H. Fu, MD, D.Sc. (Hon.), D.Ps. (Hon.)

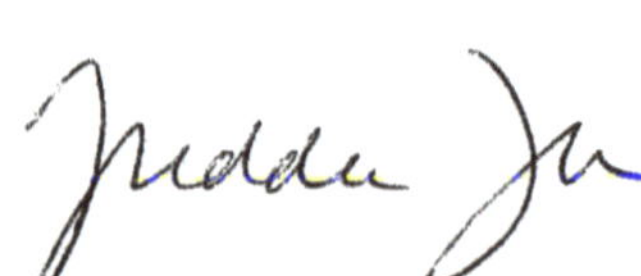

Preface

The anterior cruciate ligament (ACL) of the knee is one of the most frequently injured ligaments encountered in the field of orthopaedic sports medicine. Rupture of the ACL is a common, serious and costly injury; it is a critical event in a career, especially for top athletes, because ACL injuries usually require reconstructive surgery and many months of rehabilitation. Reconstruction of a ruptured ACL has become a common surgical treatment, and the surgical technique has evolved significantly over the last 30 years. More than 15 years ago, the gold standard for ACL reconstruction was the non-anatomic single-bundle technique. However, several reports estimated that as many as 10–20 % of patients had persistent pain and rotational instability even after the surgery. Therefore, interest in anatomic ACL reconstruction has been growing because of its higher potential to restore knee kinematics. Over the past few years, an emerging body of evidence has shown the importance of anatomic ACL reconstruction. Several biomechanical studies have demonstrated the advantage of anatomic multiple-bundle reconstruction over conventional single-bundle reconstruction. Anatomic multiple-bundle ACL reconstruction can mimic more closely the normal structure of the ACL. However, some studies show that even central anatomic single-bundle ACL reconstruction can restore normal knee function. In addition, several recent studies demonstrated the superiority of the anatomic rectangular tunnel technique with a bone–patellar tendon–bone graft. Although the optimal surgical methods for ACL injury have been controversial, it has been established that ACL reconstruction should be anatomic.

Many Japanese orthopaedic surgeons have performed great feats in the field of arthroscopy. Professor Masaki Watanabe is considered the founder of modern arthroscopy. Professor Watanabe developed the first practical arthroscope. In 1974, the International Arthroscopy Association was established and Professor Watanabe was appointed the first president of the organization. He was also awarded the title "Father of Arthroscopy". In addition, the superiority of multiple-bundle ACL reconstruction was first presented and discussed heatedly by Japanese surgeons, and Professor Freddie Fu has continuously advertised the merits of double-bundle ACL reconstruction. Moreover, several current topics including the anatomy of normal ACL, quantitative measurement of the pivot shift test and ACL augmentation (remnant-preserving ACL reconstruction) technique have become major hot topics of debate because many experimental and clinical studies have been performed by orthopaedic surgeons in our society (JOSKAS: Japanese Orthopaedic Society of Knee, Arthroscopy and Sports Medicine). Therefore, we decided to publish a book on ACL injury and its treatment in order to provide ACL surgeons in the world with the contents of the intense discussion in our society.

ACL Injury and Its Treatment provides an update on a wide variety of hot topics in the field of ACL. This book describes the latest information on the surgically relevant anatomy and histology of the ACL, biomechanics, diagnostics and ACL reconstruction. In addition, the book includes information on the future of ACL reconstruction based on the recent experimental study on the treatment of ACL injury. We would like to sincerely thank all the authors for their excellent contributions to this book. Additionally, we wish to acknowledge Dr. Atsuo Nakamae, who has helped with this project. It is our sincere hope that the book will be of interest to its readers and will serve as an educational tool to increase their knowledge of ACL in order to support their treatment decisions and to improve patient care.

Hiroshima, Japan — Mitsuo Ochi
Osaka, Japan — Konsei Shino
Sapporo, Japan — Kazunori Yasuda
Kobe, Japan — Masahiro Kurosaka

Contents

About the Editors

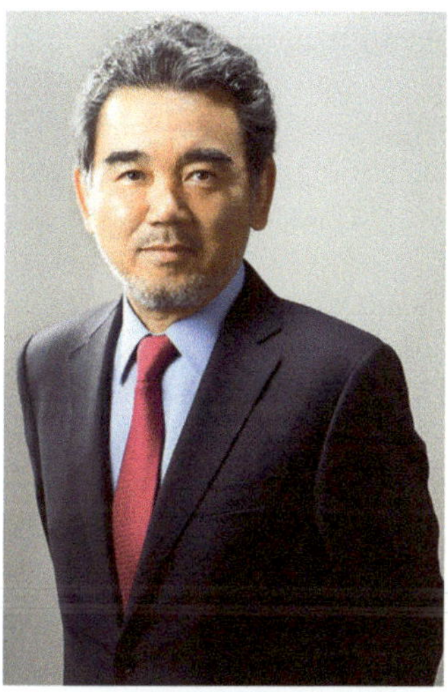

Mitsuo Ochi is currently the president of Hiroshima University. He received the John Joyce Award in 1993 and 2005 for his clinical work on knee surgeries and basic research on cartilage, ligaments and the meniscus. In 1996, he successfully performed the world's first clinical trial of second-generation ACI. Clinical trials of a less-invasive technique using magnets are already under way. Prof. Ochi has served as the first president of the Japanese Orthopaedic Society of Knee, Arthroscopy and Sports Medicine (JOSKAS) since 2009 and was appointed as the first president of the Asia-Pacific Knee, Arthroscopy and Sports Medicine Society (APKASS) from January 2013 to December 2014.

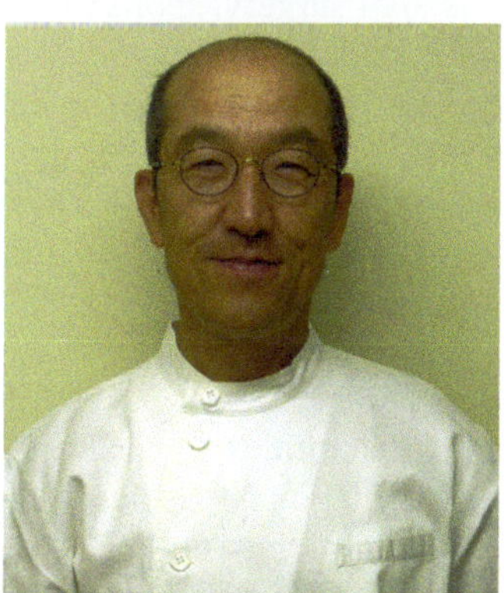

Konsei Shino is the head of the Sports Orthopaedic Center at Yukioka Hospital, Osaka, Japan. He was a pioneer in allograft ligament surgery in the last century. Currently, he is well known as a pioneer of anatomical ACL reconstructions including rectangular tunnel BTB or triple bundle hamstring tendon procedures. He developed several medical devices including the DSP (double spike plate) for those procedures. He has been honoured with three John Joyce Awards and two Albert Trillat Awards by the International Society of Arthroscopy, Knee Surgery and Orthopaedic Sports Medicine (ISAKOS), the Porto Award by the European Society for Sports Traumatology, Knee Surgery and Arthroscopy

(ESSKA), the Watanabe Award by the Japanese Orthopaedic Society of Knee, Arthroscopy and Sports Medicine (JOSKAS) and the Takagi–Watanabe Award by the Asia-Pacific Knee, Arthroscopy and Sports Medicine Society (APKASS). Also, he was elected as an honorary member by the Arthroscopy Association of North America (AANA) and ISAKOS.

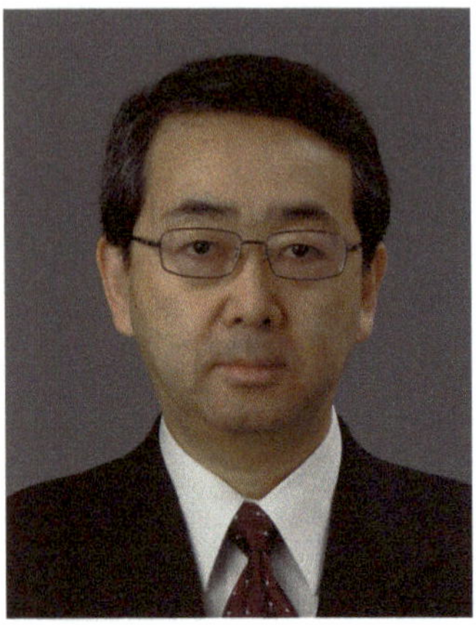

Kazunori Yasuda is the executive/vice-president of Hokkaido University, Sapporo, Japan. He has an MD degree (awarded in 1976) and a PhD degree (in 1985) from Hokkaido University. He has been a professor in and the chairman of the Department of Sports Medicine, Hokkaido University Graduate School of Medicine since 1997. Dr. Yasuda has performed a number of basic and clinical research projects in the field of sports medicine and knee joint surgery in the past 35 years. Specifically, concerning the anterior cruciate ligament, he has published approximately 100 scientific papers, which have been cited 3200 times. He has contributed to the Japanese Orthopaedic Society of Knee, Arthroscopy and Sports Medicine (JOSKAS) and the International Society of Arthroscopy, Knee Surgery and Orthopaedic Sports Medicine (ISAKOS) as president, executive, member at large, program chair and in other positions. He is now an editorial board member of several international journals, including *the American Journal of Sports Medicine*, *Arthroscopy* and *Knee Surgery, Sports Traumatology, Arthroscopy*.

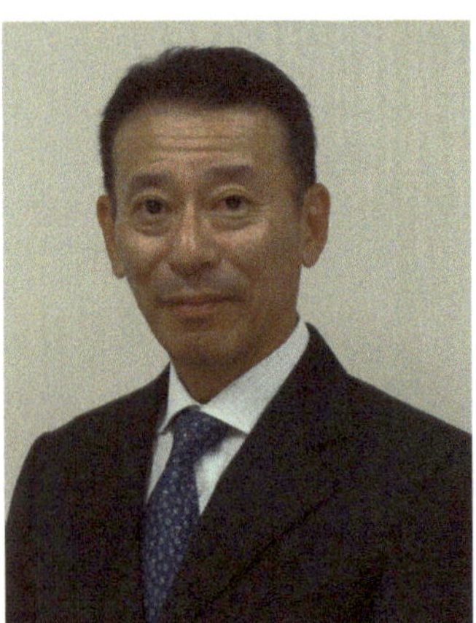

Masahiro Kurosaka is a professor and chairman of the Department of Orthopaedic Surgery, Kobe University Graduate School of Medicine. His primary research interest is joint surgery, sports medicine and regenerative medicine. During a fellowship at the Cleveland Clinic, he developed the interference fit screw which was named the "Kurosaka Screw" and his name became known worldwide for this invention. In addition to his roles as the editor-in-chief of the *Asia-Pacific Journal of Sports Medicine*, *Arthroscopy* and *Rehabilitation and Technology*, Prof. Kurosaka is a member of the Executive Committee (President, 2013–2015) of the International Society of Arthroscopy, Knee Surgery and Orthopaedic Sports Medicine (ISAKOS).

Part I
Anatomy and Histology of the ACL

Chapter 1
Functional Anatomy of the ACL Fibers on the Femoral Attachment

Tomoyuki Mochizuki and Keiichi Akita

Abstract The fanlike extension fibers of the anterior cruciate ligament (ACL) adhere to the bone surface; regardless of the knee flexion angle, the fiber location and orientation do not change, in relation to the femoral surface. However, the ACL midsubstance fiber orientation related to the femur does change during knee motion.

The ACL femoral attachment was divided into a central area of dense fibers, with direct insertion into the femur, and anterior and posterior fanlike extension areas. The central area resisted 82–90 % of the anterior drawer force with the anterior and posterior fanlike areas at 2–3 % and 11–15 %, respectively. Among the 4 central areas, most load was carried close to the roof of the intercondylar notch.

An anatomic variation of the lateral intercondylar ridge (LIR) was identified in 94.0 % of 318 femora and the distal half of LIR was not visible in 18.4 % of these femora. The LIR was situated in the anteriormost part of the lateral condyle surface in 8.8 % and in the posteriormost part in 8.5 %. The ACL attachment anterior margin was typically located anterior to the middle and distal part of LIR.

Keywords Midsubstance fibers • Fanlike extension fibers • Lateral intercondylar ridge • Resident's ridge

1.1 Introduction

The size and location of the femoral attachment of ACL are controversial points. Some studies have reported that ACL is attached to a narrow oval-shaped area on the lateral condyle [1–4], while other studies have described that ACL is attached to a wide area on the lateral condyle, and consequently, the posterior attachment margin abuts the articular cartilage margin [5–9]. We have thus performed a series

T. Mochizuki, M.D., Ph.D. (✉)
Department of Joint Reconstruction, Tokyo Medical and Dental University (TMDU), 1-5-45 Yushima, Bunkyo-ku, Tokyo 113-8519, Japan
e-mail: mochizuki.orj@tmd.ac.jp

K. Akita, M.D., Ph.D.
Department of Clinical Anatomy, Tokyo Medical and Dental University (TMDU), Tokyo, Japan

M. Ochi et al. (eds.), *ACL Injury and Its Treatment*,
DOI 10.1007/978-4-431-55858-3_1

of anatomic studies to clarify this discrepancy [10, 11]. In those studies, the femoral attachment of ACL fibers was found to be composed of two different shapes of fibers: (1) the main attachment of the midsubstance of ACL fibers and (2) the attachment of the thin fibrous tissue (from the midsubstance fibers and spread out like a fan on the posterior condyle). We termed these fibers "fanlike extension fibers" [10]. In addition, all fascicles which make up the midsubstance of ACL were found to attach to the relatively narrow oval area on the lateral condyle [11], although our previous study refers to these morphologies in a static phase, a knee extension position. The purpose of the 1st study was to evaluate the morphology of the midsubstance and fanlike extension fibers of ACL during knee motion with reference to the femoral attachment.

For ACL reconstruction, some have created femoral tunnels in the direct attachment of the midsubstance fibers [2, 12], whereas others have recommended that they should include as much as the whole area including the attachment of the fanlike extension fibers [13, 14]. This discrepancy can occur due to our lack of knowledge on the transmission of the load carried by the ACL to the femoral attachment. In some biomechanical studies in which the ACL was separated into 2 fiber bundles [15] or 3 fiber bundles [16], however, those did not use recent anatomic knowledge of the ACL attachment. The purpose of the second study was to clarify the load-bearing functions of the fibers of the femoral anterior cruciate ligament (ACL) attachment in the resistance of tibial anterior drawer and rotation.

Numerous studies have assessed the positional relationship of an osseous ridge (the resident's ridge), on the lateral roof of the intercondylar notch with ACL femoral attachment [17–19]. Hutchinson and Ash showed its clinical relevance as a landmark during ACL reconstruction; they described that it was immediately anterior to the ACL attachment [17]. In their description of the "lateral intercondylar ridge" (LIR), Farrow et al. reported that it is distinct in all males but less constant and less distinct in females [18]. Purnell et al. reported that LIR passes from the roof within 3 mm of the articular cartilage edge together with anterior fibers of the ACL attached to the posterior aspect of the ridge [19]. Unfortunately, the focus of these studies was only on the proximal part of LIR. The purpose of the third study was to determine positional variations of LIR and to clarify relationships between both the proximal and distal parts of LIR and the anterior margin of the ACL attachment.

1.2 Static and Dynamic Observation of the Fanlike Extension Fibers

At full extension, both fiber types were aligned parallel to the intercondylar roof without deviation (Figs. 1.1a and 1.2a). The midsubstance fiber attachment area was observed to be slightly protuberant, compared with that of the fanlike extension fibers (Fig. 1.2a). The seemingly thin and coarse fanlike extension fibers came into

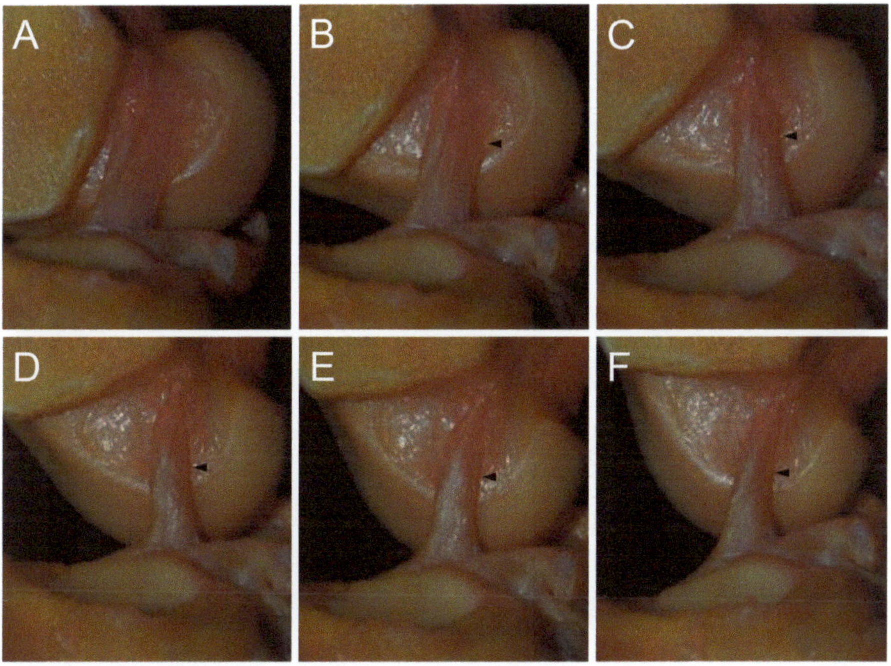

Fig. 1.1 Midsubstance and fanlike extension fibers during flexion–extension of the knee (From [20] with permission)
(**a**) Full extension: Both fiber types were aligned parallel to the intercondylar roof without curving
(**b**) 15° flexion: The midsubstance fibers were found to curve slightly (*arrowhead*) at the postero-proximal edge of the direct attachment of the midsubstance fibers (according to 30° flexion with apparent fold).
(**c**) At 30° flexion: The midsubstance fiber degree of the curving was increased.
(**d**) At 45° flexion: The ACL fiber curving showed an obvious fold.
(**e**) At 60° flexion: The midsubstance fibers showed some twisting, and the fold deepened, particularly at the postero-distal portion.
(**f**) At 90° flexion: The whole fold was deeper in the thin space between the midsubstance fibers and the femoral condyle

contact with the margin of articular cartilage (Fig. 1.2b). In the application of tension to the midsubstance fibers, the tension appeared to be distributed to the fanlike extension fibers. It was impossible to define a distinct border between the midsubstance and fanlike extension fibers.

With knee flexion of 15 and 30°, the midsubstance fibers were slightly curved anterior to the articular cartilage of the lateral condyle (Fig. 1.1b, c). The border between the midsubstance fibers and the fanlike extension fibers was then distinct (Fig. 1.2c). The location and orientation of the fanlike extension fibers, in relation to the femoral condyle surface, did not change, due to adherence to the bone surface (Fig. 1.2d).

With knee flexion of 45 and 60°, the curved area of the ACL fibers became an obvious fold on the approximate line between the postero-proximal outlet point of

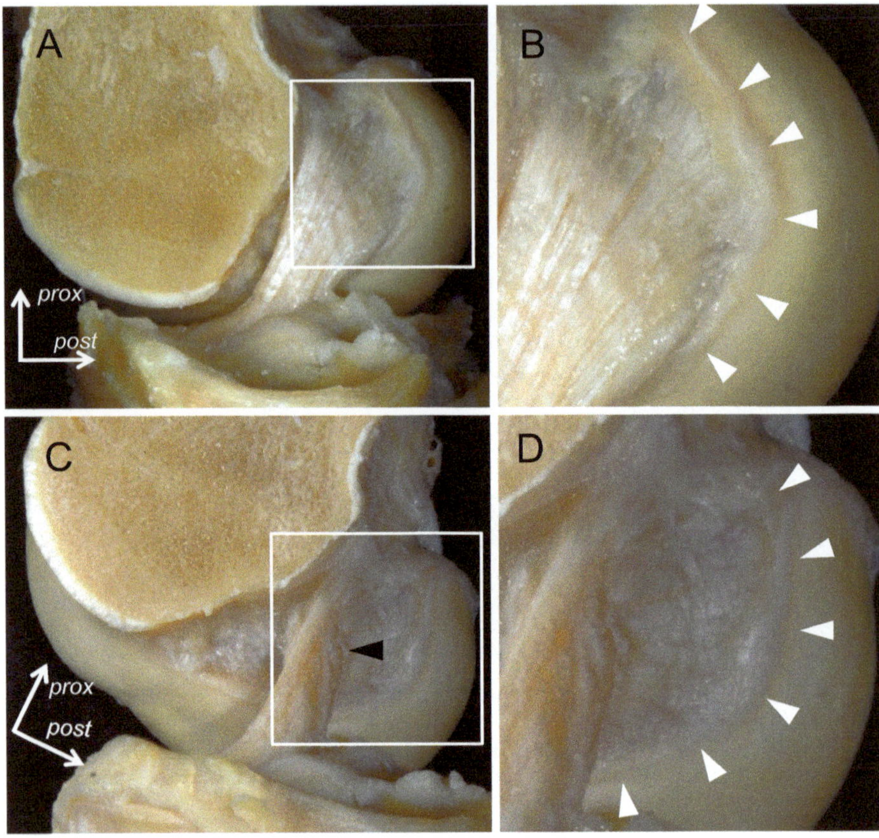

Fig. 1.2 Static observation of the midsubstance and fanlike extension fibers at full extension and at 30° of knee flexion (From [20] with permission)
(**a**) Both fiber types were aligned parallel to the intercondylar roof without curving.
(**b**) High-magnification view of ACL fibers on the lateral condyle medial wall. The fanlike extension fibers extended to the margin of articular cartilage (*arrowheads*) and tended to adhere to the medial wall; they became relatively sparse as they approached the articular cartilage.
(**c**) The midsubstance fibers were curved (*arrowhead*) and changed direction from the fanlike extension fibers
(**d**) High-magnification view of ACL fibers on the lateral condyle medial wall. The fanlike extension fibers adhered to the bone surface, with no change in fiber location or orientation in relation to the bone surface, while the orientation of midsubstance fibers did change with knee flexion. *Arrowheads* indicate the articular margin

the intercondylar edge and the postero-distal edge of the midsubstance attachment of the PL bundle (Fig. 1.1d, e). At 90°, the depth of the fold increased (Fig. 1.1f). Tension applied to the midsubstance fibers was not distributed to the fanlike extension fibers, due to the presence of the fold.

The attachment of the midsubstance fibers was significantly smaller than that of the fanlike extension fibers. The fold ratio (midsubstance attachment/whole ACL attachment) was 63.7 % (47.3–80.2 %). The attachment area of the fanlike extension fibers was approximately twofold the midsubstance fibers.

1.3 Histological Observation of Fiber Orientation

With the knee at full extension, the histological sections indicated that the AM bundle of the midsubstance fibers was attached adjacent to the proximal outlet of the intercondylar notch. The postero-proximal edge of the attachment made contact with the margin of the articular cartilage. The thin fanlike extension fibers extended from the midsubstance fibers of the PL bundle and attached to the postero-proximal aspect of the lateral condyle and extended to the articular cartilage of the lateral condyle.

With knee flexion at 120°, a fold in the midsubstance fibers was noted several millimeters from the bone surface (Fig. 1.3a–d). The thin fanlike extension fibers adhered to the bone surface in the same manner as that observed in the full extension position. The angle between the fanlike extension fibers and the midsubstance fibers was ≥90°. The area between the collagen fibers and the bone in the midsubstance fiber insertion comprised a cartilaginous zone, despite that

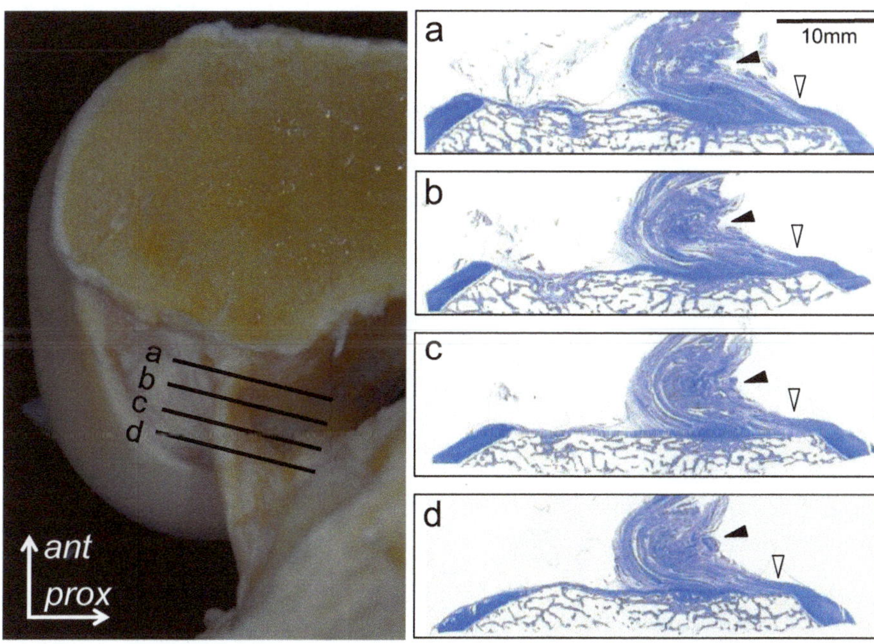

Fig. 1.3 Histological observation of fiber orientation of the two fiber types at 120° flexion (From [20] with permission)
The *left* indicates 4 oblique-axial section planes parallel to the intercondylar roof.
The fold (*black arrowheads*) was observed at the border between the midsubstance fibers and the fanlike extension fibers, several millimeters away from the bone surface (*a–d*). The thin fanlike extension fibers adhered to the bone surface of the lateral condyle. The insertion of the midsubstance fibers tends to involve the cartilaginous zone between collagen fibers and bone surface. The fanlike extension fibers tend to insert into the bone without forming transitional cartilaginous zone

almost all collagen fibers were directly attached to the bone in the fanlike extension fiber insertion and a cartilaginous tissue was rarely seen between them.

1.4 Fiber Function in the ACL Femoral Attachment

A sequential cutting study was performed on 8 fresh-frozen human knees. The femoral attachment of the ACL was divided into a central area of dense fibers which directly inserted into the femur and into the anterior and posterior fanlike extension areas (Fig. 1.4). The ACL fibers were cut sequentially from the bone in 2, 4, and 2 stages in the posterior fanlike area, the central dense area, and the anterior fanlike area, respectively. Each knee was mounted in a robotic joint testing system at 0–90 of flexion; tibial anteroposterior 6 mm translations and 10 or 15 of internal rotation were applied. The reduction in restraining force or moment was measured after each cut.

The midsubstance fibers of the ACL (the central attachment areas E, F, G, and H in Fig. 1.4) transmitted 82–90 % of the resistance to tibial displacement and that the large contribution of the central attachment fibers was biased strongly toward the roof of the femoral intercondylar notch. The fibers attached to areas G and H in Fig. 1.4, which corresponded to part of the AM bundle, provided from 66 to 84 % of the total resistance to anterior drawer across 0–90 of flexion (Fig. 1.5). The contribution of fiber attachment areas E and F in Fig. 1.4,

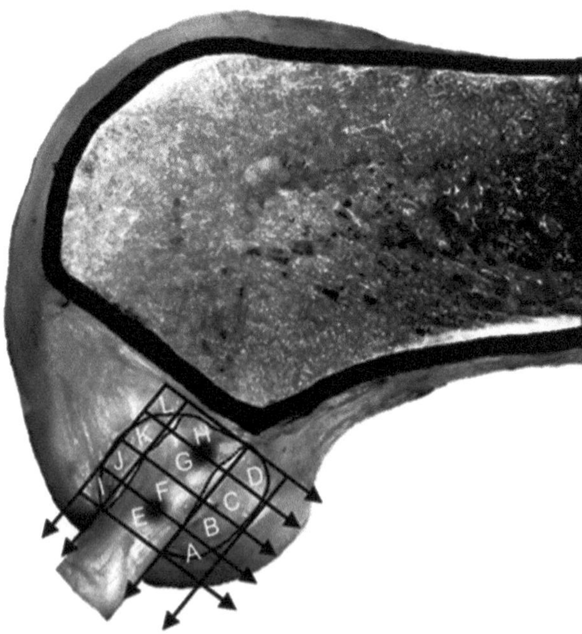

Fig. 1.4 Femoral ACL attachment partition on lateral wall of intercondylar notch. The outer lines are tangent to the ACL attachment and oriented parallel to Blumensaat's line or a line between the centers of the 2 fiber bundles of the ACL (anteromedial and posterolateral). Areas *A*, *B*, *C*, and *D* comprise the posterior fanlike extension; areas *E*, *F*, *G*, and *H* comprise the central direct attachment area; and areas *I*, *J*, *K*, and *L* comprise the anterior fanlike extension (From [26] with permission)

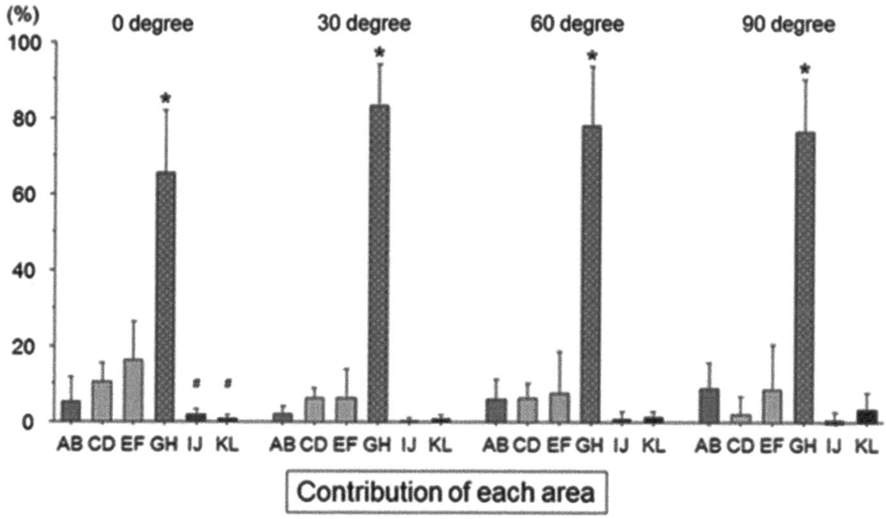

Fig. 1.5 The percentage contribution of each area to a 6 mm anterior tibial translation (force of the anterior cruciate ligament in intact knee was considered 100 %). The percentage contribution of zones E and F and zones G and H approximately shows that of the posterolateral and anteromedial bundle attachments, respectively. The percentage contribution of zones G and H was markedly greater at each angle of knee flexion ($P < .05$) compared with other angles (asterisks). # Significant differences ($P < .05$) compared with areas E and F (From [26] with permission)

which corresponded to part of the PL bundle, fell from 16 % at 0 to 9 % at 90. These changes reflected the slackening of the more posterior ACL fibers with knee flexion, which allowed more of the load to fall onto area H, which was "close to isometric." Similarly, the posterior fanlike extension attachment fibers (areas A, B, C, and D in Fig. 1.4), which form a large part of the attachment area, contributed 15 % of the resistance to tibial anterior translation in the extended knee, falling to 11 % at 90 (Figs. 1.5 and 1.6).

1.5 Anatomic Variations of the Lateral Intercondylar Ridge

A total 318 feomora were examined to determine anatomic variations of the LIR. In addition, 20 cadavers knees, in which the anterior margin was marked by radiopaque silicon markers, were examined with micro-computed tomography to evaluate the positional relationship between LIR and the anterior margin of the ACL attachment.

Although LIR was identified in 94.0 % of the 318 femora (Table 1.1), the distal half of LIR was not visible in 18.4 % of these femora. LIR was single in 96.3 %,

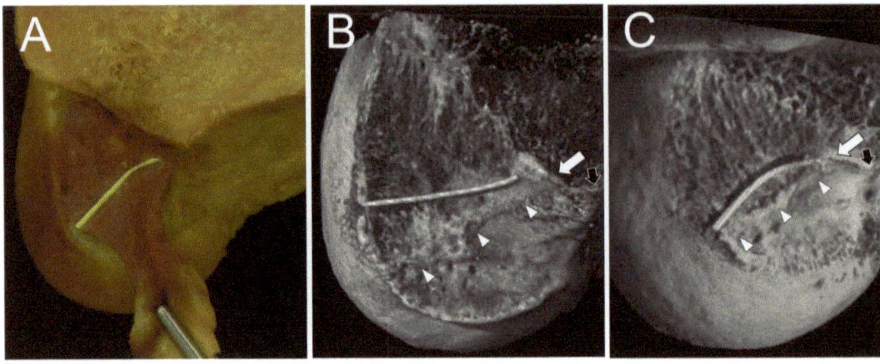

Fig. 1.6 Evaluation of the anterior margin of the ACL and LIR via micro-CT evaluation
(**a**) The medial femoral condyles and much of the notch roof have been removed. ACL is retracted posteriorly. A radiopaque silicon marker is on the anterior margin line of the femoral ACL attachment.
(**b**) In 15 of the 20 knees, the anterior margin line of the ACL, indicated by the marker, was straight (type 1) such that the marker–ridge distance was longest (mean, 4.5 mm) at the most distal part of the lateral intercondylar ridge (*LIR*). *White arrow*, resident's ridge; *white arrowheads*, LIR; *black arrow*, intercondylar notch outlet.
(**c**) In the remaining 5 knees, the anterior margin line of the ACL was curved (type 2) such that the marker–ridge distance was greatest (mean, 2.8 mm) in the middle part of LIR (From [32] with permission)

whereas 2 and 3 ridges were identified in 3.3 % and 0.3 %, respectively. Moreover, LIR was located in the anteriormost part of the lateral condyle surface in 8.8 % in comparison with the common location and in a markedly posterior part in 8.5 %. The length–height ratio (69.9 % in men, 63.6 % in women) and the length between the inlet of the notch roof and the proximal part of LIR (19.9 mm in men, 17.9 mm in women) were significantly greater in males than in females ($P = .0028$ and $P < .0001$, respectively) (Table 1.1). The anterior margin of the ACL attachment was commonly located anterior to the middle and distal part of LIR, having the mean marker–ridge distance of 4.2 mm.

1.6 Discussion

1.6.1 Anatomy of the Midsubstance and Fanlike Extension Fibers

The most important finding of the present study [20] was that because the fanlike extension fibers adhered to the bone surface, the fiber location and orientation in relation to the femoral surface did not change, regardless of the knee flexion angle, while orientation of the midsubstance fibers in relation to the femur did change

Table 1.1 Gross observation of osseous morphology of lateral intercondylar ridge (LIR)[α]

Variable	Total (N = 318)	Males (n = 200)	Females (n = 118)	*P* Value
Presence of visible LIR, no. of knees (%)				
Present	299 (94.0)	189 (94.5)	110 (93.2)	.64
Absent	19 (6.0)	11 (5.5)	8 (6.8)	
Length of the LIR, mm	18.5 ± 3.0	19.0 ± 2.9	17.7 ± 2.9	.0005
Length–height ratio, %	67.6 ± 17.6	69.9 ± 16.9	63.6 ± 18.2	.0028
Ratio > 50 %, no. of knees (%)	244 (76.7)	161 (80.5)	83 (70.3)	.036
Ratio < 50 %, no. of knees (%)	55 (17.3)	28 (14.0)	27 (22.9)	
Location of the LIR, n (%)				
Anterior (<60°)	28 (8.8)	13 (6.5)	15 (12.7)	.053
Standard (60–90°)	244 (76.7)	155 (77.5)	89 (75.4)	
Posterior (>90°)	27 (8.5)	21 (10.5)	6 (5.1)	
Length between inlet of notch and proximal part of LIR, mm	19.2 ± 2.6	19.9 ± 2.6	17.9 ± 2.0	<.0001

[α]Values are expressed as mean ± standard deviation unless otherwise indicated

during knee motion. These two different structures formed a fold, observed in knee flexion, at the border between the midsubstance fibers and the fanlike extension.

There have been no reports in which fanlike extension fibers were observed in knee flexion positions, although a few anatomic studies histologically have observed fanlike extension fibers only at the full extension position [10, 21, 22]. The insertion of the midsubstance fibers involved cartilaginous zone, which is regarded as the direct insertion [23]. On the other hand, the fanlike extension fibers were directly attached to the bone without forming a transitional cartilaginous zone, which is regarded as the indirect insertion [24]. Sasaki et al. reported similar observations concerning the femoral attachment of the ACL [22]. This study performed at various flexion positions provided new information, which is critical to the understanding of the mechanism of the above-described fold formation, but also in consideration of the function of the fanlike extension fibers.

This study demonstrated the two types of attachment margins of ACL: (1) the relatively narrow oval attachment margin of the midsubstance fibers of ACL and (2) the broader attachment margin of the fanlike extension fibers. The previous studies were thus confirmed regarding the correct information on a part of the ACL attachment. Those previous studies might have observed one or both of these two attachment margins.

This study also showed that a deep fold was formed in the postero-proximal aspect of the midsubstance fibers several millimeters from the bone surface as the knee was flexed. To date, no other study has described this phenomenon or considered its functional significance. Interestingly, some previous studies report the fold formation can be noted in a few ACL photographs, taken at a knee flexion position [4, 5, 9, 25], although no discussion of this phenomenon was included. The above-described anatomic results suggested that the load distribution mechanism from the ACL midsubstance to the femur is more complex than previously thought. At the full extension position, some of the load is widely distributed to the fanlike extension fibers. As the knee is flexed, it is the midsubstance fibers that may play a more important role than the fanlike extension fibers.

1.6.2 Fiber Function in the Femoral Attachment

This biomechanical study [26], under the specific experimental conditions, yielded the following: the central area resisted 82–90 % of the anterior drawer force; the anterior fanlike area, 2–3 %; and the posterior fanlike area, 11–15 %. Among the 4 central areas with 0–90 of flexion, most load was carried close to the roof of the intercondylar notch: the anteromedial and posterolateral bundles resisted 66–84 % and 16–9 % of the force, respectively.

Our study suggests that in ACL reconstruction, the most important fibers to resist tibial anterior displacement attach to the central/proximal part of the femoral attachment; this would correspond to the AM fiber bundle [4]. With knee flexion, the contribution of the postero-distal ACL was reduced, thereby further concentrating the load onto the anteroproximal area. This behavior is in line with ACL isometry and fiber length change patterns [16, 27, 28].

The mechanical findings of this study are in agreement with observations of the higher-density collagen fibers in the more anterior area of ACL [29, 30], which matches the variation of tensile material properties [31] as well as the microscopic morphology of direct fiber insertions into the bone in the central band of the femoral attachment [10, 11, 20–22]. In contrast, these data pose the question of the function of the fanlike extension areas, since these areas seem to carry very little load though they occupy a considerable portion of the attachment area.

1.6.3 Anatomic Variations of LIR

This study [32] highlighted the great degree of variation (both positional and dimensional) in LIR. The distal half of LIR, when present, was not visible in 18.4 %. LIR was single in 96.3 %, whereas there were 2 and 3 ridges in 3.3 % and 0.3 %, respectively. Second, there were significant positional and dimensional LIR differences between male and female femora. Third, despite that the LIR proximal area showed relative correspondence with the ACL attachment anterior margin, micro-CT analysis showed that the ACL attachment anterior margin was commonly located anterior to the LIR middle and distal parts.

Farrow et al. reported that LIR was present in 194 of 200 human femora (97 %). However, they also described that LIR was visible in only 95 of the 194 femora, whereas the remaining 99 (51 %) did not have a visibly elevated ridge [33]. Further, they revealed a significant variation in the anatomy of LIR. Thus, their 2 studies indicated that LIR, particularly the distal part, has a great degree of positional and dimensional variation [18].

Considering LIR and ACL attachments, it has been believed that LIR completely corresponds to the anterior margin line of the ACL attachment [7, 17, 19, 21]. Hutchinson and Ash, in canted cross-sectional sagittal section observations of distal femur specimens, described that the resident's ridge is located just anterior to the ACL femoral attachment [17]. However, they did not report any measurements or observe the distal part of LIR. Ferretti et al., in 3-D laser camera assessment of osseous landmarks, reported no ACL attachment anterior to LIR [7], although they did not observe LIR and the ACL attachment in the anterior border simultaneously. Purnell et al. used high-resolution CT scan simultaneous observation of LIR and the ACL attachment by Hounsfield unit scale control [19]. However, this method may incorrectly identify the anterior margin of the ACL because the ACL attaches to the femur by "direct" insertion (4 layers of bone, calcified cartilage, noncalcified cartilage, and fibrous tissues) [20–22]. Therefore, it is often difficult to simultaneously visualize the ACL attachment and LIR via control of the Hounsfield unit scale of CT. In the present study, micro-CT (a well-recognized scientific tool) was used to simultaneously visualize both LIR and ACL attachment. In addition, the radiopaque line marker (anterior margin of the ACL attachment) confirmed the relationship between the micro-CT image and the surgeon's observation. Therefore, this is the first study to employ simultaneous observation of the whole LIR and the complete ACL attachment anterior margin.

1.7 Clinical Relevance Based on These Studies

This anatomic study [20] on the fanlike extension fibers and midsubstance fibers indicated the difficulty to reconstruct the natural function of the fanlike extension fibers by creating a tunnel at the ends of each fiber bundle, although the midsubstance fibers can be reconstructed in such a fashion. It also provided critical biomechanical study data [26] which clarified fanlike extension fiber biomechanics and also facilitated the creation of mathematical models of ACL. Our biomechanical study [26] also did not support the method of covering the entire ACL attachment area with a graft [34]. Second, considering anterior laxity, the results suggest that the femoral tunnel of single-bundle ACL reconstruction in the central/proximal area would most closely mimic the natural restraint. Data do not confirm reconstruction of a central "anatomic single bundle" [35, 36]. As for double-bundle ACL reconstruction, this study indicated the creation of two femoral tunnels in the central/proximal and central/distal areas, where the ACL attachment is most dense.

Recently, though some studies recommend creation of a femoral tunnel to reconstruct the AM bundle of the ACL [13, 37], such a method may not achieve reconstruction of the normal ACL in terms of function and morphology for the following reasons. The fanlike extension fibers contributed only 15 % of the resistance to tibial anterior translation in the extended knee, and 11 % at 90. Further, it would be difficult to reconstruct the natural morphology. However, it is the midsubstance fibers of the ACL that transmitted 82–90 % of the resistance to tibial displacement; they can be reconstructed by such tunnel creation.

Regarding LIR variations, LIR may be useful as an osseous landmark for conventional single-bundle reconstruction, as previously reported [17, 18, 33]. However, even the proximal part of LIR has great variations, and thus, knowledge and skills are critical to determine the appropriate tunnel location when encountering a knee with an invisible ridge or a ridge in an untypical position. Most noteworthy is that the present study indicates that use of LIR as an osseous landmark is limited in femoral tunnel creation for anatomic single- and double-bundle reconstructions, and due to the great variations, it is often difficult for surgeons to determine an appropriate tunnel position using LIR as a bony landmark in these reconstruction procedures.

References

1. Girgis FG, Marshall JL, Monajem A (1975) The cruciate ligaments of the knee joint. Anatomical, functional and experimental analysis. Clin Orthop Relat Res 106:216–231
2. Yasuda K, Kondo E, Ichiyama H, Kitamura N, Tanabe Y, Tohyama H, Minami A (2004) Anatomic reconstruction of the anteromedial and posterolateral bundles of the anterior cruciate ligament using hamstring tendon grafts. Arthroscopy 20(10):1015–1025. doi:10.1016/j.arthro.2004.08.010
3. Takahashi M, Doi M, Abe M, Suzuki D, Nagano A (2006) Anatomical study of the femoral and tibial insertions of the anteromedial and posterolateral bundles of human anterior cruciate ligament. Am J Sports Med 34(5):787–792
4. Edwards A, Bull AMJ, Amis AA (2008) The attachments of the anteromedial and posterolateral fibre bundles of the anterior cruciate ligament. Knee Surg Sports Traumatol Arthrosc 16 (1):29–36
5. Odensten M, Gillquist J (1985) Functional anatomy of the anterior cruciate ligament and a rationale for reconstruction. J Bone Joint Surg Am 67(2):257–262
6. Harner CD, Baek GH, Vogrin TM, Carlin GJ, Kashiwaguchi S, Woo SLY (1999) Quantitative analysis of human cruciate ligament insertions. Arthroscopy 15(7):741–749
7. Ferretti M, Ekdahl M, Shen W, Fu FH (2007) Osseous landmarks of the femoral attachment of the anterior cruciate ligament: an anatomic study. Arthroscopy 23(11):1218–1225
8. Zantop T, Wellmann M, Fu FH, Petersen W (2008) Tunnel positioning of anteromedial and posterolateral bundles in anatomic anterior cruciate ligament reconstruction. Am J Sports Med 36(1):65–72
9. Otsubo H, Shino K, Suzuki D, Kamiya T, Suzuki T, Watanabe K, Fujimiya M, Iwahashi T, Yamashita T (2012) The arrangement and the attachment areas of three ACL bundles. Knee Surg Sports Traumatol Arthrosc 20(1):127–134. doi:10.1007/s00167-011-1576-z
10. Mochizuki T, Muneta T, Nagase T, Shirasawa S, Akita K, Sekiya I (2006) Cadaveric knee observation study for describing anatomic femoral tunnel placement for two-bundle anterior cruciate ligament reconstruction. Arthroscopy 22(4):356–361
11. Hara K, Mochizuki T, Sekiya I, Yamaguchi K, Akita K, Muneta T (2009) Anatomy of normal human anterior cruciate ligament attachments evaluated by divided small bundles. Am J Sports Med 37(12):2386–2391

12. Yagi M, Wong EK, Kanamori A, Debski RE, Fu FH, Woo SL (2002) Biomechanical analysis of an anatomic anterior cruciate ligament reconstruction. Am J Sports Med 30(5):660–666
13. Shino K, Nakata K, Nakamura N, Toritsuka Y, Horibe S, Nakagawa S, Suzuki T (2008) Rectangular tunnel double-bundle anterior cruciate ligament reconstruction with bone-patellar tendon-bone graft to mimic natural fiber arrangement. Arthroscopy 24(10):1178–1183. doi:10.1016/j.arthro.2008.06.010
14. Forsythe B, Kopf S, Wong AK, Martins CA, Anderst W, Tashman S, Fu FH (2010) The location of femoral and tibial tunnels in anatomic double-bundle anterior cruciate ligament reconstruction analyzed by three-dimensional computed tomography models. J Bone Joint Surg Am 92(6):1418–1426. doi:10.2106/JBJS.I.00654
15. Sakane M, Fox RJ, Woo SL, Livesay GA, Li G, Fu FH (1997) In situ forces in the anterior cruciate ligament and its bundles in response to anterior tibial loads. J Orthop Res 15 (2):285–293. doi:10.1002/jor.1100150219
16. Amis A, Dawkins G (1991) Functional anatomy of the anterior cruciate ligament. Fibre bundle actions related to ligament replacements and injuries. J Bone Joint Surg Br 73(2):260–267
17. Hutchinson MR, Ash SA (2003) Resident's ridge: assessing the cortical thickness of the lateral wall and roof of the intercondylar notch. Arthroscopy 19(9):931–935
18. Farrow LD, Gillespie RJ, Victoroff BN, Cooperman DR (2008) Radiographic location of the lateral intercondylar ridge: its relationship to Blumensaat's line. Am J Sports Med 36 (10):2002–2006. doi:10.1177/0363546508317413
19. Purnell ML, Larson AI, Clancy W (2008) Anterior cruciate ligament insertions on the tibia and femur and their relationships to critical bony landmarks using high-resolution volume-rendering computed tomography. Am J Sports Med 36(11):2083–2090
20. Mochizuki T, Fujishiro H, Nimura A, Mahakkanukrauh P, Yasuda K, Muneta T, Akita K (2014) Anatomic and histologic analysis of the mid-substance and fan-like extension fibers of the anterior cruciate ligament during knee motion, with special reference to the femoral attachment. Knee Surg Sports Traumatol Arthrosc 22(2):336–344
21. Iwahashi T, Shino K, Nakata K, Otsubo H, Suzuki T, Amano H, Nakamura N (2010) Direct anterior cruciate ligament insertion to the femur assessed by histology and 3-dimensional volume-rendered computed tomography. Arthroscopy 26(9):S13–S20
22. Sasaki N, Ishibashi Y, Tsuda E, Yamamoto Y, Maeda S, Mizukami H, Toh S, Yagihashi S, Tonosaki Y (2012) The femoral insertion of the anterior cruciate ligament: discrepancy between macroscopic and histological observations. Arthroscopy 28(8):1135–1146. doi:10.1016/j.arthro.2011.12.021
23. Schneider H (1956) Structure of tendon attachments. Z Anat Entwicklungsgesch 119:431–456 (in German)
24. Benjamin M, Evans EJ, Copp L (1986) The histology of tendon attachments to bone in man. J Anat 149:89–100
25. Ziegler CG, Pietrini SD, Westerhaus BD, Anderson CJ, Wijdicks CA, Johansen S, Engebretsen L, LaPrade RF (2011) Arthroscopically pertinent landmarks for tunnel positioning in single-bundle and double-bundle anterior cruciate ligament reconstructions. Am J Sports Med 39(4):743–752
26. Kawaguchi Y, Kondo E, Takeda R, Akita K, Yasuda K, Amis AA (2015) The role of fibers in the femoral attachment of the anterior cruciate ligament in resisting tibial displacement. Arthroscopy 31(3):435–444. doi:10.1016/j.arthro.2014.08.033
27. Hefzy MS, Grood ES, Noyes FR (1989) Factors affecting the region of most isometric femoral attachments. Part II: the anterior cruciate ligament. Am J Sports Med 17(2):208–216
28. Sidles JA, Larson RV, Garbini JL, Downey DJ, Matsen FA 3rd (1988) Ligament length relationships in the moving knee. J Orthop Res 6(4):593–610. doi:10.1002/jor.1100060418
29. Mommersteeg TJ, Blankevoort L, Kooloos JG, Hendriks JC, Kauer JM, Huiskes R (1994) Nonuniform distribution of collagen density in human knee ligaments. J Orthop Res 12 (2):238–245. doi:10.1002/jor.1100120213

30. Petersen W, Tillmann B (1999) Structure and vascularization of the cruciate ligaments of the human knee joint. Anat Embryol (Berl) 200(3):325–334
31. Butler DL, Guan Y, Kay MD, Cummings JF, Feder SM, Levy MS (1992) Location-dependent variations in the material properties of the anterior cruciate ligament. J Biomech 25 (5):511–518
32. Tsukada S, Fujishiro H, Watanabe K, Nimura A, Mochizuki T, Mahakkanukrauh P, Yasuda K, Akita K (2014) Anatomic variations of the lateral intercondylar ridge: relationship to the anterior margin of the anterior cruciate ligament. Am J Sports Med 42(5):1110–1117. doi:10.1177/0363546514524527
33. Farrow LD, Chen MR, Cooperman DR, Victoroff BN, Goodfellow DB (2007) Morphology of the femoral intercondylar notch. J Bone Joint Surg Am 89(10):2150
34. van Eck CF, Lesniak BP, Schreiber VM, Fu FH (2010) Anatomic single- and double-bundle anterior cruciate ligament reconstruction flowchart. Arthroscopy 26(2):258–268. doi:10.1016/j.arthro.2009.07.027
35. Vaiyapuri S, Vaiyapuri R, Ashokan R, Ramasamy K, Nattamaisundar K, Jeyaraj A, Chandran V, Gajjeraman P, Baksh MF, Gibbins JM, Hutchinson EG (2013) Snakebite and its socio-economic impact on the rural population of Tamil Nadu, India. PLoS ONE 8(11), e80090. doi:10.1371/journal.pone.0080090
36. Kondo E, Merican AM, Yasuda K, Amis AA (2011) Biomechanical comparison of anatomic double-bundle, anatomic single-bundle, and nonanatomic single-bundle anterior cruciate ligament reconstructions. Am J Sports Med 39(2):279–288. doi:10.1177/0363546510392350
37. Suzuki T, Shino K, Nakagawa S, Nakata K, Iwahashi T, Kinugasa K, Otsubo H, Yamashita T (2011) Early integration of a bone plug in the femoral tunnel in rectangular tunnel ACL reconstruction with a bone-patellar tendon-bone graft: a prospective computed tomography analysis. Knee Surg Sports Traumatol Arthrosc 19:S29–S35. doi:10.1007/s00167-011-1481-5

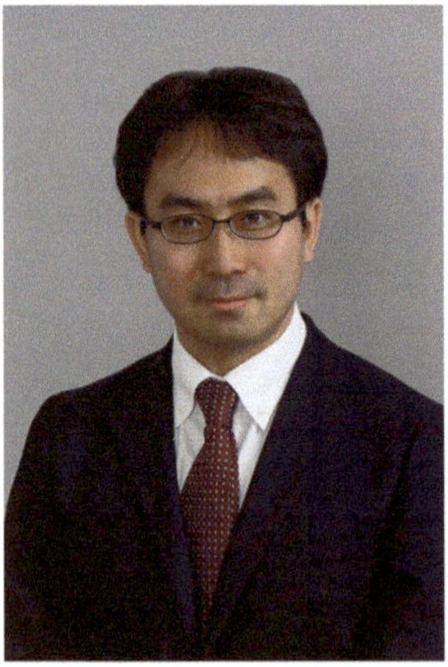

Tomoyuki Mochizuki, M.D., Ph.D, Department of Joint Reconstruction, Tokyo Medical and Dental University, Tokyo, Japan.

Chapter 2
The Anatomical Features of ACL Insertion Sites and Their Implications for Multi-bundle Reconstruction

Daisuke Suzuki and Hidenori Otsubo

Abstract The anatomical features of insertion sites of the anterior cruciate ligament (ACL) were reviewed and illustrated. The ACL generally had been divided into two bundles, i.e., the anteromedial (AM) and posterolateral (PL) bundle. However, subsequent studies suggested that the ACL could be separated into three bundles; the AM bundle was subdivided into the anteromedial bundle lateral part (AM-L bundle) and the anteromedial bundle medial part (AM-M bundle).

The ACL insertion sites were easily discernable by distribution of the calcified fibrocartilage having smooth surface. In the femoral insertion, the AM-L bundle occupies the proximo-anterior part, and the AM-M bundle occupies the proximo-posterior part. The PL bundle occupies the distal part. In the tibial insertion, the AM-M bundle occupies the anteromedial part, and the AM-L bundle occupies the anterolateral part. The PL bundle occupies the posterior part.

These positional relations of the insertion sites produce the differences of each bundle function and provide a rationale for performing multi-bundle ACL reconstruction.

Keywords ACL insertion sites • AM-M bundle • AM-L bundle • PL bundle

2.1 Introduction

The heterogeneity of the anterior cruciate ligament (ACL) was first reported by Palmer [1], who suggested that the parts of the ACL had different roles during flexion-extension movement. In 1975, the anatomical study by Girgis et al. [2] described two bundles of the ACL and observed the tensioning pattern of each

D. Suzuki, Ph.D. (✉)
Department of Musculoskeletal Biomechanics and Surgical Development, Sapporo Medical University, South 1 West 17, Chuo-ku, Sapporo, Hokkaido 060-8556, Japan
e-mail: daisuke@sapmed.ac.jp

H. Otsubo
Obithiro Kyokai Hospital, Hokkaido, Japan

M. Ochi et al. (eds.), *ACL Injury and Its Treatment*,
DOI 10.1007/978-4-431-55858-3_2

bundle from knee extension to flexion. The anteromedial (AM) bundle was taut through knee extension to flexion, while the posterolateral (PL) bundle was taut only in knee extension and slack in flexion. Since then, many researchers have examined these two bundles of the ACL. Both morphological and biomechanical studies have confirmed that the AM and PL bundles have different stress distributions in a series of knee motions [3–5]. Norwood and Cross [6] divided the ACL into three bundles, the "*AM*" bundle, the intermediate (IM) bundle, and the PL bundle. However, their description of the femoral insertion sites of each bundle was amended in later studies. The IM bundle occupied the superoanterior part of the femoral insertion by fiber analysis of subsequent studies [4, 7, 8], and it was not located at the position between the "*AM*" and PL bundles. In addition, Otsubo et al. [8] mentioned that the IM bundle was coincident with the lateral part of the "*AM*" bundle. The IM bundle could more easily be separated from the "*AM*" bundle by loading the anterior tibial drawer. Thus, the IM bundle was named the anteromedial bundle lateral part (AM-L bundle), and the other part of the AM bundle was named the anteromedial bundle medial part (AM-M bundle); we use these terms in the following section (Fig. 2.1).

Otsubo et al. [8] reported that the triple-bundle structure of the ACL was identified in all examined knees. Some of the ACL was clearly confirmed at the

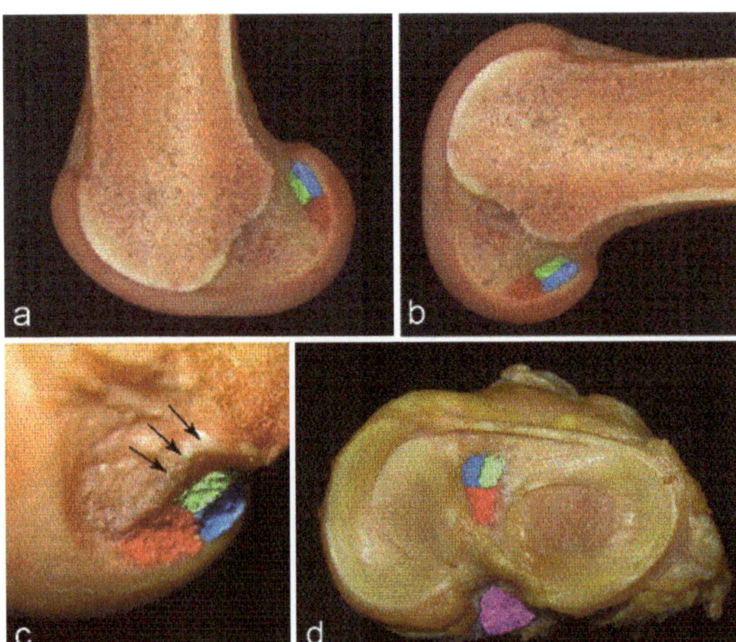

Fig. 2.1 Attachment areas of the three ACL bundles. *Blue*, anteromedial bundle medial part (AM-M), anteromedial bundle lateral part (AM-L); *red*, posterolateral (PL) bundle. (**a**) Femur sagittal view from the medial side. (**b**) 90° flexion of the femur. Each bundle insertion is changed in its positional relationship between the femur and the tibia. (**c**) Femur oblique view from the anteromedial side. *Arrow*: resident's ridge. (**d**) Tibia axial view from the proximal side

boundary between the AM-L and AM-M bundle without tension. However, in the vicinity of the femoral insertion, the boundary was unclear in most of the examined ACLs, while the boundary of the PLB was easier to demarcate. MacKay et al. [9] reported that 15 of 73 knees showed three well-separated bundles on MRI. This triple-bundle structure is seen not only in humans but also in other animals, including both herbivore and carnivore mammals [10]. Thus, the triple-bundle structure of the ACL is broadly distributed among mammals.

2.2 The Bone-Ligament Interface of the ACL

A bone-ligament/tendon interface was termed an enthesis, and entheses of the ACL were classified as direct insertions, with fibrocartilage between the ligament and bone. The direct insertion was characterized by the following four stratified structures: ligament (fibrous tissue), uncalcified fibrocartilage, calcified fibrocartilage, and bone. A line between uncalcified fibrocartilage and calcified fibrocartilage is termed a tidemark [11] (Fig. 2.2).

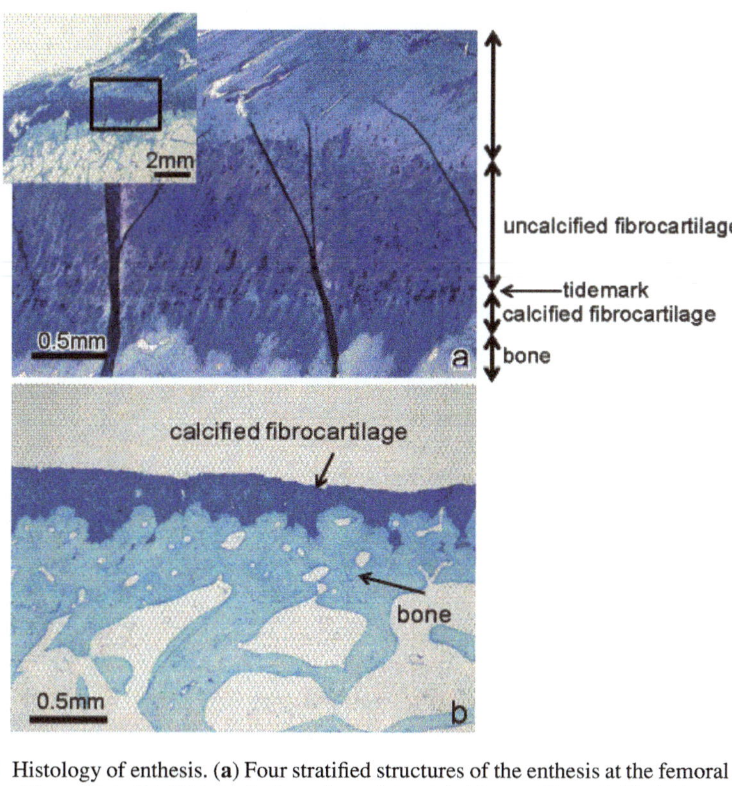

Fig. 2.2 Histology of enthesis. (**a**) Four stratified structures of the enthesis at the femoral insertion (toluidine blue stain). (**b**) Histological section of the dried bone. The calcified fibrocartilage is firmly connected to the bone, while the uncalcified fibrocartilage, which is superficial to the tidemark, is completely removed (toluidine blue stain)

The calcified fibrocartilage consisting of hard tissue is firmly connected to the bone, and it is easily discernible because of its smoother surface [12] (Fig. 2.2). Hence, the calcified fibrocartilage is helpful to assess the ACL insertion area. In observation of dried bone, the calcified fibrocartilage area shows a shallow depression with a smoother surface. The anterior part of the femoral insertion forms a small ridge at the end of calcified fibrocartilage, known as the resident's ridge, named by Clancy [13, 14] (Fig. 2.3), or the lateral intercondylar ridge proposed by

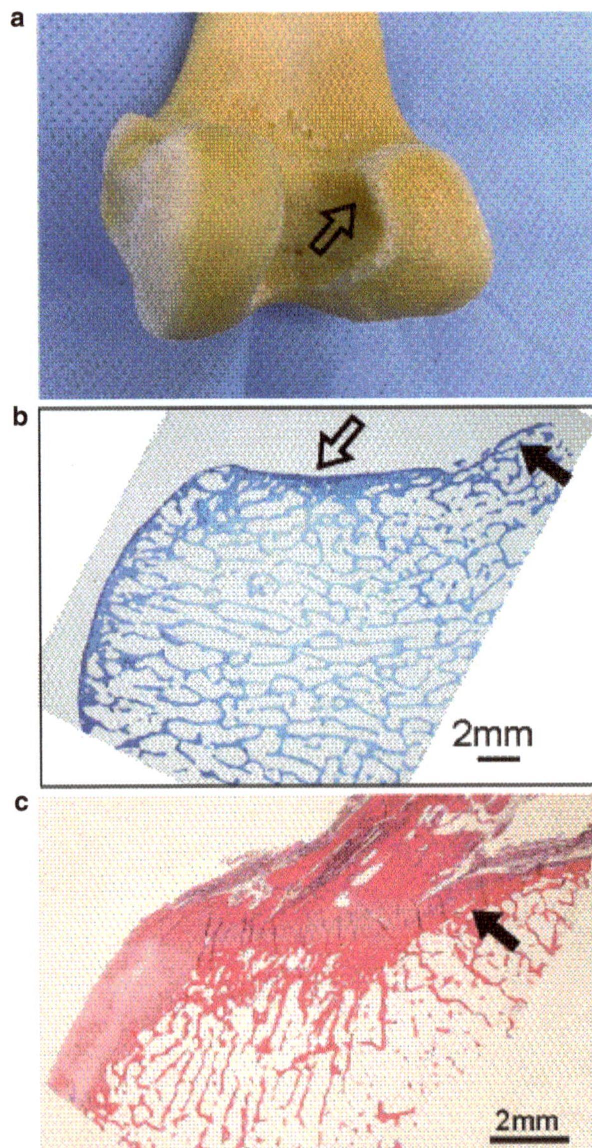

Fig. 2.3 Femoral insertion. (**a**) Macroscopic femoral ACL insertion. (**b**) Histological section of the dried bone. The calcified fibrocartilage is distributed on the insertion area (toluidine blue stain). (**c**) Histological section of the ACL femoral insertion (H&E stain). *Open arrow*, ACL insertion; *closed arrow*, resident's ridge

Ferretti et al. [15]. Thus, the resident's ridge could be an important landmark to confirm the attachment area during ACL surgery; for that reason, soft tissues around the area have to be removed. This structure including a shallow depression and ridge is also seen in the tibial insertion.

2.2.1 Femoral Insertion

The femoral insertion of the ACL is located around the posterior border of the medial wall of the lateral condyle (Fig. 2.3). The insertion part forms an ellipsoid or anterior truncated ellipsoid shape (Figs. 2.1 and 2.3). The AM bundle occupies most of the proximal part, and the PL bundle occupies the distal part. In cases of triple-bundle separation, the AM-L bundle occupies the anterior part, and the AM-M bundle occupies the posterior part of the insertion of the AM bundle.

According to Ferretti et al. [15], the femoral insertion has a ridge, named the lateral bifurcate ridge, indicating the boundary between the AM and PL bundles. However, it is not consistently present as Zauleck et al. [16] reported that the lateral bifurcate ridge was found 21.3 % of 235 human femora, and Van Eck et al. [17] reported that the lateral bifurcated ridge was present in 48 % during arthroscopic ACL reconstructive surgery. However, the resident's ridge, which delineates the anterior margin of the femoral insertion, was consistently present in 100 % [13, 15, 16] and in 93.6 % [16]. Takahashi et al. [18] reported that the resident's ridgelike structure was formed by analysis of bone remodeling based on the bony interstitial fluid flow due to the tensile force of the ACL. Thus, the resident's ridge was probably produced by the ACL itself. These suggest that the resident's ridge is a useful landmark for creating the femoral tunnel at the time of ACL reconstruction [19]. The resident's ridge is more prominent in the proximal portion where the AM-L bundle is attached, and it becomes less discernible in the distal part where the PL bundle is attached.

Iwahashi [20] identified the direct femoral ACL attachment area histologically and quantified the direct insertion area by superimposing the microscopic anatomy of the region onto the three-dimensional (3D) volume rendering CT model of the femoral condyle. According to the previous reports on the femoral insertion area by macroscopic observation, the area averaged 131 mm^2, though the value may have been obtained from incompletely dissected specimens (Table 2.1). Kudo et al. [21] reported that the mean area was 122.7 ± 0.28 mm^2 by measuring the calcified fibrocartilage area in the dried bones (Table 2.1). On the other hand, Ferretti et al. [15], using a unique 3D measurement method, reported that the mean area was 196 mm^2, which is much greater than that in the other studies (Table 2.1).

Table 2.1 Measurements of the femoral and tibial insertion areas

				Femoral insertion				Tibial insertion			
Author	Year	Reference	Sex	ACL area	AM area	PL area	n	ACL area	AM area	PL area	n
Muneta	1997	AJSM	Male	99.6 ± 25.0			16	155.0 ± 32.2			16
			Female	86.9 ± 42.2				131.7 ± 28.1			
Harner	1999	Arthroscopy			47 ± 13	49 ± 13	5		56 ± 21	53 ± 21	5
Takahashi	2006	AJSM			66.9 ± 2.3	66.9 ± 2.3	32		67.0 ± 18.4	52.4 ± 17.6	31
Feretti	2007	Arthroscopy		196.8 ± 23.1	120 ± 19.8	76.8 ± 15.6	60				
Luites	2007	KSSTA		184 ± 52	81 ± 27	103 ± 39	35	229 ± 53	136 ± 37	93 ± 33	35
Siebold	2008	Arthroscopy	male	98 ± 22	53 ± 14	45 ± 13	17				
			Female	76 ± 13	39 ± 10	39 ± 9	33				
Siebold	2008	Arthroscopy	Male					130 ± 45	72 ± 30	55 ± 16	17
			Female					106 ± 29	65 ± 31	51 ± 22	33
Kudo	2009	JOSKAS		122.7 ± 0.28			16				
Iwahashi	2010	Arthroscopy		128.3 ± 10.5			8				
Otsubo	2011	KSSTA		124.6	36.1(AMM)	53.6	1	119.1	34.5(AMM)	53.6	1
					34.9(AML)				31.0(AML)		
Iriuchishima	2013	KSSTA		72.3 ± 24.4			24	134.1 ± 32.4			24
Lee	2014	KSSTA			70.3 ± 10.9	67.4 ± 17.9	15		75.9 ± 22.4	73.3 ± 22.9	15
Zauleck	2014	Clin Anat	(dried bone)	127.21 ± 32.54			166				
			(cadaver)	119.58 ± 34.84			69				
Mean area				130.7				146			

2.2.2 Tibial Insertion

The tibial insertion of the ACL is demarcated anteriorly by the anterior ridge, posteriorly by the tibial spine, medially by the medial intercondylar ridge, and laterally by the anterior horn of the lateral meniscus (Figs. 2.1 and 2.4). The average tibial insertion area from the previous reports is 146 mm^2, which is slightly larger than that of the femoral insertion (Table 2.1). In addition, the strict insertion area was scooped posteriorly by the nutrient artery of the ACL [7, 22]

The AM bundle generally attached to the anterior part of the tibial insertion, while the PL bundle attached to the posterior part [4, 7]. Hara et al. [7] classified the tibial insertions into two patterns depending on the direction of the boundary between the AM bundle and the PL bundle: oblique type in 60 % and transverse type in 40 %. In the oblique type, the AM fibers extended from anterolateral to

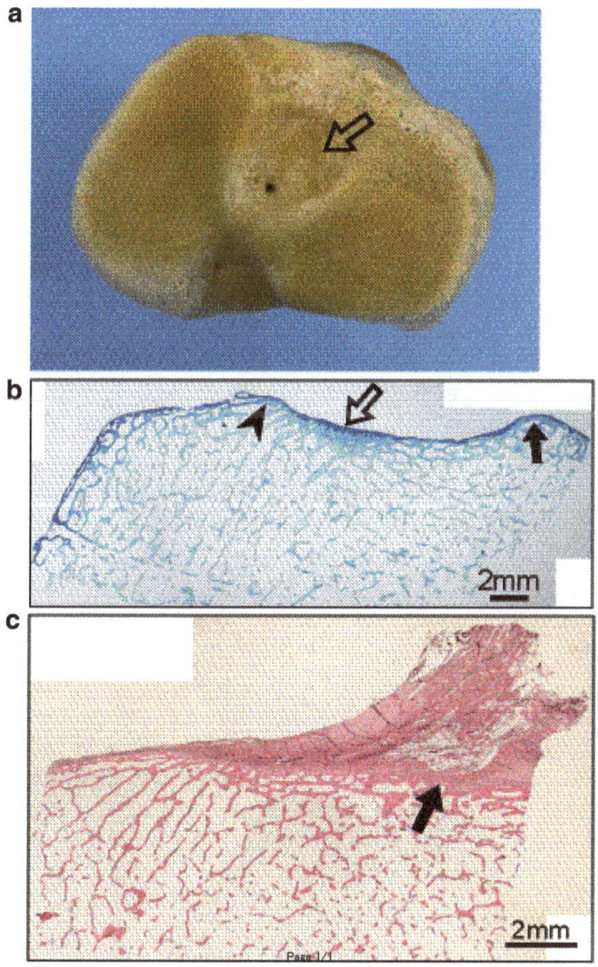

Fig. 2.4 Tibial insertion. (**a**) Macroscopic tibial ACL insertion. (**b**) Histological section of the dried bone. The calcified fibrocartilage is distributed on the insertion area (toluidine blue stain). (**c**) Histological section of the ACL femoral insertion (H&E stain). *Open arrow*, ACL insertion; *closed arrow*, small ridge; *arrow head*, Parson's knob

posteromedial, while the transverse pattern showed that the AM fibers were attached in the anterior half, and the PL fibers were attached in the posterior half. In the triple-bundle separation, the AM-M bundle occupies the medial part of the AM attachment site, and the AM-L bundle occupies the lateral part [8] (Fig. 2.1). The insertion area is smoother without any ridges, while its posterior margin forms a prominent ridge, the tibial ACL ridge/tibial spine, which might function as a pulley for the tensile force from the ACL, similar to the resident's ridge on the femoral side (Fig. 2.4).

The anterior border of the tibial insertion frequently has a projection termed the Parson's knob, which was detected in 45 % of dried bone specimens [23], suggesting that it can be helpful for proper tibial tunnel placement for ACL reconstructive surgery [24]. This knob could be considered a kind of enthesophyte, which is commonly seen in other tendon/ligament attachments [25].

2.3 Implications for Multiple-bundle Reconstruction

The purpose of ACL reconstruction is to restore knee stability without loss of motion. ACL reconstruction has improved from the traditional single-bundle reconstruction, Rosenberg's two femoral socket ("bi-socket") procedure, to anatomical double-bundle reconstruction [26–28]. The anatomical double-bundle reconstruction is performed by placing the hamstring tendon grafts at the original insertions of both the "anteromedial" and "posterolateral" bundles. This method has greater potential to restore kinematics closer to those of the normal knee than conventional methods [29, 30]. In addition, favorable short-term clinical outcomes with this procedure have been reported [28, 31, 32].

Shino et al. [33] introduced the triple-bundle ACL reconstruction technique in which the three bundles of the ACL are individually reconstructed with hamstring tendon autografts. This technique may have much greater potential to closely mimic not only the morphology but also the biomechanical behavior of the native ACL [34–36]. Clinically, immediate postoperative stability was better in the triple-bundle procedure than in the double-bundle reconstruction [37]. In addition, Suzuki et al. [38] reported that laxity match pretension at 15° knee flexion became smaller in the triple-bundle reconstruction than in double-bundle reconstruction. The enlarged contact area between the graft and the tunnel wall in the three tibial tunnels might have contributed to this improved biomechanical performance.

The anatomical and biomechanical studies reviewed in this chapter provide a rationale for performing multi-bundle ACL reconstruction. Multi-bundle reconstruction is much more advantageous to not only morphologically but also biomechanically mimic the native ACL to achieve the goal of ACL reconstruction.

References

1. Palmer I (1938) On the injuries to the ligaments of the knee joint, a clinical study. Acta Chir Scand 81(Suppl 53):1–283
2. Girgis FG, Marshall JL, Monajem A (1975) The cruciate ligaments of the knee joint. Anatomical, functional and experimental analysis. Clin Orthop Relat Res 106:216–231
3. Arnoczky SP (1983) Anatomy of the anterior cruciate ligament. Clin Orthop Relat Res 172:19–25
4. Mommersteeg TJ, Kooloos JG, Roeling FQ et al (1995) The fibre bundle anatomy of human cruciate ligaments. J Anat 187:461–471
5. Sakane M, Fox RJ, Woo SL et al (1997) In situ forces in the anterior cruciate ligament and its bundles in response to anterior tibial loads. J Orthop Res 15:285–293
6. Norwood LA, Cross MJ (1979) Anterior cruciate ligament: functional anatomy of its bundles in rotatory instabilities. Am J Sports Med 7:23–26
7. Hara K, Mochizuki T, Sekiya I et al (2009) Anatomy of normal human anterior cruciate ligament attachments evaluated by divided small bundles. Am J Sports Med 37:2386–2391
8. Otsubo H, Shino K, Suzuki D et al (2012) The arrangement and the attachment areas of three ACL bundles. Knee Surg Sports Traumatol Arthrosc 20:127–134
9. MacKay JW, Whitehead H, Toms AP (2014) Radiological evidence for the triple bundle anterior cruciate ligament. Clin Anat 27:1097–1102
10. Tantisricharoenkul G, Linde-Rosen M, Araujo P et al (2014) Anterior cruciate ligament: an anatomical exploration in humans and in a selection of animal species. Knee Surg Sports Traumatol Arthrosc 22:961–971
11. Cooper RR, Misol S (1970) Tendon and ligament insertion. J Bone Joint Surg Am 52:1–20
12. Benjamin M (1986) The histology of tendon attachments to bone in man. J Anat 149:89–100
13. Hutchinson MR, Ash SA (2003) Resident's ridge: assessing the cortical thickness of the lateral wall and roof of the intercondylar notch. Arthroscopy 19:931–935
14. Purnell ML, Larson AI, Clancy W (2008) Anterior cruciate ligament insertions on the tibia and femur and their relationships to critical bony landmarks using high-resolution volume-rendering computed tomography. Am J Sports Med 36:2083–2090
15. Ferretti M, Ekdahl M, Shen W, Fu FH (2007) Osseous landmarks of the femoral attachment of the anterior cruciate ligament: an anatomic study. Arthroscopy 11:1218–1225
16. Zauleck MK, Gabriel S, Fischmeister MF, Hirtler L (2014) Origin of the anterior cruciate ligament and the surrounding osseous landmarks of the femur. Clin Anat 27:1103–1110
17. Van Eck CF, Morse KR, Lesniak BP et al (2010) Does the lateral intercondylar ridge disappear in ACL deficient patients? Knee Surg Sports Traumatol Arthrosc 18:1184–1188
18. Takahashi Y, Fujie H, Nakada K et al (2014) Resident's ridge formation due to tensile force in the anterior cruciate ligament. Jpn J Clin Biomechanics 35:137–142. (in Japanese)
19. Shino K, Suzuki T, Iwahashi T et al (2010) The resident's ridge as an arthroscopic landmark for anatomical femoral tunnel drilling in ACL reconstruction. Knee Surg Sports Traumatol Arthrosc 18:1164–1168
20. Iwahashi T, Shino K, Nakata K et al (2010) Direct anterior cruciate ligament insertion to the femur assessed by histology and 3-dimensional volume-rendered computed tomography. Arthroscopy 26:S13–S20
21. Kudo M, Shino K, Suzuki D et al (2009) Observation of ACL femoral attachment on dried bones. The first annual meeting JOSKAS (in Japanese)
22. Siebold R, Schuhmacher P, Fernandez F et al (2015) Flat midsubstance of the anterior cruciate ligament with tibial "C"-shaped insertion site. Knee Surg Sports Traumatol Arthrosc 23:3136–3142
23. Jacobsen K (1974) Area intercondylaris tibiae: osseous surface structure and its relation to soft tissue structures and applications to radiography. J Anat 117:605–618
24. Berg EE (1993) Parsons' knob (tuberculum intercondylare tedium). A Guide to Tibial Anterior Cruciate Ligament Insertion. Clin Orthop Relat Res 292:229–231

25. Rogers J, Shepstone L, Dieppe P (1997) Bone formers: osteophyte and enthesophyte formation are positively associated. Ann Rheum Dis 56:85–90
26. Frank CB, Jackson DW (1997) Current concepts review – the science of reconstruction of the anterior cruciate ligament. J Bone Joint Surg Am 79:1556–1576
27. Maeda A, Shino K, Horibe S (1996) Anterior cruciate ligament reconstruction with multistranded autogenous semitendinosus tendon. Am J Sports Med 24:504–509
28. Toritsuka Y, Amano H, Kuwano M et al (2009) Outcome of double-bundle ACL reconstruction using hamstring tendons. Knee Surg Sports Traumatol Arthrosc 17:456–463
29. Mae T, Shino K, Matsumoto N et al (2006) Force sharing between two grafts in the anatomical two bundle anterior cruciate ligament reconstruction. Knee Surg Sports Traumatol Arthrosc 14:505–509
30. Morimoto Y, Ferretti M, Ekdahl M et al (2009) Tibiofemoral joint contact area and pressure after single- and double-bundle anterior cruciate ligament reconstruction. Arthroscopy 25:62–69
31. Kondo E, Yasuda K, Azuma H et al (2008) Prospective clinical comparisons of anatomic double-bundle versus single-bundle anterior cruciate ligament reconstruction procedures in 328 consecutive patients. Am J Sports Med 36:1675–1687
32. Otsubo H, Shino K, Nakamura N et al (2007) Arthroscopic evaluation of ACL grafts reconstructed with the anatomical two-bundle technique using hamstring tendon autograft. Knee Surg Sports Traumatol Arthrosc 15:720–728
33. Shino K, Nakata K, Nakamura N et al (2005) Anatomic anterior cruciate ligament reconstruction using two double-looped hamstring tendon grafts via twin femoral and triple tibial tunnels. Oper Tech Orthop 15:130–134
34. Amis AA, Dawkins GP (1991) Functional anatomy of the anterior cruciate ligament. Fibre bundle actions related to ligament replacements and injuries. J Bone Joint Surg Br 73:260–267
35. Hollis JM, Takai S, Adams DJ (1991) The effects of knee motion and external loading on the length of the anterior cruciate ligament (ACL): a kinematic study. J Biomech Eng 113:208–214
36. Iwahashi T, Shino K, Nakata K et al (2008) Assessment of the "functional length" of the three bundles of the anterior cruciate ligament. Knee Surg Sports Traumatol Arthrosc 16:167–174
37. Mae T, Shino K, Matsumoto N (2013) Immediate postoperative anterior knee stability: double- versus triple-bundle anterior cruciate ligament reconstructions. Arthroscopy 29:213–219
38. Suzuki T, Otsubo H, Fujie H et al (2015) Biomechanical comparison of anterior cruciate ligament reconstructions with hamstring graft. The seventh annual meeting JOSKAS (in Japanese)

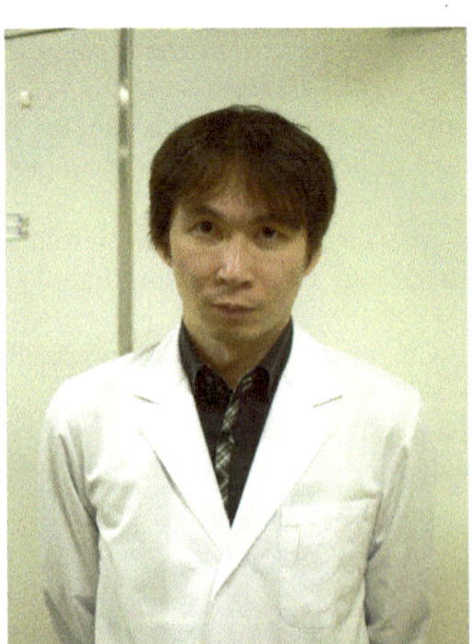

Daisuke Suzuki, PhD, Department of Musculoskeletal Biomechanics and Surgical Development, Sapporo Medical University, Hokkaido, Japan.

Chapter 3
Discrepancy Between Macroscopic and Histological Observations

Norihiro Sasaki

Abstract For better clinical results of anterior cruciate ligament (ACL) reconstruction, it is very important for surgeons to know the original femoral ACL insertion. Previously, many anatomical studies of the femoral ACL insertion have been performed. However, its position was described differently depending on the report and is still controversial. In this chapter, the position of the femoral ACL insertion is clarified from past reports and our study. Macroscopically, the femoral ACL insertion was located at the back of the lateral intercondylar ridge. The posterior margin of the femoral ACL insertion remained controversial. However, there was some distance between the posterior margin and the posterior cartilage border in microscopic observation. This difference between macroscopic and microscopic observation was considered to be due to the ACL attaching on the femoral lateral condyle in a fanlike manner. When making the femoral bone tunnel during ACL reconstruction, this information is very meaningful and of help to decide the position of the bone tunnel.

Keywords Anatomical anterior cruciate ligament insertion • Macroscopic observation • Microscopic observation

3.1 Introduction

Previously, anatomical studies have been performed to know the position of the anatomical anterior cruciate ligament (ACL) insertion [1–18], and the ACL can be divided into two parts: the anteromedial (AM) and posterolateral (PL) bundles [1]. These bundles have different functions with different lengths and force-change patterns [19–21], and some biomechanical studies described that anatomical double-bundle (DB) ACL reconstruction achieved equal knee kinematics to those of the intact knee with stability of tibial anterior translation and rotation [22–24]. As a result, anatomical DB ACL reconstruction is a widely used procedure. Femoral

N. Sasaki, M.D. (✉)
Department of Orthopaedic Surgery, Hirosaki University Graduate School of Medicine, 5 Zaifu-cho, Hirosaki, Aomori 036-8562, Japan
e-mail: norisasa@hirosaki-u.ac.jp

M. Ochi et al. (eds.), *ACL Injury and Its Treatment*,
DOI 10.1007/978-4-431-55858-3_3

tunnel positions in anatomical ACL reconstruction are considered to be one of the most important factors effecting knee kinematics and clinical results [23, 25, 26]. Therefore, to accurately identify the location of an anatomical ACL insertion is very important.

3.2 The Macroscopic Observation of the ACL

The long axis of the femoral insertion of the ACL looks toward slightly forward from the axis of the femur [1, 3] and continues from the posterior femoral cortex [27]. Several previous studies investigated the femoral insertion of the ACL [1–3, 5, 8, 14, 16] and reported the size and area of the femoral ACL insertion. For the area, some authors indicated a large insertion area that extends over the articular cartilage margin, with reported value of from 100 to 200 mm^2 [5, 6, 8, 10, 14]. On the other hand, some authors showed a relatively narrow insertion area: from 65 to 130 mm^2 [7, 12, 16]. Furthermore, Śmigielski et al. recently reported the average width of the ACL was only 3.54 mm [27]. For the shape, Girgis et al. described that the femoral ACL insertion had a straight anterior side and convex posterior side [1]. Some authors showed that the shape of the femoral ACL insertion was more oval [28, 29]. Other authors observed further detail of the area and size of the femoral ACL insertion with removal of the surface membrane and described the shape of the femoral ACL insertion as more oval and narrow and away from the posterior cartilage margin [7, 12, 16]. Recently, the shape of the ACL insertion was reported to be narrower and to have a ribbonlike appearance [27]. In this way, the area of the femoral ACL insertion was described differently depending on the researchers (Fig. 3.1). However, the presence of the lateral intercondylar ridge [10, 15, 30, 31] is widely known as the landmark to identify the ACL insertion by common

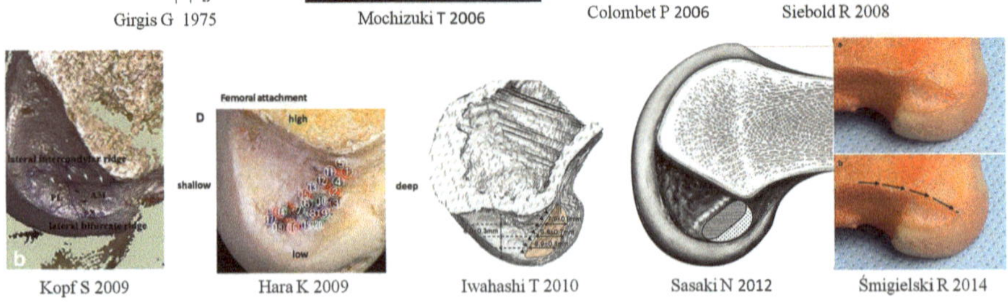

Fig. 3.1 Various ACL femoral insertions

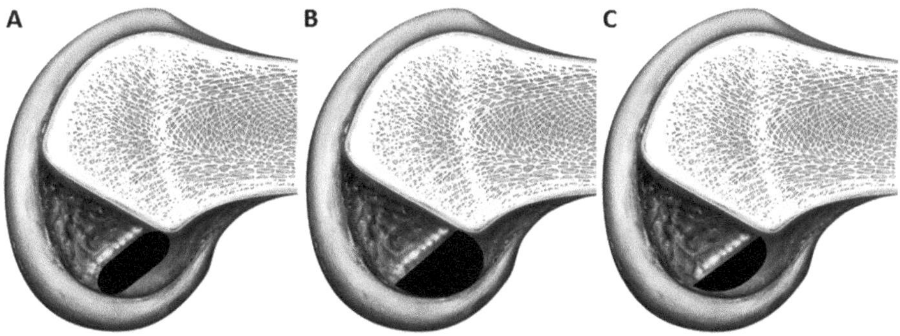

Fig. 3.2 Examples of the ACL femoral insertion. (**A**) Oval shape. The short axis of the ACL was narrow, and there was some space between the posterior cartilage and ACL insertion. (**B**) Semicircular shape. The ACL insertion was located between the lateral intercondylar ridge and posterior cartilage. (**C**) Small semicircular shape. The ACL insertion area was relatively wide and separated from the posterior cartilage [32]

consensus. The ridge—the so-called resident's ridge as coined by William Clancy Jr.—is a bony ridge in the medial wall of the lateral femoral condyle that exists throughout the ACL insertion from proximal to distal, reaching the articular cartilage. Although it is also a common recognition that the ACL attaches posteriorly to the lateral intercondylar ridge, the posterior margin of insertion remains controversial, as previously described (Fig. 3.2). In our macroscopic study, the femoral ACL insertion area was narrow and oval shaped, and the average length of the long axis was 17.7 ± 2.7 mm (range, 12–20 mm). They were some distance between the posterior margin of ACL insertion and the posterior cartilage border, and the average distance was 7.8 ± 1.2 mm [32]. For the length, width, and area of the femoral ACL insertion, previous data are shown in Table 3.1.

3.3 The Microscopic Observation of ACL

The differences of macroscopic observation may lead to surgeon disruption when deciding the femoral tunnel positions during ACL reconstruction. Therefore, microscopic investigation is absolutely imperative to better understand the ACL femoral insertion in detail.

Iwahashi et al. investigated the ACL insertion histologically and stated the direct insertion, which was constituted of ligament fibers, noncalcified fibrocartilage, calcified fibrocartilage, and bone located in a concave between the lateral intercondylar ridge and the articular cartilage border [10]. Meanwhile, in our microscopic study, the ACL insertion was found to extend between the lateral intercondylar ridge and the posterior cartilage margin by H&E staining (Fig. 3.3A). The direct insertion having four distinct layers was only positioned at

Table 3.1 The reports of measurement of the femoral anterior cruciate ligament (ACL) insertion

Literature	Study design	ACL insertion			Relationship between ACL and posterior cartilage[b]
		Length (mm ± SD)	Width (mm ± SD)	Area (mm^2 ± SD)	
Girgis FG, et al. (1975)	Macroscopical	23	–	–	Separate
Odensten M, et al. (1985)	Macroscopical	18 ± 2	11 ± 2	150[a]	Close
Amis AA, et al. (1991)	Macroscopical	–	–	–	Close
Muneta T, et al. (1997)	Macroscopical	16.0 ± 2.8	8.3 ± 2.8	93.3 ± 34.1	–
Harner CD, et al. (1999)	Macroscopical	–	–	113 ± 27	Close
Yasuda K, et al. (2004)	Macroscopical	–	–	–	Separate
Colombet P, et al. (2006)	Macroscopical	18.3 ± 2.3	10.3 ± 2.7	148[a]	Close
Takahashi M, et al. (2006)	Macroscopical	AM 11.3 ± 1.6	AM 7.5 ± 1.3	AM 66.9 ± 2.3	Separate
	Radiographical	PL 11.0 ± 1.7	PL 7.6 ± 1.0	PL 66.4 ± 2.3	
Mochizuki T, et al. (2006)	Macroscopical	AM 9.2 ± 0.7	4.7 ± 0.6	65[a]	Separate
		PL 6.0 ± 0.8			
Ferretti M, et al. (2007)	Macroscopical	17.2 ± 1.2	9.9 ± 0.8	196.8 ± 23.1	Close
	Arthroscopical				
	3D laser digitizer				
Hara K, et al. (2009)	Macroscopical	–	–	–	Separate
Iwahashi T, et al. (2010)	Microscopical	17.4 ± 0.9	8.0 ± 0.5	128.3 ± 10.5	Close
	3D Volume-rendered CT				
Kopf S, et al. (2011)	Arthroscopical	AM 9.2 ± 1.2	AM 8.9 ± 0.9	102.7[a]	–
		PL 7.1 ± 1.1	PL 6.9 ± 1.0		
Sasaki N, et al. (2012)	Macroscopical	17.7 ± 2.7	4.6 ± 0.7		Separate
	Microscopical		5.3 ± 1.1		
Smigielski R, et al. (2014)	Macroscopical	16.0	3.54	56.6	Separate

[a]Value other than one calculated from length and width
[b]Judgment from figure or measurement value of paper
Modified the table of reference No.32

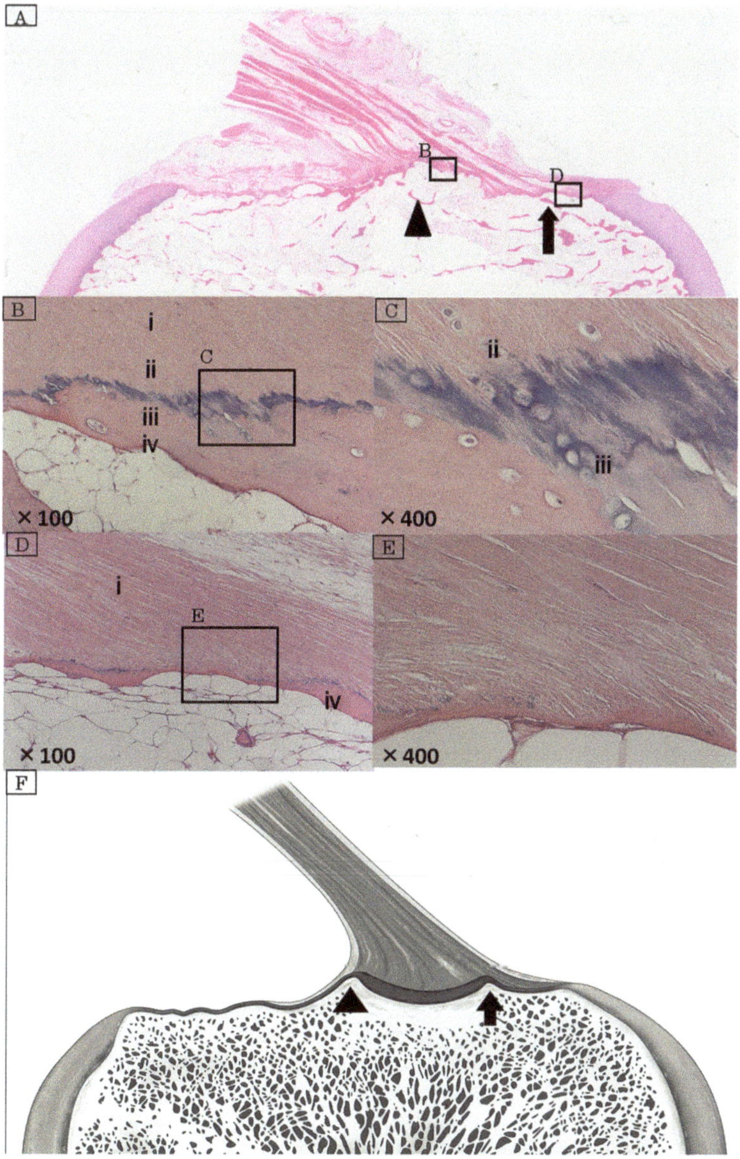

Fig. 3.3 Histology of the ACL insertion in hematoxylin and eosin staining. (**A**) The ACL insertion extended from the lateral intercondylar ridge and the posterior cartilage border. The arrowhead indicates the lateral intercondylar ridge, and the black arrow indicates the lateral intercondylar posterior ridge. The ACL attached between the lateral intercondylar ridge and the lateral intercondylar posterior ridge. (**B**) The direct insertion had a four-layered structure: ligamentous tissue, noncalcified fibrocartilage, calcified fibrocartilage, and bone (original magnification × 100). (**C**) The direct insertion with high magnification (original magnification × 400). Chondrocytes were observed. (**D**) The posterior area of direct insertion did not have a four-layered structure (original magnification × 100). The area located between the

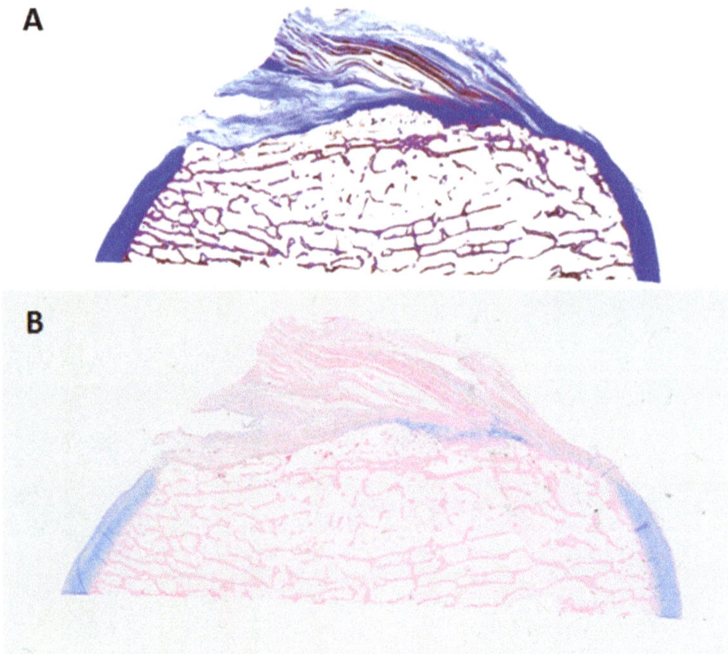

Fig. 3.4 Histology of the ACL insertion. (**A**) All collagen fibers were stained, and the cartilage layer and the ligaments appeared continuous to the posterior cartilage in azan staining. (**B**) In alcian blue staining, the fibrocartilage layers were stained. The area between the direct insertion and the posterior cartilage border was not stained, and calcified and noncalcified fibrocartilage layers were positioned a few millimeters away from the posterior cartilage [32]

the central portion of the ACL insertion, supported by the previous study (Fig. 3.3B). In the direct insertion, the chondrocytes were confirmed in noncalcified and calcified fibrocartilage layers (Fig. 3.3C). The thickness of the calcified fibrocartilage and bone layer (CFB) in the direct insertion was an average of 0.8 ± 0.3 mm. Another bony ridge, the "lateral intercondylar posterior ridge" (Fig. 3.3A black arrow), was found and positioned at the posterior margin of the direct insertion. However, the four-layered structure disappeared in the area posterior to the lateral intercondylar posterior ridge, and the ligament fibers connected with the cortical bone surface without the fibrocartilage layers and extended to the posterior cartilage border (Fig. 3.3D, E). In azan staining, all collagen fibers were stained and the cartilage layer and ligaments appeared continuous to the posterior cartilage (Fig. 3.4A). However, in alcian blue staining, there was an unstained area

---

Fig. 3.3 (continued) direct insertion and the posterior cartilage border. (**E**) The posterior area of direct insertion with high magnification (original magnification × 400). (**F**) An illustration of the lateral intercondylar ridge (arrowhead) and the lateral intercondylar posterior ridge (black arrow). i, ligaments; ii, noncalcified fibrocartilage; iii, calcified fibrocartilage; iv, bone [32]

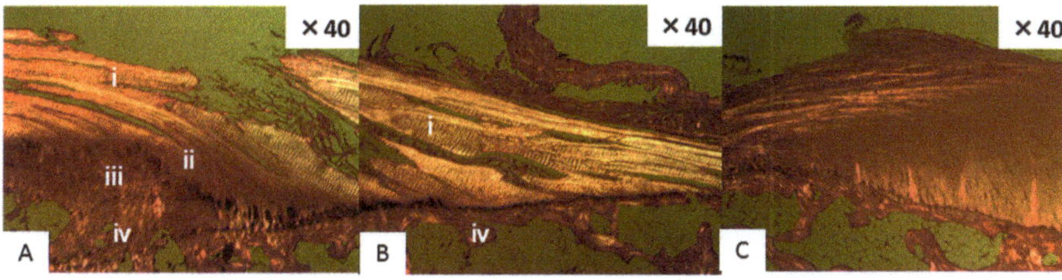

Fig. 3.5 Histology of the ACL insertion under polarizing microscope. (**A**) Observation of the direct insertion. There was a four-layered structure (original magnification × 40). (**B**) Observation of the posterior portion of the direct insertion. The ligaments attached to the bone directly without a four-layered structure (original magnification × 40). (**C**) The fibers of the ACL or the ACL membrane grew into the posterior cartilage (original magnification × 40). i, ligaments; ii, noncalcified fibrocartilage; iii, calcified fibrocartilage; iv, bone [32]

between the direct insertion and posterior cartilage border, and calcified and noncalcified cartilage layers existed a few millimeters anterior away from the posterior cartilage border (Fig. 3.4B). A polarizing microscopy also showed the direct insertion consisting of the four-layered structure (Fig. 3.5A), the ligament fiber attachment without the fibrocartilage layers posterior to the direct insertion (Fig. 3.5B), and the ligament fibers extending to the posterior joint cartilage (Fig. 3.5C).

3.4 Discrepancy Between Macroscopic and Microscopic Observations

There had been no studies comparing macroscopic and microscopic observations of the femoral ACL insertion. Our study compared macroscopic and microscopic observations of the femoral ACL insertion, and there were width differences of the ACL insertion between the macroscopic and microscopic measurements. Macroscopically, the distance from the anterior margin of the ACL insertion to the posterior cartilage border was 12.4 ± 1.7 mm, while the distance from the anterior margin of the direct insertion to the posterior cartilage border was 10.1 ± 1.3 mm microscopically. The position of the macroscopic ACL insertion was more anterior than that of the direct insertion because the distance from the posterior margin of the ACL insertion to the posterior cartilage border was 7.8 ± 1.2 mm macroscopically; however, the distance from the posterior margin of the direct insertion to the posterior cartilage border was 4.4 ± 0.5 mm microscopically. And the width of the macroscopic ACL insertion was narrower than that of the direct insertion (4.6 ± 0.7 and 5.3 ± 1.1 mm, respectively). The difference was considered to be due to the ACL appearing to be the fanlike structure at its insertion site.

3.5 The Function of Each Insertion

The major function of the direct insertion is mechanical linkage between the ligament and bone [33]. The noncalcified fibrocartilage layer has a function of bending-control reaction to the stress that occurs when a ligament and tendon change directions and acts as a stretching brake reaction to the tension that occurs when muscles contract [34, 35]. The CFB interface also had a complex interlocking pattern [36] and became deeper and more complex with greater stress [37, 38]. In cadaveric study, the fanlike area resisted 11–15 % of tibial anterior drawer force against the fiber of the direct insertion area which resisted 82–90 % of it [39]. Another study demonstrated that the debridement of fanlike area had minimum effect on the knee kinematics under anterior tibial load, and combination of valgus and internal rotatory torque [40]. These results in biomechanical studies are supported by the histological feature of the ACL femoral insertion, which was demonstrated in our study.

3.6 Clinical Relevance in ACL Reconstruction

For surgeons, it is very important to accurately identify the position of the ACL insertion during ACL reconstruction. As previously described, it would be ideal to make the femoral tunnel on the direct insertion in the native ACL. There is a bony concavity corresponding with the area of the ACL direct insertion, and the lateral intercondylar ridge exists at the anterior margin of this concavity [10] and the lateral intercondylar posterior ridge at the posterior margin of this concavity [32]. There are no ACL insertions anterior to this ridge [6]; therefore, the lateral intercondylar ridge has been used as the osseous landmark in anatomical ACL reconstruction [4, 10, 15]. And another bony ridge at the posterior ACL insertion margin has possibilities to be an osseous landmark, too. This ridge (i.e., the lateral intercondylar posterior ridge) could be called an "expert ridge" contrasted with the resident's ridge. The direct insertion was extended just between the lateral intercondylar ridge and lateral intercondylar posterior ridge. From our study, the direct insertion is located about 4 mm away from the posterior cartilage border, which has a narrow width (about 5 mm width), and the area which has no four-layered structure is positioned between the direct insertion and the posterior cartilage border; these findings are corroborated by alcian blue staining, polarizing microscopy, and the depth of the CFB [32]. After identification of the lateral intercondylar ridge, the bone tunnels were made at the back of this (Fig. 3.6).

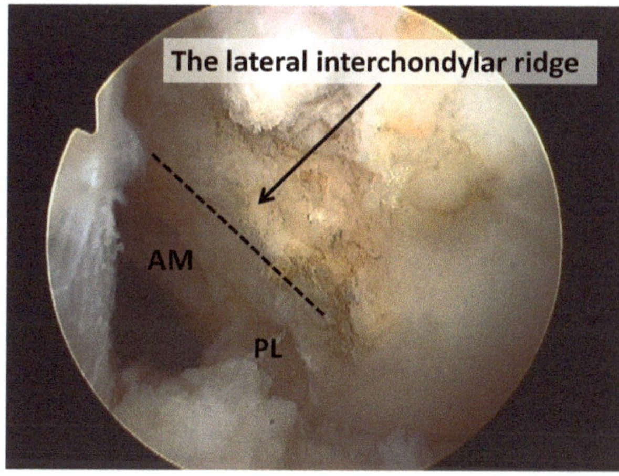

Fig. 3.6 Actual femoral bone tunnel position during ACL reconstruction in arthroscopy

References

1. Girgis FG, Marshall JL, Al Monajem ARS (1975) The cruciate ligaments of the knee joint. Anatomical, functional and experimental analysis. Clin Orthop 106:216–231
2. Amis AA, Dawkins GPC (1991) Functional anatomy of the anterior cruciate ligament. J Bone Joint Surg (Br) 73:260–267
3. Arnoczky SP (1983) Anatomy of the anterior cruciate ligament. Clin Orthop Rel Res 172:19–25
4. Cain EL Jr, Clancy WG Jr (2002) Anatomic endoscopic anterior cruciate ligament reconstruction with patella tendon autograft. Orthop Clin N Am 33:717–725
5. Colombet P, Robinson J, Christel P et al (2006) Morphology of anterior cruciate ligament attachments for anatomic reconstruction: a cadaveric dissection and radiographic study. Arthroscopy 22;984–992
6. Ferretti M, Ekdahl M, Shen W et al (2007) Osseous landmarks of the femoral attachment of the anterior cruciate ligament: an anatomic study. Arthroscopy 23:1218–1225
7. Hara K, Mochizuki T, Sekiya I et al (2009) Anatomy of normal human anterior cruciate ligament attachments evaluated by divided small bundles. Am J Sports Med 37:2386–2391
8. Harner CD, Baek GH, Vogrin TM et al (1999) Quantitative analysis of human cruciate ligament insertion. Arthroscopy 15:741–749
9. Hutchinson MR, Ash SA (2003) Resident's ridge: assessing the cortical thickness of the lateral wall and roof of the intercondylar notch. Arthroscopy 19:931–935
10. Iwahashi T, Shino K, Nakata K et al (2010) Direct anterior cruciate ligament insertion to the femur assessed by histology and 3-dimensional volume-rendered computed tomography. Arthroscopy 26:S13–S20
11. Kopf S, Musahl V, Tashman S et al (2009) A systematic review of the femoral origin and tibial insertion morphology of the ACL. Knee Surg Sports Traumatol Arthrosc 17:213–219
12. Mochizuki T, Muneta T, Nagase T et al (2006) Cadaveric knee observation study for describing anatomic femoral tunnel placement for two-bundle anterior cruciate ligament reconstruction. Arthroscopy 22:356–361
13. Muneta T, Takakuda K, Yamamoto H (1997) Intercondylar notch width and its relation to the configuration and cross-sectional area of the anterior cruciate ligament. A cadaveric knee study. Am J Sports Med 25:69–72
14. Odensten M, Gillquist J (1985) Functional anatomy of the anterior cruciate ligament and a rationale for reconstruction. J Bone Joint Surg Am 67:257–262

15. Shino K, Suzuki T, Iwahashi T et al (2010) The resident's ridge as an arthroscopic landmark for anatomical femoral tunnel drilling in ACL reconstruction. Knee Surg Sports Traumatol Arthrosc 18:1164–1168
16. Takahashi M, Doi M, Abe M et al (2006) Anatomical study of the femoral and tibial insertion of the anteromedial and posterolateral bundles of human anterior cruciate ligament. Am J Sports Med 34:787–792
17. Siebold R, Ellert T, Metz S et al (2008) Femoral insertions of the anteromedial and posterolateral bundles of the anterior cruciate ligament: morphometry and arthroscopic orientation models for double-bundle bone tunnel placement—a cadaver study. Arthroscopy 24:585–592
18. Yasuda K, Kondo E, Ichiyama H et al (2004) Anatomic reconstruction of the anteromedial and posterolateral bundles of the anterior cruciate ligament using hamstring tendon grafts. Arthroscopy 20:1015–1025
19. Sakane M, Livesay GA, Fox RJ et al (1999) Relative contribution of the ACL, MCL, and bony contact to the anterior stability of the knee. Knee Surg Sports Traumatol Arthrosc 7:93–97
20. Takai S, Woo SL, Livesay GA et al (1993) Determination of the in situ loads on the human anterior cruciate ligament. J Orthop Res 11:686–695
21. Xerogeanes JW, Takeda Y, Livesay GA et al (1995) Effect of knee flexion on the in situ force distribution in the human anterior cruciate ligament. Knee Surg Sports Traumatol Arthrosc 3:9–13
22. Mae T, Shino K, Miyama T et al (2001) Single- versus two-femoral socket anterior cruciate ligament reconstruction technique: biomechanical analysis using robotic simulator. Arthroscopy 17:708–716
23. Musahl V, Plakseychuk A, VanScyoc A et al (2005) Varying femoral tunnels between the anatomical footprint and isometric positions. Am J Sports Med 33:712–718
24. Yagi M, Wong EK, Kanamori A et al (2002) Biomechanical analysis of an anatomic anterior cruciate ligament reconstruction. Am J Sports Med 30:660–666
25. Tashman S, Collon D, Anderson K et al (2004) Abnormal rotational knee motion during running after anterior cruciate ligament reconstruction. Am J Sports Med 32:975–983
26. Zantop T, Petersen W, Sekiya JK et al (2006) Anterior cruciate ligament anatomy and function relating to anatomical reconstruction. Knee Surg Sports Traumatol Arthrosc 14:982–992
27. Śmigielski R, Zdanowicz U, Drwięga M et al (2014) Ribbon like appearance of the midsubstance fibres of the anterior cruciate ligament close to its femoral insertion site: a cadaveric study including 111 knees. Knee Surg Sports Traumatol Arthrosc 23:3143–3150
28. Petersen W, Tillmann B (2002) Anatomy and function of anterior cruciate ligament. Orthopade 31:710–718
29. Petersen W, Zantop T (2007) Anatomy of the anterior cruciate ligament with regard to its two bundles. Clin Orthop Relat Res 454:35–47
30. Bicer EK, Lustig S, Servien E et al (2010) Current knowledge in the anatomy of the human anterior cruciate ligament. Knee Surg Sports Traumatol Arthrosc 18:1075–1084
31. Tanaka Y, Shiozaki Y, Yonetani Y et al (2011) MRI analysis of the attachment of the anteromedial and posterolateral bundles of anterior cruciate ligament using coronal oblique images. Knee Surg Sports Traumatol Arthrosc 30:1–6
32. Sasaki N, Ishibashi Y, Tsuda E et al (2012) The femoral insertion of the anterior cruciate ligament: discrepancy between macroscopic and histological observations. Arthroscopy 28:1135–1146
33. Schneider H (1956) Zur struktur der sehnenansatzzonen. Z Anat Entwicklungsgesch 119:431–456
34. Kumai T, Takakura Y, Rufai A et al (2002) The functional anatomy of the human anterior talofibular ligament in relation to ankle sprains. J Anat 200:457–465
35. Evans EJ, Benjamin M, Pemberton DJ (1990) Fibrocartilage in the attachment zones of the quadriceps tendon and patellar ligament of man. J Anat 171:155–162
36. Milz S, Rufai A, Buettner A et al (2002) Three-dimensional reconstructions of the Achilles tendon insertion in man. J Anat 200:145–152

37. Evans EJ, Benjamin M, Permberton DJ (1991) Variations in the amount of calcified tissue at the attachments of the quadriceps tendon and patellar tendon in man. J Anat 174:145–151
38. Kumai T, Takakura Y (2005) Pathogenesis and treatments for enthesopathy in sporting activities. Orthop Surg Traumatol 48:527–538
39. Kawaguchi Y, Kondo E, Takeda R et al (2015) The role of fibers in the femoral attachment of the anterior cruciate ligament in resisting tibial displacement. Arthroscopy 31:435–444
40. Pathare NP, Nicholas SJ, Colbrunn R et al (2014) Kinematic analysis of the indirect femoral insertion of the anterior cruciate ligament: implications for anatomic femoral tunnel placement. Arthroscopy 30:1430–1438

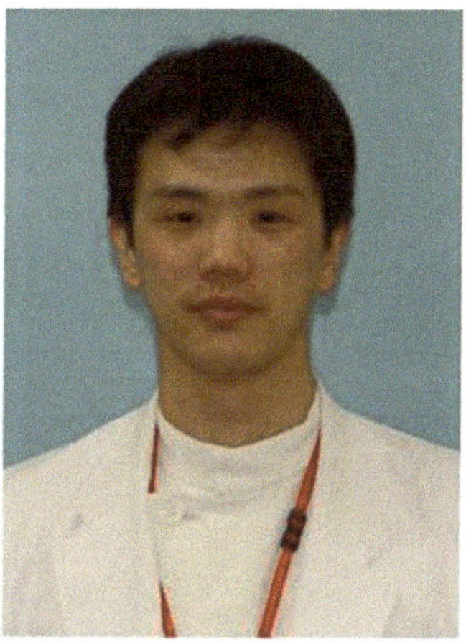

Norihiro Sasaki, M.D., Department of Orthopaedic Surgery, Hirosaki University Graduate School of Medicine, Aomori, Japan.

Chapter 4
Tibial Insertion of the ACL: 3D-CT Images, Macroscopic, and Microscopic Findings

Keiji Tensho

Abstract Accurate and detailed knowledge of ACL footprint anatomy is essential for successful anatomical ACL reconstruction. On the femoral side, the discovery of bony landmarks led to the standardization of femoral bone tunnel construction; however, the detailed morphology and location of ACL tibial footprint continue to be a topic of debate, and there are still no standardized methods for tibial tunnel construction. We previously reported the ACL tibial attachment site anatomy and bony landmarks and compared 3D images with visual and histological evaluations. The results from the study found a unique bony landmark surrounding the ACL attachment site, showing the relationship of these bony landmarks and surrounding anatomical landmarks as a useful indicator for determining tunnel positions during arthroscopic surgery. This section will clarify the detailed anatomy and bony landmark of the ACL tibial footprint necessary for reconstructive surgery by reviewing our previous research in conjunction with the available literature.

Keywords Anterior cruciate ligament (ACL) • Tibial footprint • Bony landmark • Anatomical landmark

4.1 Introduction

With the development of anatomical approach for anterior cruciate ligament (ACL) reconstruction in recent years, a more detailed anatomical research of ACL attachment has become a focus of attention. However, the morphology and location of footprint continue to be a topic of debate, and a general consensus has not yet been reached. We have presented a detailed report on the bony landmarks around the ACL tibial footprint, as well as the relationship between these bony landmarks and anatomical structures around the ACL tibial footprint [1]. This section will clarify the detailed anatomy of the ACL tibial footprint necessary for reconstructive surgery by reviewing our previous research in conjunction with the available literature.

K. Tensho, M.D., Ph.D. (✉)
Department of Orthopedic Surgery, Shinshu University School of Medicine, Asahi 3-1-1, Matsumoto, Nagano 390-8621, Japan
e-mail: kten@shinshu-u.ac.jp

M. Ochi et al. (eds.), *ACL Injury and Its Treatment*,
DOI 10.1007/978-4-431-55858-3_4

4.2 Bony Landmark Around ACL Tibial Footprint

In contrast to the femur, reports on bony landmarks of the ACL tibial footprint are rare. Purnell et al. demonstrated in their research using 3D-CT images that there is an absence of anterior/lateral bony landmarks in the tibia, though one can confirm the medial intercondylar ridge in the medial border and a tibial ridge in the posterior border of the ACL attachment [2]. Berg et al. utilized X-ray images to report an anterior bony prominence to the ACL attachment at approximately 30 % of the knee joint called the Parsons' knob [3]. Ziegler et al. also reported two bony landmarks, the ACL ridge and ACL tubercle, located at the anterior border of the ACL, in addition to the anterolateral fossa located in the lateral border [4]. Hutchinson described the "over-the-back position (ridge)" located posterior to the ACL tibial footprint as the most reliable and accurate bony reference for ACL tibial tunnel creation [5].

In our research, we found a bony protrusion that approximately corresponds to the ACL footprint, located anterior to the medial and lateral tubercle and the center of the tibial plateau (Fig. 4.1). A bony ridge (anterior ridge) medial laterally extends anterior to the aforementioned protrusion. We believed the anterior ridge might be the same bony structure as the "Parson's knob"; however, this landmark does not resemble the morphology of a knob but rather a ridgelike structure with some width. Also, this landmark joins with the medial intercondylar ridge at the anterior border to form an L-shaped ridge [1]. Furthermore, between the medial and lateral tubercle, a small depression referred to as the intertubercular fossa can be confirmed, in addition to a lateral groove that extends anteroposteriorly. Although the morphology of bony protrusions can be classified into two categories of oval and triangular types, these morphological characteristics surrounding the protrusion can be confirmed in almost all cases, demonstrating a general morphological tendency.

4.3 Anterior and Medial Side of the ACL Tibial Footprint

Soft tissues such as the synovial membrane are absent anteriorly and medially to the ACL tibial attachment, and the border between bone and ligament is distinct. A small protrusion observed by 3D-CT images, corresponding to the anterior ridge, can also be grossly observed and palpated. The anterior ridge is a small protrusion that is 1 mm in width and 10–11 mm in length, and the ACL was attached posterior to this protrusion. Additionally, this protrusion joins together the medial intercondylar ridge and anteromedial border, forming the anteromedial border of the ACL footprint. The anterior ridge can also be clearly confirmed histologically, and it can be observed that the ACL is attached posteriorly to this ridge (Fig. 4.2).

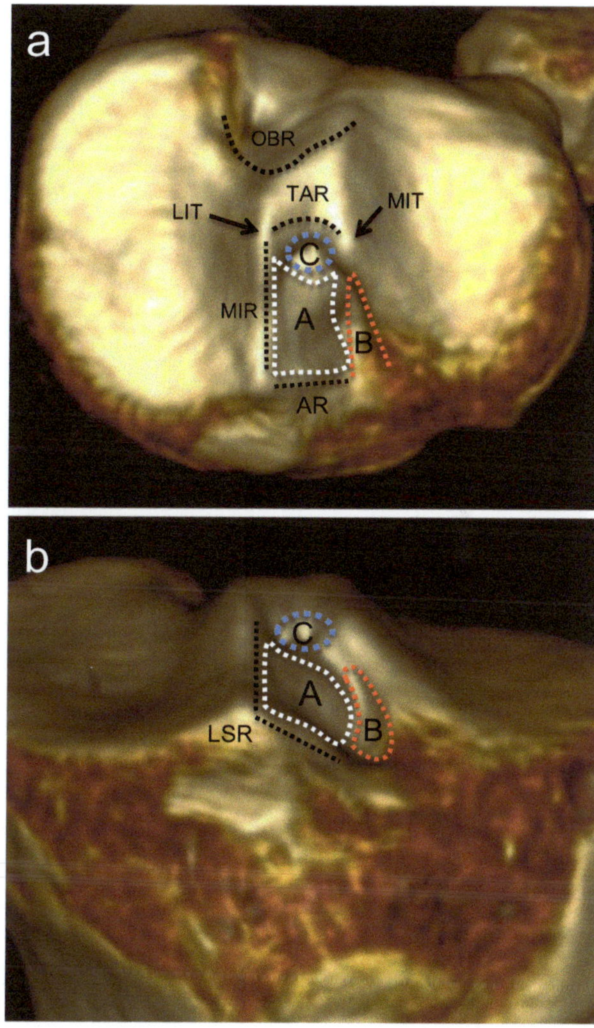

Fig. 4.1 (**a**) 3D axial images of left knee tibial plateau. (**b**) Anterosuperior view of tibial plateau. A (*white dash line*), bony protrusion of ACL tibial attachment; B (*red dash line*), lateral groove; C (*blue dash line*), intertubercular fossa; *AR* anterior ridge, *MIR* medial intercondylar ridge, *LIT* lateral intercondylar tubercle, *MIT* medial intercondylar tubercle, *TAR* tibial ACL ridge, *OBR* over-the-back ridge, *LSR* L-shaped ridge

4.4 Lateral Side of ACL Tibial Footprint

The ACL comes into adjacency with the anterior horn of the lateral meniscus under gross observation, and parts of the ACL fiber are attached to the anterior horn with an anterior width ranging from 1/3–1/2 of its surface. Moreover, fat and scar tissues cover its border, and the border between the anterior horn of the lateral meniscus and ACL attachment cannot be grossly identified. When these surface layers of soft tissues are carefully detached, both structures are overlapped anteriorly and the lateral meniscus slips under the substratum of the ACL posteriorly (Fig. 4.3). The anterior horn of the lateral meniscus was attached on the base of the lateral groove and lateral aspect of the aforementioned bony protrusion, and the attachment was

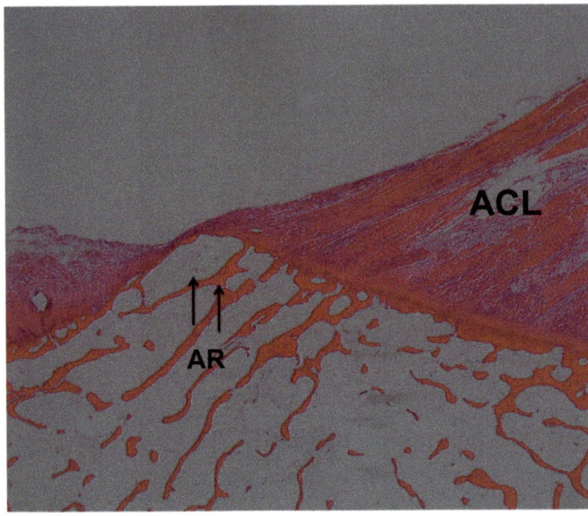

Fig. 4.2 Histological observation of anterior margin of ACL tibial footprint (original magnification × 2). ACL fiber was attached posterior to anterior ridge. *AR*: anterior ridge. *Black arrow* indicates the anterior ridge

located almost anterior to the lateral intercondylar tubercle. Although the ACL attaches anteriorly at the base of the groove, in terms of its histology, the lateral meniscus attaches to the base of lateral groove and the lateral aspect of the protrusion mediated by connective tissue as the attachment site moves posteriorly (Fig. 4.4).

4.5 Posterior Border of ACL Tibial Footprint

Under gross observation, fibrous tissue was found between the medial intercondylar tubercles, tibial ACL ridge, and ACL. A careful removal of these tissues revealed that ligaments were attached to the medial intercondylar tubercle; however, these ligaments were not attached to the ACL tibial ridge and the intertubercular fossa (Fig. 4.5). The same observation was confirmed histologically, and vascular tissues and synovial membrane were confirmed in the intertubercular fossa (Fig. 4.5). From these findings, we can extrapolate that the main fiber of the ACL is not attached posteriorly to the anterior margin of the medial and lateral intercondylar tubercle, and that its posterior border is positioned relatively anterior to what has been previously believed.

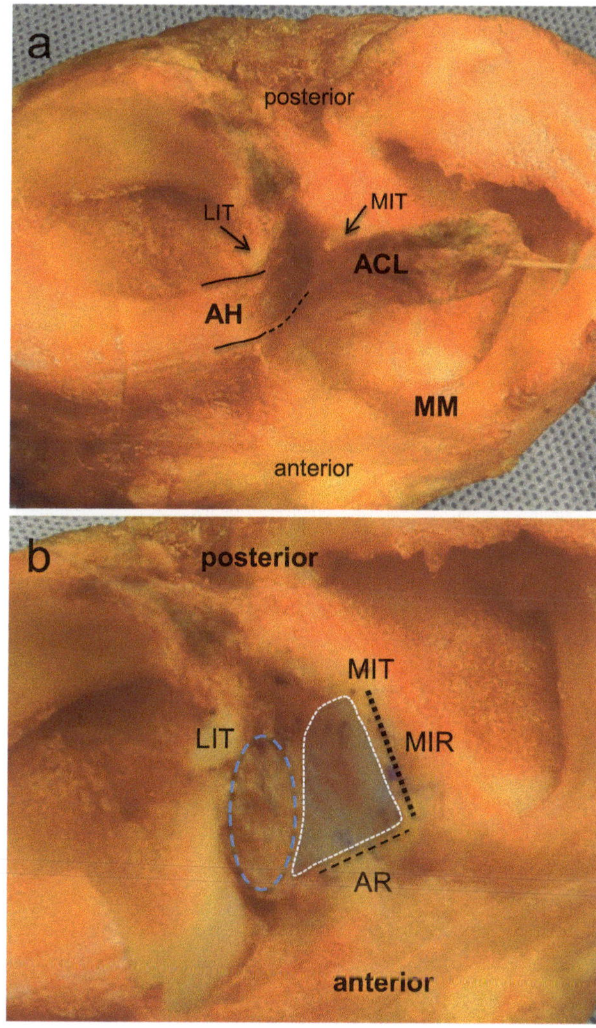

Fig. 4.3 (**a**, **b**) Macroscopic observation of ACL tibial footprint. (**a**) ACL and lateral meniscus are overlapped anteriorly, and the lateral meniscus slips under the substratum of the ACL posteriorly. (**b**) After resection of ACL and lateral meniscus attachment. *AH* anterior horn of lateral meniscus, *MM* medial meniscus, *LIT* lateral intercondylar tubercle, *MIT* medial intercondylar tubercle, *white dot area* ACL tibial footprint, *blue dot area* attachment of anterior horn of lateral meniscus

4.6 Discussion

4.6.1 Size and Morphology of ACL Tibial Footprint

A detailed anatomical knowledge of the attachment area of the ACL is essential for successful anatomical ACL reconstruction. In contrast to the femoral attachment, previous studies reported various sizes and morphologies of the tibial ACL attachment (Table 4.1). Girgis et al. reported 30 mm of length [6], Tállay et al. reported a length of 19.5 ± 2.6 mm and width of 10.3 ± 1.9 mm [7], Ferretti et al. reported a length of 18.1 ± 2.8 mm and width of 10.7 ± 1.9 mm [8], Purnell et al. reported a

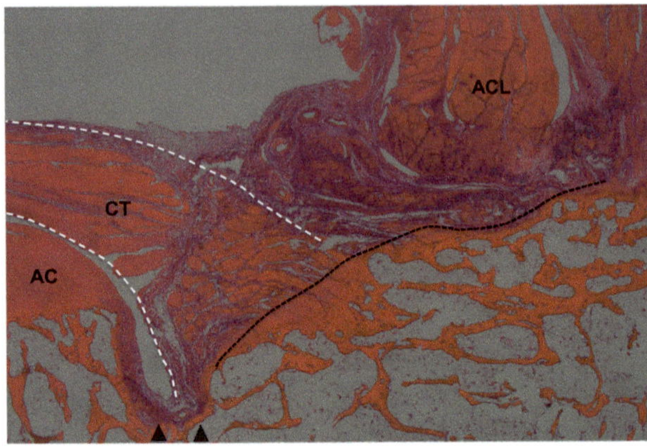

Fig. 4.4 Coronal histological section of the lateral margin of ACL tibial footprint (original magnification × 1). The lateral meniscus attaches to the base of lateral groove and the lateral aspect of the protrusion with connective tissue. *AC*: articular cartilage of lateral tibial plateau. *White dot area*: connective tissue (*CT*) of anterior horn of lateral meniscus. *Black dash line*: bony protrusion of ACL tibial footprint. *Arrowhead*: base of lateral groove

length of 10.7 ± 1.3 mm and width of 7.3 ± 1.1 mm [2], and the morphology of the attachment also varies by case, such as oval and triangular attachments [1]. There were various interpretations of ACL components including single bundle [9, 10], double bundle [11, 12], and triple bundle [13], while the arrangement of these components at the tibial footprint was widely varied. In recent years, Siebold reported that the ACL is a flat midsubstance with a ribbonlike anatomy and that the tibial attachment is C-shaped [14]. These results were not only influenced by individual difference, but also by differences in modality, age, sex, race, and body type. Moreover, because many reports grossly observed the attachment site of the ligament in order to determine its borders, the differences in the reviewers' individual interpretations greatly influenced their results. Additionally, the results may change drastically by how the synovial membrane and fat tissues are managed, resulting in a widely ranging analysis.

4.6.2 Anatomical Landmark for Tibial Tunnel Creation

An important factor in surgery is how to create bone tunnels that are accurate and reproducible amid these varied tibial footprints. Thus, when creating tibial bone tunnels, various intraoperative landmarks have been reported (Table 4.2). Tállay et al. recommended deciding the position from the anterior border of the tibia [7], Morgan et al. from the PCL [15], and Hutchinson and Edwards and Heming et al. from the distance from the over-the-back ridge [5, 10, 12]. Furthermore, there were reports that consider the intermeniscal ligament [8, 16] in the anterior and medial tibial eminence [8] in the posterior landmarks. However, these

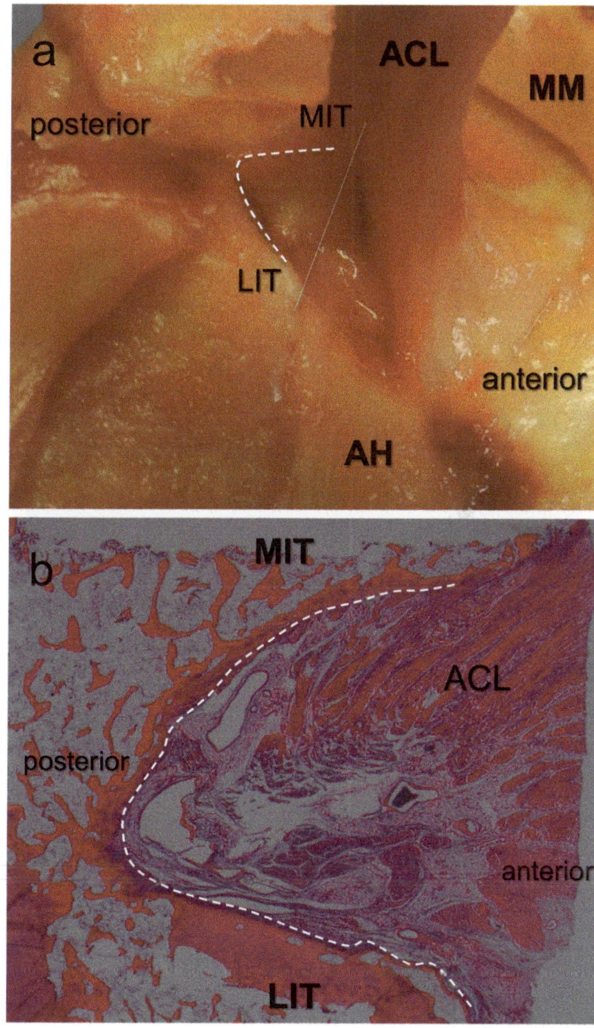

Fig. 4.5 (**a**) Macroscopic observation of ACL tibial footprint. After removal of fat and synovial tissues, the ACL is attached only to the medial intercondylar tubercle and not attached to the lateral intercondylar tubercle and intertubercular space. Main fiber of the ACL is not attached posteriorly to the anterior margin of the medial and lateral intercondylar tubercle. (**b**) Axial section of posterior border of ACL tibial footprint (original magnification × 4). Vascular tissues and synovial membrane were confirmed in the intertubercular fossa, and ACL fiber was only attached to medial intercondylar tubercle. *AH* anterior horn of lateral meniscus, *MM* medial meniscus, *LIT* lateral intercondylar tubercle, *MIT* medial intercondylar tubercle, *white solid line* anterior margin of the medial and lateral intercondylar tubercle, *white dot line* anterior margin of tibial ACL ridge

landmarks are difficult to reproduce due to the fact that they are determined by the distance from its target, making them unreliable landmarks to define an accurate position for bone tunnel construction in the varying tibial footprint. Moreover, recent detailed anatomical studies suggest that the posterior border of the ACL footprint is positioned relatively anterior to what has been previously believed with narrower bounds in the AP aspect [1, 14, 17], and a clinical application of these traditional methods to current reconstructive procedures was difficult. We utilized both macro-/microscopic observation and CT images to study the positions of the attachment boundaries and its surrounding tissues in detail, and we presented a method for bone tunnel creation with the aforementioned bony/anatomical landmarks in order to standardize surgical management. In our study, a square structure

Table 4.1 ACL tibial insertion size and anatomical landmark by previous study

Author	Mean length ± SD* (mm) (range)	Mean width ± SD* (mm) (range)	Subject/ Methodology
Girgis et al. [6]	30 mm		Cadaver/ macroscopic
Tállay et al. [7]	19.5 ± 2.6 mm	10.3 ± 1.9 mm	Human/ macroscopic
	(14.5–24.7)	(7.1–15.1)	
Purnell et al. [2]	10.7 ± 1.3 mm	7.3 ± 1.1 mm	Cadaver/3D-CT
	(9.3–13.1)	(5.9–9)	
Ferretti et al. [8]	18.1 ± 2.8 mm	10.7 ± 1.9 mm	Cadaver/ macroscopic
	(13.7–22.1)	(7.4–13.1)	
Heming et al. [10]	18.5 mm	10.3 mm	Cadaver/ macroscopic
Kopf et al. [27]	17 ± 2.0 mm	AM:9.2 ± 1.1 mm (6–11)	Human/ arthroscopic
	(AM:9.1 mm/PL:7.4 mm) (12–22)	/PL:7.0 ± 1.0 mm (4–10)	
Tensho et al. [1]	13.5 ± 1.7 mm	11.7 ± 1.7 mm	Human/3D-CT
	(10.7–18.1)	(8.6–16.8)	
Siebold et al.	12.6 ± 2.3 mm (C-shaped)	3.3 ± 0.4 mm (C-shaped)	Cadaver/ macroscopic
	(7.7–16.3)	(2.5–3.9)	

Table 4.2 Anatomical landmark for tunnel positioning

Author	Anatomical landmark for tunnel positioning
Tállay et al. [7]	Distance from anterior edge of tibia (AM, 17.2 ± 4.1 mm; PL, 25.6 ± 14.8 mm)
Morgan et al. [15]	Distance from PCL (center: 6–7 mm)
Hutchinson et al. [5]	Distance from the over-the-back position (center: 10.4 ± 2.4 mm anterior, posterior margin of ACL tibial footprint 6.7 ± 1.2 mm)
Edwards et al. [12]	Distance from the over-the-back ridge (center, 15 ± 2 mm anterior; AM, 17 ± 2 mm anterior; PL, 10 ± 1 mm anterior)
Heming et al. [10]	Tibial notch of PCL
	Center: 15.0 mm anterior
Ferretti et al. [8]	Anterior: intermeniscal ligament
	Posterior: medial tibial eminence
Tensho et al. [1]	Square model
	Anteromedial, L-shaped ridge; lateral, anterior horn of lateral meniscus; posterior, medial/lateral intercondylar tubercle

(Fig. 4.6) consisting of the following landmarks can be observed: ACL footprint, anterior; anterior ridge, medial; medial intercondylar ridge (anteromedial; L-shaped ridge), lateral; and anterior horn of the lateral meniscus, posterior; in addition, the anterior border of the medial and lateral intercondylar tubercles is invariable, regardless of size and morphology. In our anatomical study, we believe that if bone tunnels are positioned within this square structure, we can create bone tunnels with reproducibility.

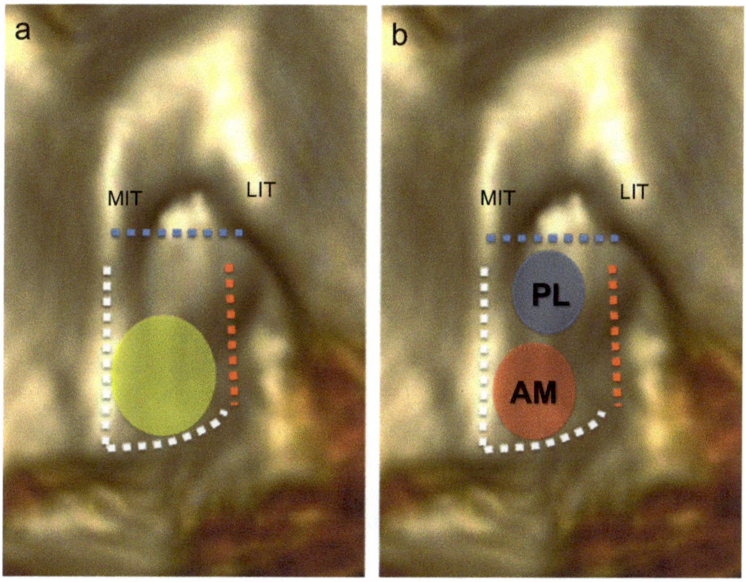

Fig. 4.6 Ideal tunnel position for (**a**) single-bundle reconstruction, (**b**) double-bundle reconstruction from our results. *White dot line*, L-shaped ridge; *red line*, attachment of anterior horn of lateral meniscus; *blue dot line*, anterior margin of the medial and lateral intercondylar tubercle; *yellow circle*, tibial tunnel for single-bundle ACL reconstruction; *red circle*, tibial tunnel of anteromedial bundle for double-bundle ACL reconstruction; *blue circle*, tibial tunnel of posterolateral bundle for double-bundle ACL reconstruction

4.6.3 Anatomical Pitfalls of Tibial Tunnel Creation

From recent studies, there are two important points that we must consider when creating tibial bone tunnels. Firstly, the tibial tunnel position greatly affects graft obliquity in the sagittal and coronal plane that is extremely important in obtaining postoperative stability for ACL reconstruction. Hatayama et al. reported that positioning the tibial tunnel anteriorly obtains better postoperative anterior knee stability [18]. Inderhaug stated that the posterior placement of the tibial tunnel had inferior rotational stability and clinical scores compared to anterior tibial tunnel placement [19]. Zampeli reported a greater rotational instability of the tibia with less oblique graft in the coronal plane and recommended a more anteromedial placement of the tunnel on the tibial side [20]. Anterior placement of the tibial tunnel was previously thought to induce the risk of graft failure or limitation in range of motion due to roof impingement. However, recent studies have proved that such risks from the anterior placement of the tibial tunnel are rather low [21–23], and we believe that the anteromedial placement of the tibial tunnel within the anatomical tibial footprint is a method we can endorse.

The second point is that the ACL attachment is extremely proximate to the anterior horn of the lateral meniscus attachment. Several articles reported the proximity of the ACL tibial attachment and the anterior horn of the lateral meniscus attachment, and in addition, that creating a bone tunnel in the center of the attachment site reduced the surface area, lowering the pullout strength [24–26]. Our detailed macroscopic/histological observation also established that the anterior horn of the lateral meniscus is positioned centrally as it runs posteriorly. The lateral meniscus is attached on the base of the lateral groove and lateral side of the bony protrusion, and the attachment is positioned more centrally at the postero-lateral margin of the ACL tibial footprint and almost anteriorly to the lateral intercondylar tubercle. Thus, surgeons should be aware that there is risk of damaging the anterior horn of the lateral meniscus attachment when creating a large bone tunnel in the center of the tibial footprint for single-bundle reconstruction and positioning the PL bone tunnel posterolaterally to the attachment site for double-bundle reconstruction. From the two aforementioned points, the bone tunnel should be created anteromedially within the square structure for single-bundle reconstruction (Fig. 4.6). Like single-bundle reconstruction, the AM bone tunnel should be positioned anteromedially within the attachment site for double-bundle reconstruction, and the PL bone tunnel should be positioned posterior, not posterolateral, to the AM bone tunnel to avoid damaging the anterior horn of the lateral meniscus attachment. To this end, we believe that the L-shaped ridge we have proposed may be an important landmark for anteromedial placement of the tibial tunnel.

4.7 Conclusion

The debate in terms of the morphology and structure of the ACL has continued to this day. The choice of graft material and tunnel position of ACL reconstruction is dependent on how various evidences from the current anatomical literature are interpreted. Our proposed method for tibial tunnel creation is greatly simplified, and we believe that our results and method for tibial tunnel creation can be usefully applied to any reconstruction technique; furthermore, we strongly believe that accurate reproducibility of tibial tunnel creation can be achieved by its standardization.

References

1. Tensho K, Shimodaira H, Aoki T, Narita N, Kato H, Kakegawa A, Fukushima N, Moriizumi T, Fujii M, Fujinaga Y, Saito N (2014) Bony landmarks of the anterior cruciate ligament tibial footprint: a detailed analysis comparing 3-dimensional computed tomography images to visual and histological evaluations. Am J Sports Med 18:1433–1440
2. Purnell ML, Larson AI, Clancy W (2008) Anterior cruciate ligament insertions on the tibia and femur and their relationships to critical bony landmarks using high-resolution volume-rendering computed tomography. Am J Sports Med 36:2083–2090

3. Berg EE (1993) Parsons' knob (tuberculum intercondylare tertium). A guide to tibial anterior cruciate ligament insertion. Clin Orthop Relat Res 292:229–231
4. Ziegler CG, Pietrini SD, Westerhaus BD, Anderson CJ, Wijdicks CA, Johansen S, Engebretsen L, LaPrade RF (2011) Arthroscopically pertinent landmarks for tunnel positioning in single-bundle and double-bundle anterior cruciate ligament reconstructions. Am J Sports Med 39:743–752
5. Hutchinson MR, Bae TS (2001) Reproducibility of anatomic tibial landmarks for anterior cruciate ligament reconstructions. Am J Sports Med 29:777–780
6. Girgis FG, Marshall JL, Monajem A (1975) The cruciate ligaments of the knee joint. Anatomical, functional and experimental analysis. Clin Orthop Relat Res 106:216–231
7. Tállay A, Lim MH, Bartlett J (2008) Anatomical study of the human anterior cruciate ligament stump's tibial insertion footprint. Knee Surg Sports Traumatol Arthrosc 16:741–746
8. Ferretti M, Doca D, Ingham SM, Cohen M, Fu FH (2012) Bony and soft tissue landmarks of the ACL tibial insertion site: an anatomical study. Knee Surg Sports Traumatol Arthrosc 20:62–68
9. Odensten M, Gillquist J (1985) Functional anatomy of the anterior cruciate ligament and a rationale for reconstruction. J Bone Joint Surg Am 67:257–262
10. Heming JF, Rand J, Steiner ME (2007) Anatomical limitations of transtibial drilling in anterior cruciate ligament reconstruction. Am J Sports Med 35:1708–1715
11. Colombet P, Robinson J, Christel P, Franceschi JP, Djian P, Bellier G, Sbihi A (2006) Morphology of anterior cruciate ligament attachments for anatomic reconstruction: a cadaveric dissection and radiographic study. Arthroscopy 22:984–992
12. Edwards A, Bull AM, Amis AA (2007) The attachments of the anteromedial and posterolateral fibre bundles of the anterior cruciate ligament: part 1: tibial attachment. Knee Surg Sports Traumatol Arthrosc 15:1414–1421
13. Otsubo H, Shino K, Suzuki D, Kamiya T, Suzuki T, Watanabe K, Fujimiya M, Iwahashi T, Yamashita T (2012) The arrangement and the attachment areas of three ACL bundles. Knee Surg Sports Traumatol Arthrosc 20:127–134
14. Siebold R, Schuhmacher P, Fernandez F, Śmigielski R, Fink C, Brehmer A, Kirsch J (2015) Flat midsubstance of the anterior cruciate ligament with tibial "C"-shaped insertion site. Knee Surg Sports Traumatol Arthrosc 23:3136–3142
15. Morgan CD, Kalman VR, Grawl DM (1995) Definitive landmarks for reproducible tibial tunnel placement in anterior cruciate ligament reconstruction. Arthroscopy 11:275–288
16. Kongcharoensombat W, Ochi M, Abouheif M, Adachi N, Ohkawa S, Kamei G, Okuhara A, Shibuya H, Niimoto T, Nakasa T, Nakamae A, Deie M (2011) The transverse ligament as a landmark for tibial sagittal insertions of the anterior cruciate ligament: a cadaveric study. Arthroscopy 27:1395–1399
17. Hara K, Mochizuki T, Sekiya I, Yamaguchi K, Akita K, Muneta T (2009) Anatomy of normal human anterior cruciate ligament attachments evaluated by divided small bundles. Am J Sports Med 37:2386–2391
18. Hatayama K, Terauchi M, Saito K, Higuchi H, Yanagisawa S, Takagishi K (2013) The importance of tibial tunnel placement in anatomic double-bundle anterior cruciate ligament reconstruction. Arthroscopy 29:1072–1078
19. Inderhaug E, Strand T, Fischer-Bredenbeck C, Solheim E (2014) Effect of a too posterior placement of the tibial tunnel on the outcome 10–12 years after anterior cruciate ligament reconstruction using the 70-degree tibial guide. Knee Surg Sports Traumatol Arthrosc 22:1182–1189
20. Zampeli F, Ntoulia A, Giotis D, Tsiaras VA, Argyropoulou M, Pappas E, Georgoulis AD (2012) Correlation between anterior cruciate ligament graft obliquity and tibial rotation during dynamic pivoting activities in patients with anatomic anterior cruciate ligament reconstruction: an in vivo examination. Arthroscopy 28:234–246

21. Plaweski S, Rossi J, Merloz P, Julliard R (2011) Analysis of anatomic positioning in computer-assisted and conventional anterior cruciate ligament reconstruction. Orthop Traumatol Surg Res 97:S80–S85
22. Iriuchishima T, Tajima G, Ingham SJ, Shen W, Smolinski P, Fu FH (2010) Impingement pressure in the anatomical and nonanatomical anterior cruciate ligament reconstruction: a cadaver study. Am J Sports Med 38:1611–1617
23. Jagodzinski M, Richter GM, Pässler HH (2000) Biomechanical analysis of knee hyperextension and of the impingement of the anterior cruciate ligament: a cinematographic MRI study with impact on tibial tunnel positioning in anterior cruciate ligament reconstruction. Knee Surg Sports Traumatol Arthrosc 8:11–19
24. Watson JN, Wilson KJ, LaPrade CM, Kennedy NI, Campbell KJ, Hutchinson MR, Wijdicks CA, LaPrade RF (2015) Iatrogenic injury of the anterior meniscal root attachments following anterior cruciate ligament reconstruction tunnel reaming. Knee Surg Sports Traumatol Arthrosc 23:2360–2366
25. LaPrade CM, Smith SD, Rasmussen MT, Hamming MG, Wijdicks CA, Engebretsen L, Feagin JA, LaPrade RF (2015) Consequences of tibial tunnel reaming on the meniscal roots during cruciate ligament reconstruction in a cadaveric model, Part 1: the anterior cruciate ligament. Am J Sports Med 43:200–206
26. LaPrade CM, Ellman MB, Rasmussen MT, James EW, Wijdicks CA, Engebretsen L, LaPrade RF (2014) Anatomy of the anterior root attachments of the medial and lateral menisci: a quantitative analysis. Am J Sports Med 42:2386–2392
27. Kopf S, Pombo MW, Szczodry M, Irrgang JJ, Fu FH (2011) Size variability of the human anterior cruciate ligament insertion sites. Am J Sports Med 39:108–113

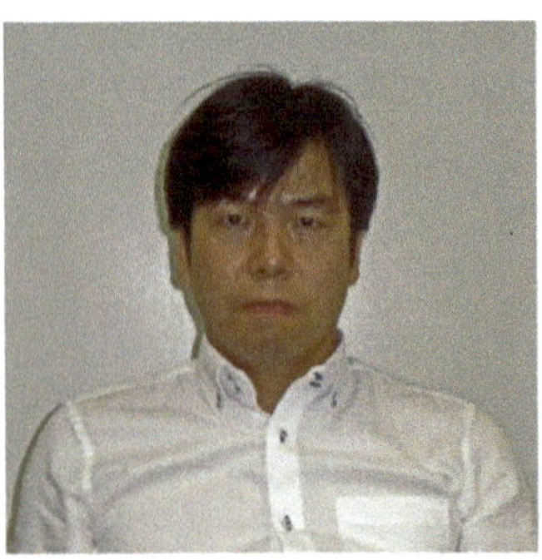

Keiji Tensho M.D., PhD, Department of Orthopedic Surgery, Shinshu University School of Medicine, Nagano, Japan.

Chapter 5
Mechanoreceptors in the ACL

Yuji Uchio

Abstract Proprioception is defined by Sherrington as cumulative neural inputs originating from joints, tendons, muscles, and associated deep tissue proprioceptors, which project to the central nervous system for processing stimuli and ultimately results in regulation of reflexes and motor control. Several anatomical and electrophysiological studies have clarified the significance of mechanoreceptors in the anterior cruciate ligament (ACL). Mechanical stimuli applied to mechanoreceptors in the ACL are converted to action potential and transferred to the cerebrum, processing all the peripheral inputs to sense joint position, detect movement and acceleration, and control voluntary movements. In ACL deficiency, impairment of proprioception is indicated by knee proprioception tests, such as reproduction of passive positioning and threshold to detect passive motion. However, it is controversial whether and when impaired proprioception associated with ACL deficiency can be recovered to normal levels following ACL reconstruction. Moreover, there is no consensus on the choice of optimal surgical method or rehabilitation program for improvement of impaired proprioception. To enable full recovery of proprioceptive function in ACL deficiency, further research on mechanoreceptors and proprioception is necessary to clarify these issues.

Keywords Mechanoreceptor • Proprioception • Neurophysiology • ACL deficiency • Rehabilitation

5.1 Definition of Proprioception

Proprioception is defined as cumulative neural inputs originating from joints, tendons, muscles, and associated deep tissue proprioceptors, which project to the central nervous system (CNS) for processing stimuli and ultimately results in regulation of reflexes and motor control [1]. Initially, proprioceptive stimuli are

---

Y. Uchio, M.D., Ph.D. (✉)
Department of Orthopaedic Surgery, Shimane University, 89-1 Enya-cho, Izumo, Shimane 693-8501, Japan
e-mail: uchio@med.shimane-u.ac.jp

M. Ochi et al. (eds.), *ACL Injury and Its Treatment*,
DOI 10.1007/978-4-431-55858-3_5

received by sensory receptors, the visual system, vestibular system, and the peripheral mechanoreceptors, which convert the mechanical stimuli to a new action potential [1]. The input is transferred to the CNS and processed at three levels: the spinal cord, the lower brain, and the cerebrum. At the spinal level, the input reacts to a fast reflex response, which regulates muscles with a closed loop efferent activity and contributes to protect joint stability. Second, the input is transferred to the lower brain, where the motor activities are learned, planned for timing of the movement, and controlled. Finally, the input is transferred to the cerebrum, which processes all the peripheral inputs to make a sense of joint position, for detection of movement and acceleration, and to control the voluntary movements. Through proprioception, we are able to perceive the sense of our body position and movement, recognize a space, and feel the shape, size, or weight of an object, even if we are blinded.

The anterior cruciate ligament (ACL) plays the key role of anterior-posterior and rotatory stability of the knee joint, as a biomechanical restraint between the femur and tibia [2]. Many studies have also shown that the ACL has a proprioceptive function by means of the mechanoreceptors in the ACL fibers [1, 3–5]. Patients with an ACL-deficient knee feel apprehension and/or a "giving way" while doing movements such as cutting, twisting, stopping at a trot, or routinely descending stairways. Surgical ACL reconstruction can restore mechanical stability of the knee joint; however, not all patients undergoing ACL reconstruction are freed from the sense of apprehension and/or giving way. These phenomena indicate ACL's role as not only a biomechanical stabilizer but also as a proprioceptive sensor.

5.2 Mechanoreceptors in the Intact ACL

Using silver staining techniques, Kennedy et al. identified rich innervation in soft tissues of the knee and a variety of specialized receptors in the ACL obtained from fresh amputated specimens [6]. They further showed that an experimentally produced knee effusion of a 60-cc volume resulted in a profound inhibition of reflexively evoked quadriceps contraction in a normal knee. In 1984, Shultz et al. demonstrated the presence of mechanoreceptors in human ACLs obtained at the time of total knee replacement and from autopsy and amputation specimens [7]. The presence of the axons and free nerve endings was noted using Bodian, Bielschowsky, and Ranvier gold chloride stains. One to three fusiform mechanoreceptor structures resembling the Golgi tendon organs were detected at the surface of the ligament. The report thus suggested that mechanical stimuli may be converted to an action potential by these mechanoreceptor structures, transferring to the CNS and contributing a proprioceptive function to inhibit injurious movement.

Ultrastructure of sensory nerve endings in the human knee joints was studied by Halata et al., and three types of nerve endings were found: free nerve endings (FNEs), Ruffini corpuscles, and Pacinian corpuscles [8]. FNEs in the joint capsule are located below the synovial layer and within the fibrous layer near blood vessels. These nerve terminals derive from myelinated A delta fibers or from unmyelinated C fibers. Halata et al. also studied the sensory innervation of the ACL of the human knee joint by light- and electron microscopy [9]. Connective tissues between the synovial membrane and the cruciate ligament contain small Ruffini corpuscles and lamellar corpuscles with several inner cores; these receptors of the ACL are indicated to influence the muscle tone via polysynaptic reflexes.

Zimny et al. used human ACLs obtained at autopsy and identified two morphologically distinct mechanoreceptors: Ruffini corpuscles and Pacinian corpuscles [10]. Following staining by a modified gold chloride method, freezing, and sectioning at 100 microns using a sliding microtome, morphometric analyses showed that populations of mechanoreceptors are greater at the femoral and tibial ends of the ACL and constitute approximately 2.5 % of the ACL. Haus et al. demonstrated nerves and nerve endings in the ACL by light microscopy, scanning electron microscopy, and transmission electron microscopy [11]. Ultrastructural examination allowed a classification of nerve endings into three types: Ruffini corpuscles, Pacinian corpuscles, and afferent and efferent FNEs. The nerve endings corresponded to those characteristics of articular capsules. These findings suggest evidence of a proprioceptive function of the ACL, in addition to its stabilizing function.

Nerve supply of ACLs and of cryopreserved bone-ACL-bone allografts were investigated by Fromm and Kummer using a rabbit model with immunohistochemical methods [12]. They demonstrated that the ACL is innervated by three different classes of nerve fibers: (1) fibers of large diameter, characterized by neurofilament immunoreactivity, which are fast-conducting mechanoreceptive sensory afferents; (2) fibers of small diameter, characterized by substance P immunoreactivity, which are slow-conducting nociceptive sensory afferents; and (3) sympathetic efferent vasomotor fibers, characterized by their immunoreactivity to the rate-limiting enzyme of noradrenaline synthesis, tyrosine hydroxylase. However, no nerve fibers were detected in the ACL allografts at 3 and 6 weeks. Sparse fibers were detected at 12 weeks, while the 24-, 36- and 52-week specimens showed many of all three fiber types. No mechanoreceptors were found in the ACL allografts.

Distribution of neurofilament-containing nerve fibers and corpuscular-like endings were shown by Krauspe et al. using human ACLs with immunofluorescence staining using a monoclonal antibody against the 68-kDa neurofilament subunit [13]. Neurofilament-containing nerve fibers were preferentially located near the bony attachments of the ACL. Two types of corpuscular-like endings were found, i.e., "spiral-like" (type I) and "spray-like" (type II) endings. Similar to nerve fibers, both types of corpuscular-like endings were found mainly near the tibial and femoral attachment sites. Most likely, the type I and type II corpuscular-like endings serve a mechanoreceptive function involved in the sensory control of normal movements and in stress protection.

Mechanoreceptors have been identified not only in the ACL but also in the other structures of the knee joint. Zimny et al. demonstrated neural elements in medial menisci obtained at autopsy by staining in bulk, using a modified gold chloride method [14]. Axons were seen penetrating from the perimeniscal tissue into the outer third of the meniscus with a heavier concentration at the horns. Assimakopoulos et al. examined innervation of human menisci from anatomic specimens stained by a modified gold chloride method and identified FNEs in the peripheral and the medial thirds of the meniscal body and three types of encapsulated mechanoreceptors in the anterior and posterior horns [15]. Haus and Halata found nerves and nerve endings in the synovium and interfascicular connective tissue besides Ruffini corpuscles and Pacinian corpuscles in the ACL [16]. De Avila et al. reported a small number of "non-Paciniform" endings identified in the human lateral collateral ligaments, although they did not detect "Paciniform" endings [17].

Mechanoreceptors can be divided into either rapidly or slowly adapting receptors [4]. Rapidly adapting receptors include the Pacinian corpuscles, nerve endings with a conical shape, and an encapsulated tip, which are found in the joint capsule, cruciate ligament, and menisci. They are extremely sensitive to a subtle change in deformation of their capsule caused by mechanically applied pressure and initiate vigorous discharge of electrical potentials that appear only during the application and removal of the stimulus, or during acceleration or deceleration of the moving joint [4].

On the other hand, slowly adapting receptors include Ruffini endings and several naked tip nerve endings encapsulated thinly emerging from a single myelinated axon, which are found in the collateral ligament and cruciate ligaments, capsule, and menisci. They are sensitive to low-level mechanical deformation such as joint angle, velocity, intraarticular pressure, and strains. Golgi tendon organs (Golgi receptors), thinly encapsulated, large corpuscles, are also slowly adapting receptors, found in the muscle tendons, the collateral and cruciate ligaments, capsule, and menisci. They have high threshold to mechanical deformation (pressure and compression) and different function existing in between the joint capsule and the muscle's tendon. Golgi receptors in the capsule signal the angle of the joint, while those in the muscle's tendon signal the force developed by the muscle [4]. Thus, various types of mechanoreceptors are distributed in the knee joint and muscles, which can convert the mechanical stimuli to new action potentials and transfer them to the CNS to make a sense of joint position, detect movement and acceleration, and control the voluntary movement. However, the relative contributions of each mechanoreceptor to proprioception remain unclear.

5.3 Innervation of the Knee Joint

Projections of inputs from the mechanoreceptors in the ACL to the CNS have been evaluated by several modalities. In 1996, Parsch et al. used rabbit ACL and clarified the sensory innervation by retrograde tracing technique using wheat germ agglutinin-horseradish peroxidase and fast blue as neuronal tracers [18]. Injection of the tracer into the ACL or into the joint cavity was followed by histo- and immunohistochemical investigation of labeled nerve cell bodies located in the dorsal root ganglia. They found the segmental distribution of retrogradely labeled neurons following injection into the ACL (L6, L7, S1) is significantly different from the distribution pattern after injection into the knee joint (L4-S2). Thus, they stated that the sensory innervation of the ACL is comprised of at least two different qualities of sensory afferent nerves: (1) small neurons immunoreactive to the inflammatory peptide substance P most likely transmitting nociceptive information centrally (44 %) and (2) large, presumably fast-conducting A-fiber afferents characterized by neurofilament proteins transmitting proprioceptive information from corpuscular mechanoreceptors (43 %). In this way, the direct neural pathway from the mechanoreceptors in the ACL to the dorsal spinal ganglia was shown.

Gómez-Barrena et al. electropysiologically demonstrated that electric activity in the articular nerves and periarticular muscles, in response to passive motion and anterior tibial displacement, is reduced in a cat's knee after ACL transection and reconstruction [19]. Further, the possibility of various patterns of periarticular muscle reaction in an ACL-deficient knee to the unconscious perception of abnormal motion was suggested. Human somatosensory evoked potentials (SEP) was measured by Pitman et al. in the cerebral cortex upon stimulation of a peripheral neuroreceptor in the ACL [20]. Under arthroscopy, the normal ACL was stimulated using electrodes applied to the femoral end, midsubstance, and tibial end, evoking recordable cortical potentials. The greatest potentials were observed upon stimulation of the midsubstance of the ligament. These findings strongly support the presence of active proprioceptive receptors within the intact ACL of the human knee.

Knee proprioception and SEPs to stimulation of the common peroneal nerve (CPN) were studied by Veleriani et al. in patients with ACL injury before and after ACL reconstruction [21]. Before surgery, all patients showed decreased knee position sense and lack of cortical P27 potential on the injured side. Arthroscopic reconstruction of the ligament was performed but knee proprioception and somatosensory central conduction did not recover to normal level. However, the loss of knee mechanoreceptors may possibly be restored by modifications of the CNS, which are not compensated by other nervous structures.

Thus, mechanoreceptors in the ACL are believed to ascend in the dorsal columns and project to the thalamus and sensory cortex to produce a kinematic perception, such as a joint position sense, velocity, pressure, and acceleration or deceleration of the moving joint. Whereas, the muscle spindle and Golgi tendon organs ascend the spinal cord and terminate in the cerebellum, though not reaching the cerebrum, which is meant to be subconscious. Input from the muscle spindle and Golgi tendon organ is utilized in the management and coordination of movements in the cerebellum, eliciting reflexes and facilitating skill and motor control [4].

With functional magnetic resonance imaging technique (using a 1.5-T scanner), Kapreli et al. investigated brain activation in patients with chronic ACL deficiency and healthy controls [22]. Compared with healthy controls, patients with ACL deficiency had diminished activation in several sensorimotor cortical areas and increased activation in three areas: pre-supplementary motor area, posterior secondary somatosensory area, and posterior inferior temporal gyrus. Kapreli et al. concluded that ACL deficiency can cause reorganization of the central nervous system, suggesting that such an injury might be regarded as a neurophysiologic dysfunction, not a simple peripheral musculoskeletal injury.

Johansson et al. stated that the knee joint ligaments contain Ruffini corpuscles, Pacinian corpuscles, Golgi organ, and FNEs with different capabilities of providing the CNS with information about movement and position, as well as about noxious events [23]. Skeletomotor neurons (alpha motoneurons) are known to be influenced only very rarely and weakly from low-threshold mechanoreceptors in the ligaments, while the effects on the tau-muscle-spindle system in the muscles around the knee are so potent that even ligament stretches at very low loads may induce major changes in the responses of the muscle spindle afferents. Since the primary muscle spindle afferents participate in the regulation of muscular stiffness, the receptors in the knee joint ligaments likely contribute, via the tau-muscle-spindle system, to preparatory adjustment (pre-setting) of the stiffness of the muscles around the knee joint and thereby to the joint stiffness and the functional joint stability.

5.4 Mechanoreceptors in Remnant of Injured ACL

Several authors have investigated the presence and significance of the mechanoreceptors in the remnant of an injured ACL. Denti et al. studied the fate of mechanoreceptors in torn and reconstructed ACL using Ruffini gold chloride staining [24]. In untreated ACL lesions in humans, morphologically normal mechanoreceptors remained in the ligament for 3 months after the injury. After that time, their number gradually decreased. By the ninth post-injury month, only a few FNEs were present. Eventually, FNEs were totally absent in the biopsy specimens from 1-year-old lesions.

Adachi et al. examined mechanoreceptors in ACL remnants using the Gairns gold chloride method [25]. They also investigated the correlation between the number of mechanoreceptors in ACL remnants and the joint position sense just before an ACL reconstruction. A positive correlation between the number of mechanoreceptors and accuracy of the joint position sense suggests that proprioceptive function of the ACL is related to the number of mechanoreceptors.

Using the gold chloride method as modified by O'Conner and Gonzares, Georgoulis et al. investigated the presence of neural mechanoreceptors in the remnants of the ruptured ACL [26]. Perioperatively, two types of ACL remnant were identified. Fifteen patients had portions of ACL adapted at the PCL. In all of these patients, mechanoreceptors (I and II) were found, and 5 patients had mushroom-like remnants which included either none or small numbers of mechanoreceptors. Free neural ends were found in both patient groups. There was a significant difference between the groups in regard to the mean number of mechanoreceptors I and II per slice. Therefore, they concluded that mechanoreceptors exist even 3 years after injury in patients with an ACL remnant adapted to the PCL.

Immunohistochemical staining of mechanoreceptors in the tibial remnants of ruptured human ACL were studied by Lee et al. [27]. They observed mechanoreceptors in the ACL remnants in 12 out of 36 cases (33 %) with a total of 17 (6 Ruffini and 11 Golgi) mechanoreceptors. No significant differences in the harvest volume, number of sections, age, or time from injury to surgery was observed between the 12 mechanoreceptor-present and the 24 mechanoreceptor-absent ones. Although the mechanoreceptors were detected relatively less frequent than they expected, it was considered not to negate the necessity of remnant-preserving ACL reconstruction.

Dhillion et al. evaluated proprioceptive potential in residual remnants from tissue harvested from ruptured ACLs in 63 consecutive patients for evidence of residual proprioceptive fibers using hematoxylin-eosin (H&E) staining and monoclonal antibodies to S-100 and NFP (neurofilament protein) [28]. Histological examination showed good subsynovial and intra-fascicular vascularity with free nerve endings in the majority. Morphologically normal mechanoreceptors (H&E staining) and proprioceptive fibers (positivity with monoclonal antibody for NFP) were found in 46 % and 52.4 % of the stumps, respectively. A statistically significant correlation between injury duration and persistence of mechanoreceptors and proprioceptive fibers was noted. More fibers were seen where ACL remnant was adherent to PCL. They stated that not shaving ACL remnants may be of benefit during ACL reconstruction, as some re-innervation and recovery of proprioceptive potential may be possible, thus improving clinical outcomes.

The histological features of the remaining fibers bridging the femur and tibia in partial ACL tears were investigated by Sonnery-Cottet et al. [29]. Competent histological structures including a well-vascularized synovial sheet, numerous fibroblasts and myofibroblasts, and mechanoreceptors were found in ACL remnants. Especially, FNEs and few Golgi or Ruffini corpuscles were detected in 41 % of the specimens of 26 ACL remnants. These histological findings suggest that the preservation of the ACL remnant is recommended in partial tears when ACL reconstruction or augmentation is to be performed.

The neural pathway from mechanoreceptors in the injured ACL remnants to cerebral cortex was proven by Ochi et al. using somatosensory evoked potentials (SEPs) after direct electrical stimulation of injured and normal ACL during arthroscopy [30]. They detected SEP in 15 out of 32 cases in the injured group, although the voltages in the injured group were significantly lower than those of the intact controls. Ochi et al. also proved this neural pathway by SEPs after direct mechanical stimulation of injured and normal ACL during arthroscopy [31]. Of the 45 injured ACLs, reproducible SEPs were detected in 26. The mean difference in anterior displacement in the SEP-positive group of the injured ACL group was significantly lower than that in the SEP-negative group.

5.5 Tests for Knee Proprioception

There have been several tests to evaluate knee proprioception, such as reproduction of passive positioning (RPP) to test the joint position sense (JPS). This requires a subject to return his or her leg actively from a free hanging position of 90° to a previously set angle [32]. During the test, a pneumatic compression boot is placed on each foot to reduce cutaneous input, and the subject is blindfolded to eliminate visual cues. An angle is randomly set from 5 to 25° as the starting position; the leg is then pulled passively by an examiner to bend the knee to a 90° angle. Accuracy in reproduced movements is recorded as the angle difference between the returning and starting positions [32]. Active motion reproduction has been also used [33, 34]. Another method is to reproduce a passive motion visually on a goniometer [35, 36]. However, the accuracy and reliability of the RPP test, though commonly used, is uncertain [5, 36].

Threshold to detect passive motion (TTDPM) is used to evaluate kinesthesia [32, 37, 38]. In TTDPM, a subject is blindfolded to eliminate visual cues and has headphones with white noise to eliminate auditory cues. When a subject's knee is passively and slowly moved over a 5–30-s period either into extension or flexion using a motor controlled device, the subject is required to respond as soon as he or she detects the motion and to inform the examiner with an on-off switch. The TTDPM, tested at slow angular velocity (0.5–2.5°/s), is considered to be the maximum to stimulate joint receptors and the minimum to stimulate muscle receptors [39].

5.6 Proprioception in ACL Deficiency

Proprioception in patients with ACL injuries has been studied by several researchers. Barrack et al. firstly quantified proprioception in a group of patients who had complete ACL tears using TTDPM and reported that threshold values for TTDPM of ACL-deficient knees were significantly higher than those of intact controls [38].

For TTDPM evaluation, Borsa et al. studied 29 ACL-deficient athletes to determine whether joint position and joint motion direction have a significant effect on proprioception [40]. Their results demonstrated statistically significant deficits of TTDPM in the deficient limb at 15° moving into extension. And the threshold was significantly more sensitive than at a starting angle of 45° moving into extension. They concluded that proprioception of deficient limbs is significantly more sensitive in the end ranges of knee extension (15°) and is significantly more sensitive when moving into the direction of extension.

Also, proprioception of ACL-deficient knees was measured in 20 subjects and compared with 17 age-matched control subjects by Corrigan et al. [41]. They found diminished position sense and threshold for movement detection in the injured patients compared with the control group. They also showed that the proprioceptive deficit recorded from the injured knee showed a significant correlation with the hamstring/quadriceps power ratio recorded from the injured leg.

Using visual estimation of passive motion on a goniometer, Carter et al. demonstrated that joint position sense (JPS) was impaired in their 50 unilateral ACL-deficient knees, although it did not correlate with functional activity tests (hop and figure eight run) [42], whereas Friden et al. showed a trend toward a higher threshold for detecting a passive motion when comparing injured knees and intact knees at 1 month, using three tests of proprioception: (1) one to determine the TTDPM from starting positions of 20 and 40°, (2) an active reproduction of a passive angular change, and (3) a visual estimation of a passive angular change [43]. An impaired ability to detect a passive motion was registered for the nearly extended knee at 1 and 2 months after a primary injury. In the active reproduction and visual estimation tests, no significant defects were found at any time during the first year in the consecutively studied patients.

Roberts et al. evaluated proprioception in two groups of patients with ACL deficiency with different severity of symptoms [44]. Their symptomatic patients had a higher threshold to TTDPM in their injured side in a flexion trial from 20° (median of 1.5° versus median of 0.5°) and in an extension trial from 40° (median of 1.0° versus median of 0.5°) than the asymptomatic patients did. No differences were found in the other threshold, active or visual reproduction tests. They concluded that patients with severe ACL deficiency symptoms have inferior proprioceptive ability in some measurements compared with patients with good knee function. Their findings indicate that proprioceptive deficits might influence the outcome of an ACL injury treated non-operatively.

5.7 Effect of Rehabilitation on Proprioception in ACL Deficiency

It has been controversial as to whether rehabilitation restores proprioception in ACL deficiency. Cater et al. examined 50 patients with unilateral ACL-deficient knees which were assessed on admission and after rehabilitation (5 h a day for 4 weeks) [42]. JPS was assessed by reproduction of passive positioning using a visual analogue incorporating a goniometer. Knee stability was analyzed by self-report questionnaire and functional activity test (single leg hop and figure eight run). Results showed that there was no improvement in JPS, although knee stability improved with exercise therapy. Using TTDPM and RPP, Pincivero et al. also demonstrated no improvement of proprioception after rehabilitation [45].

In contrast, Friden et al. showed the possibility that a 4-week rehabilitation program including proprioceptive training somewhat improve a proprioceptive deficit in the ACL deficiency; however, it is uncertain whether this program was sufficient in terms of period and content to restore the proprioception [43].

To determine how perturbation training alters muscle co-contraction and knee kinematics in potential copers, a study by Chimielewski et al. suggested that perturbation training reduced quadriceps femoris-hamstring muscle and quadriceps femoris-gastrocnemius muscle co-contractions and normalized knee kinematics in individuals with ACL rupture who were classified as potential copers [46]. They concluded that findings provide evidence for a mechanism by which perturbation training acts, as an effective intervention for promoting coordinated muscle activity in a select population of people with ACL rupture.

Roberts et al. studied the knee proprioception of 36 patients with ACL deficiency by measuring TTDPM before and after a short period of exercise on an ergometer bicycle [47]. They found trends of enhanced proprioception towards extension in the patient group after cycling, but not in the age-matched control group.

5.8 Proprioception After ACL Reconstruction

Although many studies have reported that impaired proprioception with ACL deficiency improved after ACL reconstruction, it is unclear whether ACL reconstruction fully restores the proprioception to be the same as the intact knee. It also remains unclear whether any specific rehabilitation enhances the improvement of impaired proprioception after ACL reconstruction.

In a study by Reider et al., ACL reconstructions were performed using a single-incision technique with either bone-patellar tendon-bone (BTB) or quadrupled hamstring autograft [48]. Their patients were allowed to do immediate weight-bearing as tolerated and participated in a standardized rehabilitation program, with the goal of returning to sport at approximately 6 months. Proprioception testing was carried out using an electrogoniometer, in a seated position. JPS and TTDPM were measured preoperatively and at 3 and 6 weeks and 3 and 6 months postoperatively. Preoperatively, the mean TDPM in both the injured and contralateral knees (internal controls) was significantly higher (worse) than in the age-matched healthy knees (external controls). Evaluation of changes in proprioception from preoperative to 6 months postoperative showed significant improvement in both injured and contralateral knees. At 6-month follow-up, there was no significant difference from controls.

Fremerey et al. assessed proprioception in the knee using the angle reproduction test in 20 healthy volunteers, 10 patients with acute anterior instability, and 20 patients with chronic anterior instability after ACL reconstruction with BTB [49]. Three months after operation, there remained a slight decrease in proprioception compared with the preoperative recordings, but 6 months after reconstruction, restoration of proprioception was seen at the positions of near full extension and full flexion. However, in the mid-range position, proprioception was not restored. At follow-up, an average of 3.7 years after reconstruction, there was further improvement of proprioception in the mid-range position, but not fully restored.

Other studies showed a reconstructed knee to have decreased joint position perception, a higher threshold for TTDPM, longer latency of hamstring muscles, and decreased performance in postural control at 18 months postoperatively [50]. Conversely, Mir et al. found no evidence of impaired JPS in weight-bearing positions in subjects with ACL reconstruction at a mean follow-up of 11 months after surgery compared with subjects with healthy knees [51].

Iwasa et al. evaluated proprioception of 38 patients who underwent ACL reconstruction using hamstring tendons at 3-month intervals for 24 months by RPP. Thirty patients experienced improvement in postoperative position sense in at least one of the examinations, although 8 patients had no improvement at any time. Of the 30 patients who showed improvement, 28 maintained improved position sense from 18 months to the final follow-up [52]. They also investigated the changes in anterior laxity of the knee in response to direct electrical stimulation of 8 normal and 45 reconstructed ACLs [53]. Anterior laxity was examined with the knee flexed at 20° under a force of 134 N applied anteriorly to the tibia using the KT-2000 knee arthrometer before, during, and after electrical stimulation. Anterior tibial translation in 8 normal and 17 ACL-reconstructed knees was significantly decreased during stimulation, compared with that before stimulation. Anterior tibial translation was not decreased in 22 of 28 ACL-reconstructed knees, of which the grafts were found to have detectable SEPs during stimulation. They concluded that the ACL-hamstring reflex arc in normal knees may contribute to the functional stability and that this may not be fully restored after ACL reconstruction.

Friemert et al. suggested that continuous active motion devices produced a significantly greater reduction in the proprioceptive deficit and, therefore, should be the first choice in postoperative rehabilitation immediately after ACL replacement during the first postoperative week [54].

Vathrakokilis et al. showed that a balance-training program in knee proprioception improved stability indices of balance for the reconstructed leg compared with control [55]. Brunetti et al. proposed a new protocol of postoperative treatment consisting of mechanical vibration (100 Hz frequency and < 20 microM amplitude) of the quadriceps muscle in the leg after ACL reconstruction [56]. They concluded that short-lasting proprioceptive activation by vibration may lead to a faster and more complete equilibrium recovery, probably making a permanent change in the knee posture-controlling network.

In summary, many studies suggest improvement of proprioception may be achieved in terms of joint position sense and TTPDM. However, it remains controversial whether recovery to normal levels after ACL reconstruction is possible. In addition, the effect of a graft (hamstring tendons, BTB, etc.) on proprioception is unclear. There is the possibility that specific rehabilitation enhances the improvement of impaired proprioception following ACL reconstruction.

5.9 Perspective of Research on Mechanoreceptors and Proprioception

At present, it is recognized that mechanoreceptors in the ACL contribute to proprioceptive function of the knee joint via its neural pathway to the cerebral cortex. Specifically, mechanical stimuli applied to mechanoreceptors in the ACL are converted to action potential and transferred to the cerebrum, processing all peripheral inputs to make sense of joint position, for detection of movement and acceleration, and to control voluntary movements. Patients with ACL deficiency experience not only mechanical instability due to loss of the anteroposterior and rotatory stabilizer for the femorotibial joint but also functional instability induced by impaired proprioception, causing apprehension and giving way. However, it is still uncertain whether and when impaired proprioception associated with ACL deficiency improves and recovers to normal levels following ACL reconstruction; further, the optimum choice of surgical procedure or rehabilitation program to help minimize the extent of impaired proprioception remains unclear. An augmentation technique preserving the ACL remnant may contribute to improved knee proprioception [57–59]. To enable highly skilled athletes to regain their pre-injury levels of ability, both the mechanical stability of the knee joint and adequate levels of proprioception within the knee joint are critical. To attain this mechanical and functional stability in ACL deficiency patients, continued research on mechanoreceptors and proprioception is desired in the future.

References

1. Hewett TE, Paterno MV, Myer GD (2002) Strategies for enhancing proprioception and neuromuscular control of the knee. Clin Orthop Relat Res 402:76–94
2. Woo SL, Fisher MB (2009) Evaluation of knee stability with use of a robotic system. J Bone Joint Surg Am 91(Suppl 1):78–84
3. Dhillon MS, Bali K, Prabhakar S (2012) Differences among mechanoreceptors in healthy and injured anterior cruciate ligaments and their clinical importance. Muscles Ligaments Tendons J 2(1):38–43
4. Solomonow M, Krogsgaard M (2001) Sensorimotor control of knee stability. A review. Scand J Med Sci Sports 11(2):64–80
5. Fridén T, Roberts D, Ageberg E, Waldén M, Zätterström R (2001) Review of knee proprioception and the relation to extremity function after an anterior cruciate ligament rupture. J Orthop Sports Phys Ther 31(10):567–576
6. Kennedy JC, Alexander IJ, Hayes KC (1982) Nerve supply of the human knee and its functional importance. Am J Sports Med 10(6):329–335
7. Schultz RA, Miller DC, Kerr CS, Micheli L (1984) Mechanoreceptors in human cruciate ligaments. A histological study. J Bone Joint Surg Am 66(7):1072–1076
8. Halata Z, Rettig T, Schulze W (1985) The ultrastructure of sensory nerve endings in the human knee joint capsule. Anat Embryol (Berl) 172(3):265–275
9. Halata Z, Haus J (1989) The ultrastructure of sensory nerve endings in human anterior cruciate ligament. Anat Embryol (Berl) 179(5):415–421

10. Zimny ML, Schutte M, Dabezies E (1986) Mechanoreceptors in the human anterior cruciate ligament. Anat Rec 214(2):204–209
11. Haus J, Halata Z, Refior HJ (1992) Proprioception in the anterior cruciate ligament of the human knee joint--morphological bases. A light, scanning and transmission electron microscopy study. Z Orthop Ihre Grenzgeb 130(6):484–494
12. Fromm B, Kummer W (1994) Nerve supply of anterior cruciate ligaments and of cryopreserved anterior cruciate ligament allografts: a new method for the differentiation of the nervous tissues. Knee Surg Sports Traumatol Arthrosc 2(2):118–122
13. Krauspe R, Schmitz F, Zöller G, Drenckhahn D (1995) Distribution of neurofilament-positive nerve fibres and sensory endings in the human anterior cruciate ligament. Arch Orthop Trauma Surg 114(4):194–198
14. Zimny ML, Albright DJ, Dabezies E (1988) Mechanoreceptors in the human medial meniscus. Acta Anat (Basel) 133(1):35–40
15. Assimakopoulos AP, Katonis PG, Agapitos MV, Exarchou EI (1992) The innervation of the human meniscus. Clin Orthop Relat Res 275:232–236
16. Haus J, Halata Z (1990) Innervation of the anterior cruciate ligament. Int Orthop 14 (3):293–296
17. De Avila GA, O'Connor BL, Visco DM, Sisk TD (1989) The mechanoreceptor innervation of the human fibular collateral ligament. J Anat 162:1–7
18. Parsch D, Fromm B, Kummer W (1996) Projections and fiber characteristics of sensory afferents of the anterior cruciate ligament in an animal experiment. Unfallchirurgie 22 (5):193–201
19. Gómez-Barrena E, Nuñez A, Martinez-Moreno E, Valls J, Munuera L (1997) Neural and muscular electric activity in the cat's knee. Changes when the anterior cruciate ligament is transected. Acta Orthop Scand 68(2):149–155
20. Pitman MI, Nainzadeh N, Menche D, Gasalberti R, Song EK (1992) The intraoperative evaluation of the neurosensory function of the anterior cruciate ligament in humans using somatosensory evoked potentials. Arthroscopy 8(4):442–447
21. Valeriani M, Restuccia D, Di Lazzaro V, Franceschi F, Fabbriciani C, Tonali P (1999) Clinical and neurophysiological abnormalities before and after reconstruction of the anterior cruciate ligament of the knee. Acta Neurol Scand 99(5):303–307
22. Kapreli E, Athanasopoulos S, Gliatis J, Papathanasiou M, Peeters R, Strimpakos N, Van Hecke P, Gouliamos A, Sunaert S (2009) Anterior cruciate ligament deficiency causes brain plasticity: a functional MRI study. Am J Sports Med 37(12):2419–2426
23. Johansson H, Sjölander P, Sojka P (1991) A sensory role for the cruciate ligaments. Clin Orthop Relat Res 268:161–178
24. Denti M, Monteleone M, Berardi A, Panni AS (1994) Anterior cruciate ligament mechanoreceptors. Histologic studies on lesions and reconstruction. Clin Orthop Relat Res 308:29–32
25. Adachi N, Ochi M, Uchio Y, Iwasa J, Ryoke K, Kuriwaka M (2002) Mechanoreceptors in the anterior cruciate ligament contribute to the joint position sense. Acta Orthop Scand 73 (3):330–334
26. Georgoulis AD, Pappa L, Moebius U, Malamou-Mitsi V, Pappa S, Papageorgiou CO, Agnantis NJ, Soucacos PN (2001) The presence of proprioceptive mechanoreceptors in the remnants of the ruptured ACL as a possible source of re-innervation of the ACL autograft. Knee Surg Sports Traumatol Arthrosc 9(6):364–368
27. Lee BI, Min KD, Choi HS, Kwon SW, Chun DI, Yun ES, Lee DW, Jin SY, Yoo JH (2009) Immunohistochemical study of mechanoreceptors in the tibial remnant of the ruptured anterior cruciate ligament in human knees. Knee Surg Sports Traumatol Arthrosc 17(9):1095–1101
28. Dhillon MS, Bali K, Vasistha RK (2010) Immunohistological evaluation of proprioceptive potential of the residual stump of injured anterior cruciate ligaments (ACL). Int Orthop 34 (5):737–741
29. Sonnery-Cottet B, Bazille C, Hulet C, Colombet P, Cucurulo T, Panisset JC, Potel JF, Servien E, Trojani C, Djian P, Graveleau N, Pujol N, French Arthroscopic Society (2014) Histological features of the ACL remnant in partial tears. Knee 21(6):1009–1013

30. Ochi M, Iwasa J, Uchio Y, Adachi N, Sumen Y (1999) The regeneration of sensory neurones in the reconstruction of the anterior cruciate ligament. J Bone Joint Surg (Br) 81(5):902–906
31. Ochi M, Iwasa J, Uchio Y, Adachi N, Kawasaki K (2002) Induction of somatosensory evoked potentials by mechanical stimulation in reconstructed anterior cruciate ligaments. J Bone Joint Surg (Br) 84(5):761–766
32. Barrack RL, Skinner HB, Brunet ME, Haddad RJ Jr (1983) Functional performance of the knee after intraarticular anesthesia. Am J Sports Med 11(4):258–261
33. Good L, Roos H, Gottlieb DJ, Renström PA, Beynnon BD (1999) Joint position sense is not changed after acute disruption of the anterior cruciate ligament. Acta Orthop Scand 70 (2):194–198
34. Marks R (1994) Effect of exercise-induced fatigue on position sense of the knee. Aust J Physiother 40(3):175–181
35. Barrett DS (1991) Proprioception and function after anterior cruciate reconstruction. J Bone Joint Surg (Br) 73(5):833–837
36. Fridén T, Roberts D, Zätterström R, Lindstrand A, Moritz U (1996) Proprioception in the nearly extended knee. Measurements of position and movement in healthy individuals and in symptomatic anterior cruciate ligament injured patients. Knee Surg Sports Traumatol Arthrosc 4(4):217–224
37. Barrack RL, Skinner HB, Brunet ME, Cook SD (1984) Joint kinesthesia in the highly trained knee. J Sports Med Phys Fitness 24(1):18–20
38. Barrack RL, Skinner HB, Buckley SL (1989) Proprioception in the anterior cruciate deficient knee. Am J Sports Med 17(1):1–6
39. Lephart SM, Fu FH (1995) The role of proprioception in the treatment of sports injuries. Sports, Exercise Injury 1:96–102
40. Borsa PA, Lephart SM, Irrgang JJ, Safran MR, Fu FH (1997) The effects of joint position and direction of joint motion on proprioceptive sensibility in anterior cruciate ligament-deficient athletes. Am J Sports Med 25(3):336–340
41. Corrigan JP, Cashman WF, Brady MP (1992) Proprioception in the cruciate deficient knee. J Bone Joint Surg (Br) 74(2):247–250
42. Carter ND, Jenkinson TR, Wilson D, Jones DW, Torode AS (1997) Joint position sense and rehabilitation in the anterior cruciate ligament deficient knee. Br J Sports Med 31(3):209–212
43. Fridén T, Roberts D, Zätterström R, Lindstrand A, Moritz U (1997) Proprioception after an acute knee ligament injury: a longitudinal study on 16 consecutive patients. J Orthop Res 15 (5):637–644
44. Roberts D, Fridén T, Zätterström R, Lindstrand A, Moritz U (1999) Proprioception in people with anterior cruciate ligament-deficient knees: comparison of symptomatic and asymptomatic patients. J Orthop Sports Phys Ther 29(10):587–594
45. Pincivero DM, Henry TJ, Lephart SM (1996) Kinesthetic training effects on balance and proprioception in the anterior cruciate ligament injury. J Athl Train 31:S52
46. Chmielewski TL, Hurd WJ, Rudolph KS, Axe MJ, Snyder-Mackler L (2005) Perturbation training improves knee kinematics and reduces muscle co-contraction after complete unilateral anterior cruciate ligament rupture. Phys Ther 85(8):740–754
47. Roberts D, Ageberg E, Andersson G, Fridén T (2004) Effects of short-term cycling on knee joint proprioception in ACL-deficient patients. Knee Surg Sports Traumatol Arthrosc 12 (5):357–363
48. Reider B, Arcand MA, Diehl LH, Mroczek K, Abulencia A, Stroud CC, Palm M, Gilbertson J, Staszak P (2003) Proprioception of the knee before and after anterior cruciate ligament reconstruction. Arthroscopy 19(1):2–12
49. Fremerey RW, Lobenhoffer P, Zeichen J, Skutek M, Bosch U, Tscherne H (2000) Proprioception after rehabilitation and reconstruction in knees with deficiency of the anterior cruciate ligament: a prospective, longitudinal study. J Bone Joint Surg (Br) 82(6):801–806

50. Bonfim TR, Jansen Paccola CA, Barela JA (2003) Proprioceptive and behavior impairments in individuals with anterior cruciate ligament reconstructed knees. Arch Phys Med Rehabil 84 (8):1217–1223
51. Mir SM, Hadian MR, Talebian S, Nasseri N (2008) Functional assessment of knee joint position sense following anterior cruciate ligament reconstruction. Br J Sports Med 42 (4):300–303
52. Iwasa J, Ochi M, Adachi N, Tobita M, Katsube K, Uchio Y (2000) Proprioceptive improvement in knees with anterior cruciate ligament reconstruction. Clin Orthop Relat Res 381:168–176
53. Iwasa J, Ochi M, Uchio Y, Adachi N, Kawasaki K (2006) Decrease in anterior knee laxity by electrical stimulation of normal and reconstructed anterior cruciate ligaments. J Bone Joint Surg (Br) 88(4):477–483
54. Friemert B, Bach C, Schwarz W, Gerngross H, Schmidt R (2006) Benefits of active motion for joint position sense. Knee Surg Sports Traumatol Arthrosc 14(6):564–570
55. Vathrakokilis K, Malliou P, Gioftsidou A, Beneka A, Godolias G (2008) Effects of a balance training protocol on knee joint proprioception after anterior cruciate ligament reconstruction. J Back Musculoskeletal Rehabil 21:233–237
56. Brunetti O, Filippi GM, Lorenzini M, Liti A, Panichi R, Roscini M, Pettorossi VE, Cerulli G (2006) Improvement of posture stability by vibratory stimulation following anterior cruciate ligament reconstruction. Knee Surg Sports Traumatol Arthrosc 14(11):1180–1187
57. Adachi N, Ochi M, Uchio Y, Sumen Y (2000) Anterior cruciate ligament augmentation under arthroscopy. A minimum 2-year follow-up in 40 patients. Arch Orthop Trauma Surg 120 (3–4):128–133
58. Ochi M, Adachi N, Deie M, Kanaya A (2006) Anterior cruciate ligament augmentation procedure with a 1-incision technique: anteromedial bundle or posterolateral bundle reconstruction. Arthroscopy 22(4):463.e1–463.e5
59. Ma Y, Deie M, Iwaki D, Asaeda M, Fujita N, Adachi N, Ochi M (2014) Balance ability and proprioception after single-bundle, single-bundle augmentation, and double-bundle ACL reconstruction. ScientificWorldJournal 2014:342012. doi:10.1155/2014/342012

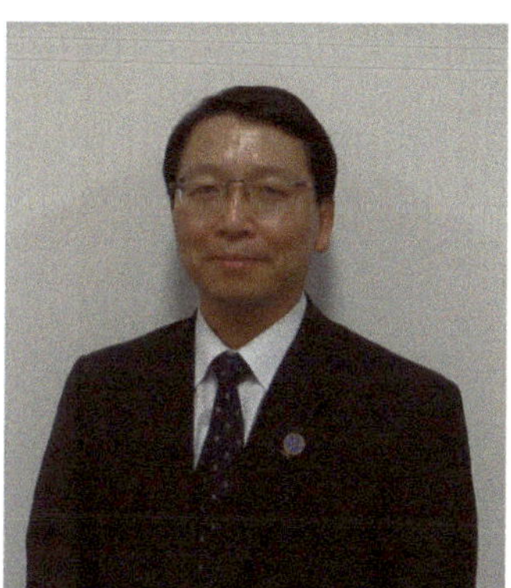

Yuji Uchio, M.D., PhD., Department of Orthopaedic Surgery, Shimane University, Shimane, Japan.

Part II
Biomechanics of the ACL

Chapter 6
Mechanical Properties and Biomechanical Function of the ACL

Hiromichi Fujie

Abstract The mechanical properties of the ACL are nonlinear, viscoelastic, and site-dependent. Large deformation may occur in the ACL up to 10 % of strain, while the load at failure exceeds 2000 N. These properties are affected by joint immobilization and maturity. With these unique properties, the ACL maintains normal knee kinematics by resisting to forces and moments applied to the knee. The ACL bears to 80 % of anterior force to the knee, while resisting to internal-external, varus-valgus, and combined rotation moments applied as a secondly restraint structure. Due to the posteroinferior slope of the tibial plateau, the ACL force is increased in ACL-intact knees, while tibial anterior subluxation occurs in ACL-deficient knees, in response to joint compressive force. Gait analysis studies revealed that the maximum anterior translation of the knee and the maximum ACL force are observed immediately after the heel strike during walking. In ACL-deficient knees, extension rotation is decreased during midsubstance, while varus and/or internal rotations are increased throughout the whole gait cycle.

Keywords Mechanical properties and functions • Knee kinematics • ACL force • Joint force and moment • Gait analysis

6.1 Mechanical Properties of the ACL

6.1.1 Material Properties

The material properties of the ACL are mainly determined from the stress-strain relationship of tensile tests. Stress is applied force per unit cross-sectional area, while strain is deformation divided by initial length. The stress-strain relationships of collagenous tissues are usually nonlinear; they increase slowly at low strain in the so-called toe region, have constant slope at middle strains in the "linear region," and then decrease at high strain in the prefailure region (Fig. 6.1). It is known that

H. Fujie, Ph.D. (✉)
Graduate School of System Design, Tokyo Metropolitan University, 6-6 Asahigaoka, Hino, Tokyo 191-0065, Japan
e-mail: fujie@tmu.ac.jp

M. Ochi et al. (eds.), *ACL Injury and Its Treatment*,
DOI 10.1007/978-4-431-55858-3_6

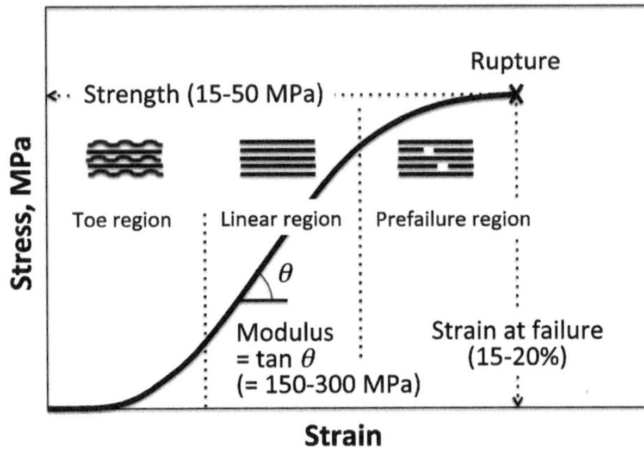

Fig. 6.1 Typical stress-strain relationship of the ACL and the definition of material properties (modulus, strength, and strain at failure) with schematic drawings of the microstructure of collagen fibers. Numerical data of the strength, modulus, and strain at failure are referred from the original work [5]

Table 6.1 Material properties (modulus, strength, and strain at failure) of the anteromedial, anterolateral, and posterior bundles of the human ACL

	Unit	Anteromedial bundle	Anterolateral bundle	Posterior bundle
Modulus	MPa	283.1 ± 114.1	285.9 ± 140.6	154.9 ± 119.5
Strength	MPa	45.7 ± 19.5	30.6 ± 11.0	15.4 ± 9.5
Strain at failure		19.1 ± 2.8	16.1 ± 3.9	15.2 ± 5.2

Data and terminology of the ACL bundles are referred from the original work [4]

such nonlinearity in collagenous tissues is due to the crimp pattern found at the fascicle level [32]. Therefore, the crimp pattern gradually disappears as strain increases during tensile testing. The modulus is the slope of the stress-strain relationship, the strength is the maximum stress, and the strain at failure is the strain when rupture occurs (Fig. 6.1). Although material properties are native to the material and independent of dimensions in general, these properties of the ACL are dependent on the scale due to its nonuniform and hierarchical structure. With respect to the human ACL, the mechanical properties were determined at the sub-ligament (bundle) level via a tensile test at a strain rate of 1 s^{-1} [5] (Table 6.1). The strength was approximately 46 MPa, 31 MPa, and 15 MPa in the anteromedial bundle, anterolateral bundle, and posterior bundle, respectively. It should be noted that the modulus (in linear region) and strength are significantly higher in the anteromedial and anterolateral bundles than in the posterior bundle, while strain at failure is almost identical in all the bundles. It was reported that the mechanical properties of the ACL deteriorate age dependently [23].

6.1.2 Structural Properties

The structural properties of the ACL are mainly determined from the load-deformation relationship of tensile tests. In the same manner as the stress-strain

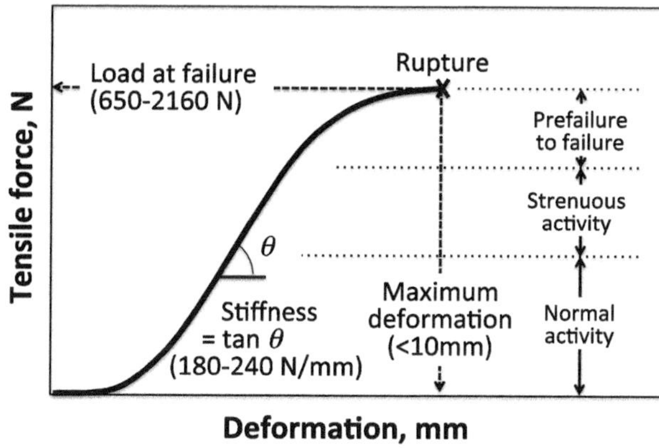

Fig. 6.2 Typical load-deformation relationship of the ACL and the definition of structural properties (stiffness, load at failure, and maximum deformation). Numerical data of the load at failure and stiffness are referred from the original work [33] while numerical datum of the maximum deformation is an approximate number

Table 6.2 Structural properties (stiffness and load at failure) of the human ACL as a function of age

	Unit	Young subjects (20–35 years old)	Middle subjects (40–50 years old)	Old subjects (60–97 years old)
Stiffness	N/mm	242 ± 28	220 ± 24	180 ± 25
Load at failure	N	2160 ± 157	1503 ± 83	658 ± 129

Data are referred from the original work [33]

relationships, the load-deformation relationships of collagenous tissues are usually nonlinear (Fig. 6.2). The stiffness is the slope of the relationship, the load at failure is the maximum load, and the maximum deformation is the deformation when rupture occurs. In contrast to the mechanical properties, the structural properties are dependent on material dimensions; for example, the load at failure doubles as the cross-sectional area doubles. With respect to the human ACL, the structural properties were determined for the whole ACL via tensile tests [34] (Table 6.2). It was reported that the load at failure is more than 2000 N for young subjects between 20 and 35 years old, decreased to approximately 1500 N for middle-aged subjects between 40 and 50 years old, and then decreased to less than 700 N for old subjects between 60 and 97 years old.

6.1.3 Viscoelastic Properties

It is known that the stress-strain and load-deformation relationships of the ACL are dependent on strain rate due to its viscoelastic property. Although perfectly elastic materials respond to loading and unloading instantaneously, viscoelastic materials have a time-dependent response to loading and unloading. Biological tissues usually exhibit remarkable viscoelastic behavior due to high water content. It is reported that the modulus of rabbit ACLs increases 30 % over a four-decade increase in strain rate [6]. It is also reported that the load at failure of rhesus monkey ACLs increases 24 % over a two-decade increase in extension rate [24]. Another aspect of the viscoelastic properties of the ACL is static/dynamic creep and stress relaxation; creep is a phenomenon of time-dependent strain increase in response to a constant stress, while stress relaxation is a phenomenon of time-dependent stress decrease in response to a constant strain. It was reported that static stress relaxation is more than 50 % over 120 min in the porcine ACL bundle [16].

6.1.4 Effects of Maturation and Exercise/Immobilization

Both the mechanical and structural properties of the ACL are affected by maturation and immobilization/exercise. In immature subjects, failure occurs at the ligament insertion rather than the ligament substance in tensile tests, because the bone-ligament junction is weaker than the ligament substance in immature subjects [34]. However, failure occurs more frequently at the ACL substance in mature subjects because the bone-ligament junction becomes stronger than ACL substance. A variety of animal studies have indicated that the strength and load at failure of ligaments rapidly decrease in response to immobilization or stress deprivation. They also suggest that the rate of recovery after mobilization is very slow. It was reported that after 5 months of recovery following 8 weeks of immobilization of the knee joint, the load at failure of the ACL of rhesus monkey recovered to 79 % of controls [22, 25]. Effects of physical exercise on the mechanical and structural properties of the ACL have not been fully determined due to the difficulty of quantifying and controlling exercise intensity.

6.2 Mechanical Function of the ACL

6.2.1 Response to Isolated and Combined Loadings

The primary motion of the knee joint is flexion-extension rotation around an axis passing through the medial and lateral femoral condyles. The three-dimensional motions of the knee other than flexion-extension rotation are constrained by ligaments, menisci, and articular surface configuration. The biomechanical functions of the ACL are mainly to resist anterior tibial translation, and secondly to resist internal and valgus tibial rotation, or combined motions.

The ACL is the primary restraint structure to anterior forces applied to the tibia because of its alignment and position with respect to the femur and tibia. More than 80 % of the anterior load is borne by the ACL [4, 29]. The force in the whole ACL

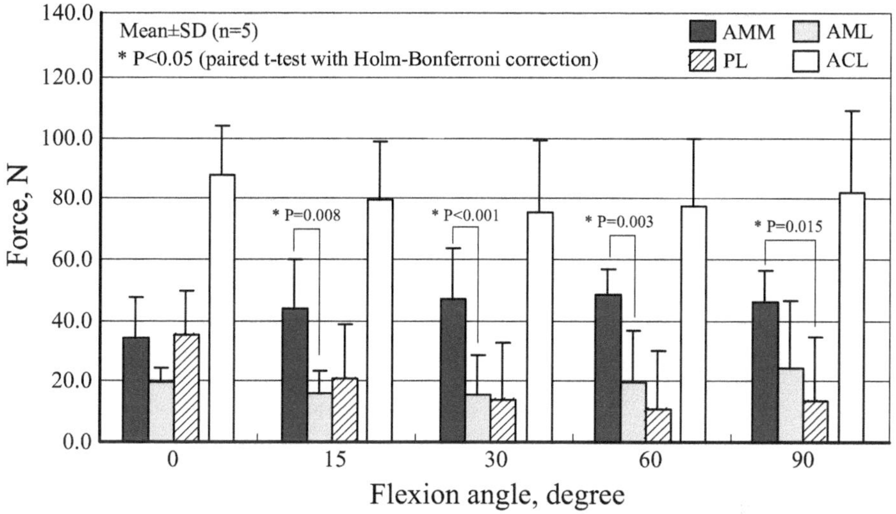

Fig. 6.3 Force sharing in the medial part (AMM) and lateral part (AML) of the anteromedial bundle and posterolateral bundle (PL) of the human ACL in response to 100 N of tibial anterior load. The figure and terminology of the ACL bundles are referred from the original work [8]

has been determined in experimental studies: approximately 80 N in response to 100 N of anterior force [8] (Fig. 6.3), between 70 N and 110 N in response to 110 N of anterior force [27], and more than 200 N in response to 200 N of anterior force [19]. In response to an anterior force, the posterolateral (PL) bundle carries more load than or same as the anteromedial (AM) bundle at low flexion angles, and the AM bundle carries more load than the PL bundle at deep flexion angles [1, 8, 27, 29]. Anterior tibial translation in response to an anterior tibial force is dependent on the magnitude of the anterior force as well as the knee flexion angle; anterior translation in response to 110 N of anterior tibial load is a couple of mm at full extension and increases to approximately 10 mm at 60° of flexion [27], the anterior-posterior translation between 100 N of anterior and posterior force is approximately 6–7 mm at flexion angles between 0 and 30° and decreases as the flexion angle increases [8] (Fig. 6.4), and the anterior-posterior translation between 200 N of anterior and posterior forces is less than 10 mm at full extension and increases more than 10 mm at depper flexion angles [19]. The translation increases more than double in ACL-transected knees [8, 9]. Anterior tibial force results in not only anterior translation of the knee but also coupled internal rotation [9, 12] with a medially shifted rotational axis [17, 20]. It is believed that the phenomenon directly or indirectly relates to the ACL because the coupled internal rotation decreases in ACL-transected knees [9].

The ACL is also the restraint structure to internal and/or valgus tibial moments. The ACL force in response to 10 Nm of internal moment applied to the tibia is approximately 70 N at full extension and decreases at flexion angles more

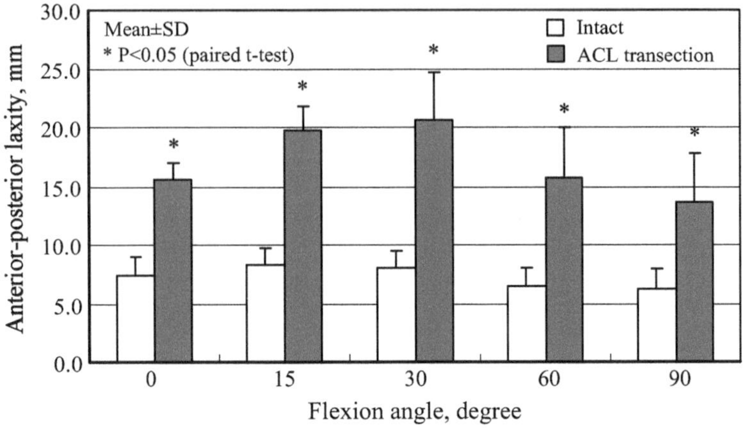

Fig. 6.4 Anterior-posterior laxity of the ACL-intact and ACL-deficient knees between 100 N of anterior and posterior forces as a function of flexion angle. The figure is referred from the original work [8]

than 60° [14]. Internal tibial rotation in response to 10 Nm of internal moment is more than 10° at full extension and increases at flexion angles more than 60°. The internal rotation and coupled anterior translation in response to an internal tibial moment significantly increase in ACL-deficient knees at low flexion angles. The ACL force in response to 10 Nm of valgus moment is approximately 90 N at full extension [19] and 40 N at 15° of flexion [15] and decreases with an increase of flexion angle. The application of valgus moment combined with internal moment to the knee results in significant increases in ACL forces as compared with an isolated loading of either internal moment or valgus moment at low flexion angles [14, 15].

Joint compressive force equivalent to body weight results in increases in ACL strain [3, 7] and ACL force [13], because anterior force is generated in association with joint compressive force due to the posteroinferior slope of the tibial plateau [11]. As a result, the neutral position of the tibia shifted anteriorly in response to joint compressive loading [7, 31]. Therefore, the anterior laxity, defined as a translation of the knee from the neutral position in response to an externally applied anterior force, decreases under the application of compressive loading. It is reported that anterior tibial subluxation of ACL-deficient knees is more significant in lateral side than in medial side in response to weight bearing [18].

6.2.2 Response to Physiological Loadings

An in vivo measurement combined with a knee model found that the tensile strain in the ACL increases over 10 % at the mid-stance during walking [30]. According to a mathematical analysis using a musculoskeletal low limb model that incorporated a 3D knee model, the ACL force increases approximately to 300 N at the beginning of stance phase during normal walking [28]. Note that the magnitude of the ACL force is much higher than that determined in an analytical study frequently referenced [21]. Relative knee motions in response to physiological loadings are determined via in vivo experimental studies. It was observed that the maximum anterior translation of the ACL-intact knee during walking is less than 10 mm and occurs immediately after heel strike [26]. In ACL-deficient knees, a significant reduction of extension is observed during midsubstance, while greater varus and internal rotations are observed throughout whole gait cycle [10]. During swing phase, reduced anterior translation and external rotation are observed in ACL-deficient knees associated with an internal rotation offset of the tibia [2].

References

1. Amis AA, Dawkins GP (1991) Functional anatomy of the anterior cruciate ligament. Fibre bundle actions related to ligament replacements and injuries. J Bone Joint Surg Br 73:260–267
2. Andriacchi TP, Dyrby CO (2005) Interactions between kinematics and loading during walking for the normal and ACL deficient knee. J Biomech 38:293–298
3. Beynnon BD, Johnson RJ, Fleming BC, Stankewich CJ, Renstrom PA, Nichols CE (1997) The strain behavior of the anterior cruciate ligament during squatting and active flexion-extension. A comparison of an open and a closed kinetic chain exercise. Am J Sports Med 25:823–829
4. Butler DL, Guan Y, Kay MD, Cummings JF, Feder SM, Levy MS (1992) Location-dependent variations in the material properties of the anterior cruciate ligament. J Biomech 25:511–518
5. Butler DL, Noyes FR, Grood ES (1980) Ligamentous restraints to anterior-posterior drawer in the human knee. A biomechanical study. J Bone Joint Surg Am 62:259–270
6. Danto MI, Woo SL (1993) The mechanical properties of skeletally mature rabbit anterior cruciate ligament and patellar tendon over a range of strain rates. J Orthop Res 11:58–67
7. Fleming BC, Renstrom PA, Beynnon BD, Engstrom B, Peura GD, Badger GJ, Johnson RJ (2001) The effect of weightbearing and external loading on anterior cruciate ligament strain. J Biomech 34:163–170
8. Fujie H, Otsubo H, Fukano S, Suzuki T, Suzuki D, Mae T, Shino K (2011) Mechanical functions of the three bundles consisting of the human anterior cruciate ligament. Knee Surg Sports Traumatol Arthrosc 19(Suppl 1):S47–S53
9. Fukubayashi T, Torzilli PA, Sherman MF, Warren RF (1982) An in vitro biomechanical evaluation of anterior-posterior motion of the knee. Tibial displacement, rotation, and torque. J Bone Joint Surg Am 64:258–264
10. Gao B, Zheng NN (2010) Alterations in three-dimensional joint kinematics of anterior cruciate ligament-deficient and -reconstructed knees during walking. Clin Biomech 25:222–229
11. Hashemi J, Chandrashekar N, Gill B, Beynnon BD, Slauterbeck JR, Schutt RC Jr, Mansouri H, Dabezies E (2008) The geometry of the tibial plateau and its influence on the biomechanics of the tibiofemoral joint. J Bone Joint Surg Am 90:2724–2734

12. Hollis JM, Takai S, Adams DJ, Horibe S, Woo SL (1991) The effects of knee motion and external loading on the length of the anterior cruciate ligament (ACL): a kinematic study. J Biomech Eng 113:208–214
13. Hosseini A, Gill TJ, Van de Velde SK, Li G (2011) Estimation of in vivo ACL force changes in response to increased weightbearing. J Biomech Eng 133:051004
14. Kanamori A, Woo SL, Ma CB, Zeminski J, Rudy TW, Li G, Livesay GA (2000) The forces in the anterior cruciate ligament and knee kinematics during a simulated pivot shift test: a human cadaveric study using robotic technology. Arthroscopy 16:633–639
15. Kanamori A, Zeminski J, Rudy TW, Li G, Fu FH, Woo SL (2002) The effect of axial tibial torque on the function of the anterior cruciate ligament: a biomechanical study of a simulated pivot shift test. Arthroscopy 18:394–398
16. Kwan MK, Lin TH, Woo SL (1993) On the viscoelastic properties of the anteromedial bundle of the anterior cruciate ligament. J Biomech 26:447–452
17. Lipke JM, Janecki CJ, Nelson CL, McLeod P, Thompson C, Thompson J, Haynes DW (1981) The role of incompetence of the anterior cruciate and lateral ligaments in anterolateral and anteromedial instability. A biomechanical study of cadaver knees. J Bone Joint Surg Am 63:954–960
18. Logan M, Dunstan E, Robinson J, Williams A, Gedroyc W, Freeman M (2004) Tibiofemoral kinematics of the anterior cruciate ligament (ACL)-deficient weightbearing, living knee employing vertical access open "interventional" multiple resonance imaging. Am J Sports Med 32:720–726
19. Markolf KL, Gorek JF, Kabo JM, Shapiro MS (1990) Direct measurement of resultant forces in the anterior cruciate ligament. An in vitro study performed with a new experimental technique. J Bone Joint Surg Am 72:557–567
20. Matsumoto H (1990) Mechanism of the pivot shift. J Bone Joint Surg Br 72:816–821
21. Morrison JB (1970) The mechanics of the knee joint in relation to normal walking. J Biomech 3:51–61
22. Noyes FR (1977) Functional properties of knee ligaments and alterations induced by immobilization: a correlative biomechanical and histological study in primates. Clin Orthop Relat Res 123:210–242
23. Noyes FR, DeLucas JL, Torvik PJ (1974) Biomechanics of anterior cruciate ligament failure: an analysis of strain-rate sensitivity and mechanisms of failure in primates. J Bone Joint Surg Am 56:236–253
24. Noyes FR, Grood ES (1976) The strength of the anterior cruciate ligament in humans and Rhesus monkeys. J Bone Joint Surg Am 58:1074–1082
25. Noyes FR, Torvik PJ, Hyde WB, DeLucas JL (1974) Biomechanics of ligament failure. II. An analysis of immobilization, exercise, and reconditioning effects in primates. J Bone Joint Surg Am 56:1406–1418
26. Obuchi S, Andrew PD, Cummings GS, Johnson BF (1999) Assessment of anteroposterior instability of the knee during gait. J Jpn Phys Ther Assoc 2:7–15
27. Sakane M, Fox RJ, Woo SL, Livesay GA, Li G, Fu FH (1997) In situ forces in the anterior cruciate ligament and its bundles in response to anterior tibial loads. J Orthop Res 15:285–293
28. Shelburne KB, Pandy MG, Anderson FC, Torry MR (2004) Pattern of anterior cruciate ligament force in normal walking. J Biomech 37:797–805
29. Takai S, Woo SL, Livesay GA, Adams DJ, Fu FH (1993) Determination of the in situ loads on the human anterior cruciate ligament. J Orthop Res 11:686–695
30. Taylor KA, Cutcliffe HC, Queen RM, Utturkar GM, Spritzer CE, Garrett WE, DeFrate LE (2013) In vivo measurement of ACL length and relative strain during walking. J Biomech 46:478–483
31. Torzilli PA, Deng X, Warren RF (1994) The effect of joint-compressive load and quadriceps muscle force on knee motion in the intact and anterior cruciate ligament-sectioned knee. Am J Sports Med 22:105–112

32. Viidik A (1973) Functional properties of collagenous tissues. Int Rev Connect Tissue Res 6:127–215
33. Woo SL, Hollis JM, Adams DJ, Lyon RM, Takai S (1991) Tensile properties of the human femur-anterior cruciate ligament-tibia complex. The effects of specimen age and orientation. Am J Sports Med 19:217–225
34. Woo SL, Orlando CA, Gomez MA, Frank CB, Akeson WH (1986) Tensile properties of the medial collateral ligament as a function of age. J Orthop Res 4:133–141

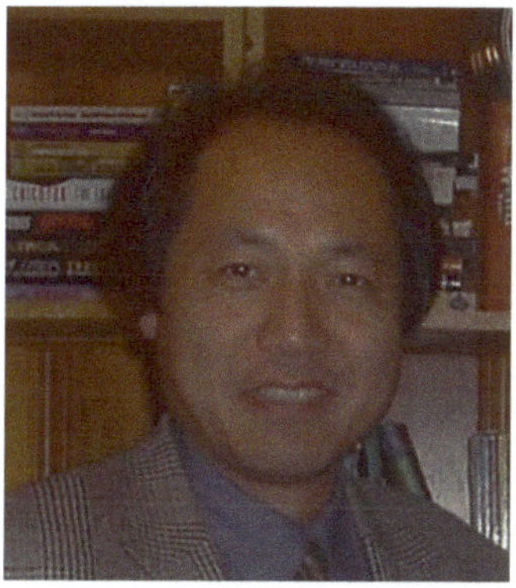

Hiromichi Fujie, PhD, Graduate School of System Design, Tokyo Metropolitan University, Tokyo, Japan.

Chapter 7
Biomechanics of the Knee with Isolated One-Bundle Tear of the Anterior Cruciate Ligament

Eiji Kondo and Kazunori Yasuda

Abstract This history of previous studies has resulted in the current confusion concerning the definition of the partial ACL tear in the clinical field. The purpose of this chapter was to introduce the changes in the kinematics of the knee that result from isolated deficiency of the anteromedial (AM) or posterolateral (PL) bundle of the anterior cruciate ligament. Anterior translation laxity under an anterior tibial load, rotational laxity under an internal tibial torque, and anterior translation laxity under pivot shift loading were significantly different between the knees with AM and PL bundle deficiencies, but the changes were small: less than 3 mm or 1.5°. An isolated AM or PL bundle tear caused a small increase in laxity. If there is a clinically identifiable increase in laxity – in addition to the isolated tear of the AM or PL bundle – there must also be a tear of the other bundle of the ACL or at least a partial tear.

Keywords Anterior cruciate ligament • Anteromedial bundle • Injury • Partial tear • Posterolateral bundle

7.1 Introduction

7.1.1 *Confusion in Definition of "Partial" ACL Tear*

There are various patterns in anterior cruciate ligament (ACL) injury [1, 2]. Many clinical studies have been conducted on partial ACL tear [3–7]. In these studies, however, the definition of the partial ACL tear has been unclear. The normal ACL

E. Kondo, M.D., Ph.D. (✉)
Department of Advanced Therapeutic Research for Sports Medicine, Hokkaido University Graduate School of Medicine, Kita-15 Nishi-7, Kita-ku, Sapporo, Hokkaido 060-8638, Japan
e-mail: eijik@med.hokudai.ac.jp

K. Yasuda, M.D., Ph.D.
Department of Sports Medicine and Joint Surgery, Hokkaido University Graduate School of Medicine, Sapporo, Hokkaido, Japan

M. Ochi et al. (eds.), *ACL Injury and Its Treatment*,
DOI 10.1007/978-4-431-55858-3_7

consists of two fiber bundles: the anteromedial (AM) and posterolateral (PL) [8, 9]. The previous studies on partial ACL tear included not only knees in which one bundle was torn and the other was intact ("isolated one-bundle tear") but also knees with other types of ACL injury, such as knees in which one bundle was torn and the other was permanently elongated and knees in which both bundles were permanently elongated. This history of previous studies has resulted in the current confusion concerning the definition of the partial ACL tear in the clinical field. Moreover, this confusion causes many controversial issues in the diagnosis and the treatment of the partial ACL tear [2, 10, 11].

7.1.2 Isolated AM or PL Bundle Tear

Recently, a few studies have reported the procedures for the isolated one-bundle tear, in which the AM or PL bundle was reconstructed with preservation of the other bundle remnant tissue, naming the procedure "selective" AM or PL bundle reconstruction [10, 12–14]. However, these studies did not describe how to clinically diagnose the isolated AM or PL bundle tear. In addition, it is unclear whether an isolated AM or PL bundle tear can be diagnosed accurately or consistently with the clinically available tools and techniques. Consequently, the clinical entity of an isolated AM or PL bundle tear has not been established as of yet. To establish how to diagnose the isolated AM or PL bundle tear, it is necessary to increase our fundamental database on kinematics of the knee with an isolated AM or PL bundle injury in comparison with kinematics of the normal knee, as well as that of a completely ACL-deficient knee.

However, only a few studies have reported kinematic information that contributes directly to our knowledge of clinical manual tests [2, 15–17]. Furman et al. [15] applied loads by hand and found a clear difference between the effects of cutting each bundle: isolated AM bundle cutting allowed increased anterior translation in the flexed knee but not in extension, whereas the reverse was found when the isolated PL bundle was cut. Zantop et al. [17] reported that isolated transection of the PL bundle significantly increased anterior tibial translation at 30° of flexion, whereas transection of the AM bundle significantly increased the translation at 60 and 90° of flexion. However, Hole et al. [16] described that isolated transection of the PL bundle did not increase the anterior translation significantly at 30° of flexion. Thus, there were conflicting conclusions among the previous studies. Therefore the diagnosis of partial tears of the ACL remains difficult, and thus there is still a need to increase the database on the kinematics of the knee with an isolated AM or PL bundle injury under various biomechanical conditions in comparison with those of the normal knee.

Recently, the authors reported a kinematic study with 14 fresh-frozen cadaveric knees to clarify the changes in the kinematics of the knee that result from the isolated tear of the AM or PL bundle [18]. In this chapter, the authors introduce the results of that study and discuss about clinical relevance of the results. Specifically, a focus of the discussion is whether the isolated tear of the AM or PL bundle can be diagnosed by measurement of the knee instability with manual tests or a KT-2000 arthrometer.

7.2 Methods

Fourteen fresh-frozen cadaveric knees were used in this study. Each knee was mounted onto the specially designed apparatus, which was reported in the previous literature in detail [19]. The kinematics of the tibiofemoral joint was measured dynamically with a Polaris stereo-optical system (Northern Digital, Waterloo, Canada) with Traxtal active optical trackers (Traxtal, Toronto, Canada), mounted on the tibia and femur (Fig. 7.1). The intact knee was moved from full extension to 110 of knee flexion and then back to extension for three cycles. Then, each of the following loads was applied to the tibia: (1) 90-N anterior drawer force, (2) 90-N posterior drawer force, (3) 5-Nm internal rotation torque, (4) 5-Nm external rotation torque, and (5) simulated pivot shift test. The pivot shift test was simulated by use of a 50-N iliotibial band tension, 5-Nm valgus moment, and 1-Nm internal rotation torque [20–22]. A nylon cable secured to the iliotibial band was attached to a precalibrated pneumatic cylinder alongside the femur to generate the 50-N tension [21, 22]. The 14 knees were separated into two groups: In seven specimens the midsubstance of the AM bundle was transected first at the midsubstance to simulate an isolated AM bundle tear (Fig. 7.2). In the remaining seven specimens, the PL

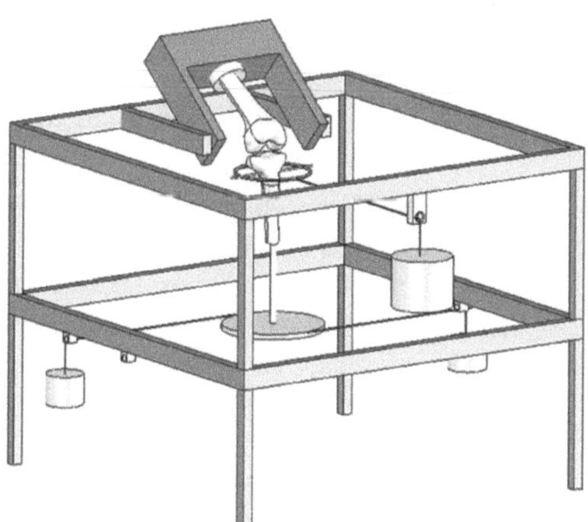

Fig. 7.1 Flexion-extension movements were applied to the femur while the tibia hung vertically below it; the motion of the hanging tibia was otherwise unconstrained. The anterior or posterior drawer force was applied with a weight and cable connected to a hoop around the proximal tibia. Internal or external rotation torque was applied with weights connected to both sides of a polyethylene disk secured at the end of the tibial rod. (From Ref. [19]. Reprinted by permission of SAGE Publications. 2007 American Orthopaedic Society for Sports Medicine)

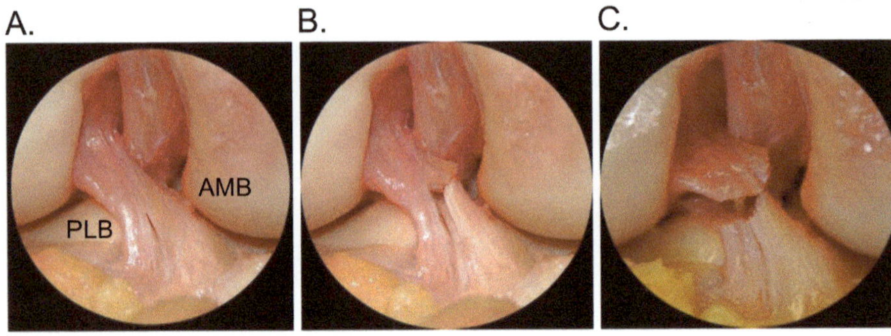

Fig. 7.2 (**a**) Arthroscopic finding of intact ACL, (**b**) AM bundle cut, and (**c**) complete ACL cut (From Ref. [18]. Reprinted by permission of SAGE Publications. 2014 Arthroscopy)

bundle was transected at the midsubstance to simulate an isolated PL bundle tear. Knee kinematic measurements were repeated for the isolated AM or PL bundle tear. Then, the remaining bundle was transected arthroscopically, and the kinematics of the ACL-deficient knee were measured in all 14 knees with the five external loading conditions described earlier.

The laxities measured when the knees were intact were in line with previously published data [18]. This study presents the changes from normal, which yields greater clarity regarding the effects of cutting the fiber bundles.

7.3 Kinematics of ACL-Injured Knees

7.3.1 Anterior Translation Under 90-N Anterior Load

Under a 90-N anterior load, ANOVA showed that there were significant differences in anterior translation laxity among the groups of ACL-deficient knees and knees with AM and PL bundle tears ($P < .001$) and that there were significant interactions with knee flexion ($P = .012$) (Fig. 7.3). Post hoc testing found that cutting the PL bundle alone did not significantly increase the anterior translation in a range between 0 and 110° of knee flexion in comparison with the normal translation ($P = .552$ to $P = .982$) (Fig. 7.3). Similarly, cutting the AM bundle alone did not significantly increase the anterior translation at 0–110° of knee flexion in comparison with the normal translation ($P = .998$ at 0° to $P = .078$ at 110°). The maximal increment caused by cutting the AM bundle was 3.7 mm ($P = .075$), at 95° of knee flexion (Fig. 7.3). After both bundles were cut, the anterior tibial translation increased at each angle of knee flexion in comparison with the normal translation; this was significant from 0 to 100° of flexion ($P < .001$ to $P = .007$) (Fig. 7.3). The maximal increment caused by cutting both of the bundles was 11 mm ($P < .001$), at 30° of knee flexion (Fig. 7.3).

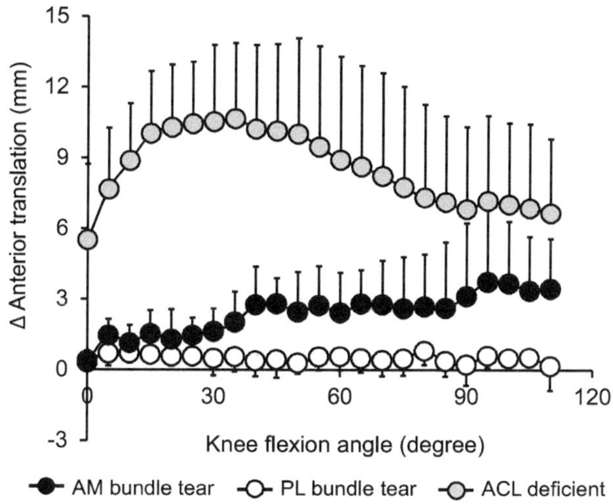

Fig. 7.3 Difference in anterior translation from intact knee under 90-N anterior load, presented as mean and standard deviation (error bars) (From Ref. [18]. Reprinted by permission of SAGE Publications. 2014 Arthroscopy)

7.3.2 Tibial Rotation Under 5-Nm Torque

Under a 5-Nm internal rotation torque, ANOVA found significant differences in tibial internal rotation laxity between the knees with partial ACL cutting and the ACL-deficient state ($P < .001$); there were also significant interactions with knee flexion ($P < .001$) (Fig. 7.3). The maximal increase in internal rotation was 1.2° by cutting either the AM or PL bundle alone, at 25° and 80° of knee flexion ($P = .330$ and $P = .218$, respectively) (Fig. 7.4). After both bundles were cut, the pathologic increase in tibial rotation increased toward the extended posture, reaching 3.8° in extension (Fig. 7.4). Post hoc testing showed that cutting both the AM and PL bundles significantly increased the tibial internal rotation near knee extension in comparison with AM bundle-deficient laxity ($P = .014$ at 0–30° of flexion), as well as in relation to PL bundle deficiency ($P = .006$ at 0–55° of flexion) (Fig. 7.4). Under a 5-Nm external rotation torque, ANOVA did not show significant differences between the ACL-deficient knees and the knees with AM and PL bundle tears.

7.3.3 Anterior Translation and Internal Rotation Under Simulated Pivot Shift Loading

Under simulated pivot shift loading, ANOVA indicated that there were significant differences in tibial anterior translation among the ACL-deficient knees, knees with isolated AM bundle deficiency, and knees with isolated PL bundle deficiency ($P < .001$) (Fig. 7.5). There were also significant interactions between anterior laxity and the angle of knee flexion ($P < .001$). Post hoc testing did not show that

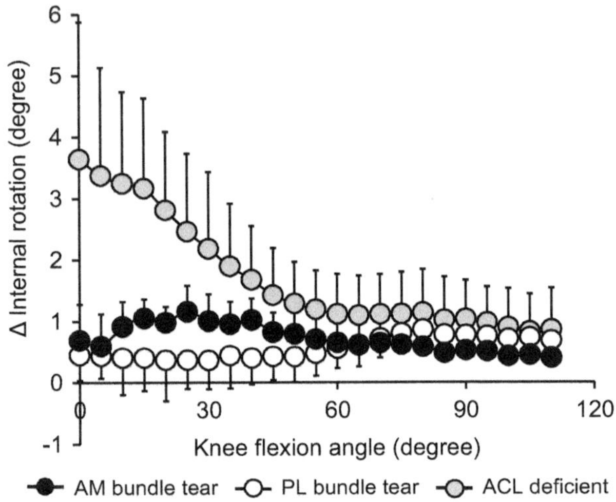

Fig. 7.4 Difference in tibial internal rotation from intact knee under 5-Nm internal tibial torque, presented as mean and standard deviation (error bars) (From Ref. [18]. Reprinted by permission of SAGE Publications. 2014 Arthroscopy)

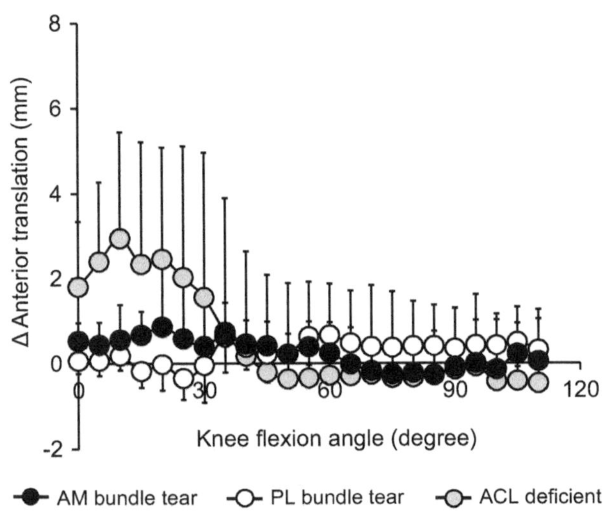

Fig. 7.5 Difference in tibial anterior translation from intact knee under pivot shift loading, presented as mean and standard deviation (error bars) (From Ref. [18]. Reprinted by permission of SAGE Publications. 2014 Arthroscopy)

cutting either the AM bundle ($P = .242$) or PL bundle ($P = .305$) in isolation increased the anterior translation significantly at any angle of knee flexion in comparison with the anterior translation during the pivot shift test when the ACL was intact (Fig. 7.5). After both bundles were cut, the anterior tibial translation increased significantly ($P < .001$) at 0 and 15° of knee flexion (Fig. 7.5), reaching 3 mm at 10°of knee flexion. On the other hand, transection of the ACL did not cause a significant change in tibial internal rotation during the simulated pivot shift test.

7.4 Discussion

7.4.1 Considerations of the Results in Comparison with the Previous Studies

The present study dealt with isolated AM or PL bundle deficiency, in which one bundle was transected and the other was intact. Therefore, we must distinguish the isolated one-bundle tear from the other types of partial ACL injury. The present study provided important information on anterior tibial translation to solve the previously described controversy that has existed in the clinical field of ACL injury.

First, under the 90-N anterior load, cutting either the PL or AM bundle alone did not significantly increase tibial anterior translation, while cutting both the AM and PL bundles dramatically increased anterior translation or rotation under the 90-N anterior load. There are controversies among the previous studies and the present study. Concerning the effect of PL bundle transection, Hole et al. [16] reported that sectioning the PL bundle alone did not significantly increase anterior translation at 30° under a 133-N anterior load. On the other hand, Zantop et al. [17] reported that when a 134-N anterior load was applied to the tibia at 30, 60, and 90° of knee flexion, isolated transection of the PL bundle significantly increased anterior tibial translation at 30°. Regarding the effect of AM bundle transection, Zantop et al. [17] reported that transection of the AM bundle alone significantly increased the translation at 60 and 90 when the robotic system in their study applied 134 N. The differences in the effect of isolated PL or AM bundle transection among the studies may be a result of the differences in the testing conditions. In general, application of larger loads will magnify any changes in laxity, but a judgment must be made in repeated measures studies because the loads must be small enough that they will not cause permanent deformations of the remaining ligament bundles.

The present study showed that, under the 5-Nm internal rotation torque, cutting either the AM or PL bundle did not significantly increase the tibial rotation at each angle of knee flexion in comparison with normal rotation. Also under pivot shift loading, cutting either the AM or PL bundle alone did not lead to a significant increase in tibial anterior translation. Then, a significant increase was found only after transection of both the bundles. On the other hand, Zantop et al. [17] applied a combined rotatory load of 10 Nm of valgus moment and 4 Nm of internal torque at a fixed angle of knee flexion without any loads on the iliotibial band, and reported that transection of the PL bundle significantly increased anterior translation at 0 and 30° of knee flexion, although transection of the AM bundle did not significantly increase coupled anterior translation. Namely, the effect of PL bundle transection was different, although the effect of AM bundle transection was similar between the two studies. The difference is considered to be due to differences in the loading conditions: in addition to the differing moments and iliotibial band tension applied, when the pivot shift occurs in the moving knee, the instant axis of rotation will differ from that which occurs at a fixed angle of flexion.

7.4.2 Clinical Relevance of the Present Study

Our study has provided important information on the clinical diagnosis of an isolated AM or PL bundle tear using manual tests such as the Lachman, anterior drawer, and pivot shift, as well as noninvasive measurement devices such as the KT-2000 arthrometer [23]. In the present study, for example, the 90-N anterior load was applied because it is similar to a biomechanical condition in the clinical tests.

Concerning the isolated PL bundle tear, there were few differences in tibial translation or rotation between the intact knee and the isolated PL bundle-deficient knee under any loading condition. It is considered that the effect of isolated PL bundle transection was not significantly detected because the intact AM bundle remained relatively tight during knee motion [24–26]. These results suggest that it is impossible to clinically diagnose an isolated PL bundle tear, using physical examinations. Hole et al. [16] reported that only 11 % of the examinations correctly diagnosed the isolated PL bundle resection, although the examiners were accurate in their interpretation of the status of the ACL in 89 % of the intact specimens and 80 % of completely sectioned ACLs. Clinical evaluation is accurate in defining intact and completely sectioned ACLs. However, it is unable to differentiate a sectioned PL bundle from an intact ACL.

Regarding the isolated AM bundle tear, there was only a tendency for the tibial translation under the anterior force to increase toward 90° of knee flexion in comparison with the normal knee, and there were no differences under simulated pivot shift test loading. Zantop et al. [17] did find a significant increase in the flexed knee under a larger force. Therefore, it is theoretically possible to clinically diagnose an isolated AM bundle tear using the anterior drawer test. However, the maximal increment by cutting the AM bundle was only 3 mm and 1.5°. Therefore, these facts imply that it may be difficult for common orthopedic surgeons to always detect the abnormal laxity of the isolated AM bundle tear only using the manual tests. Previously, Lintner et al. [3] sectioned the AM bundle of the ACL and found that clinical examination and KT-1000 arthrometer testing were unable to detect differences from the intact knee because the small (1.3 mm) increase in anterior translation that occurred was within the 2-mm normal bound of side-to-side differences. On the other hand, the tibial translation and rotation were dramatically increased by cutting both the AM and PL bundles. This fact indicated that the knee with obviously abnormal translation and rotation of the tibia and positive pivot shift phenomenon in comparison with the normal knee should be strongly suspected of having a complete tear of the two bundles.

In the previous literature, a clinical diagnosis of isolated PL or AM bundle tear was frequently made by clinically identified increases in knee laxity. The present study suggests that such knees might involve not only PL or AM bundle tear but also AM or PL bundle injury with permanent elongation. Therefore, the "isolated AM (or PL) bundle reconstruction" for such knees, which reconstructs only the PL (or AM) bundle and leaves the AM (or PL) bundle without any treatments, should be recognized as a treatment for such knees with such type insufficiency of both the

AM and PL bundles. On the other hand, some authors noted that, even with extensive clinical and imaging assessment, the exact injury pattern of an isolated bundle tear might only be established arthroscopically [10, 11, 14, 17, 24]. Therefore, there is a possibility that comprehensive examinations including arthroscopic observation may find out some degrees of one-bundle injury without any abnormalities in the other bundle. However, the present study suggests that such knees may not clinically show any abnormal laxity. However, the authors believe that such knees without any instability are not involved in the indications of ACL reconstruction surgery.

References

1. Zantop T, Brucker PU, Vidal A, Zelle BA, Fu FH (2007) Intraarticular rupture pattern of the ACL. Clin Orthop Relat Res 454:48–53
2. DeFranco MJ, Bach BR (2009) A comprehensive review of partial anterior cruciate ligament tears. J Bone Joint Surg Am 91:198–208
3. Lintner DM, Kamaric E, Moseley JB, Noble PC (1995) Partial tears of the anterior cruciate ligament: are they clinically detectable? Am J Sports Med 23:111–118
4. Noyes FR, Mooar LA, Moorman CT et al (1989) Partial tears of the anterior cruciate ligament: progression to complete ligament deficiency. J Bone Joint Surg (Br) 71:825–833
5. Odensten M, Lysholm J, Gillquist J (1985) The course of partial anterior cruciate ligament ruptures. Am J Sports Med 13:183–186
6. Sandberg R, Balkfors B (1987) Partial rupture of the anterior cruciate ligament: natural course. Clin Orthop Relat Res 220:176–178
7. Sommerlath K, Odensten M, Lysholm J (1992) The late course of acute partial anterior cruciate ligament tears. A nine to 15-year follow-up evaluation. Clin Orthop Relat Res 281:152–158
8. Girgis FG, Marshall JL, Al Monajem ARS (1976) The cruciate ligaments of the knee joint: anatomical, functional and experimental analysis. Clin Orthop Relat Res 106:216–231
9. Yasuda K, Kondo E, Ichiyama H et al (2004) Anatomic reconstruction of the anteromedial and posterolateral bundles of the anterior cruciate ligament using hamstring tendon grafts. Arthroscopy 20:1015–1025
10. Siebold R, Fu HF (2008) Assessment and augmentation of symptomatic anteromedial or posterolateral bundle tears of the anterior cruciate ligament. Arthroscopy 24:1289–1298
11. Colombet P, Dejour D, Panisset JC, Siebold R (2010) Current concept of partial anterior cruciate ligament ruptures. Orthop Traumatol Surg Res 96S:S109–S118
12. Ochi M, Adachi N, Deie M, Kanaya A (2006) Anterior cruciate ligament augmentation procedure with a 1-incision technique: anteromedial bundle or posterolateral bundle reconstruction. Arthroscopy 22:463.e1–463.e5
13. Ochi M, Adachi N, Uchio Y et al (2009) A minimum 2-year follow-up after selective anteromedial or posterolateral bundle anterior cruciate ligament reconstruction. Arthroscopy 25:117–122
14. Tjoumakaris FP, Donegan DJ, Sekiya JK (2011) Partial tears of the anterior cruciate ligament: diagnosis and treatment. Am J Orthop 40:92–97
15. Furman W, Marshall JL, Gigris FG (1976) The anterior cruciate ligament: a functional analysis based on postmortem studies. J Bone Joint Surg Am 58:179–185
16. Hole RL, Lintner DM, Kamaric E, Moseley JB (1996) Increased tibial translation after partial sectioning of the anterior cruciate ligament: the posterolateral bundle. Am J Sports Med 24:556–560

17. Zantop T, Herbort M, Raschke MJ, Fu FH, Petersen W (2007) The role of the anteromedial and posterolateral bundles of the anterior cruciate ligament in anterior tibial translation and internal rotation. Am J Sports Med 35:223–227
18. Kondo E, Merican AM, Yasuda K, Amis AA (2014) Biomechanical analysis of knee laxity with isolated anteromedial or posterolateral bundle-deficient anterior cruciate ligament. Arthroscopy 30:335–343
19. Cuomo P, Rama KR, Bull AMJ, Amis AA (2007) The effects of different tensioning strategies on knee laxity and graft tension after double-bundle anterior cruciate ligament reconstruction. Am J Sports Med 35:2083–2090
20. Bull AMJ, Andersen HN, Basso O, Targett J, Amis AA (1999) Incidence and mechanism of the pivot-shift: an in-vitro study. Clin Orthop Relat Res 363:219–231
21. Lie DTT, Bull AMJ, Amis AA (2007) Persistence of the mini pivot shift after anatomically placed anterior cruciate ligament reconstruction. Clin Orthop Relat Res 457:203–209
22. Kondo E, Merican AM, Yasuda K, Amis AA (2010) Biomechanical comparisons of knee stability after anterior cruciate ligament reconstruction between two clinically available transtibial procedures: anatomic double-bundle versus single-bundle. Am J Sports Med 38:1349–1358
23. Daniel D, Malcolm L, Losse G, Stone M, Sachs R, Burks R (1985) Instrumented measurement of anterior laxity of the knee. J Bone Joint Surg Am 67:720–726
24. Sidles JA, Larson RV, Garbini JL, Downey DJ, Matsen FA III (1988) Ligament length relationships in the moving knee. J Orthop Res 6:593–610
25. Amis AA, Dawkins GPC (1991) Functional anatomy of the anterior cruciate ligament: fiber bundle actions related to ligament replacement and injuries. J Bone Joint Surg (Br) 73:260–267
26. Fuss FK (1989) Anatomy of the cruciate ligaments and their function in extension and flexion of the human knee joint. Am J Sports Med 184:165–176

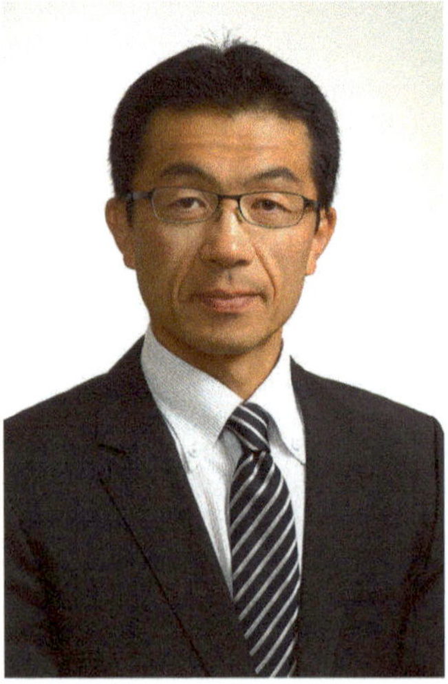

Eiji Kondo, M.D., PhD, Department of Advanced Therapeutic Research for Sports Medicine, Hokkaido University Graduate School of Medicine, Sapporo, Hokkaido, Japan.

Chapter 8
Function and Biomechanics of ACL Remnant

Junsuke Nakase and Hiroyuki Tsuchiya

Abstract Remnant-preserving anterior cruciate ligament (ACL) reconstruction recently gained popularity because it has some advantages for patients. In this paper, we discuss our assessment of preoperative images of ACL remnants, indicate intraoperative classification, and review the proprioceptive function, revascularization, and biomechanical function of remnant tissue. We describe the neural mechanoreceptors and reinnervation of the reconstructed ACL graft as well as enhancement of the revascularization process of the ACL graft based on previous reports. Finally, we discuss the biomechanical function of the ACL remnants. Attention to detail is important since there are various remnant types. The ACL has healing abilities, and its remnants are thought to be endowed with various repair factors. Surgeons should arthroscopically examine the remnants at the time of the ACL reconstruction to determine the best approach to treating ACL injury.

Keyword ACL remnant • Remnant type • Proprioceptive function • Biomechanical function

8.1 Introduction

Remnant-preserving anterior cruciate ligament (ACL) reconstruction recently gained popularity because it has proven biomechanical [1, 2], vascular [3], and proprioceptive [4] advantages; moreover, it has been shown to reduced synovial fluid leakage into the bone tunnels [5] and improve knee stability [6]. Thus, ACL reconstruction using remnant-preserving techniques has received much attention. However, few studies to date have reviewed the function and biomechanics of ACL remnants.

Differential diagnosis of partial ACL tears becomes an issue in discussions of ACL remnant function and biomechanics. A uniform definition of a partial ACL tear does not exist, and its diagnosis remains clinically challenging. Partial ACL

J. Nakase, M.D., Ph.D. (✉) • H. Tsuchiya, M.D., Ph.D.
Department of Orthopaedic Surgery, School of Medicine, Kanazawa University, 13-1 Takaramachi, Kanazawa, Ishikawa 920-0934, Japan
e-mail: nakase1007@yahoo.co.jp

M. Ochi et al. (eds.), *ACL Injury and Its Treatment*,
DOI 10.1007/978-4-431-55858-3_8

tears have reportedly been excised in their entirety together with the femur attachment site. A histological investigation of this tissue reported that the femur attachment site retained a normal structure in only 22.7 % of cases [7]. It was believed difficult to clearly classify residual ligaments after partial damage and remnant tissues after complete rupture. Kazusa summarized the current evidence that the remnant-preserving ACL reconstruction is indicated whether patients have remnants between the tibia and either the femur or the posterior cruciate ligament (PCL) after complete ACL ruptures or have only partial rupture of the anteromedial or posterolateral bundle [8]. In this paper, we primarily discuss the function and biomechanics of remnant tissue after complete rupture.

8.2 Preoperative Assessment

Magnetic resonance imaging (MRI) and computed tomography (CT) are primarily used for preoperatively evaluating remnant tissue. Preoperative awareness of remnant morphology and biomechanical function would be advantageous in the selection of an appropriate surgical method, and various reports have been published on this topic. Ng et al. reported that the addition of oblique axial imaging to standard MRI improves diagnostic accuracy for detecting either partial tears or individual bundle tears of the ACL [9]. In a like manner, Kosaka et al. reported that oblique coronal and sagittal MRI improved the accuracy of diagnosis of ACL tears and showed a reasonable level of efficacy in detecting remnant ACL tissue [10]. We occasionally see papers stating that it is possible to identify the detailed morphology of remnant tissues by recording MRI in line with ACL directionality.

On the other hand, Adachi et al. conducted some fascinating research using three-dimensional CT (3D CT) and reported a concordance rate of 77.8 % for morphological patterns of ACL remnants using 3D CT with the volume-rendering technique and patterns defined using arthroscopy without probing [11]. However, the concordance rate was reduced to 49.2 % when arthroscopic probing was used to confirm the femoral attachment of the ACL remnants.

Although ACL remnant morphology can be identified to some extent before surgery using careful photography, biomechanical function cannot be assessed quite as easily at that stage. However, in the future, the use of high-performance equipment or functional MRI and so on may resolve these problems, so further research is essential.

8.3 Arthroscopic Classification

Arthroscopic classification and evaluation methods for remnants are extremely important factors in the selection of the surgical technique and can result in conflicting opinions. As described above, presurgical imaging alone does not

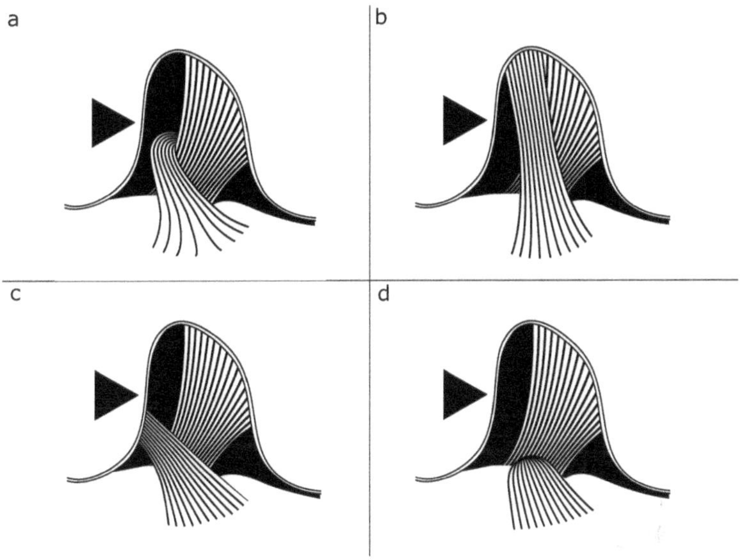

Fig. 8.1 Arthroscopic ACL remnant pattern by Crain. The normal ACL attachment on femur (*arrow head*) (from [12] with permission). (**a**) Group 1: ACL scarring to the PCL. (**b**) Group 2: ACL healing to roof of the notch. (**c**) Group 3: Attenuated ACL remnant healed to the lateral wall more anterior and distal than its anatomic origin. (**d**) Group 4. Resorption of the torn ACL

enable a complete evaluation of remnant tissue that includes an assessment of biomechanical function; as such, the remnants are mainly evaluated with arthroscopy. Many papers have reported arthroscopic classification with a focus on the proximal end of the remnant attachment site. Of them, that reported by Crain in 2005 is now one of the most commonly used classifications [12]. Crain divided ACL remnants into four categories by morphology: (1) ACL remnant with scarring to the PCL, (2) ACL remnant with scarring to the roof of the notch, (3) ACL remnant with scarring to the lateral wall of the notch or the medial aspect of the lateral femoral condyle, and (4) no identifiable ligament tissue remaining (Fig. 8.1). This classification system is widely used and works well. However, there were cases in which remnants were continuous near the ACL anatomical insertion and no cases in which evaluated the attenuated ACL remnant that had healed to the lateral wall more anteriorly and distally than its anatomic origin. Accordingly, Maeda [13] and Nakase [14] created a new classification system that included bridging between the anatomical attachments of the ACL on the lateral wall of the femoral condyle and the tibia. These classifications are suitable when surgeons consider remnant morphology (Fig. 8.2).

On the other hand, Muneta reported a remnant volume evaluation (Fig. 8.3) [15]. The ACL remnant was divided into three parts: tibial attachment (distal 20 %), midsubstance (middle 60 %), and femoral attachment (proximal 20 %). Muneta concluded that the remnant volume had a certain level of correlation with the postoperative outcome. Furthermore, the tension and anatomic position of the

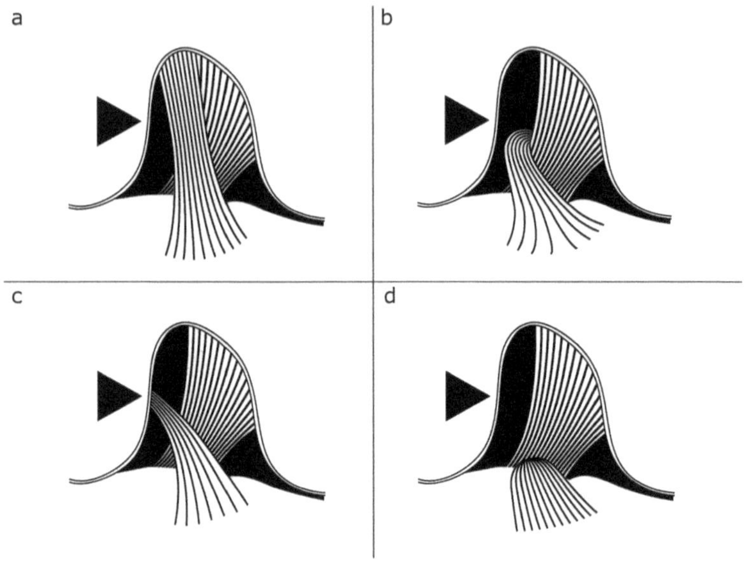

Fig. 8.2 Arthroscopic classification of remnants by Nakase. The normal ACL attachment on femur (*arrow head*) (from [14] with permission). (**a**) Type 1: Bridging between the roof of the intercondylar notch and tibia. (**b**) Type 2: Bridging between the posterior cruciate ligament and tibia. (**c**) Type 3: Bridging between the anatomical attachments of the ACL on the lateral wall of the femoral condyle and the tibia. (**d**) Type 4; No bridging ACL remnants

remnant tissue were not evaluated in their study because they were difficult to assess objectively. Future studies should be based on more objective measures of ACL remnant volume, such as 3D MRI. Even by using 3D MRI, however, remnant tension cannot be easily assessed. We will need new or improved technologies for arthroscopic examination in the future.

8.4 Proprioceptive Function

Proprioceptive function has an important role to play in regaining nearly normal function after ACL reconstruction as well as a return to sports activities. The presence of mechanoreceptors on the intact ACL has been well documented [16, 17]. Some histological studies reported that there were portions of mechanoreceptors within ACL remnants [18]. Denti et al. used Ruffini gold chloride staining to identify mechanoreceptors within ACL remnants [19]. They found that, in untreated ACL lesions in humans, morphologically normal mechanoreceptors persisted in the ACL remnant for approximately 3 months after the injury. Beyond that time, the number of receptors decreased. By the ninth month after injury, only a few nerve endings were found; by 1 year, they were completely absent. Georgoulis reported the presence of neural mechanoreceptors in ACL remnants as a possible

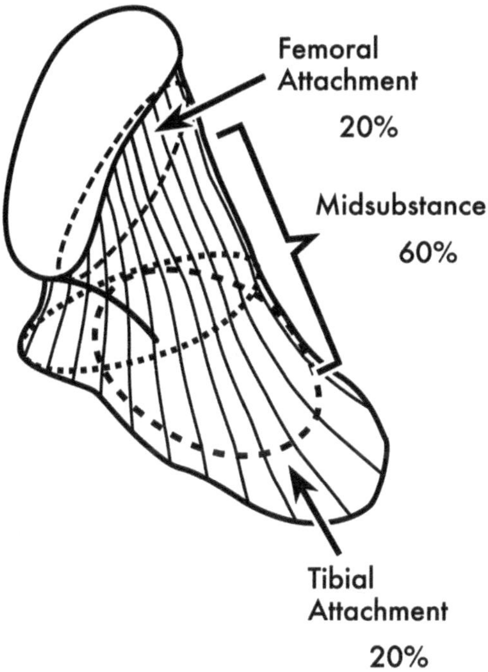

Fig. 8.3 Arthroscopical determination of the ACL remnant volume (from [15] with permission). An entire volume of the ACL was divided into three parts of tibial attachment, midsubstance, and femoral attachment. Twenty percent, 60 %, and 20 % were assigned to the tibial attachment, midsubstance, and femoral attachment, respectively

source of reinnervation of the reconstructed ACL graft [20]. They reported two types of ACL remnants. In 15 patients, the ACL was adhered to the PCL; mechanoreceptors were observed in all of these ligaments. In five patients, mushroom-like remnants were found either none or a few mechanoreceptors; however, free nerve endings were found in both patient groups. They concluded that in patients with ACL remnants that are adherent to the PCL, the mechanoreceptors existing in the ACL remnants might actually act as a possible source of graft reinnervation. Dhillon et al. evaluated the proprioceptive function in ACL remnants using immunohistological methods [21]. They harvested the remnants in 63 patients undergoing ACL reconstruction. A statistically significant negative relationship was found between injury duration and the persistence of mechanoreceptors and proprioceptive fibers. The proprioceptive potential was also higher in ACL remnants that were adherent to the PCL. The duration of persistence of viable mechanoreceptors reportedly varies. This may be due to the methods by which they are evaluated, so Bali et al. proposed standardization of the evaluative techniques [22].

Proprioceptive function of the knee has been measured in various ways, such as with the joint position sense test [23] and latency of reflex hamstring contractions [24]. It is unclear how much of the knee's proprioceptive function is due to ACL mechanoreceptors. Mechanoreceptors that control proprioception of the knee joint are distributed not only to the ACL but also to the surrounding tissues [25]. Specific and validated techniques are needed to assess the proprioceptive function of the ACL remnant. Preservation of the ACL remnant may have some advantage for proprioceptive function. Adachi reported a positive correlation between the number of mechanoreceptors in ACL remnants and the accuracy of preoperative joint position sense [4]. They concluded that leaving the ACL remnants as a source for reinnervation may be beneficial. The development of new validated methods to assess the proprioceptive function of the ACL remnant alone could contribute to evaluations of the effectiveness of the remnant-preserved ACL reconstruction compared with the conventional method. This could help answer questions such as how much remnant should be spared or whether it is necessary to retain remnant continuity.

8.5 Revascularization

Enhancing the graft revascularization process is one goal of remnant-preserving ACL reconstruction. There are several reports on the hemodynamics of the ACL and surrounding tissues. Odenstein reported a cadaveric study of uniformly placed connective tissue containing blood vessels [26]. Dodds reported a vascularized synovial envelope around the ACL and periligamentous vessels that transversely penetrated the ligament and performing anastomosis with a longitudinal network of endoligamentous vessels [27]. They also reported that the proximal and distal attachments of the ACL have greater vascular density than the mid-section, with the proximal part having greater vascularity than the distal portion. In a rabbit model, the ACL was dissected and compared with a control group 4 months after a standardized surgically induced partial ACL tear [28]. The results showed a significant increase in blood flow and vascular volume in the injured group. Other reports confirmed that cases with a good revascularization process showed better graft incorporation on follow-up MRI, which correlated with a favorable clinical outcome [29–31]. We believe that when the ACL remnant is preserved, blood vessels within the remnant are also preserved, which improves ACL graft revascularization. The gold standard for evaluating graft revascularization status should be histological assessment of graft biopsy samples. However, histological evaluation has not been widely used because of the invasive nature of the biopsy procedure.

MRI is too subjective to show true ACL graft vascularization. Therefore, Song et al. cannot conclude that the ACL remnant has an important role for ACL graft revascularization [32]. How do these processes affect graft ligamentization? In the future, we will need to consider how it correlates to the clinical outcomes. Furthermore, if we can discover a way to assess blood flow quality and volume within the remnant, research in this field progress.

8.6 Biomechanics

Remnant tissue is thought to adhere to the lateral wall of the femoral condyle and PCL at the healing point after a complete ACL tear, making it difficult to inspect remnant tissue biomechanics in cadaveric studies. For this reason, biomechanical evaluation of remnant tissue is performed during ACL reconstruction.

Crain et al. reported on the correlation between the remnant pattern and anterior laxity in 48 patients [12]. They evaluated anterior knee laxity before and after ACL remnant resection using a KT-1000 knee arthrometer. Of 48 knees, 14 (29 %) loosened by more than 2 mm after ACL remnant resection. After resection of the ACL remnant attached to the femur, a mean loosening of 3.9 mm occurred. They concluded that ACL remnants that heal while adherent to the femur effectively cross the joint and contribute a small degree to knee stability.

Maeda et al. performed a prospective study of 83 knees subjected to primary navigated ACL reconstruction [13]. Anterior tibial translation and range of internal-external rotation of the tibia at 15°, 30°, 45°, 60°, 75°, and 90° of knee flexion were measured before and after ACL remnant resection using the navigation system. The mean anterior tibial translation at 15° of knee flexion before resection significantly increased after resection in cases in which the remnants bridged the lateral wall of the intercondylar notch and the tibia. After remnant resection, 14.5 % of cases in which the remnants had bridged the lateral wall of the intercondylar notch and the tibia showed an increased anterior tibial translation by $\geq$3 mm. However, there were no significant differences in mean total rotation before versus after resection at any knee flexion angle for any of the remnant types defined by the Maeda and Nakase classification (Fig. 8.2). Thus, they concluded that ACL remnants do not play a major role in knee stabilization. However, the remnant type that bridged between the lateral wall of the intercondylar notch and the tibia significantly decreased anterior knee extension.

Nakase reported the roles of ACL remnants in knee stability using the same type of navigation system [14]. They conducted a prospective study of 50 knees subjected to primary ACL reconstruction. The ACL remnants were classified into four morphologic types as above (Fig. 8.2). Anterior tibial translation and rotatory laxity were measured before and after remnant resection at 30°, 60°, and 90° of knee flexion using a navigation system. The amount of change in anterior tibial translation and the rotatory laxity of each morphologic type was compared among the remnant types. The amount of change in anterior tibial translation and rotatory laxity at 30° of knee flexion in type 3 (bridging between the anatomical insertions of the ACL on the lateral wall of the femoral condyle and the tibia) was significantly larger than in the other types. There were no significant differences in either tibial translation or rotatory laxity at 60° or 90° of knee flexion among the types. They concluded that the remnants that bridge the anatomical attachments of the ACL on the lateral wall of the femoral condyle and the tibia contribute to anteroposterior and rotatory knee laxity evaluated at 30° of knee flexion. Further, the bridging point of the remnants is important to knee laxity. The limitation of this study was that patients with a partial ACL tear may have been included as type 3, which may have influenced the results.

The ACL does have some healing abilities, and its remnants are thought to be endowed with various repair factors [33]. Different types of remnants can affect the surgical procedure. The surgeon should perform a preoperative arthroscopic evaluation of the remnants at the time of the ACL reconstruction to determine the best ACL injury treatment approach.

References

1. Borbon CA, Mouzopoulos G, Siebold R (2012) Why perform an ACL augmentation? Knee Surg Sports Traumatol Arthrosc 20:1245–1251. doi:10.1007/s00167-011-1565-2
2. Hong L, Li X, Zhang H, Liu X, Zhang J, Shen JW, Feng H (2012) Anterior cruciate ligament reconstruction with remnant preservation: a prospective, randomized controlled study. Am J Sports Med 40:2747–2755. doi:10.1177/0363546512461481
3. Hu J, Qu J, Xu D, Zhang T, Zhou J, Lu H (2014) Clinical outcomes of remnant preserving augmentation in anterior cruciate ligament reconstruction: a systematic review. Knee Surg Sports Traumatol Arthrosc 22:1976–1985. doi:10.1007/s00167-013-2749-8
4. Adachi N, Ochi M, Uchio Y, Iwasa J, Ryoke K, Kuriwaka M (2002) Mechanoreceptors in the anterior cruciate ligament contribute to the joint position sense. Acta Orthop Scand 73:330–334
5. Junkin DM Jr, Johnson DL (2008) ACL tibial remnant, to save or not? Orthopedics 31:154–159
6. Kondo E, Yasuda K, Onodera J, Kawaguchi Y, Kitamura N (2015) Effects of remnant tissue preservation on clinical and arthroscopic results after anatomic double-bundle anterior cruciate ligament reconstruction. Am J Sports Med 11. doi:10.1177/0363546515587713
7. Sonnery-Cottet B, Bazille C, Hulet C et al (2014) Histological features of the ACL remnant in partial tears. Knee 21:1009–1013. doi:10.1016/j.knee.2014.07.020
8. Kazusa H, Nakamae A, Ochi M (2013) Augmentation technique for anterior cruciate ligament injury. Clin Sports Med 32:127–140. doi:10.1016/j.csm.2012.08.012
9. Ng AW, Lee RK, Ho EP, Law BK, Griffith JF (2013) Anterior cruciate ligament bundle measurement by MRI. Skelet Radiol 42:1549–1554. doi:10.1007/s00256-013-1705-5
10. Kosaka M, Nakase J, Toratani T, Ohashi Y, Kitaoka K, Yamada H, Komura K, Nakamura S, Tsuchiya H (2014) Oblique coronal and oblique sagittal MRI for diagnosis of anterior cruciate ligament tears and evaluation of anterior cruciate ligament remnant tissue. Knee 21:54–57. doi:10.1016/j.knee.2013.04.016
11. Adachi N, Ochi M, Takazawa K, Ishifuro M, Deie M, Nakamae A, Kamei G (2016) Morphologic evaluation of remnant anterior cruciate ligament bundles after injury with three-dimensional computed tomography. Knee Surg Sports Traumatol Arthrosc 24:148–153. doi:10.1007/s00167-014-3354-1
12. Crain EH, Fithian DC, Paxton EW, Luetzow WF (2005) Variation in anterior cruciate ligament scar pattern: does the scar pattern affect anterior laxity in anterior cruciate ligament-deficient knees? Arthroscopy 21:19–24
13. Maeda S, Ishibashi Y, Tsuda E, Yamamoto Y, Toh S (2011) Intraoperative navigation evaluation of tibial translation after resection of anterior cruciate ligament remnants. Arthroscopy 27:1203–1210. doi:10.1016/j.arthro.2011.03.080

14. Nakase J, Toratani T, Kosaka M, Ohashi Y, Tsuchiya H (2013) Roles of ACL remnants in knee stability. Knee Surg Sports Traumatol Arthrosc 21:2101–2106. doi:10.1007/s00167-012-2260-7
15. Muneta T, Koga H, Ju YJ, Horie M, Nakamura T, Sekiya I (2013) Remnant volume of anterior cruciate ligament correlates preoperative patients' status and postoperative outcome. Knee Surg Sports Traumatol Arthrosc 21:906–913. doi:10.1007/s00167-012-2023-5
16. Johansson H, Sjölander P, Sojka P (1991) A sensory role for the cruciate ligaments. Clin Orthop Relat Res 268:161–178
17. Schutte MJ, Dabezies EJ, Zimny ML, Happel LT (1987) Neural anatomy of the human anterior cruciate ligament. J Bone Joint Surg Am 69:243–247
18. Lee BI, Min KD, Choi HS, Kwon SW, Chun DI, Yun ES, Lee DW, Jin SY, Yoo JH (2009) Immunohistochemical study of mechanoreceptors in the tibial remnant of the ruptured anterior cruciate ligament in human knees. Knee Surg Sports Traumatol Arthrosc 17:1095–1101. doi:10.1007/s00167-009-0831-z
19. Denti M, Monteleone M, Berardi A, Panni AS (1984) Anterior cruciate ligament mechanoreceptors. Histologic studies on lesions and reconstruction. Clin Orthop Relat Res 308:29–32
20. Georgoulis AD, Pappa L, Moebius U, Malamou-Mitsi V, Pappa S, Papageorgiou CO, Agnantis NJ, Soucacos PN (2001) The presence of proprioceptive mechanoreceptors in the remnants of the ruptured ACL as a possible source of re-innervation of the ACL autograft. Knee Surg Sports Traumatol Arthrosc 9:364–368
21. Dhillon MS, Bali K, Vasistha RK (2010) Immunohistological evaluation of proprioceptive potential of the residual stump of injured anterior cruciate ligaments (ACL). Int Orthop 34:737–741. doi:10.1007/s00264-009-0948-1
22. Bali K, Dhillon MS, Vasistha RK, Kakkar N, Chana R, Prabhakar S (2012) Efficacy of immunohistological methods in detecting functionally viable mechanoreceptors in the remnant stumps of injured anterior cruciate ligaments and its clinical importance. Knee Surg Sports Traumatol Arthrosc 20:75–80. doi:10.1007/s00167-011-1526-9
23. Corrigan JP, Cashman WF, Brady MP (1992) Proprioception in the cruciate deficient knee. J Bone Joint Surg Br 74:247–250
24. Beard DJ, Kyberd PJ, Fergusson CM, Dodd CA (1993) Proprioception after rupture of the anterior cruciate ligament. An objective indication of the need for surgery? J Bone Joint Surg (Br) 75:311–315
25. Lee BI, Kwon SW, Kim JB, Choi HS, Min KD (2008) Comparison of clinical results according to amount of preserved remnant in arthroscopic anterior cruciate ligament reconstruction using quadrupled hamstring graft. Arthroscopy 24:560–568. doi:10.1016/j.arthro.2007.11.011
26. Odensten M, Gillquist J (1985) Functional anatomy of the anterior cruciate ligament and a rationale for reconstruction. J Bone Joint Surg Am 67:257–262
27. Dodds JA, Arnoczky SP (1994) Anatomy of the anterior cruciate ligament: a blueprint for repair and reconstruction. Arthroscopy 10:132–139
28. Bray RC, Leonard CA, Salo PT (2002) Vascular physiology and long-term healing of partial ligament tears. J Orthop Res 20:984–989
29. Ochi M, Adachi N, Uchio Y, Deie M, Kumahashi N, Ishikawa M, Sera S (2009) A minimum 2-year follow-up after selective anteromedial or posterolateral bundle anterior cruciate ligament reconstruction. Arthroscopy 25:117–122. doi:10.1016/j.arthro.2008.10.011
30. Ahn JH, Wang JH, Lee YS, Kim JG, Kang JH, Koh KH (2011) Anterior cruciate ligament reconstruction using remnant preservation and a femoral tensioning technique: clinical and magnetic resonance imaging results. Arthroscopy 27:1079–1089. doi:10.1016/j.arthro.2011.03.002
31. Ohsawa T, Kimura M, Kobayashi Y, Hagiwara K, Yorifuji H, Takagishi K (2012) Arthroscopic evaluation of preserved ligament remnant after selective anteromedial or posterolateral bundle anterior cruciate ligament reconstruction. Arthroscopy 28:807–817. doi:10.1016/j.arthro.2011.11.033

32. Song GY, Zhang H, Zhang J, Li X, Chen XZ, Li Y, Feng H (2013) The anterior cruciate ligament remnant: to leave it or not? Arthroscopy 29:1253–1262. doi:10.1016/j.arthro.2013.03.078
33. Costa-Paz M, Ayerza MA, Tanoira I, Astoul J, Muscolo DL (2012) Spontaneous healing in complete ACL ruptures: a clinical and MRI study. Clin Orthop Relat Res 470:979–985. doi:10.1007/s11999-011-1933-8

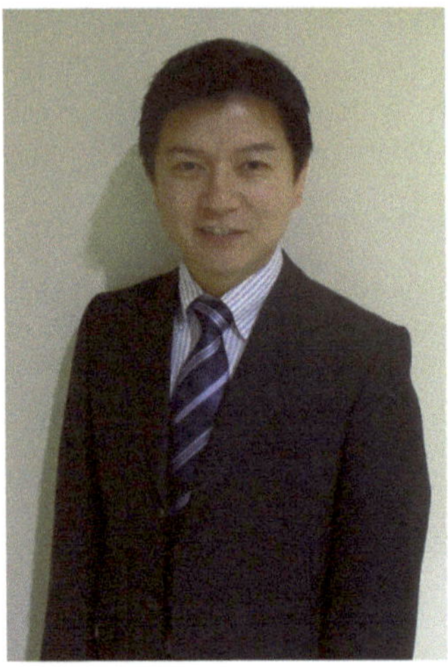

Junsuke Nakase, M.D., PhD, Department of Orthopaedic Surgery, School of Medicine, Kanazawa University, Ishikawa, Japan.

Chapter 9
Biomechanics of Single- and Double-Bundle ACL Reconstruction

Eiji Kondo and Kazunori Yasuda

Abstract The biomechanical studies showed that the anatomic single-bundle (SB) reconstruction was significantly better concerning the knee stability under a 90-N anterior force and a 5-Nm internal torque than the conventional SB reconstruction in a range between 0 and 30°. However, there were no significant differences between the two reconstructions not only in the other ranges of knee flexion under these loading conditions but also in all the ranges under the simulated pivot shift test. On the other hand, the anatomic double-bundle (DB) reconstruction was significantly better concerning the knee stability under a 90-N anterior force and a 5-Nm internal torque than the conventional SB reconstruction not only in a range between 0 and 30° but also in the range between 35 and 70°. In addition, the anatomic DB reconstruction was significantly better under the simulated pivot shift test than the conventional SB reconstruction in a range between 0 and 30°. These results showed that although both the anatomic SB and DB reconstructions were significantly better than conventional SB reconstruction, the effect of the anatomic SB reconstruction on the knee stability is not completely identical to the effect of the anatomic DB reconstruction. Preliminary in vivo data suggest that anatomic DB reconstruction can restore normal knee kinematics, but further studies including research on anatomic SB reconstruction are required before definitive conclusions can be reached.

Keywords Anterior cruciate ligament • Anteromedial bundle • Anatomic reconstruction • Double bundle • Posterolateral bundle • Single bundle

---

E. Kondo, M.D., Ph.D. (✉)
Department of Advanced Therapeutic Research for Sports Medicine, Hokkaido University Graduate School of Medicine, Kita-15 Nishi-7, Kita-ku, Sapporo, Hokkaido 060-8638, Japan
e-mail: eijik@med.hokudai.ac.jp

K. Yasuda, M.D., Ph.D.
Department of Sports Medicine and Joint Surgery, Hokkaido University Graduate School of Medicine, Sapporo, Hokkaido, Japan

M. Ochi et al. (eds.), *ACL Injury and Its Treatment*,
DOI 10.1007/978-4-431-55858-3_9

9.1 Introduction

Single-bundle (SB) reconstruction of the anterior cruciate ligament (ACL) is the standard surgical option to treat ACL-deficient knees. However, recent biomechanical studies have reported that conventionally performed SB ACL reconstruction cannot restore normal anterior translation or rotatory laxity [1, 2]. Kinematic studies have also shown that the SB reconstruction cannot completely restore the patient's rotatory stability during walking or more strenuous activities [3, 4]. The normal ACL consists of anteromedial (AM) and posterolateral (PL) bundles, which have different functions [5–8]. To improve such biomechanical disadvantages of SB reconstruction, Yasuda et al. [9, 10] reported the first practical arthroscopic procedure to anatomically reconstruct both the AM and PL bundles of the ACL in 2004. Several biomechanical studies have reported significantly better knee stability than after conventional SB reconstruction [11–13]. On the other hand, recently, an idea of anatomic SB ACL reconstruction, in which the femoral tunnel is created at the center of the AM and PL bundle attachments on the femur, has attracted notice in the clinical field [14, 15]. Thus, a following question has been arisen. Is the effect of the anatomic SB reconstruction on the knee stability completely identical to the effect of the anatomic DB reconstruction? The first aim of this chapter is to answer this question. To answer to the question, the authors compared the degrees of superiority of the anatomic SB and DB reconstructions to the conventional SB reconstruction, using the previously reported database of the knee laxity after various ACL reconstruction procedures [16].

The second aim of this chapter is to answer the following question: Can the clinically available transtibial procedure for anatomic DB reconstruction really obtain significantly better knee stability in comparison with the conventional SB reconstruction procedure? This question must be asked because the previous biomechanical studies, which reported that the former procedure can obtain significantly better knee stability than the latter procedure [11–13], widely exposed the knee joint and directly identify the anatomic attachments. Clinically, however, the authors have used an arthroscopic transtibial procedure for femoral tunnel creation. Therefore, there is a possibility that the femoral tunnel positions in the clinical are not identical to the ideal tunnel locations created in the previous biomechanical studies. To answer the following question, the authors performed the arthroscopic transtibial procedure of anatomic DB reconstruction, which had been performed in the authors' clinical practice, in cadaver specimens, and compared the results with those of the conventional SB reconstruction procedure [11].

9.2 Is the Effect of the Anatomic SB ACL Reconstruction Completely Identical to the Effect of the Anatomic DB ACL Reconstruction?

9.2.1 Methods

Eight fresh-frozen cadaveric knees were used in this study [16]. Each knee was mounted onto the specially designed apparatus, which was reported in the previous literature in detail [17]. The intact knee was moved by hand from full extension to 110° of flexion and then back to extension for three cycles. Then, the below-described measurement of the knee laxity was repeated in the normal knee and the ACL-reconstructed knees. Each of the following loads was applied to the tibia: (1) 90-N tibial anterior drawer force, (2) 5-Nm tibial internal rotation torque, (3) 5-Nm tibial external rotation torque, and (4) a combined load to simulate the pivot shift test: 50-N iliotibial tract tension, 5-Nm valgus moment, and 1-Nm tibial internal rotation torque, according to our previous works [18, 19]. The iliotibial tract was loaded by linking it with a nylon cable to a pneumatic cylinder. In each loading condition, three cycles of knee flexion-extension between 0 and 110° were repeated manually. The kinematics of the tibiofemoral joint was measured dynamically with a Polaris stereo optical system (Northern Digital Inc., Waterloo, Canada) with Traxtal active optical trackers (Traxtal Technologies Inc., Toronto, Canada) mounted on the tibia and femur.

The conventional SB reconstruction procedure was performed using the same technique as the above-described study (Fig. 9.1a) [10]. In anatomic SB reconstruction, the tibial tunnel was placed at the center of the normal ACL attachment between the medial and lateral tibial eminences, and the femoral tunnel was placed at the center between the AM and PL bundle attachments (Fig. 9.1b). The anatomic DB reconstruction was performed with the previously reported procedure with a specially designed device (Fig. 9.1c) [20, 21]. After one reconstruction was made in a cadaver knee, the knee laxity was measured. Then, after the graft was removed and the vacant tunnel was filled with polyester resin paste, the next reconstruction was performed and the knee laxity was measured. Thus, the knee laxity data after each ACL reconstruction were obtained, independent from the order of measurement. The following analyses were made using this database. The authors divided the whole range of knee flexion into three ranges, a range between 0 and 30°, a range between 35 and 70°, and a range between 75 and 110°, and comparisons were made in each range. Rather than present normal laxity data, this article displays the changes from normal, which has greater clarity regarding residual laxities after the reconstructions.

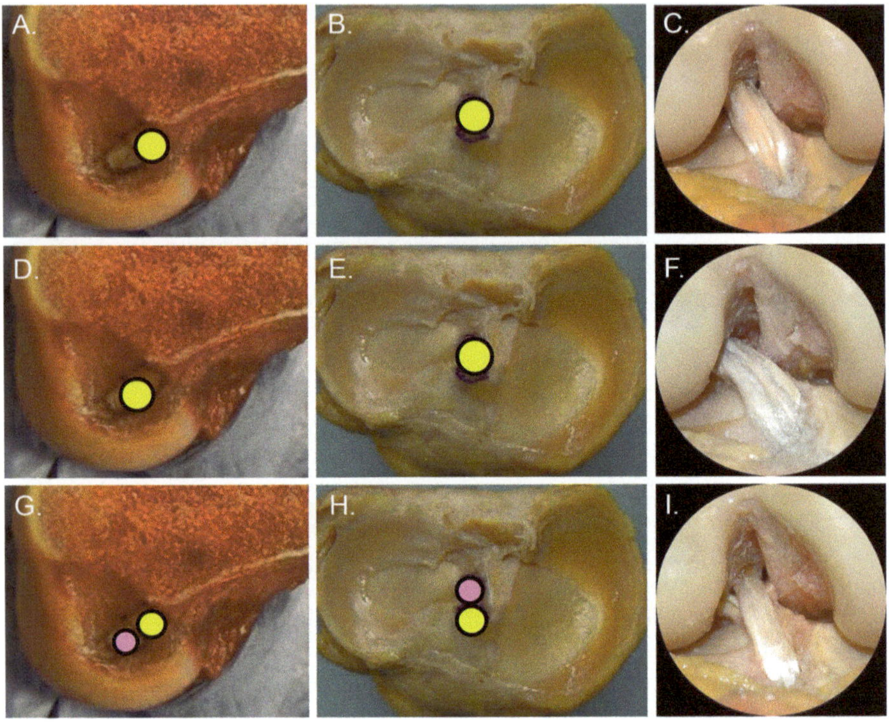

Fig. 9.1 (**a, b, c**): The conventional single-bundle procedure A, the single femoral tunnel was placed at the center of the anatomic attachment of the anteromedial bundle of the ACL; B, the tibial tunnel was placed at the center of the anatomic attachment of the ACL; C, the intra-articular autogenous tendon graft was composed of 4 strands of tendons
(**d, e, f**): The anatomic single-bundle procedure A, the femoral tunnel was placed at the center of the anatomic attachment of the ACL; B, the tibial tunnel was placed at the center of the anatomic attachment of the ACL; C, the autogenous tendon portion of the graft was composed of 4 strands of tendon
(**g. h, i**): The anatomic double-bundle procedure A, two femoral tunnels were created at the centers of the anatomic attachments of the anteromedial and posterolateral bundles; B, two tibial tunnels were created at the centers of the anatomic attachments of the anteromedial and posterolateral bundles; C, the two tendon grafts placed in the tunnels (From Ref. [16]. Reprinted by permission of SAGE Publications. 2011 American Orthopaedic Society for Sports Medicine)

9.2.2 Results

Under a 90-N anterior force (Fig. 9.2), the ANOVA demonstrates that the anatomic SB reconstruction was significantly better than the conventional SB reconstruction ($p=0.0211$) only in the range between 0 and 30° and that there were no significant differences in the other ranges of knee flexion (Table 9.1). On the other hand, the anatomic DB reconstruction was significantly better than the conventional SB reconstruction both in the range between 0 and 30° ($p=0.0027$) and in the range

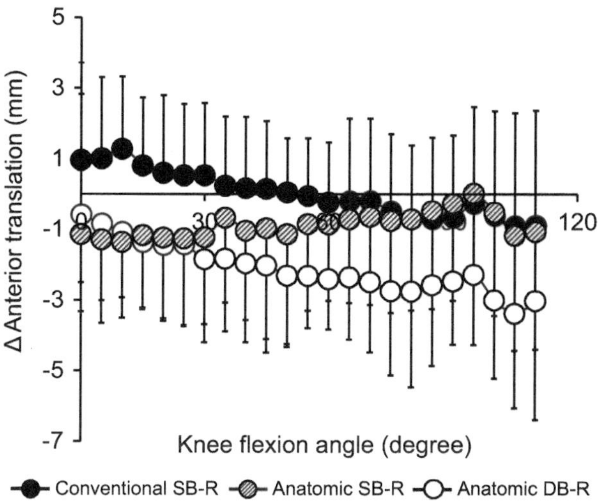

Fig. 9.2 The difference in anterior translation from the intact knee (which is the zero-datum axis) under 90-N anterior load for the intact and ACL-reconstructed knee (mean +/− standard deviation). Values above the datum axis represent greater laxity compared with the intact behavior, and vice versa. *R*, reconstruction

Table 9.1 Comparisons of the knee laxity between the anatomic SB reconstruction and the conventional SB reconstruction in a range between 0 and 30°, a range between 35 and 70°, and a range between 75 and 110°

Comparison	0–30 °	35–70°	75–110°
Under a 90-N anterior force			
ASB[a] versus CSB[b]	P = 0.0211	NS[*]	NS
ADB[c] versus CSB	P = 0.0027	P = 0.0041	NS
Under a 5-Nm internal torque			
ASB[a] versus CSB[b]	P = 0.0344	NS	NS
ADB[c] versus CSB	P = 0.0268	P = 0.0479	NS
Under the simulated pivot shift test			
ASB[a] versus CSB[b]	NS	NS	NS
ADB[c] versus CSB	P = 0.0259	NS	NS

These results were compared with the results of comparisons between the anatomic double-bundle reconstruction and the conventional SB reconstruction

[*]Not significant

[a]*ASB* anatomic SB reconstruction

[b]*CSB* conventional SB reconstruction

[c]*ADB* anatomic DB reconstruction

between 35 and 70° (p = 0.0041). Under a 5-Nm internal torque (Fig. 9.3), the ANOVA demonstrates that the anatomic SB reconstruction was significantly better than the conventional SB reconstruction (p = 0.0344) only in the range between 0 and 30° (Table 9.1). On the other hand, the anatomic DB reconstruction was significantly better than the conventional SB reconstruction both in the range between 0 and 30° (p = .0268) and in the range between 35 and 70° (p = 0.0479). Under the simulated pivot shift test (Fig. 9.4), the ANOVA demonstrates that there was no significant difference between the anatomic and conventional SB reconstructions at each range of knee flexion (Table 9.1). On the other hand, the anatomic

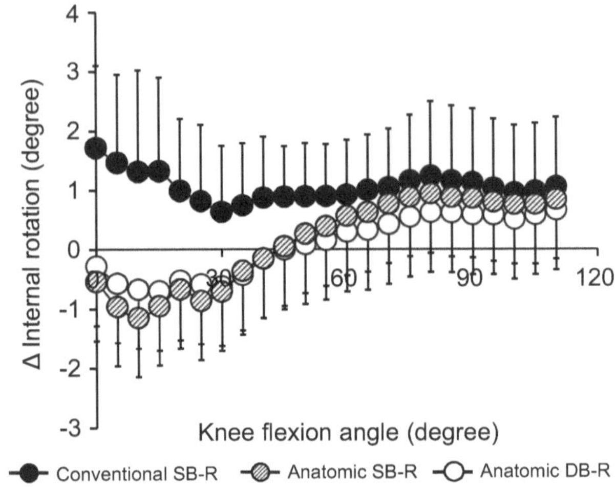

Fig. 9.3 The difference from the intact knee in tibial internal rotation under 5-Nm internal rotation torque for the ACL-reconstructed knee (mean +/− standard deviation). *R*, reconstruction (From Ref. [16]. Reprinted by permission of SAGE Publications. 2011 American Orthopaedic Society for Sports Medicine)

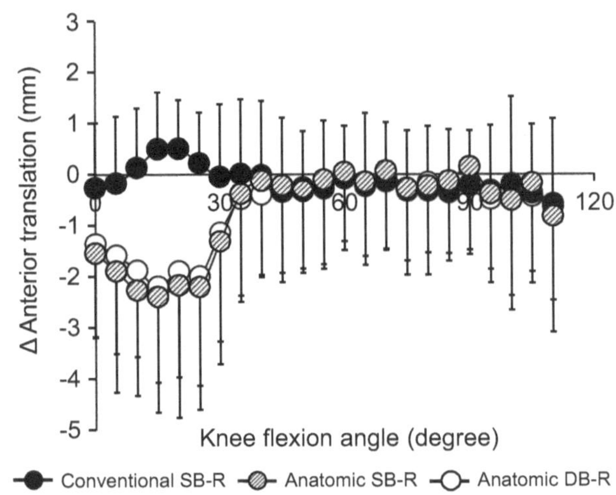

Fig. 9.4 The difference in the tibial anterior translation from the intact knee during the pivot shift for the ACL-reconstructed knee (mean +/− standard deviation). *ACL* anterior cruciate ligament, *R* reconstruction (From Ref. [16]. Reprinted by permission of SAGE Publications. 2011 American Orthopaedic Society for Sports Medicine)

DB reconstruction was significantly better than the conventional SB reconstruction only in the range between 0 and 30° ($p = 0.0259$).

9.2.3 Discussion

The first study question was whether the effect of the anatomic SB reconstruction on the knee stability is completely identical to the effect of the anatomic DB reconstruction. The present analyses showed that the anatomic SB reconstruction was significantly better concerning the knee stability under a 90-N anterior force and a 5-Nm internal torque than the conventional SB reconstruction in a range between 0 and 30°. However, it is noted that there were no significant differences between the two reconstructions not only in the other ranges of knee flexion under these loading conditions but also in all the ranges under the simulated pivot shift test. On the other hand, the anatomic DB reconstruction was significantly better concerning the knee stability under a 90-N anterior force and a 5-Nm internal torque than the conventional SB reconstruction not only in a range between 0 and 30° but also in the range between 35 and 70°. In addition, the anatomic DB reconstruction was significantly better under the simulated pivot shift test than the conventional SB reconstruction in a range between 0 and 30°. These results showed that although both the anatomic SB and DB reconstructions were significantly better than conventional SB reconstruction, the effect of the anatomic SB reconstruction on the knee stability is not completely identical to the effect of the anatomic DB reconstruction. Namely, a significant effect of anatomic DB reconstruction on the knee laxity can be found in a wider range of knee flexion under each loading condition in comparison with the anatomic SB reconstruction. From the clinical viewpoint, the authors can say that the anatomic DB reconstruction is biomechanically superior to the anatomic SB reconstruction.

The biomechanical reason of the difference between the effects of the two anatomic reconstructions is speculated. Yamamoto et al. [22] reported that the effect of "laterally placed" SB reconstruction, in which the femoral tunnel was created at the center of the PL bundle attachment on the femur, on the knee stability was not significant in a range of knee flexion, but significant only in a range near full extension. In the anatomic SB reconstruction, the femoral tunnel was created at the center between the AM and PL bundle attachments. The distance between the two femoral tunnels created in these two reconstructions was only several millimeters. Therefore, the bundle created in anatomic SB reconstruction is considered to become slack in a range of knee flexion, although the degree of the slackness may be less than the bundle created in the "laterally placed" SB reconstruction. The complex function of the ACL results from integration of the AM and PL bundle functions. Therefore, it is considered that there is a limit in reconstructing the ACL with one bundle. Thus, this study showed that, biomechanically, the anatomic DB procedure can reconstruct the ACL function closer to the normal one than the anatomic SB procedure, at least, immediately after surgery. In the anatomic DB reconstruction, anterior tibial translations were slightly over constrained immediately after surgery. However, after ACL reconstruction, stress relaxation occurs immediately after surgery even after rigorous preconditioning [23]. This should be taken into account, independent of the type of fixation device [24, 25]. Preliminary in vivo data [9, 10, 29–31] suggest that anatomic DB reconstruction can restore normal knee kinematics, but further studies including research on anatomic SB reconstruction are required before definitive conclusions can be reached.

9.3 Can the Clinically Available Transtibial Anatomic DB Procedure Really Obtain Significantly Better Knee Stability in Comparison With Conventional SB Reconstruction Procedure?

9.3.1 *Methods*

A different biomechanical study was performed to compare the anatomical DB reconstruction performed with the arthroscopic transtibial procedure, which has been clinically used, with the conventional SB reconstruction procedure using eight fresh-frozen cadaveric knees [11]. These two procedures were reported in the previous clinical study [10]. The same measurement system and loading conditions as the above-described study [16] were used in this experiment. The test regimen was repeated with the knee in three further states: (1) after arthroscopic transection of the ACL, (2) after arthroscopically assisted anatomic DB ACL reconstruction, and (3) after arthroscopically assisted SB ACL reconstruction. The bone tunnels were filled with polyester resin paste.

9.3.2 *Results*

Under a 90-N anterior force, the anterior translation versus flexion curves for SB and DB reconstruction were significantly less than in the ACL-deficient knee ($p < 0.0235$) (Fig. 9.5). Tibial anterior translation with the DB reconstruction was a mean of 3.5 mm less than with the SB reconstruction at 20° of knee flexion, and

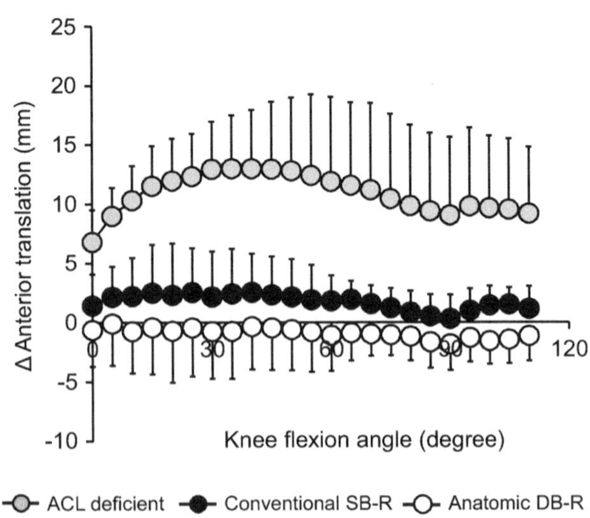

Fig. 9.5 The difference in anterior translation from the intact knee (which is the zero-datum axis) under 90-N anterior load for the intact, ACL-deficient, and ACL-reconstructed knee (mean +/− standard deviation). *ACL* anterior cruciate ligament, *R* reconstruction (From Ref. [11]. Reprinted by permission of SAGE Publications. 2010 American Orthopaedic Society for Sports Medicine)

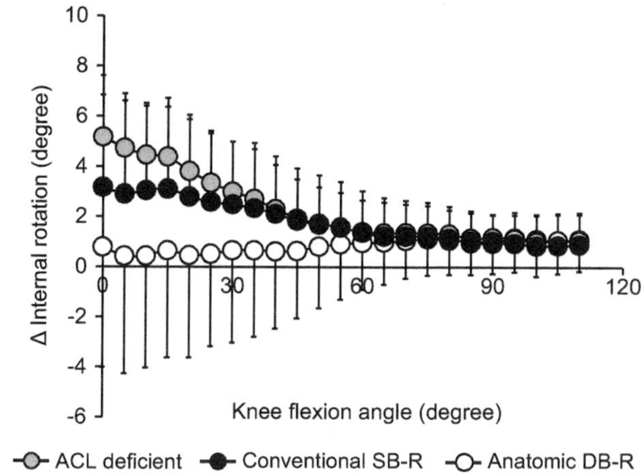

Fig. 9.6 The difference from the intact knee in tibial internal rotation under 5-Nm internal rotation torque for the ACL-deficient and ACL-reconstructed knee (mean +/− standard deviation). *ACL* anterior cruciate ligament, *R* reconstruction (From Ref. [11]. Reprinted by permission of SAGE Publications. 2010 American Orthopaedic Society for Sports Medicine)

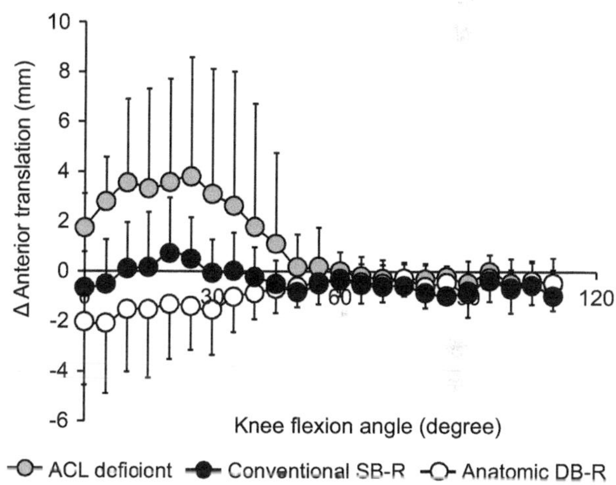

Fig. 9.7 The difference in the tibial anterior translation from the intact knee during the pivot shift for the ACL-deficient and ACL-reconstructed knee (mean +/− standard deviation). *ACL* anterior cruciate ligament, *R* reconstruction (From Ref. [11]. Reprinted by permission of SAGE Publications. 2010 American Orthopaedic Society for Sports Medicine)

post hoc testing found that this difference was significant at all flexion angles from 0 to 75° ($p < 0.0119$). Under 5-Nm internal torque (Fig. 9.6), the tibial rotation with the DB reconstruction was a mean of 2.5° less than that with the SB reconstruction near knee extension. Post hoc testing showed that this was significantly less from 0 to 45° of knee flexion ($p < 0.0347$). Significant differences were not found between the ACL-deficient knee and the SB reconstruction. Under the simulated pivot shift test (Fig. 9.7), the anterior translation versus flexion curves were significantly different among the ACL-deficient knee and the SB and DB reconstructions ($p < 0.0001$). The anterior translation with the DB reconstruction was significantly less than with the SB reconstruction ($p = 0.0006$); the post hoc tests found significant differences ($p < 0.0387$) at 20 and 25° of knee flexion, where the mean difference in the anterior shift was 2 mm. Thus, this study showed that anterior laxity under anterior tibial load, rotational laxity under internal tibial torque, and anterior laxity under pivot shift loading were significantly less after the anatomic DB reconstruction performed with the arthroscopic transtibial procedure, which has been clinically used, than after the conventional SB reconstruction.

9.3.3 Discussion

The second study question was whether the clinically available transtibial procedure for anatomic DB reconstruction can really obtain significantly better knee stability in comparison with the conventional SB reconstruction procedure. The anterior translation laxity in response to a 90-N anterior drawer force was significantly less after the anatomic DB reconstruction than after the SB reconstruction from 0 to 75° of knee flexion. Previous biomechanical studies have shown that the PL bundle of the intact ACL carries one-half to two-thirds of the total force in the ACL near full extension of the knee, when the knee is subjected to an anterior tibial load [8, 26, 27]. As the conventional SB reconstruction reproduces only the AM bundle, loss of the function of the natural PL bundle is considered to result in the insufficient function in the conventional SB reconstruction in the range between 0 and 75° of knee flexion. On the other hand, Yamamoto et al. [22] and Yasuda et al. [28] reported that the reconstructed PL bundle cannot restrain anterior tibial translation at flexion angles of the knee. This fact explains the similarity concerning the knee laxity between the two reconstructions: namely, only the reconstructed AM bundle stabilizes the knee near flexion position in response to anterior tibial load.

For tibial internal rotation torque, the anatomic DB reconstruction restored the tibial rotation of the ACL to the level of the intact knee, whereas the conventional SB reconstruction did not. Yasuda et al. [28] measured the AM and PL graft tensions intraoperatively and found that tension of the PL graft was increased significantly by internal rotation at 15 and 30° of knee flexion. On the other hand, a graft placed in the conventional SB reconstruction was more vertical than the two bundles placed in the anatomic DB reconstruction, so it could not effectively the knee near extension in response to 5-Nm internal rotation torque.

In the pivot shift loading, the conventional SB reconstruction allowed a "mini-pivot" to persist. In previous biomechanical and clinical studies [18, 19], it was reported that SB ACL reconstruction frequently leaves a residual mini-pivot. Woo et al. [1] reported that the SB reconstruction using the hamstring tendon graft or the bone-patella tendon-bone graft cannot completely restore the normal anterior laxity and that it is not effective for rotatory instability. In addition, kinematic studies [3, 4] demonstrated that SB reconstruction with the bone-patella tendon-bone or hamstring tendon graft did not have a significant effect on the rotatory instability during walking or more active activities. This study supported the evidence that the rotatory instability may persist after conventional SB reconstruction. Recent clinical studies [29–31] have reported that 32–49 % of the patients had a positive pivot shift, grade 1 or 2, at a few years after SB ACL reconstruction. These studies implied that clinical results for the pivot shift test after common SB reconstruction procedures may be worse than the previously expected result.

9.4 Clinical Relevance of These Studies

These biomechanical results cannot directly refer to selection of ACL reconstruction procedure in the clinical field, because the selection is decided from various clinical viewpoints, including not only biomechanical superiority but also surgeon's skill, frequency of postoperative graft failure, cost of the surgery, and so on. However, one of the final goals of ACL reconstruction is the complete restoration of normal knee stability in all patients. The authors believe that the biomechanical superiority in knee stability may affect the long-term clinical results concerning postoperative meniscus damage and/or osteoarthritic changes, resulting in possible superiority in future subjective and functional evaluations. To pursue the complete restoration of normal knee stability in the long-term clinical results, it is essential to select the procedure in which the biomechanical function of the reconstructed ACL is the closest to that of the normal ACL at the time of surgery. Therefore, the authors believe that the anatomic DB reconstruction is the most effective procedure to pursue the final goal of ACL reconstruction. However, surgeons should have sufficient skill to successfully perform the anatomic double-bundle reconstruction.

References

1. Woo SL, Kanamori A, Zeminski J, Yagi M, Papageorgiou C, Fu FH (2002) The effectiveness of reconstruction of the anterior cruciate ligament with hamstrings and patellar tendon: a cadaveric study comparing anterior tibial and rotational loads. J Bone Joint Surg Am 84:907–914
2. Lee MC, Seong SC, Lee S et al (2007) Vertical femoral tunnel placement results in rotational knee laxity after anterior cruciate ligament reconstruction. Arthroscopy 23:771–778
3. Georgoulis AD, Ristanis S, Chouliaras V, Moraiti C, Stergiou N (2007) Tibial rotation is not restored after ACL reconstruction with a hamstring graft. Clin Orthop Relat Res 454:89–94
4. Tashman S, Kolowich P, Collon D, Anderson K, Anderst W (2007) Dynamic function of the ACL-reconstructed knee during running. Clin Orthop Relat Res 454:66–73
5. Bach JM, Hull ML, Patterson HA (1997) Direct measurement of strain in the posterolateral bundle of the anterior cruciate ligament. J Biomech 30:281–283
6. Gabriel MT, Wong EK, Woo SL, Yagi M, Debski RE (2004) Distribution of in situ forces in the anterior cruciate ligament in response to rotatory loads. J Orthop Res 22:85–89
7. Kurosawa H, Yamakoshi K, Yasuda K, Sasaki T (1991) Simultaneous measurement of changes in length of the cruciate ligaments during knee motion. Clin Orthop Relat Res 256:233–240
8. Sakane M, Fox RJ, Woo SL, Livesay GA, Li G, Fu FH (1997) In situ forces in the anterior cruciate ligament and its bundles in response to anterior tibial loads. J Orthop Res 15:285–293

9. Yasuda K, Kondo E, Ichiyama H et al (2004) Anatomic reconstruction of the anteromedial and posterolateral bundles of the anterior cruciate ligament using hamstring tendon grafts. Arthroscopy 20:1015–1025
10. Yasuda K, Kondo E, Ichiyama H, Tanabe Y, Tohyama H (2006) Clinical evaluation of anatomic double bundle anterior cruciate ligament reconstruction procedure using hamstring tendon grafts: comparisons among 3 different procedures. Arthroscopy 22:240–251
11. Kondo E, Merican AM, Yasuda K, Amis AA (2010) Biomechanical comparisons of knee stability after anterior cruciate ligament reconstruction between two clinically available transtibial procedures: anatomic double bundle versus single bunde. Am J Sports Med 38:1349–1358
12. Mae T, Shino K, Miyama T et al (2001) Single- versus two-femoral socket anterior cruciate ligament reconstruction technique: biomechanical analysis using a robotic simulator. Arthroscopy 17:708–716
13. Markolf KL, Park S, Jackson SR, McAllister DR (2008) Simulated pivot-shift testing with single and double bundle anterior cruciate ligament reconstructions. J Bone Joint Surg Am 90:1681–1689
14. Ho JY, Gardiner A, Shah V, Steiner ME (2009) Equal kinematics between central anatomic single bundle and double bundle anterior cruciate ligament reconstructions. Arthroscopy 25:464–472
15. Lee JK, Lee S, Seong SC, Lee MC (2014) Anatomic SB ACL reconstruction is possible with use of the modified transtibial technique: a comparison with the anteromedial transportal technique. J Bone Joint Surg Am 96:664–672
16. Kondo E, Merican AM, Yasuda K, Amis AA (2011) Biomechanical comparison of anatomic double-bundle, anatomic single-bundle and non-anatomic single-bundle anterior cruciate ligament reconstructions. Am J Sports Med 39:279–288
17. Cuomo P, Rama KR, Bull AMJ, Amis AA (2007) The effects of different tensioning strategies on knee laxity and graft tension after double 171 bundle anterior cruciate ligament reconstruction. Am J Sports Med 35:2083–2090
18. Bull AMJ, Andersen HN, Basso O, Targett J, Amis AA (1999) Incidence and mechanism of the pivot shift: an in vitro study. Clin Orthop Relat Res 363:219–231
19. Lie DT, Bull AM, Amis AA (2007) Persistence of the mini pivot shift after anatomically placed anterior cruciate ligament reconstruction. Clin Orthop Relat Res 457:203–209
20. Bellier G, Christel P, Colombet P, Djian P, Franceschi JP, Sbihi A (2004) Double-stranded hamstring graft for anterior cruciate ligament reconstruction. Arthroscopy 20:890–894
21. Christel P, Franceschi JP, Sbihi A, Colombet P, Djian P, Bellier G (2005) Anatomic anterior cruciate ligament reconstruction: the French experience. Oper Tech Orthop 15:103–110
22. Yamamoto Y, Hsu WH, Woo SL, Van Scyoc AH, Takakura Y, Debski RE (2004) Knee stability and graft function after anterior cruciate ligament reconstruction: a comparison of a lateral and an anatomical femoral tunnel placement. Am J Sports Med 32:1825–1832
23. Arnold MP, Lie DTT, Verdonschot N, de Graaf R, Amis AA, van Kampen A (2005) The remains of anterior cruciate ligament graft tension after cyclic knee motion. Am J Sports Med 33:536–542
24. Numazaki H, Tohyama H, Nakano H, Kikuchi S, Yasuda K (2002) The effect of initial graft tension in anterior cruciate ligament reconstruction on the mechanical behaviors of the femur-graft-tibia complex during cyclic loading. Am J Sports Med 30:800–805
25. Yamanaka M, Yasuda K, Tohyama H, Nakano H, Wada T (1999) The effect of cyclic displacement upon the biomechanical characteristics of anterior cruciate ligament reconstructions. Am J Sports Med 27:772–777
26. Yagi M, Wong EK, Kanamori A, Debski RE, Fu FH, Woo SL (2002) Biomechanical analysis of an anatomic anterior cruciate ligament reconstruction. Am J Sports Med 30:660–666
27. Zantop T, Herbort M, Raschke MJ, Fu FH, Petersen W (2007) The role of the anteromedial and posterolateral bundles of the anterior cruciate ligament in anterior tibial translation and internal rotation. Am J Sports Med 35:223–227

28. Yasuda K, Ichiyama H, Kondo E, Miyatake S, Inoue M, Tanabe Y (2008) An in vivo biomechanical study on the tension-versus-knee flexion angle curves of two grafts in anatomic double-bundle anterior cruciate ligament reconstruction: effects of initial tension and internal tibial rotation. Arthroscopy 24:276–284
29. Aglietti P, Giron F, Cuomo P, Losco M, Mondanelli N (2007) Single- and double-incision double-bundle ACL reconstruction. Clin Orthop Relat Res 454:108–113
30. Kondo E, Yasuda K, Azuma H, Tanabe Y, Yagi T (2008) Prospective clinical comparisons of anatomic double-bundle versus single-bundle anterior cruciate ligament reconstruction procedures in 328 consecutive patients. Am J Sports Med 36:1675–1687
31. Muneta T, Koga H, Mochizuki T et al (2007) A prospective randomized study of 4-strand semitendinosus tendon anterior cruciate ligament reconstruction comparing single-bundle and double-bundle techniques. Arthroscopy 23:618–628

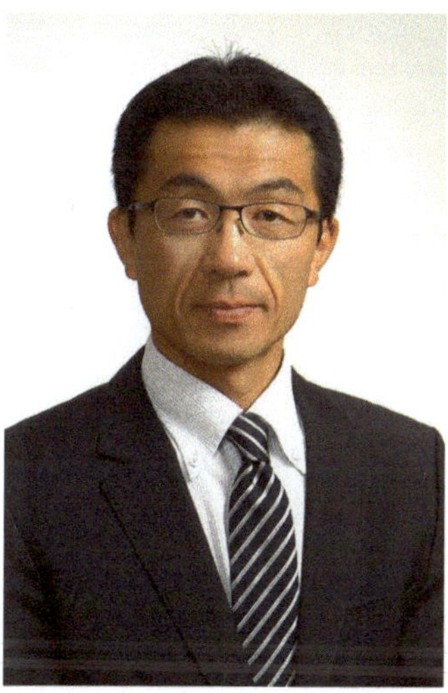

Eiji Kondo, M.D., PhD, Department of Advanced Therapeutic Research for Sports Medicine, Hokkaido University Graduate School of Medicine, Sapporo, Hokkaido, Japan.

Chapter 10
ACL Injury Mechanisms

Hideyuki Koga and Takeshi Muneta

Abstract Model-based image-matching (MBIM) technique has enabled detailed video analysis of injury situations that had been limited to simple visual inspection. We have analyzed anterior cruciate ligament (ACL) injury situations from ten analogs and one HD video sequence using the MBIM technique. The knee kinematical patterns were remarkably consistent, with immediate valgus and internal rotation (IR) motion occurring within 40 ms after initial contact (IC), and then an external rotation was observed. Peak vertical ground reaction force (GRF) occurred at 40 ms after IC. Based on these results, it is likely that the ACL injury occurred approximately 40 ms after IC. 9 mm of abrupt anterior tibial translation at the time of injury was also detected in the HD video. On the other hand, the hip kinematics was constant at abducted, flexed, and IR position during 40 ms after IC. Based on these results together with previous studies, we proposed a new hypothesis for ACL injury mechanisms that valgus loading and lateral compression generate IR motion and anterior translation of tibia, due to the joint geometry, resulting in ACL rupture. Moreover, it seems that the hip is relatively "locked" at IC and cannot absorb energy from GRF and knee is exposed to a larger force, which leads to ACL injury. These results suggest that prevention programs should focus on acquiring a good cutting and landing technique with knee flexion avoiding knee valgus and foot internal rotation and with hip flexion to absorb energy from GRF. Moreover, the fact that the ACL injury occurs 40 ms after IC suggests that "feed-forward" strategies before landing may be critical, as "feedback" strategies are too slow to prevent ACL injuries.

Keywords Anterior cruciate ligament • Video analysis • Injury mechanism

---

H. Koga, M.D., Ph.D. (✉) • T. Muneta
Department of Joint Surgery and Sports Medicine, Graduate School of Medicine, Tokyo Medical and Dental University, 1-5-45 Yushima, Bunkyo-ku, Tokyo 113-8519, Japan
e-mail: koga.orj@tmd.ac.jp

M. Ochi et al. (eds.), *ACL Injury and Its Treatment*,
DOI 10.1007/978-4-431-55858-3_10

10.1 Introduction

Anterior cruciate ligament (ACL) injuries occur mostly during sports activities, and the incidence remains high, especially in young athletes. Recent development of ACL reconstruction procedures has enabled such athletes' return to sports, and favorable clinical results have been achieved; yet it takes a relatively long period for most athletes to get back to sports activities. It has also been reported that ACL reconstruction could not prevent progression of osteoarthritis [1]. Therefore, importance of ACL injury prevention has been emphasized, and various ACL injury prevention programs have been developed successfully [2–6]; however, it is not well understood how the different elements in these multicomponent programs play particular roles in preventing the injury. The most common mechanism of ACL injuries for the sports commonly associated with this injury was noncontact, except men's contact sports, and the noncontact mechanism predominantly occurs during cutting or one-leg landing maneuvers [7–9]. Nevertheless, to develop more targeted injury preventive programs, a more detailed description of the mechanism(s) of noncontact ACL injuries is needed.

10.1.1 Research Approaches to Injury Mechanisms

As mentioned above, it is important to understand the detailed injury mechanisms in order to develop specific prevention methods for ACL injuries. A number of different methodological approaches have been used to investigate ACL injury mechanisms. These include athlete interviews, clinical studies, laboratory motion analysis, video analysis, cadaver studies, and mathematical simulations [10].

10.1.2 Previously Proposed ACL Injury Mechanisms

Noncontact ACL injury mechanisms have been investigated using the abovementioned approaches, and several theories have been proposed; however, it is still a matter of controversy, with the main opponents favoring either sagittal or non-sagittal plane knee joint loading. DeMorat et al. proposed that aggressive quadriceps loading was responsible, based on a cadaver study which demonstrated that aggressive quadriceps loading could take the ACL to failure [11,12]. In contrast, Mclean et al., based on a mathematical simulation model, argued that sagittal plane loading alone could not produce such injuries [13,14]. A prospective cohort study among female athletes, showing that increased dynamic valgus and high valgus loads increased injury risk, leads Hewett et al. to suggest valgus loading as an important component [15,16]. Some video analyses also showed that valgus collapse seemed to be the main mechanism among female athletes [8,9]. However, cadaver studies and mathematical simulation have shown that pure valgus motion would not produce ACL injuries without tearing the medial collateral ligament (MCL) first [17,18].

Nevertheless, other simulation studies have suggested that valgus loading would substantially increase ACL force in situations where an anterior tibial shear force is applied [19]. In the MRI findings, Speer et al. reported that bone bruises of the lateral femoral condyle or posterolateral portion of tibial plateau occurred in more than 80 % of acute ACL noncontact injuries. They concluded that valgus in combination with internal rotation and/or anterior tibial translation occurred at the time of ACL injuries [20]. Furthermore, it has been shown that valgus loading induces a coupled motion of valgus and internal tibial rotation [21,22].

Although both cadaver studies and MRI studies have suggested that internal rotation is present in ACL injury situations, video analyses have suggested that valgus in combination with external rotation is the most frequent motion pattern [9,23].

10.1.3 Development of Model-Based Image-Matching Technique

Among several different approaches to investigate ACL injury mechanisms, video analysis of injury tapes is the only method available to extract kinematic data from actual injury situations. However, video analyses have so far been limited to simple visual inspection [7,9,24], and the accuracy of this method has been shown to be poor, even among experienced researchers [25]. In addition, simple visual inspection is not sufficient to extract a time course for joint angles, velocities, and accelerations; therefore, it is difficult to determine the point of ACL rupture. The analyses are also compromised with poor video qualities.

Therefore, model-based image matching (MBIM) technique has been developed as an alternative to simple visual inspection, in order to extract joint kinematics from video recordings using one or more uncalibrated cameras [26–29]. Detailed procedure of the MBIM technique has been described in the literatures; the idea of this technique is that matching a model to the background video sequences gives an estimate of the actual three-dimensional body kinematics using the commercially available program Poser® and Poser® Pro Pack (Curious Labs Inc., Santa Cruz, California, USA). This technique has been validated in noninjury situations in a laboratory environment. The MBIM technique has shown to be much more accurate than the simple visual inspection approach, and the validation study has shown that root-mean-square (RMS) differences for knee flexion, abduction, and rotation with two or three cameras were less than 10°, 6°, and 11°, respectively [25,26]. Another study also found this technique to be feasible for use in actual ACL injury situations [29]. Therefore, videotapes of noncontact ACL injury situations were analyzed using the MBIM technique to describe detailed kinematics of ACL injuries, in order to identify ACL injury mechanisms.

10.2 Biomechanics in Noncontact ACL Injuries

Ten ACL injury situations from women's team handball (n = 7) and basketball (n = 3), recorded with at least two analog cameras during TV broadcasts, were analyzed using MBIM technique (Fig. 10.1); all of them occurred during game situations [27]. All the players were handling the ball in the injury situation; seven were in possession of the ball at the time of injury, two had shot, and one had passed the ball. In six cases, there was player-to-player contact with an opponent at the time of injury, all of them to the torso being pushed or held. There was no direct contact to the knee. The injury situations could be classified into two groups; seven cases occurred when cutting and three during one-leg landings.

The knee kinematical patterns were remarkably constant among the ten cases (Fig. 10.2). The knee was relatively straight, with a flexion angle of 23° (range,

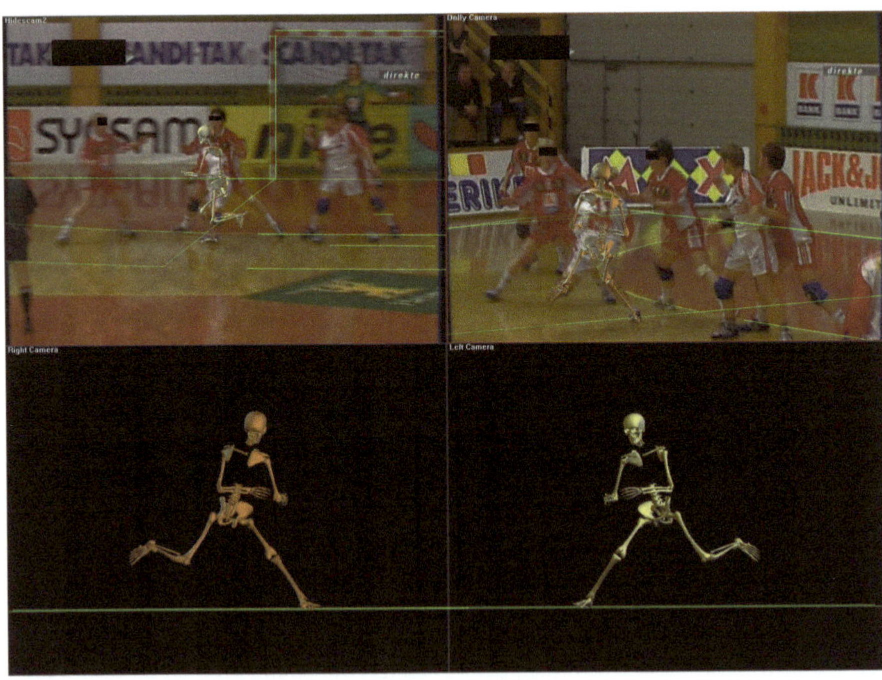

Fig. 10.1 An example of a video matched in Poser, two-camera handball injury situation 40 ms after initial contact (IC). The two *top panels* show the customized skeleton model and the handball court model superimposed on and matched with the background video image from two cameras with different angles. The two *bottom panels* show the skeleton model from back and side views created in Poser

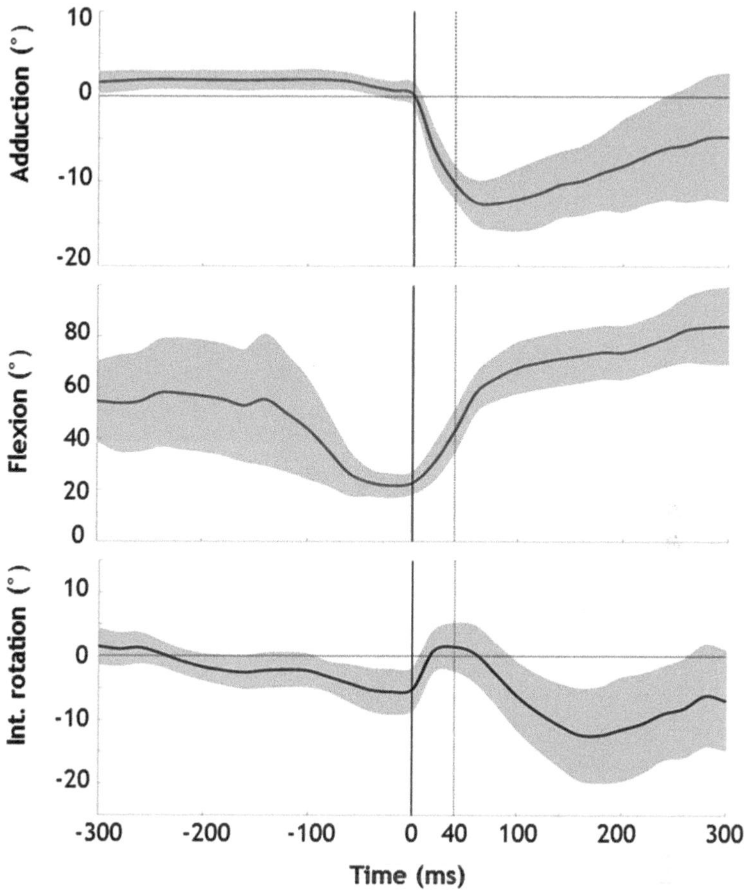

Fig. 10.2 Time sequences of the mean knee angles (°) (*black line*) of the ten cases with 95 % confidence intervals (CI) (*gray area*). Time 0 indicates IC and the *dotted vertical line* indicates the time point 40 ms after IC

11–30°) at initial contact (IC) and had increased by 24° (95 % CI, 19–29°, $p < 0.001$) 40 ms later. The knee abduction angle was neutral, 0° (range, −2–3°) at IC, but had increased by 12° (95 % CI, 10–13°, $p < 0.001$) 40 ms later. As for knee rotation angle, the knee was externally rotated 5° (range, −5–12°) at IC, but abruptly rotated internally by 8° (95 % CI, 2–14°, $p = 0.037$) during the first 40 ms. From 40 ms to 300 ms after IC, however, we observed an external rotation of 17° (95 % CI, 13–22°, $p < 0.001$). In addition, the estimated peak vertical ground reaction force (GRF) was 3.2 times body weight (95 % CI, 2.7–3.7) and occurred at 40 ms (range, 0–83) after IC. On the other hand, the hip kinematics was constant at 20° abducted, 50° flexed, and 30° IR position during 40 ms after IC (Fig. 10.3).

However, limitations of the abovementioned analysis were how accurate the joint kinematics and timing of peak GRF could be estimated from the relatively low

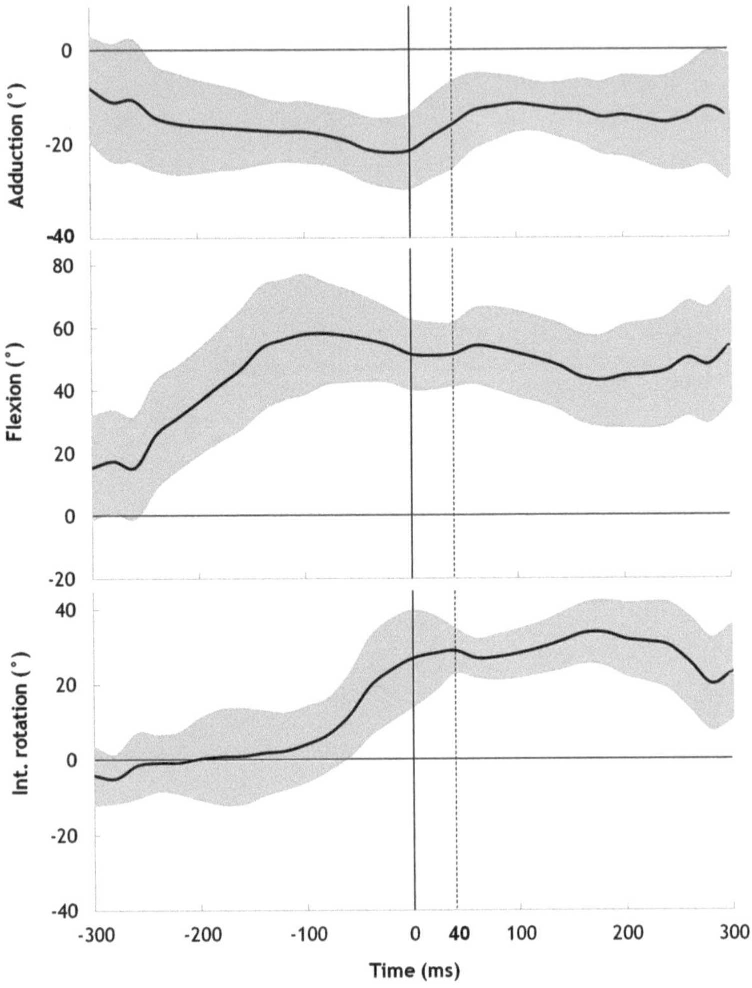

Fig. 10.3 Time sequences of the mean hip angles (°) (*black line*) of the ten cases with 95 % CI (*gray area*). Time 0 indicates IC and the *dotted vertical line* indicates the time point 40 ms after IC

frame rate (50 or 60 Hz) and low-quality images (768 × 576 pixels) in analog video sequences, and therefore we were unable to assess the anterior translation of the tibia. However, a noncontact ACL injury situation in a male footballer was available which had been recorded using four high-definition (HD) cameras including two high-speed recordings (100 and 300 Hz) [28]. In this case, the 26-year-old male elite football player suffered a noncontact ACL injury to his right knee during a national team match, when he tried to stop after having passed the ball with his right leg. This case was analyzed using the MBIM technique to describe the more detailed joint kinematics, including tibial translations (Fig. 10.4). Knee kinematics in this case was strikingly consistent with the previous analyses of the ten cases

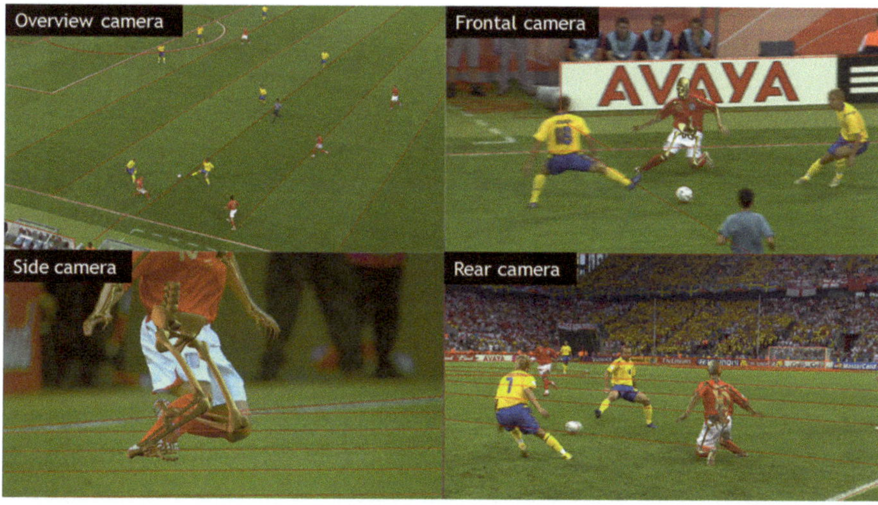

Fig. 10.4 A soccer injury situation recorded using HD cameras. Each panel shows the customized skeleton model and the football pitch model superimposed on and matched with the background video image from each camera. *Overview camera* and *rear camera* had an effective frame rate after being deinterlaced of 50 Hz, *frontal camera* 100 Hz, and *side camera* 300 Hz

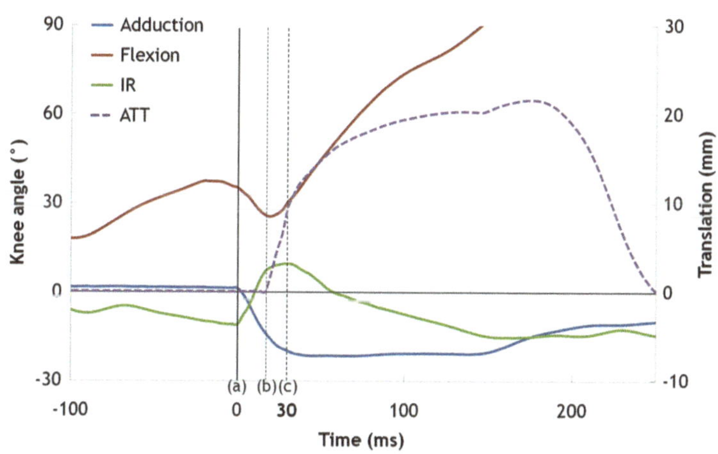

Fig. 10.5 Time sequences of knee joint angles (*left axis*) and anterior tibial translation (*right axis*) in the soccer case. Time 0 (*a*) indicates IC and the dotted vertical lines (*b*) and (*c*) indicate the time point 20 and 30 ms after IC, respectively

(Fig. 10.5). The knee was flexed 35° at IC, with initial extension (26° of flexion) until 20 ms after IC, after which flexion angle continued to increase. The knee abduction angle was neutral at IC, but had increased by 21° 30 ms later. The knee was externally rotated 11° at IC, but abruptly rotated internally by 21° during the first 30 ms, and then changed its direction to external rotation after this. In addition, anterior tibial translation was able to be detected; it started to occur at 20 ms after IC, where the knee was the most extended, and by 30 ms after IC approximately 9 mm of anterior translation had occurred. The translations plateaued by 150 ms and then shifted back to a reduced position between 200 ms and 240 ms after IC.

10.3 Timing of Noncontact ACL Injuries

It has not been possible to determine the exact timing of ACL injury from video analysis based on simple visual inspection [7–9]. However, this may be possible by using the MBIM technique, by assessing abnormal joint configurations, sudden changes in joint angular motion, and timing of GRFs. The extracted knee kinematics during ACL injuries using MBIM technique showed that sudden increase of valgus and internal rotation angle occurred within the first 40 ms after IC. These periods also correspond to the average peak vertical GRF in these cases. Moreover, in the case recorded using HD cameras, abrupt anterior tibial translation reached 9 mm in 30 ms after IC, which corresponds to the maximum anterior translation in intact knees [30,31]. Based on these results, together with the previous studies showing that the ACL was strained shortly (approximately 40 ms) after IC in simulated landing [19,32], it seems likely that the injury occurs within 40 ms for the majority of these cases.

10.4 Mechanisms for Noncontact ACL Injury

As already mentioned, valgus collapse in combination with external rotation (i.e., knee in, toe out) has been frequently identified as an ACL injury mechanism in simple visual inspection of injury videotapes. However, it has been discussed as to whether this kinematics actually represents the cause for ACL injuries or simply is a result of the ACL being torn [9,23]. Our results using the MBIM technique showed that immediate valgus motion occurred within 40 ms after IC. The abrupt internal rotation also occurred during the first 40 ms after IC, and then external rotation was observed, which seems to have occurred after the ACL was torn. In addition, anterior tibial translation started a little later after IC and increased abruptly until when the injury might have occurred. The discrepancy between the previous studies and our results could be that the abrupt internal rotation and anterior tibial translation observed using the MBIM technique analysis are likely not easily detected from visual inspection alone; the external rotation that occurs afterwards is more pronounced and therefore easier to observe. The internal-to-external rotation sequence with anterior tibial translation has also been reported previously. In a recent cadaver study, the application of pure compressive loads led to anterior tibial translation and internal tibial rotation of up to 8°, followed by a sudden external rotation of 12°[31]. The combination of internal tibial rotation and anterior tibial

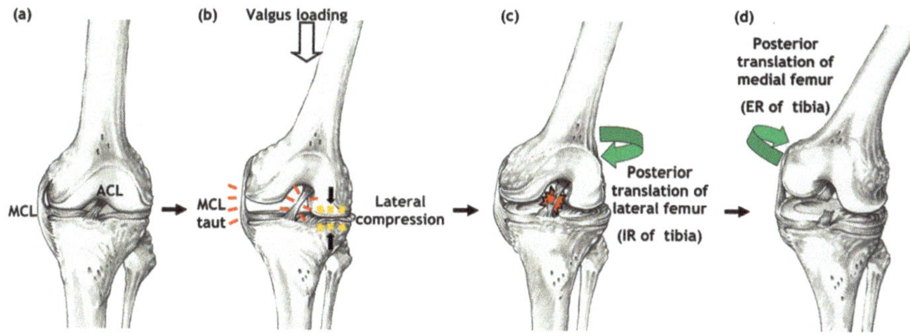

Fig. 10.6 The proposed noncontact ACL injury mechanism. (**a**) An unloaded knee. (**b**) When valgus loading is applied, the MCL becomes taut and lateral compression occurs. (**c**) This compressive load causes a lateral femoral posterior displacement, probably due to the posterior slope of lateral tibial plateau, and the tibia translates anteriorly and rotates internally, resulting in ACL rupture. (**d**) After the ACL is torn, the primary restraint to anterior translation of the tibia is gone. This causes the medial femoral condyle to also be displaced posteriorly, resulting in external rotation of the tibia

translation is probably caused by the joint surface geometry. The concave geometry of the medial tibia facet combined with the slightly convex lateral tibia facet may cause the lateral femoral condyle to slip back. This may also explain why ACL-injured patients tend to have greater posterior lateral tibial plateau slopes than uninjured controls [33–35].

Combining the results obtained using the MBIM technique with previous findings, the following hypothesis for the mechanism of noncontact ACL injury is proposed (Fig. 10.6): (1) when valgus loading is applied, the MCL becomes taut and lateral compression occurs. (2) This compressive load causes a lateral femoral posterior displacement, probably due to the posterior slope of lateral tibial plateau, and the tibia translates anteriorly and rotates internally, resulting in ACL rupture. (3) After the ACL is torn, the primary restraint to anterior translation of the tibia is gone. This causes the medial femoral condyle to also be displaced posteriorly, resulting in external rotation of the tibia. This external rotation may be exacerbated by the typical movement pattern when athletes plant and cut, where the foot typically rotates externally relative to the trunk.

10.5 Hip's Role in ACL Injury Mechanisms

Lower extremities act as a kinetic chain during dynamic tasks and the control of hip motion largely affects the knee motion. Researchers have studied the relationships between hip biomechanics and ACL injury. In terms of risk factor of ACL injury in hip biomechanics, Decker et al. [36] reported that, in drop landing, energy absorption at hip joint and hip flexion angle at IC were less in females than in males. Schmitz et al. [37] reported that, in single-leg landing, energy absorption at hip and total hip flexion displacement were smaller in female, whereas peak vertical GRF was larger in female. Yu et al. [38] also reported that hip flexion angular velocity at IC was negatively correlated with peak vertical GRF in stop-jump task. When it comes to ACL injury mechanisms, Heshemi et al. [39] reported that, in a cadaver study, a restricted flexion of the hip at 20° combined with low quadriceps and hamstring force levels in simulated single-leg landing were found to be conductive to ACL injury. A video analysis has shown that ACL-injured subjects' hip flexion and abduction angle was constant during 100 ms after IC, whereas uninjured control subjects' hip flexion increased by 15° in cutting/landing maneuvers [40]. Our study using MBIM technique also showed that hip kinematics was constant during 40 ms after IC at abducted, flexed, and internally rotated position, which seems to play a significant role in the mechanism of ACL injury. In this regard, Hashemi et al. [41] have proposed a mechanism called "hip extension, knee flexion paradox," i.e., mismatch between hip and knee flexion in landing is the cause of ACL injury. In normal condition, both the knee and hip flex together in landing, whereas in unbalanced landing, the knee is forced to flex but hip is forced to extend, and tibia will undergo anterior translation, which will increase the risk of ACL injury.

There are some possible causes of hip/knee mismatch: (1) in sagittal plane, upright or backward-leaning trunk position at IC makes center of mass posterior to the knee, and increased GRF may encourage more knee flexion than hip flexion and relatively act to extend the hip. (2) In the other plane, insufficient hip abductor/external rotator strength or activation would lead to adducted/internally rotated position of the hip, causing knee valgus. (3) Large hip internal rotation at IC seen in our video analysis could also be an explanation; ACL-injured patients could have limited range of motion in internal rotation [42], and hip joint may be locked at a large internally rotated position. As a matter of fact, hip dysplasia has also been reported to be a risk factor of ACL injury [43]. It has also been reported that decreased range of internal femoral rotation results in greater ACL strain [44].

For these reasons, it seems that hip joint is relatively locked at IC and cannot absorb energy from GRF, and knee joint is exposed to larger force, which leads to ACL injury. Therefore, it is important that prevention efforts should focus not only on knee joint but also on hip joint.

10.6 Tips for ACL Injury Prevention Based on the Proposed Mechanisms

Based on the mechanisms clarified using MBIM technique, prevention strategy for ACL injury can be proposed as follows: (1) as the kinematics when ACL injury is happening is knee valgus and internal rotation with the hip being locked, it is important to acquire a good cutting and landing technique with knee flexion avoiding knee valgus and foot internal rotation and with hip flexion to absorb energy from GRF, avoiding hip internal rotation. (2) As ACL injuries occur approximately 40 ms after IC, it is likely that a "feedback" strategy, i.e., ACL prevention program focusing on training after landing, cannot prevent ACL injury; it takes at least 150–200 ms to react after landing at risk. Prevention efforts should focus on a "feed-forward" strategy before landing, i.e., training muscular pre-activation and neural control during the pre-landing phase.

References

1. Oiestad BE, Engebretsen L, Storheim K, Risberg MA (2009) Knee osteoarthritis after anterior cruciate ligament injury: a systematic review. Am J Sports Med 37(7):1434–1443
2. Caraffa A, Cerulli G, Projetti M, Aisa G, Rizzo A (1996) Prevention of anterior cruciate ligament injuries in soccer. A prospective controlled study of proprioceptive training. Knee Surg Sports Traumatol Arthrosc 4(1):19–21
3. Gilchrist J, Mandelbaum BR, Melancon H, Ryan GW, Silvers HJ, Griffin LY, Watanabe DS, Dick RW, Dvorak J (2008) A randomized controlled trial to prevent noncontact anterior cruciate ligament injury in female collegiate soccer players. Am J Sports Med 36 (8):1476–1483
4. Mandelbaum BR, Silvers HJ, Watanabe DS, Knarr JF, Thomas SD, Griffin LY, Kirkendall DT, Garrett W Jr (2005) Effectiveness of a neuromuscular and proprioceptive training program in preventing anterior cruciate ligament injuries in female athletes: 2-year follow-up. Am J Sports Med 33(7):1003–1010
5. Myklebust G, Engebretsen L, Braekken IH, Skjolberg A, Olsen OE, Bahr R (2003) Prevention of anterior cruciate ligament injuries in female team handball players: a prospective intervention study over three seasons. Clin J Sport Med 13(2):71–78
6. Olsen OE, Myklebust G, Engebretsen L, Holme I, Bahr R (2005) Exercises to prevent lower limb injuries in youth sports: cluster randomised controlled trial. BMJ 330(7489):449
7. Boden BP, Dean GS, Feagin JA Jr, Garrett WE Jr (2000) Mechanisms of anterior cruciate ligament injury. Orthopedics 23(6):573–578
8. Krosshaug T, Nakamae A, Boden BP, Engebretsen L, Smith G, Slauterbeck JR, Hewett TE, Bahr R (2007) Mechanisms of anterior cruciate ligament injury in basketball: video analysis of 39 cases. Am J Sports Med 35(3):359–367
9. Olsen OE, Myklebust G, Engebretsen L, Bahr R (2004) Injury mechanisms for anterior cruciate ligament injuries in team handball: a systematic video analysis. Am J Sports Med 32(4):1002–1012
10. Krosshaug T, Andersen TE, Olsen OE, Myklebust G, Bahr R (2005) Research approaches to describe the mechanisms of injuries in sport: limitations and possibilities. Br J Sports Med 39 (6):330–339
11. DeMorat G, Weinhold P, Blackburn T, Chudik S, Garrett W (2004) Aggressive quadriceps loading can induce noncontact anterior cruciate ligament injury. Am J Sports Med 32 (2):477–483
12. Yu B, Garrett WE (2007) Mechanisms of non-contact ACL injuries. Br J Sports Med 41(Suppl 1):i47–i51
13. McLean SG, Andrish JT, van den Bogert AJ (2005) Aggressive quadriceps loading can induce noncontact anterior cruciate ligament injury. Am J Sports Med 33(7):1106; author reply 1106–1107
14. McLean SG, Huang X, Su A, Van Den Bogert AJ (2004) Sagittal plane biomechanics cannot injure the ACL during sidestep cutting. Clin Biomech (Bristol, Avon) 19(8):828–838
15. Hewett TE, Myer GD, Ford KR, Heidt RS Jr, Colosimo AJ, McLean SG, van den Bogert AJ, Paterno MV, Succop P (2005) Biomechanical measures of neuromuscular control and valgus

loading of the knee predict anterior cruciate ligament injury risk in female athletes: a prospective study. Am J Sports Med 33(4):492–501
16. Quatman CE, Hewett TE (2009) The anterior cruciate ligament injury controversy: is "valgus collapse" a sex-specific mechanism? Br J Sports Med 43(5):328–335
17. Mazzocca AD, Nissen CW, Geary M, Adams DJ (2003) Valgus medial collateral ligament rupture causes concomitant loading and damage of the anterior cruciate ligament. J Knee Surg 16(3):148–151
18. Shin CS, Chaudhari AM, Andriacchi TP (2009) The effect of isolated valgus moments on ACL strain during single-leg landing: a simulation study. J Biomech 42(3):280–285
19. Withrow TJ, Huston LJ, Wojtys EM, Ashton-Miller JA (2006) The effect of an impulsive knee valgus moment on in vitro relative ACL strain during a simulated jump landing. Clin Biomech (Bristol, Avon) 21(9):977–983
20. Speer KP, Spritzer CE, Bassett FH 3rd, Feagin JA Jr, Garrett WE Jr (1992) Osseous injury associated with acute tears of the anterior cruciate ligament. Am J Sports Med 20(4):382–389
21. Matsumoto H (1990) Mechanism of the pivot shift. J Bone Joint Surg (Br) 72(5):816–821
22. Matsumoto H, Suda Y, Otani T, Niki Y, Seedhom BB, Fujikawa K (2001) Roles of the anterior cruciate ligament and the medial collateral ligament in preventing valgus instability. J Orthop Sci 6(1):28–32
23. Ebstrup JF, Bojsen-Moller F (2000) Anterior cruciate ligament injury in indoor ball games. Scand J Med Sci Sports 10(2):114–116
24. Cochrane JL, Lloyd DG, Buttfield A, Seward H, McGivern J (2007) Characteristics of anterior cruciate ligament injuries in Australian football. J Sci Med Sport 10(2):96–104
25. Krosshaug T, Nakamae A, Boden B, Engebretsen L, Smith G, Slauterbeck J, Hewett TE, Bahr R (2007) Estimating 3D joint kinematics from video sequences of running and cutting maneuvers–assessing the accuracy of simple visual inspection. Gait Posture 26(3):378–385
26. Krosshaug T, Bahr R (2005) A model-based image-matching technique for three-dimensional reconstruction of human motion from uncalibrated video sequences. J Biomech 38(4):919–929
27. Koga H, Nakamae A, Shima Y, Iwasa J, Myklebust G, Engebretsen L, Bahr R, Krosshaug T (2010) Mechanisms for noncontact anterior cruciate ligament injuries: knee joint kinematics in 10 injury situations from female team handball and basketball. Am J Sports Med 38 (11):2218–2225
28. Koga H, Bahr R, Myklebust G, Engebretsen L, Grund T, Krosshaug T (2011) Estimating anterior tibial translation from model-based image-matching of a noncontact anterior cruciate ligament injury in professional football: a case report. Clin J Sport Med 21(3):271–274
29. Krosshaug T, Slauterbeck JR, Engebretsen L, Bahr R (2007) Biomechanical analysis of anterior cruciate ligament injury mechanisms: three-dimensional motion reconstruction from video sequences. Scand J Med Sci Sports 17(5):508–519
30. Jakob RP, Staubli HU, Deland JT (1987) Grading the pivot shift. Objective tests with implications for treatment. J Bone Joint Surg (Br) 69(2):294–299
31. Meyer EG, Haut RC (2008) Anterior cruciate ligament injury induced by internal tibial torsion or tibiofemoral compression. J Biomech 41(16):3377–3383
32. Shin CS, Chaudhari AM, Andriacchi TP (2007) The influence of deceleration forces on ACL strain during single-leg landing: a simulation study. J Biomech 40(5):1145–1152
33. Brandon ML, Haynes PT, Bonamo JR, Flynn MI, Barrett GR, Sherman MF (2006) The association between posterior-inferior tibial slope and anterior cruciate ligament insufficiency. Arthroscopy 22(8):894–899
34. Stijak L, Herzog RF, Schai P (2008) Is there an influence of the tibial slope of the lateral condyle on the ACL lesion? A case-control study. Knee Surg Sports Traumatol Arthrosc 16 (2):112–117
35. Hashemi J, Chandrashekar N, Mansouri H, Gill B, Slauterbeck JR, Schutt RC Jr, Dabezies E, Beynnon BD (2010) Shallow medial tibial plateau and steep medial and lateral tibial slopes: new risk factors for anterior cruciate ligament injuries. Am J Sports Med 38(1):54–62

36. Decker MJ, Torry MR, Wyland DJ, Sterett WI, Richard Steadman J (2003) Gender differences in lower extremity kinematics, kinetics and energy absorption during landing. Clin Biomech (Bristol, Avon) 18(7):662–669
37. Schmitz RJ, Kulas AS, Perrin DH, Riemann BL, Shultz SJ (2007) Sex differences in lower extremity biomechanics during single leg landings. Clin Biomech (Bristol, Avon) 22 (6):681–688
38. Yu B, Lin CF, Garrett WE (2006) Lower extremity biomechanics during the landing of a stop-jump task. Clin Biomech (Bristol, Avon) 21(3):297–305
39. Hashemi J, Chandrashekar N, Jang T, Karpat F, Oseto M, Ekwaro-Osire S (2007) An alternative mechanism of non-contact anterior cruciate ligament injury during jump-landing: in-vitro simulation. Exp Mech 47:347–354
40. Boden BP, Torg JS, Knowles SB, Hewett TE (2009) Video analysis of anterior cruciate ligament injury: abnormalities in hip and ankle kinematics. Am J Sports Med 37(2):252–259
41. Hashemi J, Breighner R, Chandrashekar N, Hardy DM, Chaudhari AM, Shultz SJ, Slauterbeck JR, Beynnon BD (2011) Hip extension, knee flexion paradox: a new mechanism for non-contact ACL injury. J Biomech 44(4):577–585
42. Gomes JL, de Castro JV, Becker R (2008) Decreased hip range of motion and noncontact injuries of the anterior cruciate ligament. Arthroscopy 24(9):1034–1037
43. Yamazaki J, Muneta T, Ju YJ, Morito T, Okuwaki T, Sekiya I (2011) Hip acetabular dysplasia and joint laxity of female anterior cruciate ligament-injured patients. Am J Sports Med 39 (2):410–414
44. Beaulieu ML, Oh YK, Bedi A, Ashton-Miller JA, Wojtys EM (2014) Does limited internal femoral rotation increase peak anterior cruciate ligament strain during a simulated pivot landing? Am J Sports Med 42(12):2955–2963

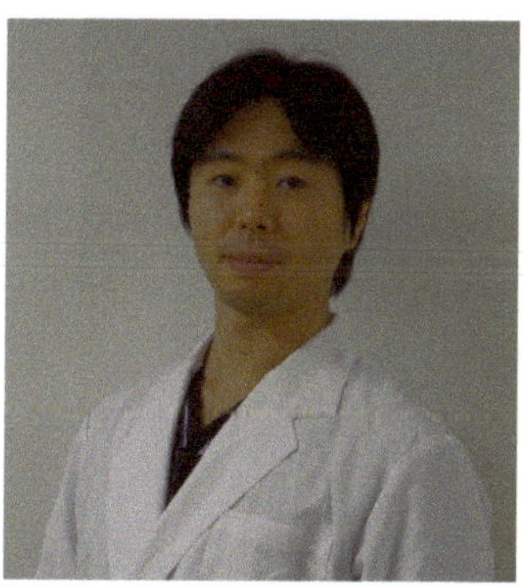

Hideyuki Koga, M.D., Ph.D., Department of Joint Surgery and Sports Medicine, Tokyo Medical and Dental University, Tokyo, Japan.

Part III
Diagnostics of ACL Injury

Chapter 11
Physical Examinations and Device Measurements for ACL Deficiency

Ryosuke Kuroda, Takehiko Matsushita, and Daisuke Araki

Abstract Anterior cruciate ligament (ACL) injury is one of the most common knee traumas, particularly during sport activities. "Giving way" is a subjective symptom of the knee with ACL insufficiency. A number of clinical tests for ACL laxity have been proposed since it was first described by Stark in 1850. To quantitatively evaluate knee laxity, several knee ligament measurement devices have been also developed. The results of the manual tests and quantitative measurement are described in a grading system for further clinical evaluations, most commonly using the IKDC (International Knee Documentation Committee) evaluation form. Recently the importance of pivot-shift test as a detector of a dynamic rotational instability has been reported. In recent years, with new technologies, dynamic three-dimensional knee instability measurement devices also have been developed.

Keywords ACL injury • Diagnosis • Physical examinations • Lachman test • Pivot-shift test

11.1 Introduction

Anterior cruciate ligament (ACL) injury is one of the most common knee traumas and is one cause of anterior knee instability, particularly during sport activities. A number of clinical tests for detecting the laxity of ACL have been proposed [1–5] since Stark first described the manual test for ACL injury in 1850 [6]. For example, to evaluate anterior knee instability, Torg and colleagues [7, 8] advocated the Lachman test. Other methods for assessing rotational knee instability have included the pivot-shift test [9], the jerk test [2], the anterolateral rotatory instability test, the Losee test [3], and the crossover test [1]. Though these tests are useful to detect ACL injuries and to evaluate the laxity, one of the problems in those manual tests is a lack of objectivity. Therefore to quantitatively evaluate knee laxity, several knee ligament measurement devices have been developed. Among these, the KT-1000

R. Kuroda, M.D, Ph.D. (✉) • T. Matsushita • D. Araki
Department of Orthopaedic Surgery, Kobe University Graduate School of Medicine,
7-5-1 Kusunoki-cho, Chuo-ku Kobe, Hyogo 650-0017, Japan
e-mail: kurodar@med.kobe-u.ac.jp

M. Ochi et al. (eds.), *ACL Injury and Its Treatment*,
DOI 10.1007/978-4-431-55858-3_11

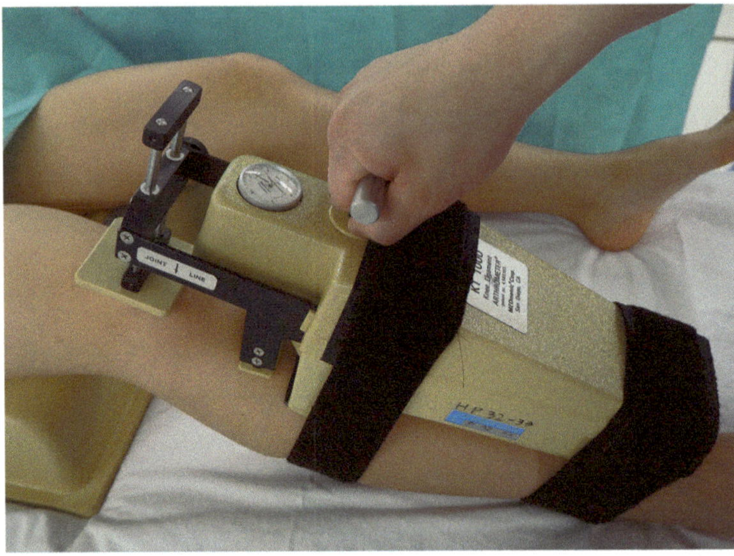

Fig. 11.1 The KT-1000 arthrometer has been widely used for diagnosis and preoperative and postoperative evaluation of ACL-deficient knees, because of its accuracy and reproducibility in the measurements of tibial anterior/posterior translation

arthrometer has been widely used for diagnosis and preoperative and postoperative evaluation of ACL-deficient knees, because of its accuracy and reproducibility in the measurements of tibial anterior/posterior translation (Fig. 11.1) [10, 11]. In recent years, new measurement devices for evaluating dynamic knee instability have been developed.

This section describes the current concepts of physical examinations and device measurements for ACL insufficiency in ACL-injured and ACL-reconstructed knees.

11.2 Lachman Test

To evaluate anterior knee instability accurately, Torg and colleagues [7, 8] advocated the Lachman test that evaluates the greatest difference in anterior/posterior translation of the tibia between injured and intact knees, with the patient's knee joint at 10–25° of knee flexion angle (Fig. 11.2) [12–16]. It has been shown that the Lachman test is highly sensitive for detecting ACL deficiency [12, 17–20], while the anterior drawer sign, which evaluates anterior/posterior tibial translation at 90° of knee flexion, has been reported to be a poor diagnostic indicator of ACL injuries, especially in an acute setting [12]. Ostrowski [15] and Benjaminse et al. [13] suggested that the Lachman test is the most sensitive and the pivot-shift test is the most specific for detecting ACL rupture. Many authors have shown the integrity

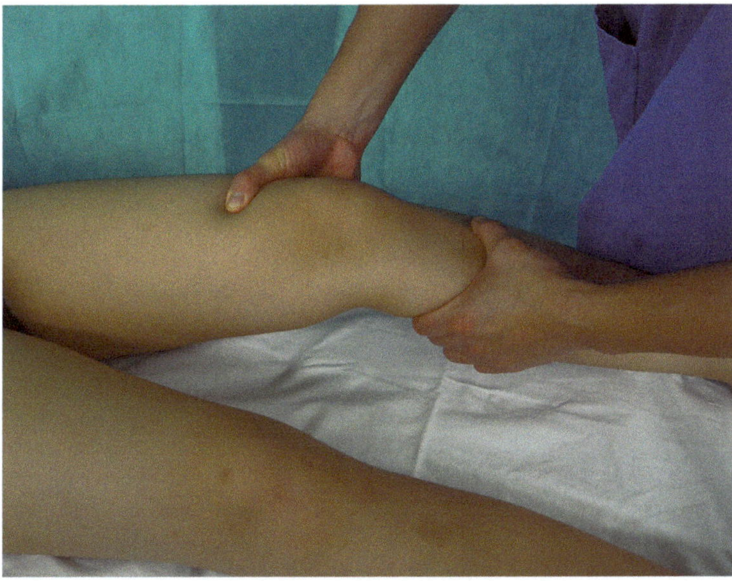

Fig. 11.2 Lachman test that evaluates the difference in anterior/posterior translation of the tibia between injured and intact knees, with the patient's knee joint at 10–25° of knee flexion angle

of the Lachman test for assessing ACL-deficient knees. Although the Lachman test has been used as a simple, reliable, and reproducible method for demonstrating ACL deficiency with clinical grades (Table 11.1) [7], this maneuver is still performed by a subjective nonparametric classification [2]. Kuroda et al. examined the similarities and differences in manual tests for ACL deficiency among international orthopedic surgeons using questionnaires and electromagnetic measurement system (EMS) and found that a relatively similar technique was used for the Lachman test across the world, whereas the actual knee kinematics of the Lachman tests was highly diverse between examiners [21]. Therefore objective assessments of anterior/posterior translation during the Lachman test are still required to accurately evaluate the knee laxity.

11.3 Static Anterior Instability Measurement

Several studies have attempted to objectively evaluate the Lachman test by subjective assessment. Lerat et al. [22] examined the anterior/posterior displacement in 563 normal knees and 487 ACL-deficient knees using stress radiography with an anterior load of 9 kg at 20° knee flexion angle, which mimicked the Lachman test. They used the posterior femoral condyle and posterior tibial plateau as reference points on radiography and measured the anterior/posterior translation in both the medial and lateral compartments. Logan et al. [23] investigated the Lachman test

Table 11.1 Lachman test and its clinical grades

Four grades	Normal	Nearly normal	Abnormal	Severely abnormal
Lachman (25° flex) manual max	−1 to 2 mm	3 to 5 mm	6 to 10 mm	>10 mm
Anterior endpoint	Firm		Soft	

using magnetic resonance imaging (MRI). They showed that the ruptures of the ACL led to anterior tibial translation coupled with tibial internal rotation and suggested that performing the Lachman test with MR scanning would be useful for evaluating ACL-deficient knees. However, it is difficult to perform this test by the use of MRI in daily practice. To quantitatively evaluate knee laxity, several knee ligament measurement devices have been developed including the KT-1000 knee ligament arthrometer (MED metric, San Diego, CA) [10, 24], Genucom knee analysis system (FARO Technologies Inc., Lake Mary, FL) [25], and Rolimeter (Aircast Europe, Neubeuern, Germany) [26, 27]. Daniel et al. [24, 28] developed the KT-1000 arthrometer as a measurement instrument for anterior tibial translation. The KT-1000 measures anterior/posterior tibial displacement by tracking the tibial tubercle in relation to the patella while applying a maximum manual force or a constant force to the tibia. Many studies have supported the utility of the KT-1000 arthrometer showing a relatively high accuracy and reproducibility in the measurement of tibial anterior/posterior laxity [29, 30]. To date, the KT-1000 arthrometer is the most widely used device to diagnose ACL deficiency and to evaluate the pre- and postoperative anterior laxity of the ACL-injured knees.

11.4 Pivot-Shift Test

The pivot-shift phenomenon [9, 31], which consists of a tibial anterior dislocation and a subsequent reduction of lateral compartment of the knee joint, is a dynamic instability [3, 9]. Losee reported the pivot-shift test in which the hip was abducted and the knee was passively flexed from full extension with internal tibial torque, axial load, and valgus stress applied manually to induce the pivot-shift phenomenon (Fig. 11.3) [3]. The pivot-shift test is usually positive in ACL-deficient knees but sometimes positive in ACL-reconstructed knees in which anterior stability has been successfully restored. The pivot-shift test has been reported to be associated with subjective symptoms and knee functions [32]; therefore, this test has been considered as an important test to assess knee stability. The grade of the pivot-shift phenomenon can be graded by the examiner subjectively as none (−), glide (+), clunk (++), or gross (+++) according to the International Knee Documentation Committee (IKDC) form (Table 11.2) [33].

Kuroda et al. examined the similarities and differences in the pivot-shift test among international orthopedic surgeons using questionnaires and reported the

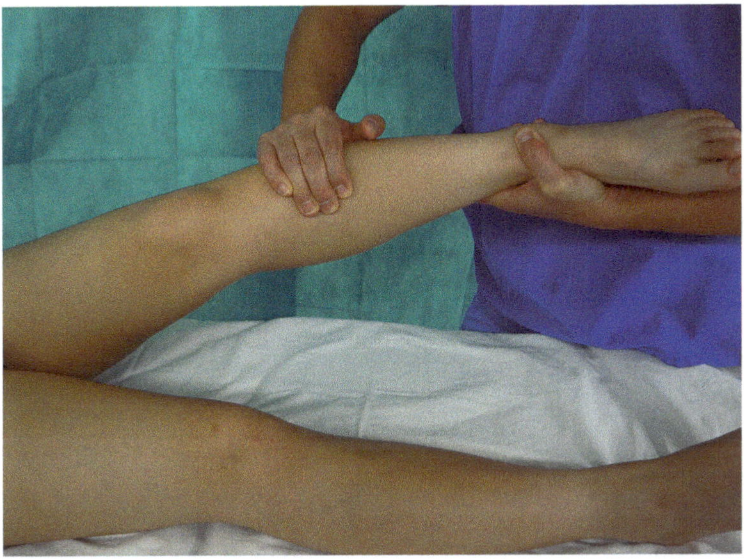

Fig. 11.3 The pivot-shift test: the hip was abducted and the knee was passively flexed from full extension with internal tibial torque, axial load, and valgus stress applied manually to induce the pivot-shift phenomenon

Table 11.2 Pivot-shift test and its clinical grades

Four grades	Normal	Nearly normal	Abnormal	Severely abnormal
Pivot shift	Equal	+ glide	++ clunk	+++ gross

detail of pivot-shift test. As for the pivot-shift test, most of the orthopedic sports surgeons recommend advocating the "flexion from extended position" maneuver, while "extension from flexed position" was still supported by a few doctors. Although valgus stress was applied during the pivot-shift test almost exclusively, there was a mixed opinion as to which, internal or external, rotational stress is applied for the pivot-shift test, while internal rotational stress was more advocated than external rotational stress. In addition, axial loading was commonly employed to examine the pivot shift [21].

11.5 Quantitative Measurement of Dynamic Rotational Instability

It is reported that patients' ability to return to their preinjury activity level after anterior cruciate ligament (ACL) reconstruction is still low [34]. One of the possible reasons is that abnormal knee joint kinematics remain despite anterior knee laxity has been improved by the ACL reconstruction. Indeed abnormal joint kinematics in ACL-reconstructed knees were detected in laboratory settings and reported in many research trials [35–38]. However, these laboratory tests cannot be easily performed in daily clinical practice because of their invasiveness, cost, and space issues.

The pivot-shift test [3, 9] is commonly performed in a clinical setting [33], and it has been reported to be associated with subjective symptoms and knee functions [32]. Therefore, the pivot-shift test could detect abnormal knee kinematics and is a convenient test in the evaluation of results of ACL reconstructions. As mentioned in the previous section, the results of the manual tests are often described in a grading system for further clinical comparisons, most commonly using the IKDC evaluation form [39]. However, the clinical evaluation of the manual tests is subjectively determined by the examiners' hands due to the lack of objective measurement systems resulting in inconsistency across examiners [40].

Some objective measurement systems have been developed and used in research and clinical practice to monitor the three-dimensional (3D) position displacement of the tibial dislocation during the pivot-shift test [40–42]. However, the measurement of the 3D position displacement in those research can be regarded as a static measurement that is assumed to be insufficient to quantify the dynamic instability and to have little relationship to subjective knee functions [32, 43]. Therefore, to quantitatively evaluate dynamic instability such as pivot-shift test in ACL-deficient and ACL-reconstructed knees is crucial for more accurately assessing clinical results after ACL reconstruction.

Several objective measurement parameters have been introduced to monitor the 3D position displacement of the tibia in relation to the femur during the pivot-shift test [40, 42]. It has been suggested that a more dynamic parameter, such as 3D acceleration, should represent the dynamism of the pivot-shift phenomenon and can be more related to the dynamic rotatory knee laxity [21, 44–48]. 3D-kinematic assessments of the pivot-shift phenomenon have been attempted in in vitro studies [42, 49–51] and in intraoperatively using a sensor measurement system [41]. However, those measurement systems cannot be utilized in current clinical setting due to the invasiveness and/or the obstructiveness to the pivot-shift testing maneuver.

Based on the background, noninvasive measurement systems have been developed. Electromagnetic measurement system, noninvasive in vivo measurement system, was developed [44, 48, 52], using an electromagnetic sensors. This system can measure the 6° of freedom of the knee during the pivot-shift test with a high sampling rate (240 Hz). It enables monitoring of 3D position displacement instantaneously and calculates a 3D acceleration of posterior translation (APT) of the tibia and coupled anterior tibial translation (c-ATT) during pivot-shift test. Mushal and Hoshino et al. developed a noninvasive image measurement system using iPad. The abnormal lateral translation during pivot-shift phenomenon in ACL-deficient knees was detected by the iPad application [53]. Lopomo et al. developed an accelerometer system using a commercial triaxial accelerometer [46]. They reported the accelerometer mounted on the patient's tibia could detect 3D acceleration during the pivot-shift test and that the values in the ACL-deficient knees were significantly higher than those in the contralateral healthy limbs. These newly developed noninvasive measurement systems can be useful to measure dynamic knee stability in clinical settings.

References

1. Arnold JA, Coker TP, Heaton LM, Park JP, Harris WD (1979) Natural history of anterior cruciate tears. Am J Sports Med 7:305–313
2. Hughston JC, Andrews JR, Cross MJ, Moschi A (1976) Classification of knee ligament instabilities. Part i. The medial compartment and cruciate ligaments. J Bone Joint Surg Am 58:159–172
3. Losee RE (1983) Concepts of the pivot shift. Clin Orthop Relat Res 172:45–51
4. Noyes FR, Bassett RW, Grood ES, Butler DL (1980) Arthroscopy in acute traumatic hemarthrosis of the knee. Incidence of anterior cruciate tears and other injuries. J Bone Joint Surg Am 62:687–695, 757
5. Slocum DB, James SL, Larson RL, Singer KM (1976) Clinical test for anterolateral rotary instability of the knee. Clin Orthop Relat Res 118:63–69
6. Snook GA (1983) A short history of the anterior cruciate ligament and the treatment of tears. Clin Orthop Relat Res 172:11–13
7. Gurtler RA, Stine R, Torg JS (1990) Lachman test revisited. Contemp Orthop 20:145–154
8. Torg JS, Conrad W, Kalen V (1976) Clinical diagnosis of anterior cruciate ligament instability in the athlete. Am J Sports Med 4:84–93
9. Galway HR, MacIntosh DL (1980) The lateral pivot shift: a symptom and sign of anterior cruciate ligament insufficiency. Clin Orthop Relat Res 147:45–50
10. Daniel DM, Malcom LL, Losse G, Stone ML, Sachs R, Burks R (1985) Instrumented measurement of anterior laxity of the knee. J Bone Joint Surg Am 67:720–726
11. Malcom LL, Daniel DM, Stone ML, Sachs R (1985) The measurement of anterior knee laxity after acl reconstructive surgery. Clin Orthop Relat Res 196:35–41
12. Katz JW, Fingeroth RJ (1986) The diagnostic accuracy of ruptures of the anterior cruciate ligament comparing the lachman test, the anterior drawer sign, and the pivot shift test in acute and chronic knee injuries. Am J Sports Med 14:88–91
13. Benjaminse A, Gokeler A, van der Schans CP (2006) Clinical diagnosis of an anterior cruciate ligament rupture: a meta-analysis. J Orthop Sports Phys Ther 36:267–288
14. Frank C (1986) Accurate interpretation of the lachman test. Clin Orthop Relat Res 213:163–166
15. Ostrowski JA (2006) Accuracy of 3 diagnostic tests for anterior cruciate ligament tears. J Athl Train 41:120–121
16. Scholten RJ, Opstelten W, van der Plas CG, Bijl D, Deville WL, Bouter LM (2003) Accuracy of physical diagnostic tests for assessing ruptures of the anterior cruciate ligament: a meta-analysis. J Fam Pract 52:689–694
17. DeHaven KE (1980) Diagnosis of acute knee injuries with hemarthrosis. Am J Sports Med 8:9–14
18. Jonsson T, Althoff B, Peterson L, Renstrom P (1982) Clinical diagnosis of ruptures of the anterior cruciate ligament: a comparative study of the lachman test and the anterior drawer sign. Am J Sports Med 10:100–102
19. Kim SJ, Kim HK (1995) Reliability of the anterior drawer test, the pivot shift test, and the lachman test. Clin Orthop Relat Res 317:237–242
20. Liu SH, Osti L, Henry M, Bocchi L (1995) The diagnosis of acute complete tears of the anterior cruciate ligament. Comparison of mri, arthrometry and clinical examination. J Bone Joint Surg 77:586–588

21. Kuroda R, Hoshino Y, Kubo S, Araki D, Oka S, Nagamune K, Kurosaka M (2012) Similarities and differences of diagnostic manual tests for anterior cruciate ligament insufficiency: a global survey and kinematics assessment. Am J Sports Med 40:91–99
22. Lerat JL, Moyen BL, Cladiere F, Besse JL, Abidi H (2000) Knee instability after injury to the anterior cruciate ligament. Quantification of the lachman test. J Bone Joint Surg 82:42–47
23. Logan MC, Williams A, Lavelle J, Gedroyc W, Freeman M (2004) What really happens during the lachman test? A dynamic mri analysis of tibiofemoral motion. Am J Sports Med 32:369–375
24. Daniel DM, Stone ML, Sachs R, Malcom L (1985) Instrumented measurement of anterior knee laxity in patients with acute anterior cruciate ligament disruption. Am J Sports Med 13:401–407
25. McQuade KJ, Sidles JA, Larson RV (1989) Reliability of the genucom knee analysis system. A pilot study. Clin Orthop Relat Res 245:216–219
26. Balasch H, Schiller M, Friebel H, Hoffmann F (1999) Evaluation of anterior knee joint instability with the rolimeter. A test in comparison with manual assessment and measuring with the kt-1000 arthrometer. Knee Surg Sports Traumatol Arthrosc 7:204–208
27. Ganko A, Engebretsen L, Ozer H (2000) The rolimeter: a new arthrometer compared with the kt-1000. Knee Surg Sports Traumatol Arthrosc 8:36–39
28. Rangger C, Daniel DM, Stone ML, Kaufman K (1993) Diagnosis of an acl disruption with kt-1000 arthrometer measurements. Knee Surg Sports Traumatol Arthrosc 1:60–66
29. Bach BR Jr, Warren RF, Flynn WM, Kroll M, Wickiewiecz TL (1990) Arthrometric evaluation of knees that have a torn anterior cruciate ligament. J Bone Joint Surg Am 72:1299–1306
30. Staubli HU, Jakob RP (1991) Anterior knee motion analysis. Measurement and simultaneous radiography. Am J Sports Med 19:172–177
31. Matsumoto H (1990) Mechanism of the pivot shift. J Bone Joint Surg 72:816–821
32. Kocher MS, Steadman JR, Briggs KK, Sterett WI, Hawkins RJ (2004) Relationships between objective assessment of ligament stability and subjective assessment of symptoms and function after anterior cruciate ligament reconstruction. Am J Sports Med 32:629–634
33. Hefti F, Muller W, Jakob RP, Staubli HU (1993) Evaluation of knee ligament injuries with the ikdc form. Knee Surg Sports Traumatol Arthrosc 1:226–234
34. Ardern CL, Taylor NF, Feller JA, Webster KE (2014) Fifty-five per cent return to competitive sport following anterior cruciate ligament reconstruction surgery: an updated systematic review and meta-analysis including aspects of physical functioning and contextual factors. Br J Sports Med 48:1543–1552
35. Brandsson S, Karlsson J, Sward L, Kartus J, Eriksson BI, Karrholm J (2002) Kinematics and laxity of the knee joint after anterior cruciate ligament reconstruction: pre- and postoperative radiostereometric studies. Am J Sports Med 30:361–367
36. Georgoulis AD, Papadonikolakis A, Papageorgiou CD, Mitsou A, Stergiou N (2003) Three-dimensional tibiofemoral kinematics of the anterior cruciate ligament-deficient and reconstructed knee during walking. Am J Sports Med 31:75–79
37. Ristanis S, Giakas G, Papageorgiou CD, Moraiti T, Stergiou N, Georgoulis AD (2003) The effects of anterior cruciate ligament reconstruction on tibial rotation during pivoting after descending stairs. Knee Surg Sports Traumatol Arthrosc 11:360–365
38. Schuster AJ, McNicholas MJ, Wachtl SW, McGurty DW, Jakob RP (2004) A new mechanical testing device for measuring anteroposterior knee laxity. Am J Sports Med 32:1731–1735
39. Irrgang JJ, Anderson AF, Boland AL, Harner CD, Kurosaka M, Neyret P, Richmond JC, Shelborne KD (2001) Development and validation of the international knee documentation committee subjective knee form. Am J Sports Med 29:600–613
40. Jakob RP, Staubli HU, Deland JT (1987) Grading the pivot shift. Objective tests with implications for treatment. J Bone Joint Surg 69:294–299
41. Bull AM, Earnshaw PH, Smith A, Katchburian MV, Hassan AN, Amis AA (2002) Intraoperative measurement of knee kinematics in reconstruction of the anterior cruciate ligament. J Bone Joint Surg 84:1075–1081

42. Gillquist J, Messner K (1995) Instrumented analysis of the pivot shift phenomenon after reconstruction of the anterior cruciate ligament. Int J Sports Med 16:484–488
43. Snyder-Mackler L, Fitzgerald GK, Bartolozzi AR 3rd, Ciccotti MG (1997) The relationship between passive joint laxity and functional outcome after anterior cruciate ligament injury. Am J Sports Med 25:191–195
44. Kubo S, Muratsu H, Yoshiya S, Mizuno K, Kurosaka M (2007) Reliability and usefulness of a new in vivo measurement system of the pivot shift. Clin Orthop Relat Res 454:54–58
45. Labbe DR, de Guise JA, Mezghani N, Godbout V, Grimard G, Baillargeon D, Lavigne P, Fernandes J, Ranger P, Hagemeister N (2010) Feature selection using a principal component analysis of the kinematics of the pivot shift phenomenon. J Biomech 43:3080–3084
46. Lopomo N, Zaffagnini S, Signorelli C, Bignozzi S, Giordano G, Marcheggiani Muccioli GM, Visani A (2012) An original clinical methodology for non-invasive assessment of pivot-shift test. Comput Methods Biomech Biomed Engin 15:1323–1328
47. Maeyama A, Hoshino Y, Debandi A, Kato Y, Saeki K, Asai S, Goto B, Smolinski P, Fu FH (2011) Evaluation of rotational instability in the anterior cruciate ligament deficient knee using triaxial accelerometer: a biomechanical model in porcine knees. Knee Surg Sports Traumatol Arthrosc 19:1233–1238
48. Hoshino Y, Kuroda R, Nagamune K, Yagi M, Mizuno K, Yamaguchi M, Muratsu H, Yoshiya S, Kurosaka M (2007) In vivo measurement of the pivot-shift test in the anterior cruciate ligament-deficient knee using an electromagnetic device. Am J Sports Med 35:1098–1104
49. Allum R, Jones D, Mowbray MA, Galway HR (1984) Triaxial electrogoniometric examination of the pivot shift sign for rotatory instability of the knee. Clin Orthop Relat Res 183:144–146
50. Andersson C, Gillquist J (1990) Instrumented testing for evaluation of sagittal knee laxity. Clin Orthop Relat Res 256:178–184
51. Bull AM, Andersen HN, Basso O, Targett J, Amis AA (1999) Incidence and mechanism of the pivot shift. An in vitro study. Clin Orthop Relat Res 363:219–231
52. Kuroda R, Hoshino Y, Araki D, Nishizawa Y, Nagamune K, Matsumoto T, Kubo S, Matsushita T, Kurosaka M (2012) Quantitative measurement of the pivot shift, reliability, and clinical applications. Knee Surg Sports Traumatol Arthrosc 20:686–691
53. Hoshino Y, Araujo P, Ahlden M, Samuelsson K, Muller B, Hofbauer M, Wolf MR, Irrgang JJ, Fu FH, Musahl V (2013) Quantitative evaluation of the pivot shift by image analysis using the ipad. Knee Surg Sports Traumatol Arthrosc 21:975–980

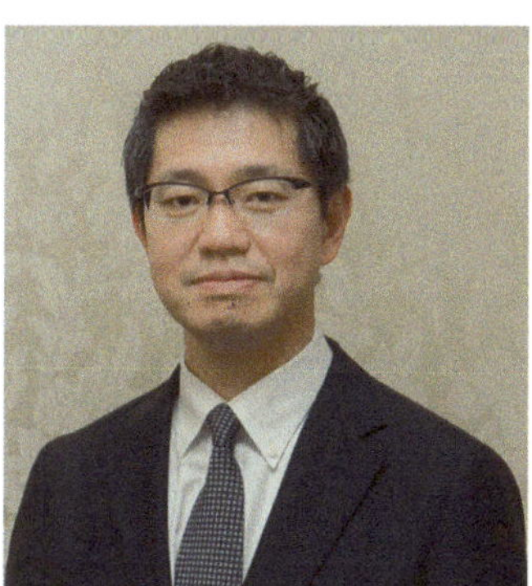

Ryosuke Kuroda, M.D., PhD, Department of Orthopaedic Surgery, Kobe University Graduate School of Medicine, Hyogo, Japan.

Chapter 12
Diagnostics of ACL Injury Using Magnetic Resonance Imaging (MRI)

Yasukazu Yonetani and Yoshinari Tanaka

Abstract Magnetic resonance imaging (MRI) is the most commonly used diagnostic tool for anterior cruciate ligament (ACL) injuries with reported sensitivities and specificities of 87–95 % and 50–100 %, respectively. The detection of differences in the appearance of not only the ACL (direct signs) but also of the surrounding tissues (indirect signs), between a normal and injured ACL, is a key element in the diagnosis of ACL injuries. Standard orthogonal MRI views have generally been used to understand normal ACL anatomy and the mechanisms of ACL injury. Although it is easy to detect the indirect signs of ACL injury using standard orthogonal MRI view, it is often impossible to visualize the entire ACL on a single image because of the oblique orientation of the ACL across the knee. Therefore, additional oblique views that slice along the plane parallel to the long axis of the ACL are recommended to achieve full-length visualization of the ACL. Knowledge of normal ACL anatomy allows for the differentiation of the appearance of a normal ligament from that of an injured ACL. Both standard orthogonal and oblique MRI views help in this differentiation. MRI findings of normal and injured ACLs are reviewed in this chapter.

Keywords Magnetic resonance imaging (MRI) • Anterior cruciate ligament (ACL) • Sagittal and coronal oblique images • Direct sign • Indirect sign

12.1 Introduction

Most ACL tears occur in the middle portion of the ligament, with less frequent tears at the femoral or tibial attachment sites [1, 2].

MRI is the most commonly used diagnostic tool for ACL injuries. Knee MRI for ACL injuries has been shown to have high sensitivity and specificity (87–95 % and

Y. Yonetani, M.D., Ph.D. (✉)
Department of Orthopedics surgery, Hoshigaoka Medical Center, 4-8-1 Hoshigaoka, Hirakata, Osaka 573-8511, Japan
e-mail: yonechan-osk@umin.ac.jp

Y. Tanaka
Department of Sports Orthopedics, Osaka Rosai Hospital, Osaka, Japan

M. Ochi et al. (eds.), *ACL Injury and Its Treatment*,
DOI 10.1007/978-4-431-55858-3_12

50–100 %, respectively) [3–9]. This diagnostic efficiency is based on the proper understanding of normal ACL anatomy and the mechanisms of ACL injury. With this understanding, it is possible to detect the differences in the appearance of the ACL and surrounding tissues between a normal and injured ACL. This comparison is made using not only standard orthogonal MRI views, which detect the secondary signs but not the direct signs of injury, but also oblique views, which allow for a full-length visualization of the ACL by slicing along the plane parallel to the long axis of the ACL. The aim of this chapter is to describe normal ACL and torn ACL MRI findings, using both standard orthogonal and oblique views.

12.2 MRI Findings of a Normal ACL (Table 12.1)

MRI is the most noninvasive method for investigating ACL fiber arraignments. The normal ACL is usually imaged in the sagittal plane using a T2-weighted pulse sequence [10]. However, axial and coronal imaging planes are also useful in the evaluation of the proximal and distal attachment sites, respectively. With the knee imaged in full extension, normal ACL fibers appear taut, with no substantial posterior drooping, and parallel to, but not touching, the roof of the intercondylar notch (Fig. 12.1A). However, a standard orthogonal MRI cannot visualize the complete ACL with a single image because of the oblique angle of the ACL which originates from the posteromedial aspect of the lateral femoral condyle and courses through the lateral intercondylar notch. Poor visualization is reported in 5–10 % of normal ACLs analyzed using images acquired from standard sagittal MRI [11]. Because of artifacts from the popliteal artery and partial volume effects, a complete diagnosis of ACL injuries is not generally possible with a single standard orthogonal image.

To improve the efficacy of visualization for ACL diagnosis, it is necessary to achieve full-length visualization of the ACL by slicing along the plane parallel to the long axis of the ACL (Fig. 12.1B–D). Using additional oblique images makes it

Table 12.1 MRI appearance of a normal ACL

Sagittal oblique view in full extension: (Fig. 12.2a**)**
Only one slice could obtained
The ACL appears taut and parallel to the roof of the intercondylar notch
Coronal oblique view in full extension: (Fig. 12.2c, d**)**
Several slices could be obtained
The ACL bundles are running from the medial aspect of the lateral femoral condyle to the tibial spine
No impingement of the PCL is shown
The ACL is attached to the MIR at the tibial insertion site
The ACL is attached to the posterior femoral cortex

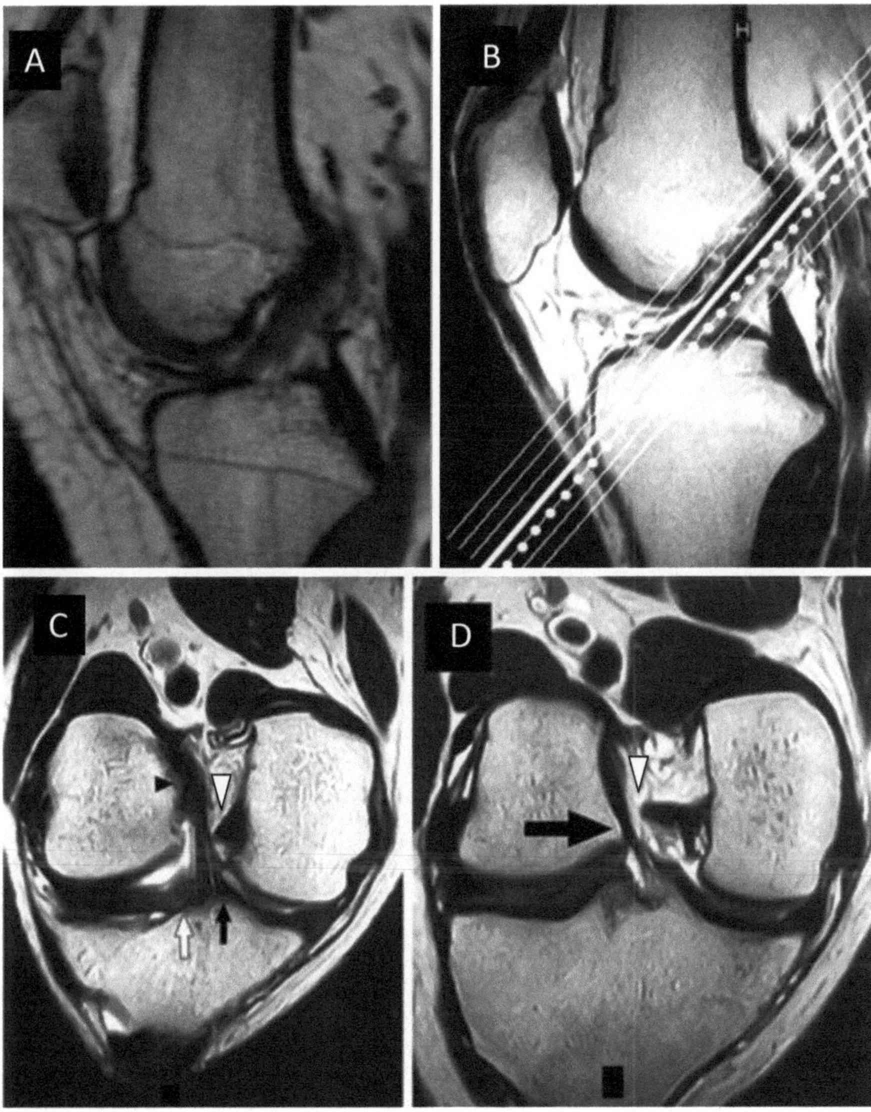

Fig. 12.1 Sagittal and coronal oblique images of the anterior cruciate ligament
(**a**) Sagittal oblique and (**b**) scout view: slices of the anteromedial (AM) bundles (*solid line*) and the posterolateral (PL) bundles (*dotted line*). Representative coronal oblique images of (**c**) the AM bundles and (**d**) the PL bundles showing the apex of the medial intercondylar ridge (*small black arrow*), the lateral meniscus (*white arrow*), the resident's ridge (*arrowhead*), and the bony eminence at the inner articular margin of the lateral femoral condyle (*large black arrow*) (C, D). No impingement to the posterior cruciate ligament (PCL) or femoral condyle was observed in each bundle (*white arrow head*)
Modified figure, reprinted from Knee Surgery, Sports Traumatology, Arthroscopy, 19, Tanaka Y, Shiozaki Y, Yonetani Y, Kanamoto T, Tsujii A, Horibe S, MRI analysis of the attachment of the anteromedial and posterolateral bundles of anterior cruciate ligament using coronal oblique images., S54–59, 2011, with permission from Springer

easier to investigate the individual course of the AM and PL bundles and to see their relationship with the surrounding structures in the notch space, such as the posterior cruciate ligament (PCL) and the femoral condyle (Fig. 12.1B–D). Because the width of the ACL is between 11.43 and 16.18 mm [12], it is easier to evaluate the entire fiber course of the two individual bundles with several coronal oblique image slices (Fig. 12.1C, D). Compared to that on coronal oblique images, the assessment of the entire course of the ACL on sagittal oblique images is slightly more difficult because the thickness of the ACL is only 2.54–3.38 mm [12] (Fig. 12.1A). Both standard orthogonal MRI and oblique images are quite useful in the evaluation of the ACL. Previous MRI studies using coronal oblique views of normal ACLs showed that not only did no impingement of the posterior cruciate ligament (PCL) or the medial wall of the lateral condyle occur [13] but AM bundles attached to the medial border of the medial intercodylar ridge (MIR) and 74 % of the PL bundles inserted between the apex and the slope of the MIR (Fig. 12.1C, D) [14].

12.3 Direct Signs of a Complete ACL Tear

Several direct MRI signs indicate a complete disruption of the ACL [15] (Table 12.2).

Discontinuity of the ACL fibers seen in any of the five imaging planes is evidence of a complete tear. The appearance of an acute disrupted ACL has been described as an edematous mass with an increased T2 signal and abnormal morphology (Fig. 12.2A). Following the acute phase, the injured ACL sometimes loses the edematous mass-like appearance and takes on a less linear, fragmented appearance, such as the loss of a parallel orientation to the intercondylar notch. In chronic cases, ACL damage tends to show an absence of the ACL fibers. The edematous mass in the subacute phase sometimes gives rise to a severe loss of extension and pain, which may require the debridement of the ACL remnant before reconstruction to achieve full range of motion. The so-called empty notch sign refers to an MRI finding in which a fluid signal rather than normal ACL fibers is seen at the proximal attachment site. It is usually best depicted on axial T2-weighted images.

The diagnostic accuracy of these direct signs for detecting an ACL tear is over 90 % [15, 16]. However, a standard orthogonal MRI cannot visualize the complete ACL on a single image because of the oblique alignment of the ACL. To improve the diagnostic efficacy for ACL injuries, it is necessary to achieve full-length visualization of the ACL by slicing along the plane parallel to the long axis of the ACL (Fig. 12.2B). Oblique coronal MR images oriented parallel to the intercondylar roof are excellent to clearly visualize the anatomical course of the ACL and its relationship to the intercondylar notch and the PCL [13, 14] (Fig. 12.1B–D). Oblique coronal images clearly visualize ACL continuity, tension, and changes in width and signal intensity (Fig. 12.2C, D), and a higher diagnostic efficacy of using an oblique coronal view of the ACL has been reported [17–19].

Table 12.2 MRI findings of ACL tear

Direct signs (Fig. 12.3**a)**
Anterior cruciate ligament discontinuity or an abnormal course
A loss of parallel orientation to the intercondylar notch
Empty notch sign
Indirect signs (Secondary) (Fig. 12.4)
Buckling of the posterior cruciate ligament
Anterior translation of the tibia
Bone bruise pattern (femoral/tibial)
Segond fracture

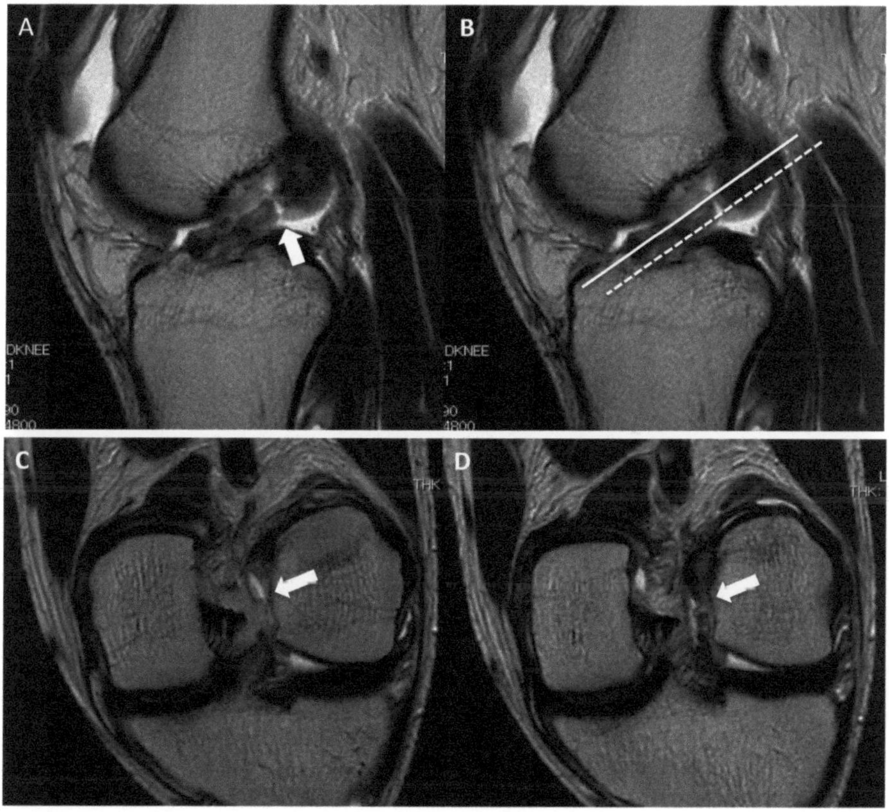

Fig. 12.2 Direct signs of anterior cruciate ligament (ACL) injury
(**a**) Oblique sagittal view showing discontinuity of the ACL (*white arrow*). (**b**) Scout view slices of the anteromedial (AM) bundles (*solid line*) and the posterolateral (PL) bundles (*dotted line*). Coronal oblique images of (**c**) the AM bundles and (**d**) the PL bundles showing a complete tear of the ACL (*white arrow*)

12.4 Indirect Signs of a Complete ACL Tear

Several secondary signs of a complete ACL tear have been described with a low sensitivity (34–90 %) but a high specificity (91–100 %) which can be a helpful hint to the diagnosis of an ACL tear (Table 12.2). The most useful secondary signs are the PCL buckle (Fig. 12.3A); an "uncovering" of the posterior horn of the lateral meniscus; the entire lateral collateral ligament (LCL) seen on one coronal image; anterior displacement of the tibia (more than 5–7 mm, more pronounced laterally) which is indicated by a line drawn at 45° to the posterosuperior end of Blumensaat's line that does not intersect with the flat part of the tibial plateau (Fig. 12.3B); the posterior PCL line, which is a line drawn parallel to the posterior margin of the distal portion of the PCL and extended proximally (Fig. 12.3C); a deep lateral femoral sulcus (deeper than 2 mm) (Fig. 12.4A); and a translational bone contusion in the lateral compartment (lateral femoral condyle and posterolateral tibial plateau) (Fig. 12.4B) [16, 20–23]. Furthermore, hemarthrosis is often associated with ACL rupture [24, 25].

The most common secondary sign is a characteristic bone bruise pattern, seen in up to 80 % of ACL tears [26]. The pivot shift mechanism creates an impact between LFC and the posterior LTP, which shows an increased signal on T2-weighted images (Fig. 12.4B). These bone bruises evolve over time following the occurrence of the acute injury and resolve after varying periods of time. Previous studies show that bone bruises are seen within 4–6 weeks after ACL injury [16, 26]. However, it should be noted that the presence of the translational bone marrow edema pattern created by the pivot shift is indicative of recent tibial translation, but not necessarily of the presence of an acute ACL injury, as these injuries may also be seen in cases

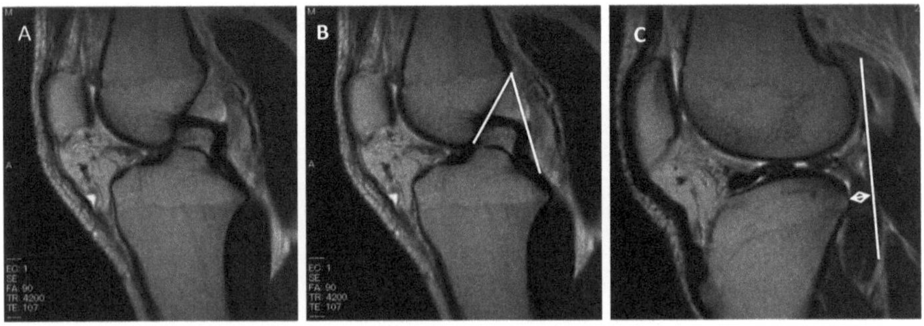

Fig. 12.3 Indirect signs of anterior cruciate ligament (ACL) injury
(**a**) Anterior tibial translation leading to posterior cruciate ligament (PCL) buckling. Thus, the PCL buckling indicates an ACL tear. (**b**) Anterior tibial translation is indicated by a line drawn at 45° to the posterosuperior end of Blumensaat's line that does not intersect with the flat part of the tibial plateau. (**c**) "Anterior draw sign": An anterior translocation of the femur on the tibia is positive in the case of an anterior distance greater than 5 mm between the posterior tibial border and a line dropped perpendicularly from the posterior aspect of the femoral condyle

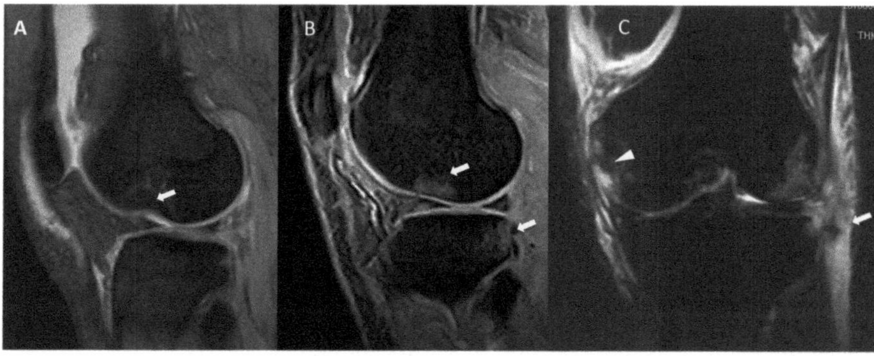

Fig. 12.4 Indirect signs of anterior cruciate ligament injury
(**a**) Deep lateral femoral sulcus (deeper than 2 mm) (*white arrow*). Impact on the lateral femoral condyle (LFC) decompressed the femoral condyle with or without a bone bruise. (**b**) Bone bruise (*white arrow*). The pivot shift mechanism created an impact between the LFC and the posterior lateral tibial plateau (LTP), which increased the signal on T2-weighted images. (**c**) ACL tears are often associated with injuries to additional structures, such as the medial collateral ligament meniscal tears (*white arrow head*) and Segond fractures (*white arrow*), which is a capsular avulsion fracture of the LTP

of chronic ACL insufficiency. The time dependency and location of bone bruises on the femoral condyle seen in ACL injuries are also similar to the patterns seen in a patellar dislocation, which can mislead the diagnosis. However, the bone bruise pattern from patellar dislocation does not involve a tibial component, and femoral contusions will be more anterior than those seen in ACL-related femoral contusions.

Furthermore, ACL tears are often associated with injuries to additional structures, such as the medial collateral ligament, meniscal tears, and Segond fractures, which are capsular avulsion fractures of the lateral tibial plateau, found in 6–13 % of ACL ruptures [27] (Fig. 12.4C).

12.5 Summary

MRI allows for the reliable assessment of knee structure and the diagnosis ACL injuries. In this chapter, the MRI signal characteristics of the ACL were demonstrated based on the anatomy of the ACL. Depending on the mechanism of ACL injury, attention should be directed toward not only the ligament but also the characteristics of the surrounding knee structures, such as bone bruises and anterior tibial translation. Both standard orthogonal and additional oblique MRI views should be utilized to ensure accurate and reproducible image interpretation.

References

1. Potter HG, Weinstein M, Allen AA, Wickiewicz TL, Helfet DL (2002) Magnetic resonance imaging of the multiple-ligament injured knee. J Orthop Trauma 16(5):330–339
2. Remer EM, Fitzgerald SW, Friedman H, Rogers LF, Hendrix RW, Schafer MF (1992) Anterior cruciate ligament injury: MR imaging diagnosis and patterns of injury. Radiographics 12 (5):901–915. doi:10.1148/radiographics.12.5.1529133
3. Moore SL (2002) Imaging the anterior cruciate ligament. Orthop Clin North Am 33 (4):663–674
4. Vahey TN, Meyer SF, Shelbourne KD, Klootwyk TE (1994) MR imaging of anterior cruciate ligament injuries. Magn Reson Imaging Clin N Am 2(3):365–380
5. Tsai KJ, Chiang H, Jiang CC (2004) Magnetic resonance imaging of anterior cruciate ligament rupture. BMC Musculoskelet Disord 5:21. doi:10.1186/1471-2474-5-21
6. Fayad LM, Parellada JA, Parker L, Schweitzer ME (2003) MR imaging of anterior cruciate ligament tears: is there a gender gap? Skeletal Radiol 32(11):639–646. doi:10.1007/s00256-003-0694-1
7. Delin C, Silvera S, Coste J, Thelen P, Lefevre N, Ehkirch FP, Le Couls V, Oudjit A, Radier C, Legmann P (2013) Reliability and diagnostic accuracy of qualitative evaluation of diffusion-weighted MRI combined with conventional MRI in differentiating between complete and partial anterior cruciate ligament tears. Eur Radiol 23(3):845–854. doi:10.1007/s00330-012-2633-9
8. Lee JK, Yao L, Phelps CT, Wirth CR, Czajka J, Lozman J (1988) Anterior cruciate ligament tears: MR imaging compared with arthroscopy and clinical tests. Radiology 166(3):861–864. doi:10.1148/radiology.166.3.3340785
9. Vellet AD, Lee DH, Munk PL, Hewett L, Eliasziw M, Dunlavy S, Vidito L, Fowler PJ, Miniaci A, Amendola A (1995) Anterior cruciate ligament tear: prospective evaluation of diagnostic accuracy of middle- and high-field-strength MR imaging at 1.5 and 0.5 T. Radiology 197(3):826–830. doi:10.1148/radiology.197.3.7480763
10. Milewski MD, Sanders TG, Miller MD (2011) MRI-arthroscopy correlation: the knee. J Bone Joint Surg Am 93(18):1735–1745. doi:10.2106/JBJS.9318icl
11. Buckwalter KA, Pennes DR (1990) Anterior cruciate ligament: oblique sagittal MR imaging. Radiology 175(1):276–277. doi:10.1148/radiology.175.1.2315495
12. Smigielski R, Zdanowicz U, Drwiega M, Ciszek B, Ciszkowska-Lyson B, Siebold R (2014) Ribbon like appearance of the midsubstance fibres of the anterior cruciate ligament close to its femoral insertion site: a cadaveric study including 111 knees. Knee Surg Sports Traumatol Arthrosc. doi:10.1007/s00167-014-3146-7
13. Staeubli HU, Adam O, Becker W, Burgkart R (1999) Anterior cruciate ligament and intercondylar notch in the coronal oblique plane: anatomy complemented by magnetic resonance imaging in cruciate ligament-intact knees. Arthroscopy 15(4):349–359
14. Tanaka Y, Shiozaki Y, Yonetani Y, Kanamoto T, Tsujii A, Horibe S (2011) MRI analysis of the attachment of the anteromedial and posterolateral bundles of anterior cruciate ligament using coronal oblique images. Knee Surg Sports Traumatol Arthrosc 19(Suppl 1):S54–S59. doi:10.1007/s00167-011-1515-z
15. Robertson PL, Schweitzer ME, Bartolozzi AR, Ugoni A (1994) Anterior cruciate ligament tears: evaluation of multiple signs with MR imaging. Radiology 193(3):829–834. doi:10.1148/radiology.193.3.7972833
16. Tung GA, Davis LM, Wiggins ME, Fadale PD (1993) Tears of the anterior cruciate ligament: primary and secondary signs at MR imaging. Radiology 188(3):661–667. doi:10.1148/radiology.188.3.8351329
17. Kwon JW, Yoon YC, Kim YN, Ahn JH, Choe BK (2009) Which oblique plane is more helpful in diagnosing an anterior cruciate ligament tear? Clin Radiol 64(3):291–297. doi:10.1016/j.crad.2008.10.007

18. Hong SH, Choi JY, Lee GK, Choi JA, Chung HW, Kang HS (2003) Grading of anterior cruciate ligament injury. Diagnostic efficacy of oblique coronal magnetic resonance imaging of the knee. J Comput Assist Tomogr 27(5):814–819
19. Kosaka M, Nakase J, Toratani T, Ohashi Y, Kitaoka K, Yamada H, Komura K, Nakamura S, Tsuchiya H (2014) Oblique coronal and oblique sagittal MRI for diagnosis of anterior cruciate ligament tears and evaluation of anterior cruciate ligament remnant tissue. Knee 21(1):54–57. doi:10.1016/j.knee.2013.04.016
20. Boeree NR, Ackroyd CE (1992) Magnetic resonance imaging of anterior cruciate ligament rupture. A new diagnostic sign. J Bone Joint Surg (Br) 74(4):614–616
21. Al-Dadah O, Shepstone L, Marshall TJ, Donell ST (2011) Secondary signs on static stress MRI in anterior cruciate ligament rupture. Knee 18(4):235–241. doi:10.1016/j.knee.2010.06.001
22. Hill PF, Vedi V, Williams A, Iwaki H, Pinskerova V, Freeman MA (2000) Tibiofemoral movement 2: the loaded and unloaded living knee studied by MRI. J Bone Joint Surg (Br) 82 (8):1196–1198
23. Gentili A, Seeger LL, Yao L, Do HM (1994) Anterior cruciate ligament tear: indirect signs at MR imaging. Radiology 193(3):835–840. doi:10.1148/radiology.193.3.7972834
24. DeHaven KE (1980) Diagnosis of acute knee injuries with hemarthrosis. Am J Sports Med 8 (1):9–14
25. Noyes FR, Bassett RW, Grood ES, Butler DL (1980) Arthroscopy in acute traumatic hemarthrosis of the knee. Incidence of anterior cruciate tears and other injuries. J Bone Joint Surg Am 62(5):687–695, 757
26. Patel SA, Hageman J, Quatman CE, Wordeman SC, Hewett TE (2014) Prevalence and location of bone bruises associated with anterior cruciate ligament injury and implications for mechanism of injury: a systematic review. Sports Med 44(2):281–293. doi:10.1007/s40279-013-0116-z
27. Goldman AB, Pavlov H, Rubenstein D (1988) The Segond fracture of the proximal tibia: a small avulsion that reflects major ligamentous damage. AJR Am J Roentgenol 151 (6):1163–1167. doi:10.2214/ajr.151.6.1163

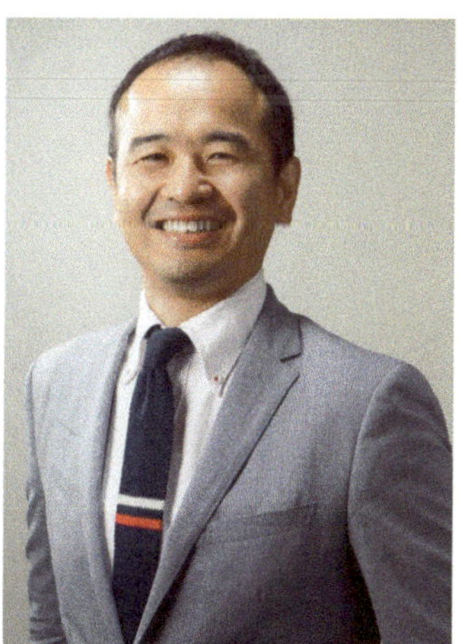

Yasukazu Yonetani M.D., PhD, Department of Orthopedics surgery, Hoshigaoka Medical Center, Osaka, Japan.

Chapter 13
Diagnosis of Injured ACL Using Three-Dimensional Computed Tomography: Usefulness for Preoperative Decision Making

Nobuo Adachi

Abstract Recently, remnant-preserving anterior cruciate ligament reconstruction has been widely performed in the world. It was reported that ACL remnant can contribute to the joint stability, proprioceptive function, and vascularity of the ACL graft. It is very important to evaluate the status of ACL remnant for better preoperative planning and informed consent to the patients. Standard evaluation, such as manual tests or MRI, cannot evaluate the three-dimensional morphology of the ACL remnant. We have used three-dimensional computed tomography with volume rendering technique for diagnosing ACL remnant. 3DCT can depict the three-dimensional morphology of the ACL remnant very clearly.

In this chapter, we describe the method of 3DCT evaluation of ACL remnant and its results.

Keywords Anterior cruciate ligament • Three-dimensional computed tomography • Remnant

13.1 Three-Dimensional Computed Tomography for Soft Tissue Evaluation

Recently, three-dimensional computed tomography (3DCT) with volume rendering has been used for diagnosing several soft tissues, such as the muscles, hand, and wrist tendons, or anterior talofibular ligament (ATFL) of the ankle [1–3].

In 2003 and 2005, Sunagawa et al. [1, 2] used 3DCT imaging with volume rendering for diagnosing extensor and flexor tendon in the hand and wrist and clearly demonstrated those tendons' rupture and stump of the tendons. In 2006, Nakasa et al. [3] used this technique for the diagnosis of ATFL injury. They reported that ATFL was depicted clearly using 3DCT in all patients with chronic

N. Adachi, M.D. (✉)
Department of Orthopaedic Surgery, Institute of Biomedical & Health Sciences, Hiroshima University, 1-2-3 Kasumi, Minami-ku, Hiroshima 734-8551, Japan
e-mail: nadachi@hiroshima-u.ac.jp

M. Ochi et al. (eds.), *ACL Injury and Its Treatment*,
DOI 10.1007/978-4-431-55858-3_13

ATFL tear and that 3DCT could evaluate the condition of ATFL remnant much better than MRI. As for the hamstring tendons in anterior cruciate ligament (ACL) surgery, in 2005, Nakamae et al. [4] evaluated the regeneration of semitendinosus tendons harvested ACL reconstruction using 3DCT imaging and compared the degree of regeneration with hamstring tendons. They reported that regeneration of hamstring tendons was depicted very clearly with 3DCT technique and there was positive correlation between the peak torque ratio of hamstring muscle strength and the proximal shift of muscle-tendon junction 6 months after surgery. More recently, in 2012, Nakamae et al. [5] evaluated the effect of immobilization on morphological changes in the semitendinosus muscle-tendon complex using 3DCT. The study clearly demonstrated the structure of regenerated tendons in 97.4 % cases after ACL reconstruction, and prolonged knee immobilization could not prevent morphological changes in the semitendinosus muscle-tendon complex. Thus, 3DCT with volume rendering technique has been widely used for diagnosing several soft tissues.

13.2 Importance of Preoperative Evaluation of ACL Remnant

There have been several reconstruction techniques for ACL reconstruction, such as single-bundle, double-bundle, or ACL remnant-preserving reconstruction [6–11]. We, ACL surgeons, sometimes encounter patients whose relatively thick ACL remnant was preserved in certain conditions. Those remnants had been removed for the newly reconstructed ACL in the past, regardless of the morphology of the remnant. However, several studies showed that certain conditioned ACL remnant can contribute biomechanical stability of the knee joint and proprioceptive function of the joint. Crain et al. [12] reported that ACL remnants healed to the lateral wall of the notch or the medial aspect of the lateral femoral condyle in a position anterior and distal to the ACL anatomic footprint contributed to the joint stability to some extent. Adachi et al. [13] identified several mechanoreceptors in the ACL remnants. Very interestingly, the number of mechanoreceptors in the ACL remnant was significantly correlated to the proprioceptive function. The ACL remnant also has highly vascularized synovium which may contribute to the vascular regeneration of the tissues [14, 15]. With the recent progress in arthroscopic ACL surgery, remnant-preserving ACL reconstruction has been taken much attention in the ACL surgery.

Although, in the remnant-preserving ACL reconstruction, it is very important to evaluate injured ACL preoperatively for better operative planning, the diagnosis of the ACL remnant has been difficult with manual tests, such as Lachman test or anterior drawer test [16, 17]. MRI can depict injured ACL remnant clearly. However, it is very difficult for evaluating three-dimensional morphology of

ACL remnants even with the advanced technique of MRI. Therefore, we focus on the 3DCT with volume rendering technique for diagnosis of ACL remnant morphology.

13.3 Condition Setting of 3DCT for ACL Remnant

Multidetector row CT scanner (LightSpeed Ultra 16; General Electric Medical Systems, Milwaukee, WI, USA) was used for 3DCT imaging. The patient was placed in a supine position with the knee joint at a 90° flexed position. 3D volume data sets of the knee joint were obtained. The scanning parameters were as follows: a gantry rotation speed of 0.6 s/rotation, 1.25 mm collimation width × 16 detectors, CT pitch factor of 0.562, and field of view of 25–30 cm. The CT dose index volume was 7.67 mGy. Then, 2D images were reconstructed with 12–25 cm field of view, 1.25 mm retrospective slice thickness, and 0.63 mm overlap. The total table motion was 20–30 cm, and finally 200–400 slices were obtained. Images were rendered qualitatively with the volume rendering technique by using a commercially available workstation (Virtual Place; AZE, Tokyo, Japan) to take the 3D images. The scanning time ranged from 40 to 60 s, and another 10–15 min was necessary for processing [18] (Fig. 13.1).

13.4 Patents' Data and Classification of 3DCT Imaging and Arthroscopic Findings of ACL Remnant

We have enrolled 63 patients whose preoperative 3DCT scan of the ACL injured knee was available. We excluded patients with multiligamentous injuries such as medial collateral ligament, posterior cruciate ligament, or posterolateral corner injuries. The patients consisted of 33 males and 30 females with the average age of 25.2 (13–52) years at the time of the operation. The cause for all ACL injuries was trauma, such as a sports-related injury or a traffic accident. The average durations between traumas and 3DCT and between 3DCT and surgery were 101.7 days and 38.2 days, respectively.

The ACL remnants on 3DCT and arthroscopic findings were classified into four morphological patterns according to the classification by Crain et al. [12] (Fig. 13.2):

Type I, bridging between the posterior cruciate ligament and tibia
Type II, bridging between roof of the intercondylar notch and tibia
Type III, bridging between the lateral wall of the intercondylar notch and tibia
Type IV, no substantial ACL remnants

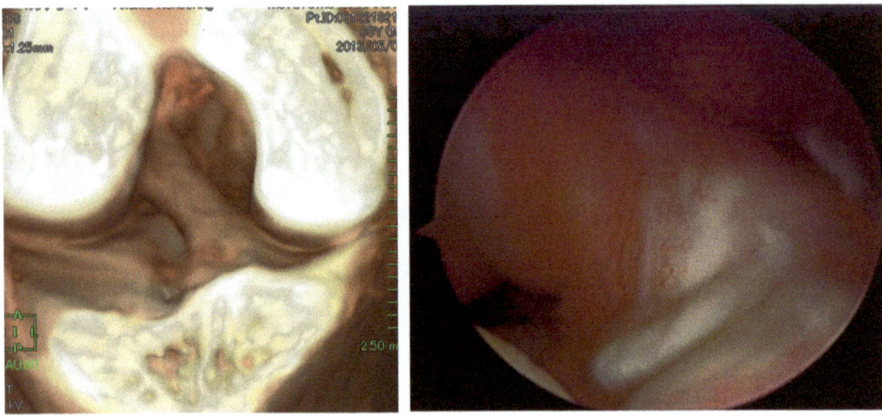

Fig. 13.1 ACL remnant on 3DCT and under arthroscopy in the same patients

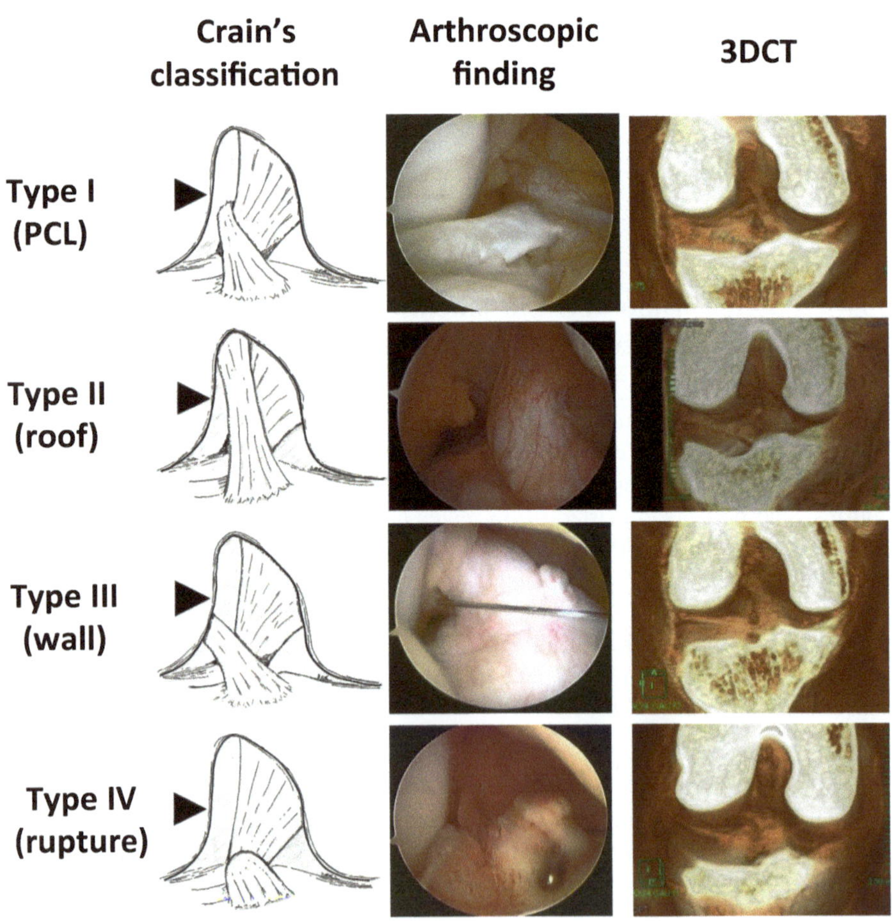

Fig. 13.2 ACL remnants and 3DCT on arthroscopy were classified into four morphological patterns according to the classification by Crain et al. (From Ref. [12, 18])

The 3DCT findings were compared with the arthroscopic findings with and without probing. The coincidence rates were calculated and statistically analyzed with χ^2 test for independence. A p-value of <0.05 was considered statistically significant. All statistical analyses were conducted using StatView 5.0 (SAS Institute, Cary, NC, USA).

13.5 Comparison of 3DCT Imaging and Arthroscopic Findings of ACL Remnant

On 3DCT, 11.1 % of the ACL remnants were classified as type I, 17.5 % type II, 46.0 % type III, and 25.4 % type IV.

Correlations between the morphological patterns on 3DCT and those on arthroscopy without and with probing are summarized in Tables 13.1 and 13.2, respectively. The morphological patterns of the ACL remnants on 3DCT were well matched with those on arthroscopy without probing in 77.8 % of the patients. However, the coincidence rate was reduced significantly to 49.2 % when arthroscopic probing was used to confirm the femoral attachment of the ACL remnants ($p < 0.05$).

Table 13.1 Correlation between the morphological patterns of ACL remnant on 3DCT and on arthroscopy without probing

	3DCT				
Scopic finding	Type I (PCL)	Type II (roof)	Type III (wall)	Type IV (rupture)	Total
Type I (PCL)	4				4
Type II (roof)	2	9	2	4	17
Type III (wall)		2	27	3	32
Type IV (rupture)	1			9	10
Total	7	11	29	16	63

The coincidence rate is 77.8 %

Table 13.2 Correlation between the morphological patterns of ACL remnant on 3DCT and on arthroscopy with probing

	3DCT				
Scopic finding	Type I (PCL)	Type II (roof)	Type III (wall)	Type IV (rupture)	Total
Type I (PCL)	5	3	4		12
Type II (roof)	1	5	13	3	22
Type III (wall)		3	11	3	17
Type IV (rupture)	1		1	10	12
Total	7	11	29	16	63

The coincidence rate is 49.2 %

13.6 Advantages and Disadvantages of 3DCT for Evaluating ACL Remnant

It has been widely accepted that MRI is the most reliable preoperative imaging tool for assessing the injured ACL. Although there were several reports that demonstrated successfully the partial rupture of ACL using special technique or sequence of MRI, van Dyck et al. [19] stated that MR imaging at 3.0 T represents a highly accurate method for the diagnosis of the ACL tears, but it was difficult to differentiate between complete and partial tears of the ACL. It is usually believed that it is difficult to evaluate partial tear of ACL or three-dimensional morphology of ACL using MRI [20–22].

3DCT with volume rendering technique has advantages for depicting injured ACL three dimensionally, especially in one image. Definitely, three-dimensional morphology, such as bulk or running route of the injured ACL remnant, is very useful information for preoperative planning and obtaining informed consent from the patients if ACL reconstruction with a remnant-preserving procedure could be performed. However, because 3DCT cannot depict the status of ACL attachment clearly, the ACL surgeons have to take attention for assessing it.

For the future study, we have to evaluate relation between the morphological status of ACL remnant on 3DCT and joint laxity for decision making for the indication of remnant-preserving ACL surgery preoperatively.

References

1. Sunagawa T, Ochi M, Ishida O, Ono C, Ikuta Y (2003) Three-dimensional CT imaging of flexor tendon ruptures in the hand and wrist. J Comput Assist Tomogr 27:169–174
2. Sunagawa T, Ishida O, Ishiburo M, Suzuki O, Yasunaga Y, Ochi M (2005) Three-dimensional computed tomography imaging: its applicability in the evaluation of extensor tendons in the hand and wrist. J Comput Assist Tomogr 29:94–98
3. Nakasa T, Fukuhara K, Adachi N, Ochi M (2006) Evaluation of anterior talofibular ligament lesion using 3-dimensional computed tomography. J Comput Assist Tomogr 30:543–547
4. Nakamae A, Deie M, Yasumoto M, Adachi N, Kobayashi K, Yasunaga Y, Ochi M (2005) Three-dimensional computed tomography imaging evidence of regeneration of the semitendinosus tendon harvested for anterior cruciate ligament reconstruction: a comparison with hamstring muscle strength. J Comput Assist Tomogr 29:241–245
5. Nakamae A, Ochi M, Deie M, Adachi N (2012) Unsuccessful regeneration of the semitendinosus tendon harvested for anterior cruciate ligament reconstruction: report of two cases. Orthop Traumatol Surg Res 98:932–935
6. Samuelsson K, Desai N, McNair E, van Eck CF, Petzold M, Fu FH, Bhandari M, Karlsson J (2013) Level of evidence in anterior cruciate ligament reconstruction research: a systematic review. Am J Sports Med 41:924–934

7. van Eck CF, Schreiber VM, Mejia HA, Samuelsson K, van Dijk CN, Karlsson J, Fu FH (2010) "Anatomic" anterior cruciate ligament reconstruction: a systematic review of surgical techniques and reporting of surgical data. Arthroscopy 26:S2–S12
8. Adachi N, Ochi M, Uchio Iwasa J, Kuriwaka M, Ito Y (2004) Reconstruction of the anterior cruciate ligament: single- versus double-bundle multistranded hamstring tendons. J Bone Joint Surg (Br) 86:515–552
9. Adachi N, Ochi M, Uchio Y, Sumen Y (2000) Anterior cruciate ligament augmentation under arthroscopy: a minimum 2-year follow-up in 40 patients. Arch Orthop Trauma Surg 120:128–133
10. Ochi M, Adachi N, Deie M, Kanaya A (2006) Anterior cruciate ligament augmentation procedure with a 1-incision technique: anteromedial bundle or posterolateral bundle reconstruction. Arthroscopy 22:463.e1–463.e5
11. Ochi M, Adachi N, Uchio Y, Deie M, Kumahashi N, Ishikawa M, Sera S (2009) A minimum 2-year follow-up after selective anteromedial or posterolateral bundle anterior cruciate ligament reconstruction. Arthroscopy 25:117–122
12. Crain EH, Fithian DC, Paxton EW, Luetzow WF (2005) Variation in anterior cruciate ligament scar pattern: does the scar pattern affect anterior laxity in anterior cruciate ligament-deficient knees? Arthroscopy 21:19–24
13. Adachi N, Ochi M, Uchio Y, Iwasa J, Ryoke K, Kuriwaka M (2002) Mechanoreceptors in the anterior cruciate ligament contribute to the joint position sense. Acta Orthop Scand 73:330–334
14. Ahn JH, Lee SH, Choi SH, Lim TK (2010) Magnetic resonance imaging evaluation of anterior cruciate ligament reconstruction using quadrupled hamstring tendon autografts: comparison of remnant bundle preservation and standard technique. Am J Sports Med 38:1768–1777
15. Gohil S, Annear PO, Breidahl W (2007) Anterior cruciate ligament reconstruction using autologous double hamstrings: a comparison of standard versus minimal debridement techniques using MRI to assess revascularisation. A randomised prospective study with a one-year follow-up. J Bone Joint Surg (Br) 89:1165–1171
16. Lintner DM, Kamaric E, Moseley JB, Noble PC (1995) Partial tears of the anterior cruciate ligament: are they clinically detectable? Am J Sports Med 23:111–118
17. Christel PS, Akgun U, Yasar T, Karahan M, Demirel B (2012) The contribution of each anterior cruciate ligament bundle to the Lachman test: a cadaver investigation. J Bone Joint Surg (Br) 94:68–74
18. Adachi N, Ochi M, Takazawa K, Ishifuro M, Deie M, Nakamae A, Kamei G (2016) Morphologic evaluation of remnant anterior cruciate ligament bundles after injury with three-dimensional computed tomography. Knee Surg Sports Traumatol Arthrosc 24:148–153
19. Van Dyck P, Vanhoenacker FM, Gielen JL, Dossche L, Van Gestel J, Wouters K, Parizel PM (2011) Three tesla magnetic resonance imaging of the anterior cruciate ligament of the knee: can we differentiate complete from partial tears? Skelet Radiol 40:701–707
20. Delin C, Silvera S, Coste J, Thelen P, Lefevre N, Ehkirch FP, Le Couls V, Oudjit A, Radier C, Legmann P (2013) Reliability and diagnostic accuracy of qualitative evaluation of diffusion-weighted MRI combined with conventional MRI in differentiating between complete and partial anterior cruciate ligament tears. Eur Radiol 23:845–854
21. Lefevre N, Naouri JF, Bohu Y, Klouche S, Herman S (2014) Partial tears of the anterior cruciate ligament: diagnostic performance of isotropic three-dimensional fast spin echo (3D-FSE-Cube) MRI. Eur J Orthop Surg Traumatol 24:85–91

22. Ng AW, Griffith JF, Hung EH, Law KY, Yung PS (2013) MRI diagnosis of ACL bundle tears: value of oblique axial imaging. Skelet Radiol 42:209–217

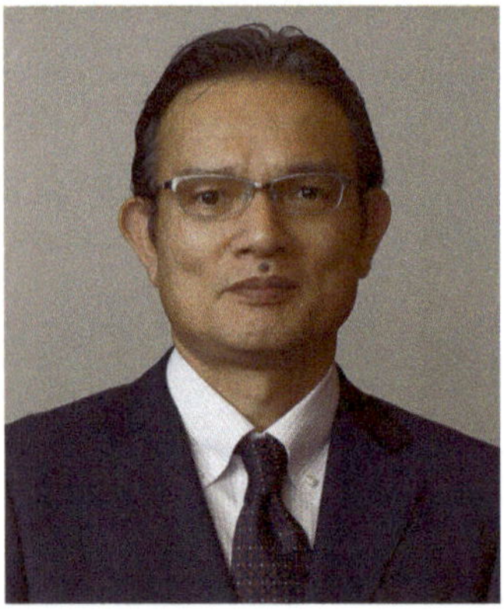

Nobuo Adachi, M.D., Department of Orthopaedic Surgery, Institute of Biomedical & Health Sciences, Hiroshima University, Hiroshima, Japan.

Part IV
Basic Knowledge of ACL Reconstruction

Chapter 14
Graft Selection

Eiichi Tsuda and Yasuyuki Ishibashi

Abstract Requirements for an ideal graft substitute in ACL reconstruction surgery are proper biomechanical strength, sufficient size, reliable fixation, rapid biological healing, no biologically adverse reaction, no donor-site morbidity, and excellent long-term outcomes. Although many types of graft have been used in a history of ACL reconstruction, it is still a question under never-ending debate as to what is the best graft. Surgeons have to understand that every type of graft available today has advantages and disadvantages. Factors in the patient side, such as age, sex, physique, activity, lifestyle, and preference, are also the issues which affect the graft selection. In most case, autologous graft is the first choice for primary reconstruction. The popular autografts are hamstring tendon graft, which is applicable for multi-bundle reconstruction and has less donor-site morbidity, and bone-patellar tendon-bone graft which has lower risk of revision surgery. Since harvest technique is another factor to affect surgical outcomes, surgeons should be acquainted with anatomy and harvesting procedures of each graft.

Keywords Auto graft • Hamstring tendon • Bone-patellar tendon-bone

14.1 Introduction

From the first half of the 1900s, anterior cruciate ligament (ACL) reconstruction surgery has been started using a pedunculated graft, of which the one side of bony or muscular attachment was left intact, prepared with an iliotibial band [1], a medial hamstring tendon [2], or a patellar tendon [3, 4]. Although these techniques provided secure fixation on the attached side, it caused prolonged running route and relatively shortened graft length and thus resulted in decreased graft strength or

E. Tsuda, M.D. (✉)
Department of Rehabilitation Medicine, Hirosaki University Graduate School of Medicine, 5 Zaifu-cho, Hirosaki, Aomori 036-8562, Japan
e-mail: eiichi@hirosaki-u.ac.jp

Y. Ishibashi, M.D.
Department of Orthopaedic Surgery, Hirosaki University Graduate School of Medicine, 5 Zaifu-cho, Hirosaki, Aomori 036-8562, Japan

M. Ochi et al. (eds.), *ACL Injury and Its Treatment*,
DOI 10.1007/978-4-431-55858-3_14

nonphysiological graft placement. In association with the development of several fixation devices, the distally attached tendon graft has taken the place of a free tendon graft from the 1980s [5, 6].

In the second half of the 1900s, several synthetic ligaments were developed and commercially available as a prosthesis, a scaffold, or an augmentation device. While the synthetic ligament swept over the biological substitutes from ACL reconstruction in the 1980s, many clinical studies disappointed orthopedic surgeons with frequent failure of transplanted synthetic ligament and presence of osteoarthritis in the 1990s [7, 8]. It was not long before the mainstream of graft choice returned back to natural tendon graft.

Allograft has several advantages of no size limitation and no donor-site morbidity over the autograft, and successful results in ACL reconstruction, which was comparable to the autograft, have been demonstrated in animal and clinical studies [9, 10]. However, the clinical availability is limited except in a few countries, due to a lack of established human tissue banking system, conservative cultures, and religious reasons. Increased cost for storage and preparation, potential risk of immunogenic reaction and disease transmission, and inferior biomechanical properties caused by sterilization process are also negative aspects of allograft tissues.

In modern ACL surgery, bone-patellar tendon-bone, hamstring tendon, and quadriceps tendon are the strong candidates for the first choice autograft for primary reconstruction. Although all the grafts have been reported to provide stably good clinical results, surgeons should make the best choice for a patient individually, based on updated and evidence-based knowledge of benefit and complication related to each graft. Patient factors including skeletal maturation, gender, activity, and preference are also taken into account for graft selection. Of course the most affecting factor for the graft selection by a patient is physician recommendation [11, 12]. Surgeons have to be well acquainted with the characteristics of all graft options and provide expert opinions based on scientific evidences to lead each individual patient to making a reasonable final decision.

14.2 Biomechanics of Graft

The structural and material properties similar to native ACL are one of the essential factors for the graft substitute in reconstruction surgery. The ultimate tensile load of native ACL reported in literature was varied 1725–2160 N. It might be affected by difference in the size of tested specimens, the age of donor, and the setting of biomechanical testing [13, 14].

The several biomechanical studies also demonstrated the tensile properties of widely used tendon graft (Table 14.1) [15–18]. When using appropriate surgical techniques, harvesting the central portion of autologous patellar tendon or quadriceps tendon with 10 mm width is a safe procedure to prevent mechanical failure of the remaining portion of tendon during the postoperative rehabilitation and after return to sports. Ultimate tensile load of 10 mm width patellar tendon is 2977 N

Table 14.1 Biomechanical properties of anterior cruciate ligament and grafts

Tissue	Ultimate strength (N)	Stiffness (N/mm)	Cross-sectional area (mm^2)
Anterior cruciate ligament [13]	2160	242	44
Bone-patellar tendon-bone graft (10 mm width) [15]	2977	620	35
Quadrupled hamstring [16]	4090	776	53
Semitendinosus tendon (single strand) [16]	1060	213	11
Semitendinosus tendon (double strand) [16]	2330	469	23
Gracilis tendon (single strand) [16]	837	160	7
Gracilis tendon (double strand) [16]	1550	336	16
Iliotibial band (18 mm) [14]	769		
Quadriceps tendon (10 mm width) [17]	2185	466	91
Tibialis anterior tendon (double strand) [18]	4122	460	48
Tibialis posterior tendon (double strand) [18]	3594	379	42

indicating superior to native ACL [15]. Because of the sufficient strength and ribbonlike appearance similar to ACL [19], the patellar tendon graft is preferably used in single-bundle reconstruction. On the other hand, both single-strand semitendinosus tendon and gracilis tendon have the ultimate tensile load inferior to native ACL and are not suitable to be used as single-strand ACL graft [16]. However, the hamstring tendon is commonly transplanted as a quadruple-strand graft for single-bundle reconstruction or a double-strand graft for anteromedial and posterolateral bundle in double-bundle reconstruction, and it provides sufficient tensile strength [16]. Quadriceps tendon graft has unique composition with a bone plug on one side and without a bone plug on the other side. The bone-free end allows surgeon to longitudinally split the tendinous portion for double-bundle reconstruction [20]. Ultimate tensile load of 10 mm width quadriceps tendon is 2185 N, which is comparable to native ACL [17]. Both tibialis anterior tendon and tibialis posterior tendons are the most popular allograft option under the established human tissue banking system. Ultimate tensile loads of the double-strand graft of tibialis anterior tendon and tibialis posterior tendon are 4122 and 3594, respectively, and it is comparable to the quadrupled hamstring tendon graft [18].

Regeneration of the hamstring tendon after harvesting for ACL reconstruction was reported as "lizard tail phenomenon." Recent systematic review showed that regenerated tendon was identified in more than 70 % of hamstring tendons using imaging and histologic methodologies [21, 22]. The animal study demonstrated that ultimate tensile load of regenerated hamstring tendon recovered to 62 % of the original tendon strength at 28 weeks after harvest [23]. However, the biomechanical properties of human regenerated hamstring tendon have not been fully investigated, and thus it is questionable whether it can be re-harvested and re-transplanted for multiple reinjured ACL.

Stiffness of the graft construct is a factor affecting the joint laxity of ACL-reconstructed knee. Lower graft stiffness yields increased anterior knee laxity compared to the intact knee. There is, however, nothing to worry about graft stiffness, since all tendon grafts widely used today have the stiffness higher than the native ACL (Table 14.1). Although the combination of extremely higher stiffness of graft and the fixation with over initial tensioning might tighten joint laxity nonphysiologically, the effect of graft stiffness on the postoperative clinical results has not been elucidated.

14.3 Graft Size

Length and diameter mismatch between the graft construct and running route forces to alter the surgical techniques and affects the initial fixation strength of transplanted graft and healing process of the graft-tunnel interface.

In case using the bone-patellar tendon-bone graft, extremely long tendon portion precludes intraosseous fixation of bone plug with an interference screw on one side. Adjusting the bone tunnel direction to lengthening the graft running route is one of the solutions that enable to secure both bone plugs intraosseously. Alternative fixation technique, such as inlay or onlay fixation of bone plug out of the tunnel, is another solution, and the surgical instruments should be backed up. Preoperative MRI measurement of the patellar tendon length is required to prevent length mismatch.

When using the hamstring tendon graft, in contrast, there is a risk of insufficient length and diameter for preparing the ACL graft especially in small Asian female patients. The minimum required length and diameter of hamstring tendon graft vary dependent on the graft configuration (single bundle or multi-bundle) and the fixation technique. A systematic review concluded that the quadrupled-strand hamstring autograft with a diameter equal to or larger than 8 mm decreases failure rates in single-bundle reconstruction [24]. It is difficult to preoperatively identify the proximal end of tendinous portion available for the graft substitute in MRI evaluation of the musculotendinous junction. For the surgical planning whether only semitendinosus tendon or additional gracilis tendon is prepared, the predictive equations for the size of hamstring tendon graft based on anthropometric measurements are proposed as a preoperative information (Tables 14.2 and 14.3) [25, 26].

14.4 Biology of Healing

Biological healing process of transplanted graft after ACL reconstruction is still one of the unsolved issues which surgeons have no established way to control in the clinical setting. It has been well investigated whether the type of graft substitutes affects the histological features during maturation process of graft-bone interface. The soft tissue graft tethered with suture materials is anchored to the tunnel wall with Sharpey-like fibers from 3 weeks postoperatively, and the indirect-type

Table 14.2 Predictive equations for semitendinosus and gracilis tendon length

For Caucasian patients [25]		
Tissue	Predicted length (mm)	Correlation with actual length
Semitendinosus	−55.3 + 2.09 (height in cm)	r = 0.69; R^2 = 0.48; P < .001
	23.3 + 3.06 (leg length in cm)	r = 0.67; R^2 = 0.45; P < .001
Gracilis	−37.5 + 1.9 (height in cm)	r = 0.58; R^2 = 0.33; P < .001
	62.5 + 2.4 (leg length in cm)	r = 0.49; R^2 = 0.24; P < .001
For Mongoloid patients [26]		
Tissue	Predicted length (mm)	Correlation with actual length
Semitendinosus	8.7 + 1.577 (height in cm)	r = 0.61; R^2 = 0.37; P < .001
	235.4 + 0.626 (weight in kg)	r = 0.42; R^2 = 0.17; P < .001
Gracilis	32.2 + 1.27 (height in cm)	r = 0.48; R^2 = 0.24; P < .001
	211.5 + 0.56 (weight in kg)	r = 0.37; R^2 = 0.14; P < .001

Table 14.3 Predictive equations for quadrupled graft diameter

For Caucasian patients [25]		
Tissue	Predicted length (mm)	Correlation with actual length
Semitendinosus and gracilis	5.7 + 0.025 (weight in kg)	r = 0.64; R^2 = 0.41; P < .001
	3.7 + 0.86 (thigh circumference)	r = 0.60; R^2 = 0.36; P < .001
	5.17 + 0.95 (BMI)	r = 0.62; R^2 = 0.38; P < .001
	3.6 + 0.024 (height in cm)	r = 0.49; R^2 = 0.24; P < .001
For Mongoloid patients [26]		
Tissue	Predicted length (mm)	Correlation with actual length
Semitendinosus	0.78 + 0.038 (height in cm)	r = 0.44; R^2 = 0.19; P < .001
	5.68 + 0.002 (weight in kg)	r = 0.47; R^2 = 0.22; P < .001
Gracilis	1.408 + 0.026 (height in cm)	r = 0.37; R^2 = 0.13; P < .001
	5.035 + 0.001 (weight in kg)	r = 0.30; R^2 = 0.09; P < .001

insertion is formed by 12 weeks in experimental animal models [27]. On the other hand, bone to bone integration between the bone plug of bone-patellar tendon-bone graft and the tunnel wall started from 3 weeks and completes by 12 weeks after transplantation. The bone-patellar tendon-bone graft has an advantage of greater failure load at fixation site until the weakest point moves to the graft midsubstance. The direct-type insertion at the patellar tendon-bone plug junction is preserved in early phase after surgery, while main linkage shifts to the indirect-type insertion newly formed between the tendinous portion and the tunnel wall in late phase [28].

The intraarticular segment of transplanted graft is placed in serious biological situation under less blood supply environment, compared to the intraosseous portion. The long maturation process consists of four phases, which are acute inflammatory response, revascularization, proliferative phase, and collage remodeling. An animal study showed that the random oriented newly formed collagen fibers were aligned with longitudinal direction in the soft tissue graft by 12 weeks [29]. However, the further histological maturation still progressed after

1 year, so that the shape and number of cell nuclei and the crimp pattern changed close to those of normal ACL. Similar maturation process was found in the bone-patellar tendon-bone graft [30]. Several trials to accelerate the graft maturation and enhance the biomechanical properties have been investigated. The potentially beneficial effect of administration of growth factors and cell transplantation has been proved in in vitro and in vivo animal models [31].

14.5 Fixation Technique

The biomechanical properties of femur-graft-tibia complex are more important rather than that of the graft itself, from the view of clinical situation. Since the graft fixation site is the weakest portion until completion of the graft-tunnel healing, the insufficient fixation strength compromises the physical exercises in early-phase rehabilitation after ACL reconstruction to be decelerated. Table 14.4 shows the failure load and stiffness of various fixation devices, which are commercially available [32–35].

Fixation techniques used for ACL reconstruction are mainly divided to two types, such as the direct-type fixation and the suspension-type fixation. The

Table 14.4 Initial graft fixation strength and stiffness in various techniques

Fixation technique	Failure load (N)	Stiffness (N/mm)
Patellar tendon [32]		
Metal interference screw	558	
Bioabsorbable interference screw	552	
Soft tissue (femoral site) [33, 34]		
EndoButton CL	1456	201
Bone Mulch Screw	1112	115
EndoButton	1086	79
RigidFix	868	77
TightRope	859	201
SmartScrew ACL	794	96
BioScrew	589	66
RCI Screw	546	68
Soft tissue (tibial site) [35]		
Intrafix	1332	223
WasherLoc	975	87
Tandem spiked washer	769	69
SmartScrew ACL	665	115
BioScrew	612	91
SoftSilk	471	61

direct-type fixation secures the graft with a fixation device without any intermediate materials connecting the graft and the fixation device. There is an advantage to secure the graft at the level close to original insertion when using an intraosseous fixation device such as the interference screw. This type of fixation can shorten the distance between femoral and tibial point of fixation, increase the stiffness of femur-graft-tibia complex, and thus restrain anterior tibial translation effectively [36].

In the suspension-type fixation, the cortical fixation devices are placed out of the femoral and tibial tunnel, and a suture material tethers the soft tissue graft to the fixation device. This type of fixation less invasively secures the graft in an inside-out fashion when using a cortical button at the femoral site and enables to control the initial graft tension when used at the tibial site [37]. Since the elastic suture material is interposed between the fixation device and the graft, the decreased stiffness of the graft construct compromises the anterior knee laxity of reconstructed knee. And it yields the larger graft-tunnel motion telescoping parallel to the bone tunnel under repetitive loading [38], even though the effect on clinical outcomes is unknown. The adjustable-loop cortical button system developed recently has an advantage, which allows surgeons to control the graft length placed within the bone tunnel during fixation procedures. It has been cautioned in biomechanical laboratory studies that the adjustable loop causes larger graft displacement compared with fixed loop under cyclic loading [34, 39], despite a no significant effect on postoperative knee stability in retrospective clinical study [40].

14.6 Graft Harvest

14.6.1 Bone-Patellar Tendon-Bone Graft

The bone-patellar tendon-bone graft was harvested using the two-longitudinal-incision technique (Fig. 14.1). A 2-cm proximal longitudinal incision was distally made from the inferior edge of the patella along the medial border of patellar tendon. The medial infrapatellar portal was placed through this incision for arthroscopic procedures later. A 2-cm distal longitudinal incision was made on 1 cm medial from medial border of the tibial tuberosity. The distal incision was used for reaming the tibial tunnel. Also, this placement of the longitudinal incision enables to approach the pes anserinus and harvest the hamstring tendon at revision ACL reconstruction in the future. The deep retinacular layer and the peritenon were dissected sharply and horizontally at the proximal and distal attachment to expose the patellar tendon and its insertions on the patella and the tibia. Using custom-made parallel knife consisting of two no. 11 blades with a 10-mm-wide interval, two longitudinal incisions parallel to the tendon fibers were placed on the patellar tendon from the patellar origin to the tibial insertion. A rectangular bone plug having 10 mm in width, 15–20 mm in length, and 10–15 mm in depth was removed

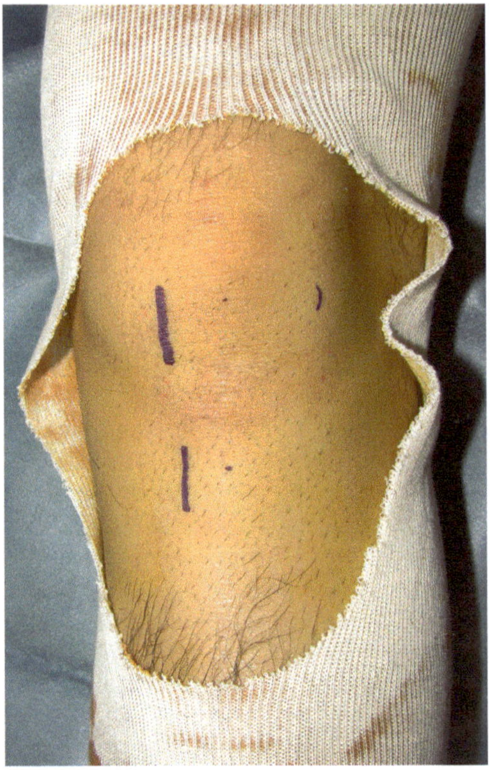

Fig. 14.1 Two longitudinal skin incisions for harvesting bone-patellar tendon-bone graft

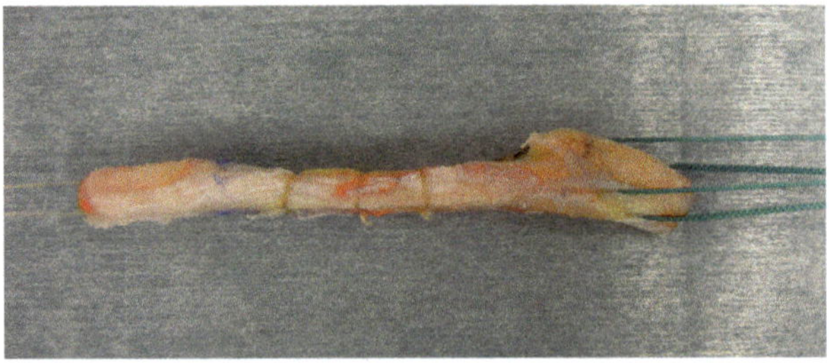

Fig. 14.2 Bone-patellar tendon-bone graft for rectangular tunnel reconstruction

from the tibial tuberosity with an oscillating bone saw and an osteotome. Subsequently, the bone plug was pulled under the peritenon and out through the proximal incision. To completely harvest a 10-mm-wide graft, another bone plug with 10 mm in width, 10–15 mm in length, and 7–10 mm in depth was cut from the distal patella in the same manner (Fig. 14.2). Bone defect on the donor site is repaired with cancellous bone graft collected by reaming the tibial tunnel later, and the periosteum is closed over the bone graft.

14.6.2 Hamstring Tendon Graft

The semitendinosus tendons were harvested from a 2-cm longitudinal incision. After identifying the tibial attachment of hamstring tendon by palpating the pes anserinus, the incision was placed on 1 cm medial from medial border of the tibial tuberosity. This incision is utilized to approach tibial tuberosity for harvesting bone-patellar tendon-bone graft at revision ACL reconstruction in the future. The sartorius fascia is incised along the fiber direction on the proximal margin of semitendinosus tendon. The tibial insertion of semitendinosus tendon is identified and sharply detached, and then the distal end of tendon is stitched with #2 nonabsorbable suture (Fig. 14.3). After complete release of fascial band extending to the gastrocnemius fascia, the semitendinosus tendon is pulled out by cutting the musculotendinous junction using a closed tendon stripper. In case a requirement arises, the gracilis tendon is harvested with the same manner (Fig. 14.4). The sartorius fascia is suture repaired before wound closure.

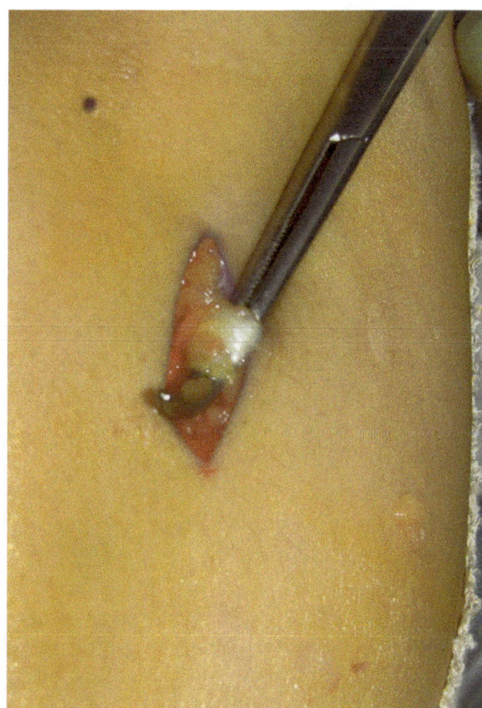

Fig. 14.3 Semitendinosus tendon beneath sartorius fascia

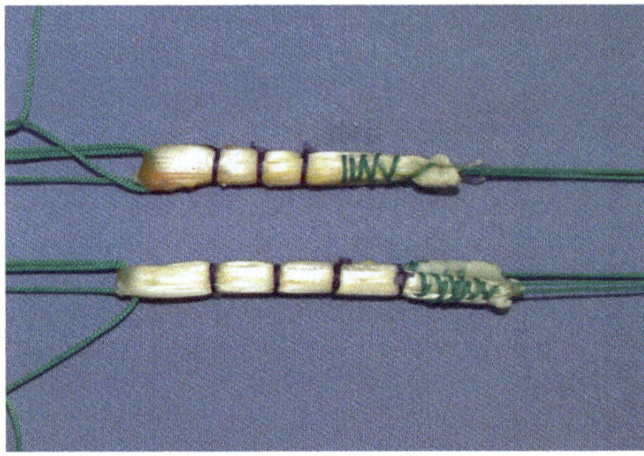

Fig. 14.4 Semitendinosus tendon graft for double-bundle reconstruction

14.7 Donor-Site Morbidity

Donor-site morbidity is a serious complication which deteriorates patient's satisfaction after ACL reconstruction with an autograft. It has been pointed out that ACL-reconstructed knees with the bone-patellar tendon-bone graft experienced anterior knee pain and kneeling pain more frequently compared to those with hamstring tendon graft [41, 42]. This is one of the major reasons that some orthopedic surgeons flinch from using the bone-patellar tendon-bone graft. On the other hand, it has been reported in clinical studies that the incidence of anterior knee pain is equal between those two grafts [43, 44]. In case using the bone-patellar tendon-bone graft, it is important to take meticulous care and make much effort to eliminate all risks of anterior knee pain and kneeling pain, such as preserving infrapatellar branch of saphenous nerve intact by using short longitudinal or transverse incisions, removing the bone plugs in requisite minimum size, restoring the patellar and tibial bone defect with bone graft, and covering over the bone graft by repair of periosteum [45, 46].

Insufficient recovery of quadriceps and hamstring strength decelerate rehabilitation progress and delay return to sports. In general, prolonged muscle strength deficit is dependent on the location of graft donor site, and then specific muscle exercises designed based on the graft choice are required especially in early rehabilitation phase. In a systematic review including eight randomized control studies, the significantly greater extension and flexion deficit at 24 months postoperatively was observed in the bone-patellar tendon-bone graft group of one study and the hamstring tendon graft group in two studies, respectively [47]. For evaluation of the hamstring muscle strength, attention should be paid to not only measure the flexion peak torque but assess the torque curve pattern. Tashiro et al. reported that the flexion peak torque angle shifted to lower flexion angle in ACL-reconstructed knees with the hamstring tendon graft, even though the value of peak torque is fully recovered [48]. This hamstring muscle weakness in deep flexion angle was emphasized when harvesting both the semitendinosus and gracilis tendon rather than the gracilis tendon alone.

Anatomical studies have previously cautioned for high injury risk of infrapatellar branch of saphenous nerve when the bone-patellar tendon-bone graft is harvested through a long longitudinal incision along the patellar tendon [49, 50]. Graft harvest through two short longitudinal or transverse incisions has been recommended to diminish a risk of the iatrogenic nerve injury [45, 46]. The incidence of damage to infrapatellar branch and sartorius branch of saphenous nerve during the hamstring tendon harvest through an anteromedial incision has been reported as more than 50 %, and it is higher than surgeons expect [51, 52]. To reduce the nerve injury, the transverse posteromedial incision placed over the semitendinosus tendon has been proposed from anatomical and clinical studies [53, 54]. In this technique, the subcutaneous branches of saphenous nerve are protected by sartorius muscle and fascia during detaching the tibial insertion of semitendinosus and gracilis tendon.

Patella fractures are one of the most serious complications intraoperatively or following ACL reconstruction when using the bone-patellar tendon-bone and quadriceps tendon graft [55, 56]. For cutting the thick and hard anterior cortex of the patella, hammering an osteotome in the patella makes a greater risk for cracking the patella. Using an oscillating bone saw with a thin blade, the patellar bone plug should be harvested in a minimum thickness leaving the subchondral bone intact. Bone grafting into the patellar bone defect also helps to avoid late patellar fracture during aggressive rehabilitation and after return to sports.

The surgical techniques for graft harvest, of course, are a crucial factor affecting donor-site morbidity for ACL reconstruction using any types of autograft. Meanwhile, it is quite difficult to clearly distinguish the causes of anterior knee symptoms and prolonged muscle weakness between graft harvest and other surgical procedures, when using the ipsilateral autograft. To reveal the really adverse effect of graft harvest on postoperative problems, several studies investigated the donor-site morbidity in ACL reconstruction with the contralateral autograft. Rubinstein et al. reported no complaint of anterior knee pain and quadriceps strength recovery to 93 % of preoperative value in the knees harvested the bone-patellar tendon-bone graft at 1 year after surgery [57]. Yasuda et al. reported that there was no significant difference in hamstring muscle strength between ACL-reconstructed knees with the ipsilateral hamstring tendon graft and those with the contralateral hamstring tendon graft after 3 months postoperatively [58]. These results suggested that postoperative problems so-called donor-site morbidity could not be attributed to the graft harvest itself as frequently as surgeons were afraid of. Less invasive tissue management should be addressed throughout all arthroscopic and extra-articular procedures. Recently, Kanamoto et al. reported a clinical study with ultrasonographic examinations and demonstrated interesting findings that increased blood flow in the infrapatellar fat pad was associated with anterior knee symptoms after ACL reconstruction with hamstring tendon graft [59]. Not only the surgical techniques, appropriate rehabilitation encouraging earlier recovery of full knee extension and patellar mobility is also a key factor to prevent anterior knee symptoms caused by patellofemoral problems.

14.8 Clinical Outcomes

Previous systematic reviews showed similar overall outcomes after ACL reconstruction between the bone-patellar tendon-bone graft and the hamstring tendon graft. Also some differences have been reported favoring the bone-patellar tendon-bone graft for stability and flexion strength and the hamstring tendon graft for anterior knee pain, range of motion, and extension strength [60]. However, the results are not consistent between original studies, and general consensus has not been reached on superiority against each other.

Recent innovation in surgical techniques might affect the long-accepted opinions in clinical results of ACL reconstruction. The hamstring tendon has an advantage to be adapted to multi-bundle ACL reconstruction reproducing the ACL anatomy. Several systematic reviews demonstrated that the double-bundle reconstruction provided significantly better postoperative knee stability evaluated with KT arthrometry and pivot-shift test than single-bundle reconstruction, whereas clinical outcomes are similar between techniques [61–63]. On the other hand, although the bone-patellar tendon-bone graft is inadequate for multi-bundle reconstruction, the rectangular tunnel technique with graft placement resembling native ACL in the fiber orientation improves biomechanical graft behavior [64]. The recent randomized prospective study, which compared the clinical outcomes between the double-bundle reconstruction with hamstring tendon graft and the single-bundle reconstruction with the bone-patellar tendon-bone graft transplanted in the rectangular tunnels, showed no significant difference in any objective knee functions or patient-based assessments [65]. Further improvement and sophistication of surgical techniques will impact on the graft selection in future.

Complete return to preinjury or higher activity level is one of the goals for patients who desire to participate in sports after ACL reconstruction. However, the best graft choice for return to sports has not been addressed because not only the reconstructed knee function but many other factors, such as fear of reinjury, attenuated motivation in competitive sports, change in lifestyle, and difference in criteria for return affect the postoperative activities. Some prospective comparative studies showed the bone-patellar tendon-bone graft was superior for return to higher levels of activity compared with the hamstring tendon graft [41]; however, only a limited number of evidences are available.

It is noteworthy that recent several publications from Scandinavian national registries reported the hamstring tendon graft was associated with an increased risk of ACL revision surgery compared to bone-patellar tendon-bone graft [66–68]. Although the graft failure and reinjury after ACL reconstruction are multifactorial, a special attention should be paid in graft selection for the patient group with a high risk of revision surgery. Further big data analysis of national registries from other countries and regions could provide a clue to a question on how surgeons decide the optimum graft for individual patient.

References

1. Hey Grove EW (1917) Operation for the repair of the cruciate ligament. Lancet 2:674–675
2. Macey HB (1939) A new operative procedure for repair of ruptured cruciate ligaments of the knee joint. Surg Gynecol Obstet 69:108–109
3. Campbell WC (1939) Reconstruction of the ligaments of the knee. Am J Surg 43:473–480
4. Jones KG (1963) Reconstruction of the anterior cruciate ligament. J Bone Joint Surg Am 45:925–932
5. Clancy WG Jr (1983) Anterior cruciate ligament functional instability: a static intra-articular and dynamic extra-articular procedure. Clin Orthop Relat Res 172:102–106
6. Zaricznyj B (1983) Reconstruction of the anterior cruciate ligament using free tendon graft. Am J Sports Med 11:164–176
7. Wilk RM, Richmond JC (1993) Dacron ligament reconstruction for chronic anterior cruciate ligament insufficiency. Am J Sports Med 21:374–379
8. Maletius W, Gillquist J (1997) Long-term results of anterior cruciate ligament reconstruction with a Dacron prosthesis. The frequency of osteoarthritis after seven to eleven years. Am J Sports Med 25:288–293
9. Shino K, Kawasaki T, Hirose H, Gotoh I, Inoue M, Ono K (1984) Replacement of the anterior cruciate ligament by an allogenic tendon graft: an experimental study in the dog. J Bone Joint Surg (Br) 66:672–681
10. Shino K, Kimura T, Hirose H, Inoue M, Ono K (1986) Reconstruction of the anterior cruciate ligament by allogeneic tendon graft: an operation for chronic ligamentous insufficiency. J Bone Joint Surg (Br) 68:739–746
11. Cohen SB, Yucha DT, Ciccotti MC, Goldstein DT, Ciccotti MA, Ciccotti MG (2009) Factors affecting patient selection of graft type in anterior cruciate ligament reconstruction. Arthroscopy 25:1006–1010
12. Cheung SC, Allen CR, Gallo RA, Ma CB, Feeley BT (2012) Patients' attitudes and factors in their selection of grafts for anterior cruciate ligament reconstruction. Knee 19:49–54
13. Woo SL, Hollis JM, Adam DJ, Lyon RM, Takai S (1991) Tensile properties of the human femur-anterior cruciate ligament-tibia complex: the effect of specimen age and orientation. Am J Sports Med 19:217–225
14. Noyes FR, Butler DL, Grood ES, Zernicke RF, Hefzy MS (1984) Biomechanical analysis of human ligament grafts used in knee ligament repairs and reconstructions. J Bone Joint Surg Am 66:344–352
15. Cooper DE (1998) Biomechanical properties of the central third patellar tendon graft: effect of rotation. Knee Surg Sports Traumatol Arthrosc 6(Suppl 1):S16–S19
16. Hamner DL, Brown CH Jr, Steiner ME, Hecker AT, Hayes WC (1999) Hamstring tendon grafts for reconstruction of the anterior cruciate ligament: biomechanical evaluation of the use of multiple strands and tensioning techniques. J Bone Joint Surg Am 81:549–557
17. Slone HS, Romine SE, Premkumar A, Xerogeanes JW (2015) Quadriceps tendon autograft for anterior cruciate ligament reconstruction: a comprehensive review of current literature and systematic review of clinical results. Arthroscopy 31:541–554
18. Haut Donahue TL, Howell SM, Hull ML, Gregersen C (2002) A biomechanical evaluation of anterior and posterior tibialis tendons as suitable single-loop anterior cruciate ligament grafts. Arthroscopy 18:589–597
19. Śmigielski R, Zdanowicz U, Drwięga M, Ciszek B, Ciszkowska-Łysoń B, Siebold R (2015) Ribbon like appearance of the midsubstance fibers of the anterior cruciate ligament close to its femoral insertion site: a cadaveric study including 111 knees. Knee Surg Sports Traumatol Arthrosc 23:3143–3150
20. Sonnery-Cottet B, Chambat P (2006) Anatomic double bundle: a new concept in anterior cruciate ligament reconstruction using the quadriceps tendon. Arthroscopy 22:1249.e1–1249.e4
21. Suijkerbuijk MA, Reijman M, Lodewijks SJ, Punt J, Meuffels DE (2015) Hamstring tendon regeneration after harvesting: a systematic review. Am J Sports Med 43:2591–2598

22. Papalia R, Franceschi F, D'Adamio S, Balzani LD, Maffulli N, Denaro V (2015) Hamstring tendon regeneration after harvest for anterior cruciate ligament reconstruction: a systematic review. Arthroscopy 31:1169–1183
23. Leis HT, Sanders TG, Larsen KM, Lancaster-Weiss KJ, Miller MD (2003) Hamstring regrowth following harvesting for ACL reconstruction: the lizard tail phenomenon. J Knee Surg 16:159–164
24. Conte EJ, Hyatt AE, Gatt CJ Jr, Dhawan A (2014) Hamstring autograft size can be predicted and is a potential risk factor for anterior cruciate ligament reconstruction failure. Arthroscopy 30:882–890
25. Treme G, Diduch DR, Billante MJ, Miller MD, Hart JM (2008) Hamstring graft size prediction: a prospective clinical evaluation. Am J Sports Med 36:2204–2209
26. Xie G, Huangfu X, Zhao J (2012) Prediction of the graft size of 4-stranded semitendinosus tendon and 4-stranded gracilis tendon for anterior cruciate ligament reconstruction: a Chinese Han patient study. Am J Sports Med 40:1161–1166
27. Tomita F, Yasuda K, Mikami S, Sakai T, Yamazaki S, Tohyama H (2001) Comparisons of intraosseous graft healing between the doubled flexor tendon graft and the bone-patellar tendon-bone graft in anterior cruciate ligament reconstruction. Arthroscopy 17:461–476
28. Ishibashi Y, Toh S, Okamura Y, Sasaki T, Kusumi T (2001) Graft incorporation within the tibial bone tunnel after anterior cruciate ligament reconstruction with bone-patellar tendon-bone autograft. Am J Sports Med 29:473–479
29. Goradia VK, Rochat MC, Kida M, Grana WA (2000) Natural history of a hamstring tendon autograft used for anterior cruciate ligament reconstruction in a sheep model. Am J Sports Med 28:40–46
30. Ballock RT, Woo SLY, Lyon RM, Hollis JM, Akeson WH (1989) Use of patellar tendon autograft for anterior cruciate ligament reconstruction in the rabbit: a long-term histologic and biomechanical study. J Orthop Res 7:474–485
31. Fu SC, Cheuk YC, Yung SH, Rolf CG, Chan KM (2014) Systematic review of biological modulation of healing in anterior cruciate ligament reconstruction. Orthop J Sports Med 2:2325967114526687
32. Caborn DN, Urban WP Jr, Johnson DL, Nyland J, Pienkowski D (1997) Biomechanical comparison between BioScrew and titanium alloy interference screws for bone-patellar tendon-bone graft fixation in anterior cruciate ligament reconstruction. Arthroscopy 13:229–232
33. Kousa P, Järvinen TL, Vihavainen M, Kannus P, Järvinen M (1997) The fixation strength of six hamstring tendon graft fixation devices in anterior cruciate ligament reconstruction. Part I: femoral site. Am J Sports Med 31:174–181
34. Petre BM, Smith SD, Jansson KS, de Meijer PP, Hackett TR, LaPrade RF, Wijdicks CA (2013) Femoral cortical suspension devices for soft tissue anterior cruciate ligament reconstruction: a comparative biomechanical study. Am J Sports Med 41:416–422
35. Kousa P, Järvinen TL, Vihavainen M, Kannus P, Järvinen M (1997) The fixation strength of six hamstring tendon graft fixation devices in anterior cruciate ligament reconstruction. Part II: tibial site. Am J Sports Med 31:182–188
36. Ishibashi Y, Rudy TW, Livesay GA, Stone JD, Fu FH, Woo SLY (1997) The effect of anterior cruciate ligament graft fixation site at the tibia on knee stability: evaluation using a robotic testing system. Arthroscopy 13:177–182
37. Shino K, Mae T, Maeda A, Miyama T, Shinjo H, Kawakami H (2002) Graft fixation with predetermined tension using a new device, the double spike plate. Arthroscopy 18:908–911
38. Tsuda E, Fukuda Y, Loh JC, Debski RE, Fu FH, Woo SLY (2002) The effect of soft-tissue graft fixation in anterior cruciate ligament reconstruction on graft-tunnel motion under anterior tibial loading. Arthroscopy 18:960–967
39. Johnson JS, Smith SD, LaPrade CM, Turnbull TL, LaPrade RF, Wijdicks CA (2015) A biomechanical comparison of femoral cortical suspension devices for soft tissue anterior cruciate ligament reconstruction under high loads. Am J Sports Med 43:154–160
40. Boyle MJ, Vovos TJ, Walker CG, Stabile KJ, Roth JM, Garrett WE Jr (2015) Does adjustable-loop femoral cortical suspension loosen after anterior cruciate ligament reconstruction? A retrospective comparative study. Knee 22:304–308

41. Xie X, Liu X, Chen Z, Yu Y, Peng S, Li Q (2015) A meta-analysis of bone-patellar tendon-bone autograft versus four-strand hamstring tendon autograft for anterior cruciate ligament reconstruction. Knee 22:100–110
42. Li S, Su W, Zhao J, Xu Y, Bo Z, Ding X, Wei Q (2011) A meta-analysis of hamstring autografts versus bone-patellar tendon-bone autografts for reconstruction of the anterior cruciate ligament. Knee 18:287–293
43. Ejerhed L, Kartus J, Sernert N, Köhler K, Karlsson J (2003) Patellar tendon or semitendinosus tendon autografts for anterior cruciate ligament reconstruction? A prospective randomized study with a two-year follow-up. Am J Sports Med 31:19–25
44. Samuelsson K, Andersson D, Karlsson J (2009) Treatment of anterior cruciate ligament injuries with special reference to graft type and surgical technique: an assessment of randomized controlled trials. Arthroscopy 25:1139–1174
45. Tsuda E, Okamura Y, Ishibashi Y, Otsuka H, Toh S (2001) Techniques for reducing anterior knee symptoms after anterior cruciate ligament reconstruction using a bone-patellar tendon-bone autograft. Am J Sports Med 29:450–456
46. Kartus J, Ejerhed L, Sernert N, Brandsson S, Karlsson J (2000) Comparison of traditional and subcutaneous patellar tendon harvest: a prospective study of donor site-related problems after anterior cruciate ligament reconstruction using different graft harvesting techniques. Am J Sports Med 28:328–335
47. Xergia SA, McClelland JA, Kvist J, Vasiliadis HS, Georgoulis AD (2011) The influence of graft choice on isokinetic muscle strength 4–24 months after anterior cruciate ligament reconstruction. Knee Surg Sports Traumatol Arthrosc 19:768–780
48. Tashiro T, Kurosawa H, Kawakami A, Hikita A, Fukui N (2003) Influence of medial hamstring tendon harvest on knee flexor strength after anterior cruciate ligament reconstruction. A detailed evaluation with comparison of single- and double-tendon harvest. Am J Sports Med 31:522–529
49. Kartus J, Ejerhed L, Eriksson BI, Karlsson J (1999) The localization of the infrapatellar nerves in the anterior knee region with special emphasis on central third patellar tendon harvest: a dissection study on cadaver and amputated specimens. Arthroscopy 15:577–586
50. Tifford CD, Spero L, Luke T, Plancher KD (2000) The relationship of the infrapatellar branches of the saphenous nerve to arthroscopy portals and incisions for anterior cruciate ligament surgery: an anatomic study. Am J Sports Med 28:562–567
51. Figueroa D, Calvo R, Vaisman A, Campero M, Moraga C (2008) Injury to the infrapatellar branch of the saphenous nerve in ACL reconstruction with the hamstrings technique: clinical and electrophysiological study. Knee 15:360–363
52. Sanders B, Rolf R, McClelland W, Xerogeanes J (2007) Prevalence of saphenous nerve injury after autogenous hamstring harvest: an anatomic and clinical study of sartorial branch injury. Arthroscopy 23:956–963
53. Roussignol X, Bertiaux S, Rahali S, Potage D, Duparc F, Dujardin F (2015) Minimally invasive posterior approach in the popliteal fossa for semitendinosus and gracilis tendon harvesting: an anatomic study. Orthop Traumatol Surg Res 101:167–172
54. Franz W, Baumann A (2016) Minimally invasive semitendinosus tendon harvesting from the popliteal fossa versus conventional hamstring tendon harvesting for ACL reconstruction: a prospective, randomised controlled trial in 100 patients. Knee 23(1):106–110
55. Papageorgiou CD, Kostopoulos VK, Moebius UG, Petropoulou KA, Georgoulis AD, Soucacos PN (2001) Patellar fractures associated with medial-third bone-patellar tendon-bone autograft ACL reconstruction. Knee Surg Sports Traumatol Arthrosc 9:151–154
56. Lee S, Seong SC, Jo CH, Han HS, An JH, Lee MC (2007) Anterior cruciate ligament reconstruction with use of autologous quadriceps tendon graft. J Bone Joint Surg Am 89 (suppl 3):116–126
57. Rubinstein RA Jr, Shelbourne KD, VanMeter CD, McCarroll JC, Rettig AC (1994) Isolated autogenous bone-patellar tendon-bone graft site morbidity. Am J Sports Med 22:324–327
58. Yasuda K, Tsujino J, Ohkoshi Y, Tanabe Y, Kaneda K (1995) Graft site morbidity with autogenous semitendinosus and gracilis tendons. Am J Sports Med 23:706–714

59. Kanamoto T, Tanaka Y, Yonetani Y, Kita K, Amano H, Kusano M, Hirabayashi S, Horibe S (2015) Anterior knee symptoms after double-bundle ACL reconstruction with hamstring tendon autografts: an ultrasonographic and power Doppler investigation. Knee Surg Sports Traumatol Arthrosc 23:3324–3329
60. Poolman RW, Abouali JA, Conter HJ, Bhandari M (2007) Overlapping systematic reviews of anterior cruciate ligament reconstruction comparing hamstring autograft with bone-patellar tendon-bone autograft: why are they different? J Bone Joint Surg Am 89:1542–1552
61. Mascarenhas R, Cvetanovich GL, Sayegh ET, Verma NN, Cole BJ, Bush-Joseph C, Bach BR Jr (2015) Does double-bundle anterior cruciate ligament reconstruction improve postoperative knee stability compared with single-bundle techniques? A systematic review of overlapping meta-analyses. Arthroscopy 31:1185–1196
62. Björnsson H, Desai N, Musahl V, Alentorn-Geli E, Bhandari M, Fu F, Samuelsson K (2015) Is double-bundle anterior cruciate ligament reconstruction superior to single-bundle? A comprehensive systematic review. Knee Surg Sports Traumatol Arthrosc 23:696–739
63. Li YL, Ning GZ, Wu Q, Wu QL, Li Y, Hao Y, Feng SQ (2014) Single-bundle or double-bundle for anterior cruciate ligament reconstruction: a meta-analysis. Knee 21:28–37
64. Suzuki T, Shino K, Otsubo H, Suzuki D, Mae T, Fujimiya M, Yamashita T, Fujie H (2014) Biomechanical comparison between the rectangular-tunnel and the round-tunnel anterior cruciate ligament reconstruction procedures with a bone-patellar tendon-bone graft. Arthroscopy 30:1294–1302
65. Sasaki S, Tsuda E, Hiraga Y, Yamamoto Y, Maeda S, Sasaki E, Ishibashi Y (2016) Prospective randomized study of objective and subjective clinical results between double-bundle and single-bundle anterior cruciate ligament reconstruction. Am J Sports Med (in press)
66. Rahr-Wagner L, Thillemann TM, Pedersen AB, Lind M (2014) Comparison of hamstring tendon and patellar tendon grafts in anterior cruciate ligament reconstruction in a nationwide population-based cohort study: results from the Danish registry of knee ligament reconstruction. Am J Sports Med 42:278–284
67. Persson A, Fjeldsgaard K, Gjertsen JE, Kjellsen AB, Engebretsen L, Hole RM, Fevang JM (2014) Increased risk of revision with hamstring tendon grafts compared with patellar tendon grafts after anterior cruciate ligament reconstruction: a study of 12,643 patients from the Norwegian cruciate ligament registry, 2004–2012. Am J Sports Med 2:285–291
68. Gifstad T, Foss OA, Engebretsen L, Lind M, Forssblad M, Albrektsen G, Drogset JO (2014) Lower risk of revision with patellar tendon autografts compared with hamstring autografts: a registry study based on 45,998 primary ACL reconstructions in Scandinavia. Am J Sports Med 42:2319–2328

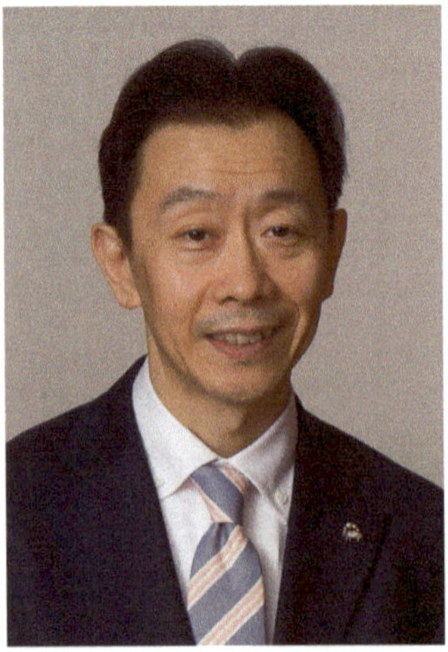

Eiichi Tsuda, MD, Department of Rehabilitation Medicine, Hirosaki University Graduate School of Medicine, Aomori, Japan.

Chapter 15
Portal Placement

Makoto Nishimori

Abstract During anterior cruciate ligament (ACL) reconstruction surgery, creating the tunnels precisely at the correct location within the very limited anatomical femoral and tibial attachments is very important for reproducing the ACL function of the anteromedial bundle and posterolateral bundle. Making such tunnels in the exact position necessary is technically demanding, but it is critical for the success of the procedure. In particular, during anatomical ACL reconstructions using the far anteromedial portal technique, the placement of the far anteromedial portal is very important. The optimum locations for specific portals and how to establish the portals needed for anatomical ACL reconstruction are discussed in this chapter. Specifically, establishing the optimum location for the far anteromedial portal will lead to a successful surgery, and that port is typically created just above the medial meniscus and about 2.5 cm medial to the medial border of the patellar tendon. This chapter provides useful information for ACL surgeons detailing how portals should be created for anatomical double-bundle ACL reconstructions.

Keywords Double-bundle ACL reconstruction • Portal placement • Far anteromedial portal

15.1 Introduction

During anatomical anterior cruciate ligament (ACL) reconstruction surgery, creating the tunnels precisely at the correct location within the anatomical femoral and tibial attachments is very important for reproducing the anatomical ACL function of the anteromedial bundle (AMB) and posterolateral bundle (PLB). Creating such tunnels at the exact position necessary is technically demanding in anatomical double-bundle ACL reconstructions. Many bone tunnel-drilling procedures have been proposed to exactly position the femoral tunnels as needed, including a transtibial technique, outside-in technique, and techniques using far anteromedial and standard

M. Nishimori, M.D., Ph.D. (✉)
Department of Orthopaedic Surgery, Hiroshima City Asa Hospital, 2-1-1 Kabeminami, Asakita-ku, Hiroshima 731-0293, Japan
e-mail: mako7119@yahoo.co.jp

M. Ochi et al. (eds.), *ACL Injury and Its Treatment*,
DOI 10.1007/978-4-431-55858-3_15

anteromedial portals [4, 5, 19]. Achieving a successful anatomical ACL reconstruction is facilitated by the use of three arthroscopic portals: the anterolateral, anteromedial, and far anteromedial portals. The proper placement of these portals is critical to the success of the procedure. In particular, the placement of the far anteromedial portal is very important for anatomical ACL reconstructions using the far anteromedial portal technique. Despite the importance of portal location, only a few papers have described the optimum locations for the specific portals used in ACL reconstructions [1, 3, 4, 14]. In this chapter, the optimum locations for specific portals and how to establish the portals for anatomical ACL reconstruction will be discussed, with emphasis on the far anteromedial portal technique.

15.2 Anterolateral Portal

15.2.1 Placement of the Anterolateral Portal

During conventional knee arthroscopy, the anterolateral portal (AL) is positioned approximately 1 cm above the joint line and about 1 cm lateral to the lateral border of the patellar tendon. During ACL reconstruction surgery, the AL portal is positioned approximately 1 cm above the joint line and just lateral to the lateral border of the patellar tendon because the ability to see the lateral notch from the AL portal using a 30° arthroscope is beneficial (Fig. 15.1). This AL portal is usually used as a viewing portal to perform the diagnostic arthroscopy and meniscal surgery.

15.2.2 Establishing the Anterolateral Portal

First, inject 50–80 cc of physiological saline from the lateral suprapatellar puncture with the knee in an extended position. After the saline injection, position the knee at 90° of flexion to confirm the AL portal position. In the ACL reconstruction procedure, the AL portal is created first. Before establishing the AL portal, confirm the lateral border of the patellar tendon and the lateral tibial plateau. After confirming those anatomical landmarks, mark the 7-mm AL portal on the skin with marker about 1 cm above the level of the lateral tibial plateau and as close as possible to the lateral border of the patellar tendon. After marking, cut the skin with a number 11 scalpel blade. When creating the AL portal, the blade should be oriented with the cutting surface positioned in the superior position to avoid damaging the lateral meniscus and cartilage. After creating the AL portal, insert a 30° arthroscope into the AL portal and perform a diagnostic arthroscopy.

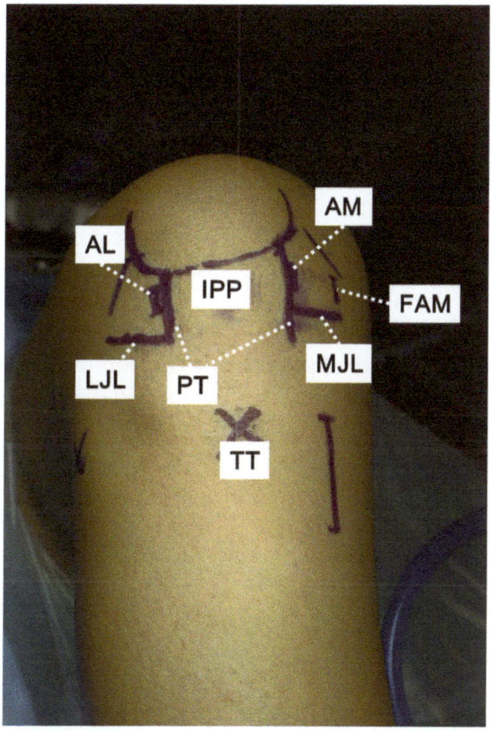

Fig. 15.1 Locations of the three portals and landmarks on the right knee joint for ACL reconstruction using the far anteromedial portal technique. *AL* anterolateral portal, *AM* anteromedial portal, *FAM* far anteromedial portal, *PT* patellar tendon, *IPP* inferior pole of the patella, *LJL* lateral joint line, *MJL* medial joint line, *TT* tibial tuberosity

15.3 Anteromedial Portal

15.3.1 Placement of the Anteromedial Portal

During conventional knee arthroscopy, the anteromedial (AM) portal is positioned about 1 cm above the joint line and nearly 1 cm medial to the medial border of the patellar tendon. During far anteromedial portal anterior cruciate ligament (ACL) reconstruction surgery, the AM portal is placed just medial to the medial border of the patellar tendon to avoid damaging the patellar tendon and about 1 cm above the medial joint line to avoid damaging the medial meniscus (Fig. 15.1). During ACL surgery, this AM portal is usually used as a working or viewing portal.

15.3.2 Establishing the Anteromedial Portal

With visualization from the anterolateral (AL) portal, insert a 23-gauge spinal needle from just medial to the medial border of the patellar tendon and about 1 cm above the joint line. Insert the 23-gauge spinal needle into the knee joint toward the intercondylar notch while visualizing the direction of the needle using a

30° arthroscope from the AL portal. Check the insertion position and direction of the spinal needle using a 30° arthroscope from the AL portal. Take care that the inserted position of the spinal needle is still placed above the medial meniscus because the insertion position of this spinal needle will be used as the lowest portion of the AM portal. After recognizing the direction of the spinal needle based on its appearance, insert a number 11 scalpel blade with the edge oriented upward instead of extruding the spinal needle while taking care to avoid damaging the cartilage of the trochlea and the medial meniscus. After cutting the joint capsule, the penetration of the blade into the joint can be confirmed by arthroscopy from the view of the AL portal.

To avoid damaging the medial femoral condyle and the medial meniscus, the blade should be advanced while confirming visually with arthroscopy. If the portal incision is not deep enough through the joint capsule, the perfusion solution will not be sufficiently discharged, making it difficult to move surgical instruments in and out of the portal. Ensure that a sufficient incision through the joint capsule is made. Begin arthroscopic confirmation by inserting the probe and forceps from the AM portal.

15.4 Far Anteromedial Portal

15.4.1 Placement of the Far Anteromedial Portal

During anatomical ACL reconstruction surgery using the far anteromedial (FAM) portal technique, the placement of the FAM portal may be one of the most important factors for achieving a successful ACL reconstruction. The optimum placement of the FAM portal will lead to a successful surgery. This portal is usually created just above the medial meniscus and about 2.5 cm medial to the medial border of the patellar tendon (Fig. 15.1). The FAM portal is usually used as a working portal for inserting instruments into the intercondylar notch and for creating the ACL femoral tunnels in the natural ACL insertion area.

15.4.2 Establishing the Far Anteromedial Portal

Under arthroscopy with the knee in 120° of flexion, insert a 23-gauge spinal needle at the optimum position for the FAM portal, aiming toward the original femoral attachment of the ACL (Fig. 15.2a, b).

The optimum location for the FAM portal during ACL reconstruction should avoid cartilage damage to the medial femoral condyle. This portal is usually created just above the medial meniscus and approximately 2.5 cm medial to the medial border of the patellar tendon. Using preoperative three-dimensional computed

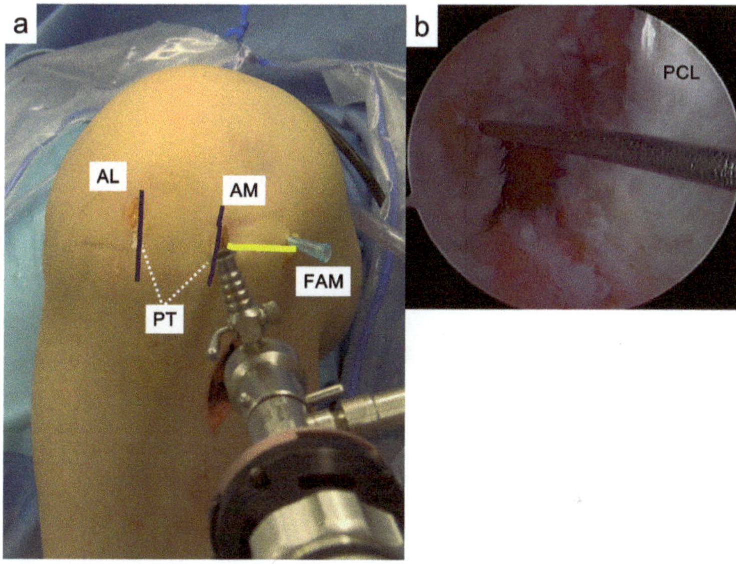

Fig. 15.2 (**a**) Creation of the far anteromedial portal. Under arthroscopic guidance, a 23-gauge spinal needle is inserted from the optimum position for the far anteromedial portal with the knee in 120° of flexion. This portal is usually created just above the medial meniscus and about 2.5 cm (*yellow line*) medial to the medial border of the patellar tendon. The FAM portal location should be as low as possible above the medial meniscus while avoiding the medial meniscus and without blowing out of the posterior wall of the lateral femoral condyle. *AL* anteromedial portal, *AM* anteromedial portal, *FAM* far anteromedial portal, *PT* patellar tendon. (**b**) Arthroscopic view of the intercondylar notch from the AM portal. A spinal needle is inserted from the FAM portal, and the distance between the spinal needle and the articular cartilage of the medial femoral condyle should be assessed with the knee in 120° of flexion to avoid the articular cartilage of the medial femoral condyle when reaming the femoral tunnels. Rotate the arthroscope to determine whether the spinal needle is positioned too closely to the medial femoral condyle

tomography (3D CT) scans, determine the optimum placement for the FAM portal. We found the optimum FAM portal location to be less than 30 mm from the medial border of the patellar tendon in male patients and less than 25 mm in female patients. Furthermore, in female patients less than 160 cm tall, it should be placed 20 mm from the medial border of the patellar tendon (Fig. 15.3a, b) [14].

The FAM portal location should be as low as possible above the medial meniscus while avoiding the medial meniscus and without blowing out of the posterior wall of the lateral femoral condyle. At this time, assess the distance between the spinal needle and the articular cartilage of the medial femoral condyle with the knee in 120° of flexion, and avoid the articular cartilage of the medial femoral condyle while reaming the femoral tunnels. Rotate the arthroscope to determine whether the spinal needle is positioned too closely to the medial femoral condyle (Fig. 15.2b). Once the position of the FAM portal is determined, advance a number 11 scalpel blade toward the ACL insertion of the femur under arthroscopic

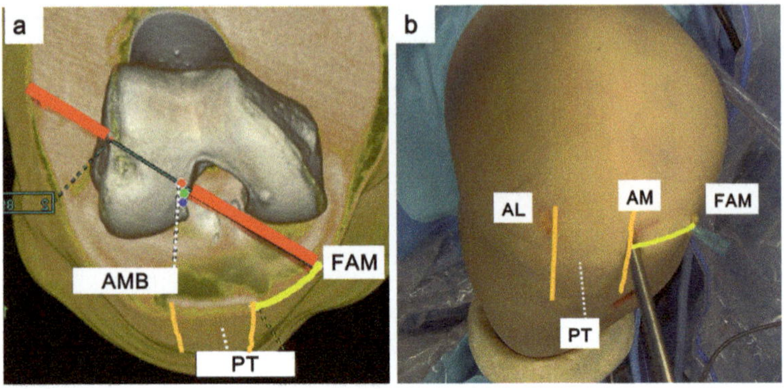

Fig. 15.3 (**a**) Preoperative three-dimensional computed tomography (3D CT). A CT scan was performed with the knee in 120° of flexion, the same knee position used intraoperatively when drilling the femoral tunnels. The distance between the optimum far anteromedial portal location and the medial border of the patellar tendon was measured on preoperative 3D CT scans. The yellow line indicates the distance from the medial border of the patellar tendon to the far anteromedial portal. (**b**) An intraoperative image taken from directly above during ACL reconstruction. A 23-gauge needle was inserted from the optimum far anteromedial portal location, which was determined using preoperative ACL reconstruction planning. *AMB*, anteromedial bundle, *PT* patellar tendon, *AL* anterolateral portal, *AM* anteromedial portal, *FAM* far anteromedial portal

visualization to create the FAM portal. It is also important to avoid the anterior horn of the medial meniscus with the surgical blade when creating the low FAM portal.

15.5 Discussion

Various bone tunnel-drilling procedures have been proposed for use during ACL reconstruction surgery to create the femoral tunnels precisely at the correct position, including a transtibial technique, outside-in technique, and techniques using FAM and standard AM portals [4, 5, 19]. Among these options, the femoral tunnels are created independently of the tibial tunnel in the FAM portal technique and the outside-in technique. This allows the surgeons to more easily create accurate femoral ACL insertions and also create more anatomical femoral tunnels. In particular, the FAM portal allows the ACL femoral attachment site to be visualized from the AM portal as tunnels are created through the FAM portal. Therefore, anatomical ACL reconstruction surgery is facilitated by the use of three arthroscopic portals, which also help the surgeon achieve an ACL insertion that more accurately mimics the ACL insertional anatomy on both the femoral and tibial sides [6–9, 15–21].

When using the FAM portal technique, the surgeons must aim toward the anatomical femoral insertion of the ACL through the FAM portal to create femoral tunnels in the very limited natural ACL attachment area. Because of this, potential risks of damaging the lateral and medial femoral condyles or the surrounding structures have been reported when reaming through the portals [2, 10–13, 22]. If the far anteromedial portal is positioned in an extreme medial position, there is a large risk of damaging the articular cartilage of the medial femoral condyle when reaming through the portal. Therefore, the position of the FAM portal may be one of the most important factors in this surgery.

The optimum FAM portal position was previously studied using preoperative 3D CT [14]. Based on the results of that study, the optimum location for the FAM portal was less than 30 mm from the medial border of the patellar tendon in male patients and less than 25 mm in female patients. Furthermore, in female patients less than 160 cm tall, it should be placed 20 mm from the medial border of the patellar tendon. This optimum location for the FAM portal during ACL reconstruction using the FAM portal technique should be used to avoid damaging the medial femoral condyle cartilage (Fig. 15.3a, b).

This chapter provided information useful to ACL surgeons when creating the FAM portal for anatomical double-bundle ACL reconstructions. Knowing the safe and optimum location for the FAM portal before surgery will allow ACL surgeons to perform safer and more anatomical ACL reconstructions.

References

1. Araujo PH, van Eck CF, Macalena JA, Fu FH (2011) Advances in the three-portal technique for anatomical single- or double-bundle ACL reconstruction. Knee Surg Sports Traumatol Arthrosc 19(8):1239–1242
2. Basdekis G, Abisafi C, Christel P (2008) Influence of knee flexion angle on femoral tunnel characteristics when drilled through the anteromedial portal during anterior cruciate ligament reconstruction. Arthroscopy 24(4):459–464
3. Brown CH Jr, Spalding T, Robb C (2013) Medial portal technique for single-bundle anatomical anterior cruciate ligament (ACL) reconstruction. Int Orthop 37(2):253–269
4. Cohen SB, Fu FH (2007) Three-portal technique for anterior cruciate ligament reconstruction: use of a central medial portal. Arthroscopy 23(3):325.e1–325.e5
5. Giron F, Cuomo P, Edwards A, Bull AM, Amis AA, Aglietti P (2007) Double-bundle "anatomic" anterior cruciate ligament reconstruction: a cadaveric study of tunnel positioning with a transtibial technique. Arthroscopy 23(1):7–13
6. Harner CD, Honkamp NJ, Ranawat AS (2008) Anteromedial portal technique for creating the anterior cruciate ligament femoral tunnel. Arthroscopy 24(1):113–115
7. Jarvela T (2007) Double-bundle versus single-bundle anterior cruciate ligament reconstruction: a prospective, randomized clinical study. Knee Surg Sports Traumatol Arthrosc 15 (5):500–507
8. Kongcharoensombat W, Ochi M, Abouheif M, Adachi N, Ohkawa S, Kamei G et al (2011) The transverse ligament as a landmark for tibial sagittal insertions of the anterior cruciate ligament: a cadaveric study. Arthroscopy 27(10):1395–1399
9. Lubowitz JH (2009) Anteromedial portal technique for the anterior cruciate ligament femoral socket: pitfalls and solutions. Arthroscopy 25(1):95–101
10. Nakamae A, Ochi M, Adachi N, Deie M, Nakasa T (2012) Clinical comparisons between the transtibial technique and the far anteromedial portal technique for posterolateral femoral

tunnel drilling in anatomic double-bundle anterior cruciate ligament reconstruction. Arthroscopy 28(5):658–666
11. Nakamae A, Ochi M, Adachi N, Deie M, Nakasa T, Kamei G et al (2014) Far anteromedial portal technique for posterolateral femoral tunnel drilling in anatomic double-bundle anterior cruciate ligament reconstruction: a cadaveric study. Knee Surg Sports Traumatol Arthrosc 22 (1):181–187
12. Nakamura M, Deie M, Shibuya H, Nakamae A, Adachi N, Aoyama H et al (2009) Potential risks of femoral tunnel drilling through the far anteromedial portal: a cadaveric study. Arthroscopy 25(5):481–487
13. Neven E, D'Hooghe P, Bellemans J (2008) Double-bundle anterior cruciate ligament reconstruction: a cadaveric study on the posterolateral tunnel position and safety of the lateral structures. Arthroscopy 24(4):436–440
14. Nishimori M, Deie M, Adachi N, Nakamae A, Ishifuro M, Ochi M (2014) Simulated anterior cruciate ligament reconstruction using preoperative three-dimensional computed tomography. Knee Surg Sports Traumatol Arthrosc 22(5):1175–1181
15. Nishimori M, Furuta T, Deie M (2014) Parsons' knob, the bony landmark of the tibial insertion of the anterior cruciate ligament, evaluated by three-dimensional computed tomography. AP-SMART 1(4):126–131
16. Nishimoto K, Kuroda R, Mizuno K, Hoshino Y, Nagamune K, Kubo S et al (2009) Analysis of the graft bending angle at the femoral tunnel aperture in anatomic double bundle anterior cruciate ligament reconstruction: a comparison of the transtibial and the far anteromedial portal technique. Knee Surg Sports Traumatol Arthrosc 17(3):270–276
17. Ochi M, Abouheif MM, Kongcharoensombat W, Nakamae A, Adachi N, Deie M (2011) Double bundle arthroscopic anterior cruciate ligament reconstruction with remnant preserving technique using a hamstring autograft. Sports Med Arthrosc Rehabil Ther Technol 3(1):30
18. Pinczewski LA, Lyman J, Salmon LJ, Russell VJ, Roe J, Linklater J (2007) A 10-year comparison of anterior cruciate ligament reconstructions with hamstring tendon and patellar tendon autograft: a controlled, prospective trial. Am J Sports Med 35(4):564–574
19. Shino K, Horibe S, Hamada M, Nakata K, Toritsuka Y, Mae T (2002) Allograft anterior cruciate ligament reconstruction. Tech Knee Surg 1(2):78–85
20. Siebold R, Benetos IS, Sartory N, He Z, Hariri N, Passler HH (2010) How to avoid the risk of intraoperative cartilage damage in anatomic four tunnel double bundle anterior cruciate ligament reconstruction. Knee Surg Sports Traumatol Arthrosc 18(1):64–67
21. Siebold R, Webster KE, Feller JA, Sutherland AG, Elliott J (2006) Anterior cruciate ligament reconstruction in females: a comparison of hamstring tendon and patellar tendon autografts. Knee Surg Sports Traumatol Arthrosc 14(11):1070–1076
22. Zantop T, Haase AK, Fu FH, Petersen W (2008) Potential risk of cartilage damage in double bundle ACL reconstruction: impact of knee flexion angle and portal location on the femoral PL bundle tunnel. Arch Orthop Trauma Surg 128(5):509–513

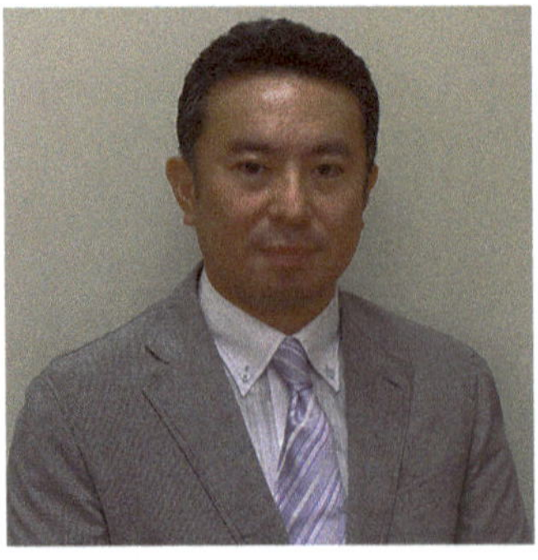

Makoto Nishimori, M.D., PhD., Department of Orthopaedic Surgery, Hiroshima City Asa Hospital, Hiroshima, Japan.

Chapter 16
Femoral Bone Tunnel Placement

Ken Okazaki

Abstract Identification of the anatomical anterior cruciate ligament (ACL) footprint is essential in femoral tunnel preparation. The lateral intercondylar ridge (LIR), which is termed the anterior border of the femoral ACL footprint, can be used as a landmark during surgery. The entire ACL footprint consists of the direct insertion of the ACL located behind the LIR and the attachment of fanlike extension fibers extended to the posterior cartilage margin. The lateral bifurcate ridge can be observed between the attached anteromedial (AM) and posterolateral (PL) bundles in 80 % of cases.

Options for drilling the femoral tunnel consist of the trans-tibial tunnel technique, the transmedial portal technique, and the outside-in technique. Although it is sometimes difficult to drill the desired point when using the conventional trans-tibial technique, modifications, such as using of a special angle guide, applying an external rotation and varus force to the tibia, or drilling the femoral AM tunnel through the tibial PL tunnel, enable consistent creation of the tunnels at the anatomical position. The transmedial portal technique requires deep knee flexion during drilling to avoid posterior wall blowout. Both the knee flexion angle and location of the working portal affect the location of the tunnel outlet on the lateral femoral surface. Retrograde reaming devices for the outside-in technique enable the use of the cortical fixation buttons for any diameter grafts. The tunnel direction relative to the cortical surface affects the shape and size of tunnel apertures at both outlets on the ACL footprint side and lateral femoral side.

Keywords Anterior cruciate ligament reconstruction • Femoral tunnel • Surgical technique

---

K. Okazaki, M.D., PhD (✉)
Department of Orthopaedic Surgery, Graduate School of Medical Sciences, Kyushu University, 3-1-1 Maidashi, Higashi-ku, Fukuoka 812-8582, Japan
e-mail: okazaki@med.kyushu-u.ac.jp

M. Ochi et al. (eds.), *ACL Injury and Its Treatment*,
DOI 10.1007/978-4-431-55858-3_16

16.1 Rationale for Anatomical Placement of Grafts

Placement of grafts within the anatomical footprint of the anterior cruciate ligament (ACL) is the primary issue in ACL reconstruction. Several studies have demonstrated the advantages of anatomical graft placements over nonanatomical placements with respect to biomechanical stability, graft impingement, and clinical outcomes [1–3]. Zantop et al. performed a biomechanical study on cadaveric knees that had undergone double-bundle ACL reconstruction using an anatomically placed femoral anteromedial (AM) tunnel and either an anatomically placed posterolateral (PL) tunnel or a nonanatomically placed PL tunnel [4]. The intact kinematics of knees with anatomical PL tunnel placement were restored and showed significantly lower anterior tibial translation under anterior tibial and combined rotatory loads than knees with nonanatomical PL tunnel placement. Kondo et al. reported a biomechanical study on cadaveric knees that had undergone anatomical double-bundle ACL reconstruction, nonanatomical single-bundle reconstruction, or anatomical single-bundle reconstruction [5]. Rotational laxity with internal tibial torque and anterior laxity in a simulated pivot shift was significantly lesser in double-bundle reconstruction and anatomical single-bundle reconstruction than in nonanatomical single-bundle reconstruction. Mae et al. used an intraoperative kinematic analysis and reported that anatomical double-bundle reconstruction showed lower tension in the grafts for restoration of the normal anterior–posterior laxity of the knee than Rosenberg's isometric bi-socket reconstruction [6]. In a clinical study, Toritsuka et al. reported that a bi-socket reconstruction with high femoral tunnel placement group received a lower subjective evaluation according to the International Knee Documentation Committee (IKDC) Knee Examination Form than low femoral tunnel placement (close to the anatomical placement) [7]. Yasuda et al. reported a prospective comparable cohort study that consists of anatomical double-bundle, nonanatomical double-bundle, and nonanatomical single-bundle reconstructions [8]. The postoperative knee laxity assessed by KT-2000 measurement and the pivot shift test were significantly less in anatomical double-bundle group than nonanatomical single-bundle group. Izawa et al. investigated clinical results of anatomical double-bundle ACL reconstruction and nonanatomical (isometric placement) single-bundle ACL reconstruction [9]. Anatomical double-bundle reconstruction showed better results in rotatory stability assessed by anterior displacement of the lateral compartment during Slocum's test measured on magnetic resonance imaging.

16.2 How to Identify the Anatomical Footprint

16.2.1 *Intraoperative Landmark*

Identification of the insertion area of the native ACL during surgery is essential in ACL reconstruction. The lateral intercondylar ridge (LIR), the so-called resident's

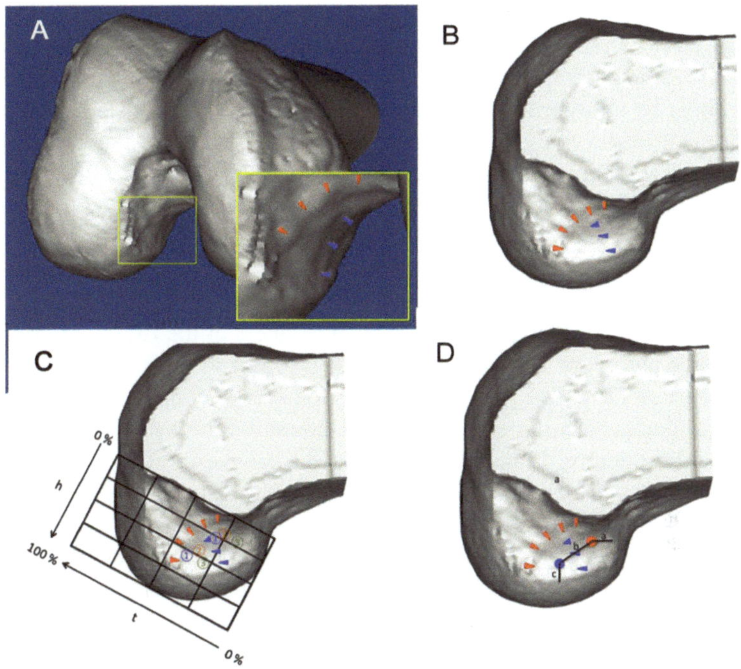

Fig. 16.1 (**a**) Femoral notch of a 3DCT model of the *right knee*. *Red arrowhead*: Lateral interchondylar ridge. *Blue arrowheads*: Bifurcate ridge. (**b**) Medial view of the lateral intercondylar notch. *Red arrowheads*: Lateral intercondylar ridge. *Blue arrowheads*: Bifurcate ridge. (**c**) Lateral intercondylar notch with the grid of quadrant method. Positions of AM and PL bundles in previous literatures were superimposed. ①: Takahashi, 2006 [23]. ②: Tsukada, 2008 [22]. ③: Zantop, 2008 [19]. (**d**) Distances between centers of AM and PL bundles and the cartilage margin are indicated with *black lines*. The position of AM and PL bundles reported by Zantop et al. were superimposed. *a*: Distance from the AM bundle and deep cartilage margin. *b*: Distance between the AM and PL bundles. *c*: Distance from the PL bundle and inferior cartilage margin

ridge, is one of the landmarks that can be used during surgery (Fig. 16.1). Iwahashi et al. performed a histological study of the ACL femoral insertion area and showed that the dense collagen fiber inserted into a concave area that was located just behind the liner bony prominence on the lateral intercondylar notch [10]. The shape of the ACL footprint was semilunar, and the mean length, width, and area of the footprint were 17.4 mm, 8.0 mm, and 128.3 mm^2, respectively. Shino et al. reported that the LIR was visible during surgery, and the femoral tunnel could be placed behind the LIR in all of their 50 consecutive cases [11]. Postoperative three-dimensional computed tomography (3DCT) showed that the ridge and apertures of femoral tunnels created behind the ridge were located at the anatomical ACL insertion site in all cases, a finding that suggested the reliability of the ridge as a landmark of ACL insertion. Ferretti et al. reported the existence of another osseous ridge between the femoral attachment of the AM and PL bundles running in an anterior-to-posterior direction behind the LIR, named the "lateral bifurcate ridge" [12] (Fig. 16.1). They showed that the lateral bifurcate ridge could be identified, particularly at the anterior part of the ACL footprint in approximately 80 % of the subjects either by arthroscopic evaluation during surgery or by histological or gross examination in cadavers. Furthermore, some recent reports have shown that the ACL femoral attachment behind the LIR could be divided into direct insertion connecting the mid-substance of the ACL with fibrocartilage layers and indirect insertion of fanlike extension fibers located between the direct insertion area and posterior cartilage [13, 14]. The area of the direct insertion was 17.7 mm in length and 5.3 mm in width, a width that is narrower than that reported in previous studies. Smigielski et al. reported that the mid-substance fibers of the ACL were ribbonlike in appearance and were 16 mm in width and 3.5 mm in thickness at the level of femoral insertion [15]. The ACL direct insertion was in continuity with the posterior femoral cortex. Similar study had been already done by Mochizuki et al. in 2006 [16]. Additionally, Tsukada et al. reported a cadaveric study that showed that although the LIR was identified in 94 % of femora, the distal half of the LIR was not visible in 18.4 % [17]. There were significant variations in the position and dimensions of the LIR, particularly in the distal part of the LIR. Moreover, the macroscopic anterior margin of the ACL attachment was located anterior to the middle and distal parts of the LIR. Therefore, they advocated that the utility of the LIR as a landmark for femoral tunnel creation was limited for the PL bundle of the ACL.

Another landmark for identification of the optimal drilling point in creating the femoral tunnels is the distance from the articular cartilage or the roof of the notch [16, 18]. Zantop et al. reported that the mean distance from the center of the AM bundle to the roof of the notch was 5.3 mm and to the shallow cartilage margin was 18.9 mm when the knee was in 90° flexion [19]. The mean distance from the center of the PL bundle to the shallow cartilage margin was 6.5 mm and to the inferior cartilage margin was 5.8 mm. These distances may be used during surgery. Tashiro et al. measured similar distances, in 3DCT femoral models of 50 Japanese subjects, for the centers of the AM and PL bundles, defined by the quadrant method reported by Zantop et al. [20] (Fig. 16.1d). The mean distances from the center of the AM bundle to the deep cartilage margin were 4.9 mm in males and 4.6 mm in females. The mean distances from the center of the PL bundle to the shallow cartilage margin were 7.3 mm in males and 7.1 mm in females and to the inferior cartilage margin were 3.7 mm in males and 3.2 mm in females. The mean distances between the centers of the AM and PL bundles were 10.2 mm in males and 9.4 mm in females. However, it should be noted that the points reported by Zantop et al. as the centers of the AM and PL bundles were those that contained the fanlike extension fibers, as discussed above. Therefore, the ideal anatomical position to create the femoral tunnel remains controversial.

16.2.2 Radiographic Assessment of the Tunnel Location

The method used to express the tunnel locations on radiographs is important for clinical study as well as for understanding the location of the anatomical footprint on the lateral intercondylar notch. This information may be useful for surgery using fluoroscopic images or navigation systems. A number of studies have used the "quadrant method" reported by Bernard et al. for assessment of tunnel locations [19, 21–23] (Fig. 16.1c). On the lateral radiograph of the femoral condyle, a line along Blumensaat's line is drawn, and the distances from the most anterior contour and most proximal contour on this line are defined as t. The distance from the Blumensaat's line to the farthest contour of the posterior condyle is defined as h, which expresses the notch height. A rectangle with side length of t and h is drawn to cover the lateral condylar notch. The location of the femoral tunnel is projected onto the anterior side (along Blumensaat's line) and proximal side of the rectangle, and the distances from the most proximal corner are measured, respectively (distance a along the anterior side and distance b along the proximal side). The ratio of a to t represents the deep–shallow position, and the ratio of b to h represents the high–low position of the tunnel in the intercondylar notch. Bernard et al. reported in 1997 that the center of the femoral insertion of the ACL was 24.8 % for the ratio of a to t and was 28.5 % for the ratio of b to h [24].

Subsequently, a number of anatomical studies have been reported showing the centers of the femoral insertion of the AM and PL bundles determined using the quadrant method (Table 16.1, Fig. 16.1c). The numerical variations in each study may have a variety of causes. The morphology of the notch may differ because of differences in individuals or race. The definition of the rectangle to cover the notch may vary because the Blumensaat's line is not always straight [25], and inclusion or exclusion of the articular cartilage within the rectangle is influenced by the method used to show the notch, i.e., plain radiography, 3DCT, or photography. Furthermore, as Iriuchishima et al. reported, the location of the center of the ACL

Table 16.1 Location of the femoral insertion centers of the anteromedial and posterolateral bundles of the ACL determined using the quadrant method

	Anteromedial bundle		Posterolateral bundle	
	Deep–shallow (a/t, %)	High–low (b/h, %)	Deep–shallow (a/t, %)	High–low (b/h, %)
Takahashi, 2006 [23]	31.9	26.9	39.8	53.2
Tsukada, 2008 [22]	25.9	17.8	34.8	42.1
Zantop, 2008 [19]	18.5	22.3	29.3	53.6
Forsythe, 2010 [21]	21.7	33.2	35.1	55.3
Iriuchishima, 2014 [26]				
Without fanlike	35	36	43	69
With fanlike	29	37	37	73

footprints could change depending on if the footprints include the fanlike extension fibers [26].

16.3 Options for Femoral Tunnel Drilling

16.3.1 Trans-tibial Tunnel Technique

Drilling the femoral tunnel through the tibial tunnel is the classic method and has been used for a long time. The method is relatively safe, the femoral drilling itself is easy, and the method may be familiar to many surgeons. However, it has been reported to be difficult to create the tunnel within the anatomical femoral insertion site of the ACL [27]. Kopf et al. reported that in cases of double-bundle ACL reconstruction, the anatomical insertion site of the AM bundle of the ACL could be targeted through the tibial tunnel of the AM bundle only in 4.4 % of the cases and through that of the PL bundle in 60 % of the cases [28]. A meta-analysis, including six studies, showed that the femoral tunnel positions were significantly higher and shallower for trans-tibial methods than for other tibial tunnel-independent methods, such as transportal or outside-in methods [29].

Yasuda et al. used a specially made angle guide for creating the tibial tunnel to indicate the direction of the tunnel that was oriented to the femoral ACL insertion site (Fig. 16.2) [30]. They reported successful tunnel creations within the femoral and tibial footprints of the ACL in anatomical double-bundle ACL reconstruction [31]. In addition, several recent studies have reported that anatomical tunnel placement could be achieved using the modified trans-tibial method in which an anterior drawer force, a varus force, or an external rotation force were applied to the proximal tibia during the femoral tunnel drilling through the tibial tunnels [32, 33].

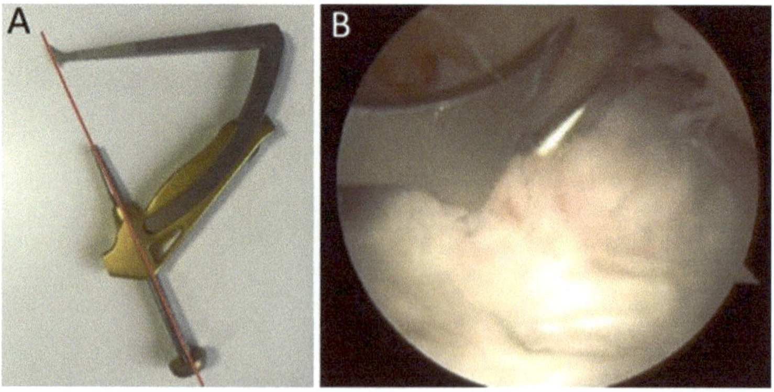

Fig. 16.2 (**a**) Angle guide with a tip indicating the direction of guide wire ("Wire navigator," Smith & Nephew Endoscopy KK, Tokyo, Japan). *Red line* shows the direction of guide wire. Note the tip of the guide indicates the same direction of the *red line*. (**b**) Arthroscopic view of double-bundle ACL reconstruction using the angle guide

Therefore, tunnels can be placed at the anatomical femoral ACL footprint using the trans-tibial method. However, some kinds of devices or tips may be necessary to consistently achieve anatomical tunnel placement. It is recommended that surgeons try several methods, such as the use of a special angle guide, application of various forces to the tibia, or aiming of the femoral AM tunnel through the tibial PL tunnel, to drill the femoral tunnel at their desired anatomical position, but alternative methods, such as the transportal method, should be considered if it is difficult to aim the anatomical site through the tibial tunnel. In addition, Tashiro et al. reported that the apertures of the femoral tunnel created by the trans-tibial method had a tendency to become an eccentric oval shape with 120–130 % elongation in the diameter of the tunnel because of the low incident angle of drilling to the wall of the intercondylar notch, which may have a risk of coalition of tunnels for the AM and PL bundles [34].

16.3.2 Transmedial Portal Technique

Drilling the femoral tunnel through the medial portal is a method that enables targeting of the drilling site freely at the surgeon's desired point. The use of the two-medial portal technique that uses the standard AM viewing portal for the arthroscope and another far medial and low working portal for a radiofrequency device or for drilling is advocated. A number of clinical studies have reported high success rates of tunnel placement within the anatomical ACL footprint using this method [11, 21, 28, 32, 35]. However, high flexion ($\geq$110°) of the knee is necessary during the tunnel drilling to avoid complications, such as posterior condyle blow-out, insufficiently long tunnels, or peroneal nerve injury [36, 37]. Nakamae et al. reported a cadaveric study that showed that a flexion angle between 110 and 120° was recommended to avoid the risk of damage to the articular cartilage and lateral collateral ligament during drilling [38]. Osaki et al. reported that the tunnel outlet on the lateral femoral surface, when using this method, was often located under the attachment of the lateral head of the gastrocnemius at the posterolateral area of the femoral condyle; thus, an interposition of thick soft tissue between the lateral cortex and cortical fixation button for the graft frequently occurred, a situation that may cause fixation failure of the graft [39] (Fig. 16.3). They showed that both the lower placement of the drilling portal and higher knee flexion angles >120° had the effect of moving the location of the tunnel outlet more anteriorly on the lateral cortex, which avoids interference with the attachment of the gastrocnemius. In contrast, medialization of the drilling portal moved the lateral tunnel outlet posteriorly. Therefore, although more medial placement of the drilling portal has a favorable effect on the shape of the tunnel aperture on the ACL footprint and avoids a predominant oval shape, it also has a tradeoff in that the location of the tunnel outlet is located at the posterior area of the lateral femoral condyle.

If the surgeon prefers a deep flexion angle >120° during femoral drilling, the position of the knee during surgery should be considered (Fig. 16.4). It may be

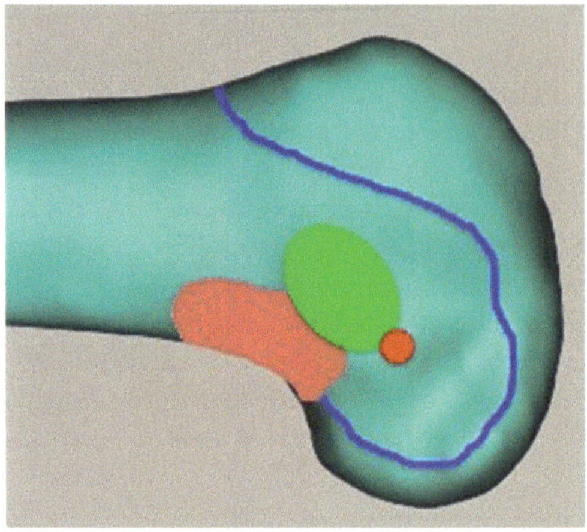

Fig. 16.3 Schema of lateral surface of the femoral condyle. The proximal and posterior area is covered by the attachment of lateral head of the gastrocnemius (*pink area*). Tunnel outlets are often located at this area with the transmedial portal technique. Deep knee bend > 135° is needed to move the tunnel outlets to the area that is not covered with thick soft tissues (*green area*). *Red dot*: Lateral epicondyle. *Blue line*: Attachment of the joint capsule

difficult to flex the knee >120° when the knee is hung on the leg holder during surgery. The use of a low profile leg holder or surgery on an operating table should be considered if the surgeon intends to drill the femoral tunnel with the knee flexed ≥130°.

The location of the tunnel outlet on the femoral surface is more lateral and posterior in the transportal technique than in the trans-tibial technique [40]. This could be a benefit with regard to reducing the graft bending angle at the femoral tunnel aperture throughout the full range of motion of the knee. Significant graft bending at the tunnel aperture might cause increased stress on the graft or tunnel aperture, which could result in the damage of the graft or tunnel widening. Nishimoto et al. reported that the graft bending angle was significantly smaller in the transportal technique than in the trans-tibial technique [41]. However, no clinical study has been reported in which either clinical results or tunnel widening was more favorable for the transportal technique than for the trans-tibial technique.

16.3.3 Outside-In Technique

The advantage of the outside-in method is that it is relatively easy to target the ACL footprint and has a good visualization for 90° flexion of the knee, which provides a familiar view of the footprint. Because this technique allows more freedom in manipulating the direction of tunnels, the surgeon can avoid complications in creating tunnels, such as posterior wall blowout and injuries of the cartilage, lateral collateral ligament, or iliotibial band. Amano et al. reported results of their case

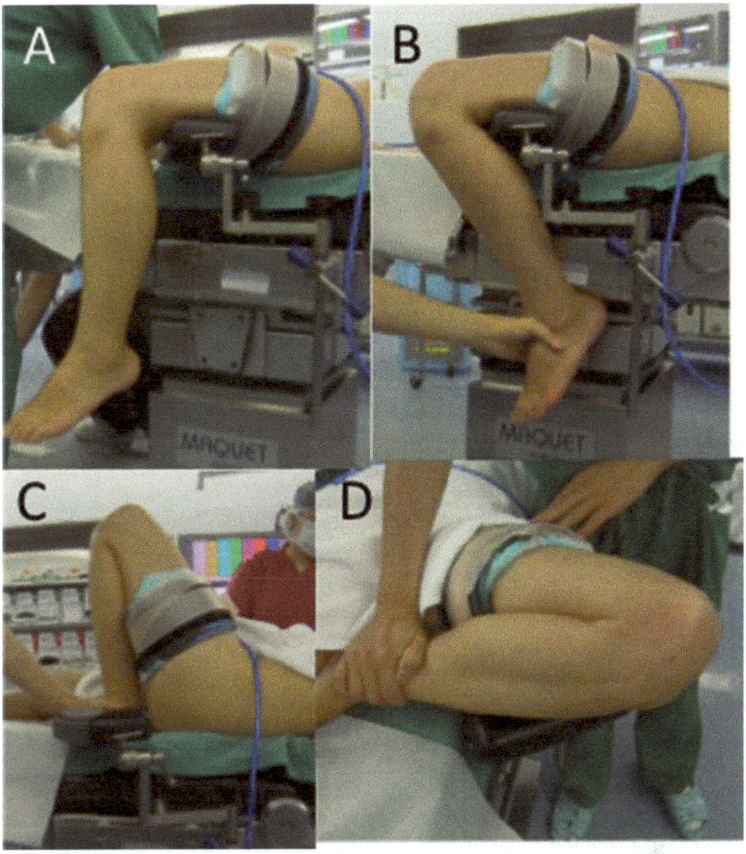

Fig. 16.4 Options of knee position during the ACL reconstruction. (**a**) The knee can be hung on a leg holder at the side or the end of the table. (**b**) Deep knee bend > 120°may be difficult on the regular leg holder. A low profile leg holder is needed to obtain the deep knee bend > 120°. (**c**) Operating on the table enables the deep knee bend up to full flexion if desired. (**d**) The deep knee bend can also be obtained with a figure-four position on the table or the regular leg holder

series of patients treated by the double-bundle ACL reconstruction with outside-in method and showed that >90 % of the patients exhibited satisfactory results regarding anterior stability, range of motion, and IKDC evaluations [42]. Although this technique requires another incision on the lateral femur, recent development of a retrograde reaming device enabled reaming of the femoral tunnel socket of any diameter through a narrow tunnel under a small incision and fixation of the graft using a suspension cortical button. Therefore, this technique may also be attractive to surgeons performing anatomical single-bundle reconstruction. Surgeons may consider manipulation of the tunnel direction using this method with an oval-shaped tunnel aperture to cover the anatomical femoral footprint of the ACL as much as possible in single-bundle reconstruction (Fig. 16.5a, b). Hensler

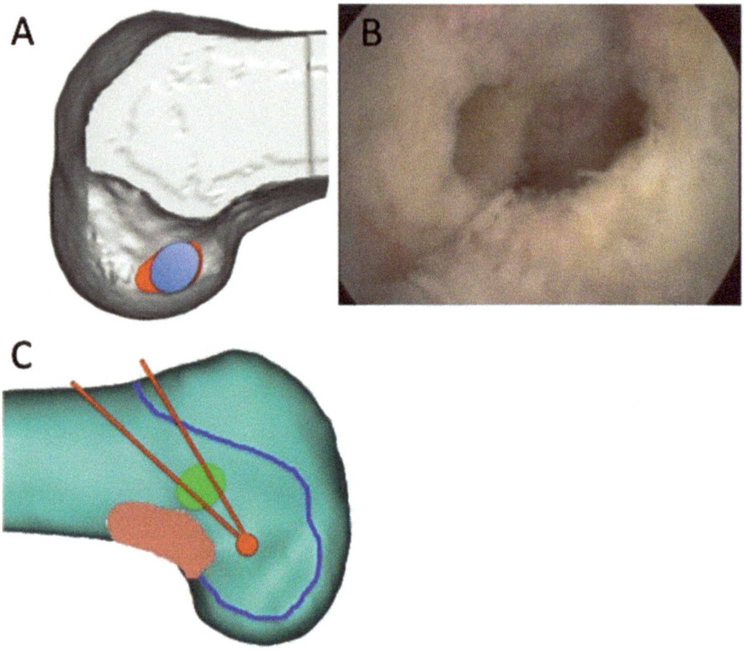

Fig. 16.5 (**a**) Simulation of aperture for 9-mm diameter tunnel (*blue oval*) placed on the ACL footprint (*red area*) to cover the footprint area as much as possible. (**b**) Arthroscopic view of single-bundle reconstruction covering the ACL footprint with the oval-shaped tunnel aperture. The diameter of the socket is 8 mm. (**c**) Schema of lateral view of the femoral condyle. Lines of 45 and 60° anterior from the proximal–distal axis are drawn from the lateral epicondyle (*red dot*). An area around 2 cm from the lateral epicondyle on the lines is indicated (*green area*). *Pink area*: Attachment of the lateral head of gastrocnemius. *Blue line*: Attachment of the joint capsule

et al. investigated the optimal flexion angle of the knee during the transmedial portal drilling to restore the anatomical ACL footprint by the tunnel aperture [43]. However, the outside-in technique is easier to manipulate the tunnel direction than the transmedial portal technique. Lubowitz et al. reported that a guide pin entrance angle of 60° to a line perpendicular to the femoral anatomical axis combined with a guide pin entrance angle of 20° to the transepicondylar axis resulted in the closest approximation of the normal anatomical morphology of the ACL femoral footprint [44]. In contrast, Matsubara et al. reported that the tunnel direction reported by Lubowitz would place the cortical fixation button on the posterior area of the lateral femoral condyle that was covered by the attachment of the lateral head of the gastrocnemius [45]. They concluded that a single-bundle tunnel connecting the center of the anatomical footprint of the ACL and an entry drilling point 2 cm from the lateral epicondyle on a line between 45 and 60° anterior from the proximal–distal axis provided an oval-shaped socket aperture at the ACL footprint that optimally covered and restored the native ACL footprint (Fig. 16.5c).

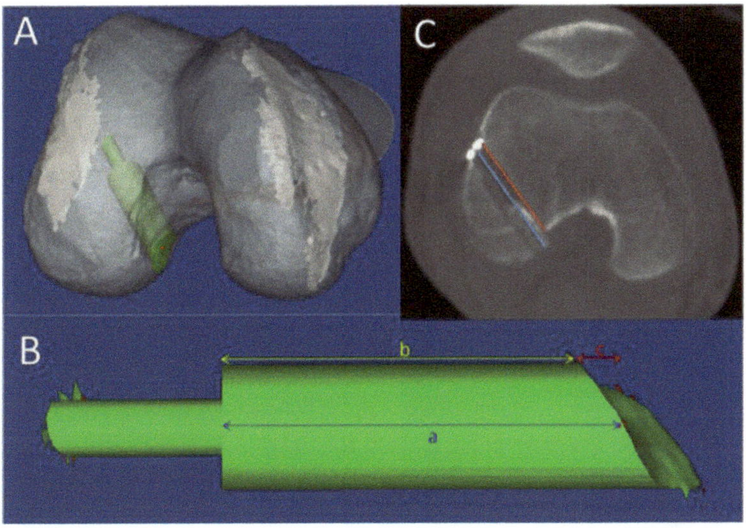

Fig. 16.6 (**a**) Simulation of the outside-in technique creating a 9-mm diameter socket with retrograde reaming. A tunnel with an oblique direction to the intercondylar wall is simulated. (**b**) The shape of the simulated tunnel and socket is shown. The socket length at the periphery (*b*) is shorter than that at the center of the tunnel (*a*). *c* Difference of the tunnel length between at the center and the shortest periphery. (**c**) A case of single-bundle reconstruction with a BTB graft. Note the tunnel length at the anterior periphery of the socket (*red line*) was shorter than the graft length adjusted to the tunnel length at the center of the tunnel (*blue line*)

A more oblique tunnel can be created if the surgeon increases the angle of the guide when performing outside-in drilling. Consequently, the tunnel outlet on the lateral femoral surface (entry point for outside-in drilling) would be located in a more anterior and proximal area of the femoral condyle. It should be noted that as the entry point for outside-in drilling moves anteriorly and proximally, the incidence angle of drilling to the femoral surface increases. Consequently, the tunnel aperture on the lateral femoral cortex becomes more oval shaped with an elongated axis. It has been reported that the long axis of an oval-shaped tunnel aperture on the lateral femoral cortex becomes more than half the size of the cortical button when the drilling entry point is located >2 cm away from the lateral epicondyle even though the tunnel diameter is 5 mm [46]. Therefore, those who make 5- to 6-mm diameter tunnels using the outside-in method for double-bundle ACL reconstruction should be aware of the risk of fixation failure of cortical buttons for grafts if the buttons are placed to align with the major axis of the oval-shaped tunnel aperture on the lateral femoral cortex.

Another concern is that the tunnel length measured in this technique represents the length at the center of the tunnel. In this technique, tunnel length is measured using a guide pin before the socket is reamed around the pin. However, when the tunnel is oblique to the intercondylar wall, the tunnel length at the periphery of the socket is shorter or longer than the length measured at the center of the tunnel (Fig. 16.6). This causes overestimation of the tunnel length and may cause a problem in graft preparation particularly in single-bundle reconstruction with a bone–patellar tendon–bone (BTB) graft. A simulation study showed that a significant oblique tunnel made using the outside-in method could cause considerable overestimation of tunnel length up to 5 mm [47]. If the surgeon intends to prepare the length of BTB graft to set the bone–tendon junction on the aperture of the socket, consideration should be given to the mismatch between the guide pin length and the actual tunnel length at the periphery of the socket (Fig. 16.6c).

16.3.4 Rectangular Socket for Grafts with a Bone Plug

Shino et al. introduced a method to place the BTB graft in an anatomically oriented fashion to cover the anatomical ACL footprint and to mimic the ribbonlike shape of the mid-substance of the native ACL. In this technique, a 5 mm × 10 mm rectangular socket is created just behind the LIR to cover the anatomical femoral footprint [48, 49]. The bone plug of the BTB graft is prepared to be 10-mm wide and 5-mm thick. To make the rectangular femoral socket, two 5-mm diameter round sockets are created, aligned side by side using the transportal method, followed by connection of the two sockets and dilation using a rectangular-shaped dilator. The outside-in technique can also be used to create the femoral rectangular tunnel, and the graft can be fixed using an interference screw [50]. Suzuki et al. reported that excellent integration of the bone plug of a BTB graft within the rectangular socket was confirmed by CT in 80 % of the patients within 8 weeks after surgery [51].

16.4 Femoral Tunnel Widening and Translation After Anatomical ACL Reconstruction

A number of studies have demonstrated that the volume and position of femoral tunnels change after surgery. Tunnel widening was often observed when measured at 1 year after ACL reconstruction using hamstring tendon grafts, with the tunnel aperture area increasing by 10–30 % relative to that of the initial area [52–55]. Some studies have reported that widening of the tunnel was more significant for a PL bundle than for an AM bundle [55]. It also has been reported that femoral tunnels had a tendency to translate in the anterior and distal directions when measured using the quadrant method [52, 53, 55]. However, whether or not this postoperative tunnel translation should be considered for the initial tunnel position is controversial because no reported studies have shown clinical differences related to the tunnel translation.

References

1. Koga H, Muneta T, Yagishita K, Watanabe T, Mochizuki T, Horie M, Nakamura T, Sekiya I (2014) Effect of femoral tunnel position on graft tension curves and knee stability in anatomic double-bundle anterior cruciate ligament reconstruction. Knee Surg Sports Traumatol Arthrosc 22(11):2811–2820. doi:10.1007/s00167-013-2693-7
2. Suzuki T, Shino K, Otsubo H, Suzuki D, Mae T, Fujimiya M, Yamashita T, Fujie H (2014) Biomechanical comparison between the rectangular-tunnel and the round-tunnel anterior cruciate ligament reconstruction procedures with a bone-patellar tendon-bone graft. Arthroscopy 30(10):1294–1302. doi:10.1016/j.arthro.2014.05.027
3. Udagawa K, Niki Y, Enomoto H, Toyama Y, Suda Y (2014) Factors influencing graft impingement on the wall of the intercondylar notch after anatomic double-bundle anterior cruciate ligament reconstruction. Am J Sports Med 42(9):2219–2225. doi:10.1177/0363546514536872
4. Zantop T, Diermann N, Schumacher T, Schanz S, Fu FH, Petersen W (2008) Anatomical and nonanatomical double-bundle anterior cruciate ligament reconstruction: importance of femoral tunnel location on knee kinematics. Am J Sports Med 36(4):678–685. doi:10.1177/0363546508314414
5. Kondo E, Merican AM, Yasuda K, Amis AA (2011) Biomechanical comparison of anatomic double-bundle, anatomic single-bundle, and nonanatomic single-bundle anterior cruciate ligament reconstructions. Am J Sports Med 39(2):279–288. doi:10.1177/0363546510392350
6. Mae T, Shino K, Matsumoto N, Hamada M, Yoneda M, Nakata K (2007) Anatomical two-bundle versus Rosenberg's isometric bi-socket ACL reconstruction: a biomechanical comparison in laxity match pretension. Knee Surg Sports Traumatol Arthrosc 15(4):328–334. doi:10.1007/s00167-006-0172-0
7. Toritsuka Y, Amano H, Yamada Y, Hamada M, Mitsuoka T, Horibe S, Shino K (2007) Bi-socket ACL reconstruction using hamstring tendons: high versus low femoral socket placement. Knee Surg Sports Traumatol Arthrosc 15(7):835–846. doi:10.1007/s00167-007-0304-1
8. Yasuda K, Kondo E, Ichiyama H, Tanabe Y, Tohyama H (2006) Clinical evaluation of anatomic double-bundle anterior cruciate ligament reconstruction procedure using hamstring tendon grafts: comparisons among 3 different procedures. Arthroscopy 22(3):240–251. doi:10.1016/j.arthro.2005.12.017
9. Izawa T, Okazaki K, Tashiro Y, Matsubara H, Miura H, Matsuda S, Hashizume M, Iwamoto Y (2011) Comparison of rotatory stability after anterior cruciate ligament reconstruction between single-bundle and double-bundle techniques. Am J Sports Med 39(7):1470–1477. doi:10.1177/0363546510397172
10. Iwahashi T, Shino K, Nakata K, Otsubo H, Suzuki T, Amano H, Nakamura N (2010) Direct anterior cruciate ligament insertion to the femur assessed by histology and 3-dimensional volume-rendered computed tomography. Arthroscopy 26(9 Suppl):S13–S20. doi:10.1016/j.arthro.2010.01.023
11. Shino K, Suzuki T, Iwahashi T, Mae T, Nakamura N, Nakata K, Nakagawa S (2010) The resident's ridge as an arthroscopic landmark for anatomical femoral tunnel drilling in ACL reconstruction. Knee Surg Sports Traumatol Arthrosc 18(9):1164–1168. doi:10.1007/s00167-009-0979-6
12. Ferretti M, Ekdahl M, Shen W, Fu FH (2007) Osseous landmarks of the femoral attachment of the anterior cruciate ligament: an anatomic study. Arthroscopy 23(11):1218–1225. doi:10.1016/j.arthro.2007.09.008
13. Sasaki N, Ishibashi Y, Tsuda E, Yamamoto Y, Maeda S, Mizukami H, Toh S, Yagihashi S, Tonosaki Y (2012) The femoral insertion of the anterior cruciate ligament: discrepancy between macroscopic and histological observations. Arthroscopy 28(8):1135–1146. doi:10.1016/j.arthro.2011.12.021

14. Mochizuki T, Fujishiro H, Nimura A, Mahakkanukrauh P, Yasuda K, Muneta T, Akita K (2014) Anatomic and histologic analysis of the mid-substance and fan-like extension fibres of the anterior cruciate ligament during knee motion, with special reference to the femoral attachment. Knee Surg Sports Traumatol Arthrosc 22(2):336–344. doi:10.1007/s00167-013-2404-4
15. Smigielski R, Zdanowicz U, Drwiega M, Ciszek B, Ciszkowska-Lyson B, Siebold R (2014) Ribbon like appearance of the midsubstance fibres of the anterior cruciate ligament close to its femoral insertion site: a cadaveric study including 111 knees. Knee Surg Sports Traumatol Arthrosc. doi:10.1007/s00167-014-3146-7
16. Mochizuki T, Muneta T, Nagase T, Shirasawa S, Akita KI, Sekiya I (2006) Cadaveric knee observation study for describing anatomic femoral tunnel placement for two-bundle anterior cruciate ligament reconstruction. Arthroscopy 22(4):356–361. doi:10.1016/j.arthro.2005.09.020
17. Tsukada S, Fujishiro H, Watanabe K, Nimura A, Mochizuki T, Mahakkanukrauh P, Yasuda K, Akita K (2014) Anatomic variations of the lateral intercondylar ridge: relationship to the anterior margin of the anterior cruciate ligament. Am J Sports Med 42(5):1110–1117. doi:10.1177/0363546514524527
18. Kai S, Kondo E, Kitamura N, Kawaguchi Y, Inoue M, Amis AA, Yasuda K (2013) A quantitative technique to create a femoral tunnel at the averaged center of the anteromedial bundle attachment in anatomic double-bundle anterior cruciate ligament reconstruction. BMC Musculoskelet Disord 14:189. doi:10.1186/1471-2474-14-189
19. Zantop T, Wellmann M, Fu FH, Petersen W (2008) Tunnel positioning of anteromedial and posterolateral bundles in anatomic anterior cruciate ligament reconstruction: anatomic and radiographic findings. Am J Sports Med 36(1):65–72. doi:10.1177/0363546507308361
20. Tashiro Y, Okazaki K, Iwamoto Y (2015) Evaluating the distance between the femoral tunnel centers in anatomic double-bundle anterior cruciate ligament reconstruction using a computer simulation. Open Access J Sports Med 6:219–224. doi:10.2147/OAJSM.S80809
21. Forsythe B, Kopf S, Wong AK, Martins CA, Anderst W, Tashman S, Fu FH (2010) The location of femoral and tibial tunnels in anatomic double-bundle anterior cruciate ligament reconstruction analyzed by three-dimensional computed tomography models. J Bone Joint Surg Am 92(6):1418–1426. doi:10.2106/JBJS.I.00654
22. Tsukada H, Ishibashi Y, Tsuda E, Fukuda A, Toh S (2008) Anatomical analysis of the anterior cruciate ligament femoral and tibial footprints. J Orthop Sci 13(2):122–129. doi:10.1007/s00776-007-1203-5
23. Takahashi M, Doi M, Abe M, Suzuki D, Nagano A (2006) Anatomical study of the femoral and tibial insertions of the anteromedial and posterolateral bundles of human anterior cruciate ligament. Am J Sports Med 34(5):787–792. doi:10.1177/0363546505282625
24. Bernard M, Hertel P, Hornung H, Cierpinski T (1997) Femoral insertion of the ACL. Radiographic quadrant method. Am J Knee Surg 10(1):14–21, discussion 21-12
25. Iriuchishima T, Ryu K, Aizawa S, Fu FH (2015) Blumensaat's line is not always straight: morphological variations of the lateral wall of the femoral intercondylar notch. Knee Surg Sports Traumatol Arthrosc. doi:10.1007/s00167-015-3579-7
26. Iriuchishima T, Ryu K, Aizawa S, Fu FH (2014) The difference in centre position in the ACL femoral footprint inclusive and exclusive of the fan-like extension fibres. Knee Surg Sports Traumatol Arthrosc. doi:10.1007/s00167-014-3373-y
27. Kopf S, Forsythe B, Wong AK, Tashman S, Irrgang JJ, Fu FH (2012) Transtibial ACL reconstruction technique fails to position drill tunnels anatomically in vivo 3D CT study. Knee Surg Sports Traumatol Arthrosc 20(11):2200–2207. doi:10.1007/s00167-011-1851-z
28. Kopf S, Pombo MW, Shen W, Irrgang JJ, Fu FH (2011) The ability of 3 different approaches to restore the anatomic anteromedial bundle femoral insertion site during anatomic anterior cruciate ligament reconstruction. Arthroscopy 27(2):200–206. doi:10.1016/j.arthro.2010.07.010

29. Lee DH, Kim HJ, Ahn HS, Bin SI (2015) Comparison of femur tunnel aperture location in patients undergoing transtibial and anatomical single-bundle anterior cruciate ligament reconstruction. Knee Surg Sports Traumatol Arthrosc. doi:10.1007/s00167-015-3657-x
30. Yasuda K, Kondo E, Ichiyama H, Kitamura N, Tanabe Y, Tohyama H, Minami A (2004) Anatomic reconstruction of the anteromedial and posterolateral bundles of the anterior cruciate ligament using hamstring tendon grafts. Arthroscopy 20(10):1015–1025. doi:10.1016/j.arthro.2004.08.010
31. Yasuda K, Tanabe Y, Kondo E, Kitamura N, Tohyama H (2010) Anatomic double-bundle anterior cruciate ligament reconstruction. Arthroscopy 26(9 Suppl):S21–S34. doi:10.1016/j.arthro.2010.03.014
32. Lee JK, Lee S, Seong SC, Lee MC (2014) Anatomic single-bundle ACL reconstruction is possible with use of the modified transtibial technique: a comparison with the anteromedial transportal technique. J Bone Joint Surg Am 96(8):664–672. doi:10.2106/JBJS.M.00088
33. Youm YS, Cho SD, Lee SH, Youn CH (2014) Modified transtibial versus anteromedial portal technique in anatomic single-bundle anterior cruciate ligament reconstruction: comparison of femoral tunnel position and clinical results. Am J Sports Med 42(12):2941–2947. doi:10.1177/0363546514551922
34. Tashiro Y, Okazaki K, Uemura M, Toyoda K, Osaki K, Matsubara H, Hashizume M, Iwamoto Y (2014) Comparison of transtibial and transportal techniques in drilling femoral tunnels during anterior cruciate ligament reconstruction using 3D-CAD models. Open Access J Sports Med 5:65–72. doi:10.2147/OAJSM.S59297
35. Taketomi S, Inui H, Nakamura K, Hirota J, Sanada T, Masuda H, Takeda H, Tanaka S, Nakagawa T (2014) Clinical outcome of anatomic double-bundle ACL reconstruction and 3D CT model-based validation of femoral socket aperture position. Knee Surg Sports Traumatol Arthrosc 22(9):2194–2201. doi:10.1007/s00167-013-2663-0
36. Nakamura M, Deie M, Shibuya H, Nakamae A, Adachi N, Aoyama H, Ochi M (2009) Potential risks of femoral tunnel drilling through the far anteromedial portal: a cadaveric study. Arthroscopy 25(5):481–487. doi:10.1016/j.arthro.2008.11.010
37. Basdekis G, Abisafi C, Christel P (2009) Effect of knee flexion angle on length and orientation of posterolateral femoral tunnel drilled through anteromedial portal during anatomic double-bundle anterior cruciate ligament reconstruction. Arthroscopy 25(10):1108–1114. doi:10.1016/j.arthro.2009.05.018
38. Nakamae A, Ochi M, Adachi N, Deie M, Nakasa T, Kamei G, Okuhara A, Niimoto T, Ohkawa S (2014) Far anteromedial portal technique for posterolateral femoral tunnel drilling in anatomic double-bundle anterior cruciate ligament reconstruction: a cadaveric study. Knee Surg Sports Traumatol Arthrosc 22(1):181–187. doi:10.1007/s00167-012-2346-2
39. Osaki K, Okazaki K, Tashiro Y, Matsubara H, Iwamoto Y (2015) Influences of knee flexion angle and portal position on the location of femoral tunnel outlet in anterior cruciate ligament reconstruction with anteromedial portal technique. Knee Surg Sports Traumatol Arthrosc 23(3):777–784. doi:10.1007/s00167-013-2705-7
40. Nakamae A, Ochi M, Adachi N, Deie M, Nakasa T (2012) Clinical comparisons between the transtibial technique and the far anteromedial portal technique for posterolateral femoral tunnel drilling in anatomic double-bundle anterior cruciate ligament reconstruction. Arthroscopy 28(5):658–666. doi:10.1016/j.arthro.2011.10.025
41. Nishimoto K, Kuroda R, Mizuno K, Hoshino Y, Nagamune K, Kubo S, Yagi M, Yamaguchi M, Yoshiya S, Kurosaka M (2009) Analysis of the graft bending angle at the femoral tunnel aperture in anatomic double bundle anterior cruciate ligament reconstruction: a comparison of the transtibial and the far anteromedial portal technique. Knee Surg Sports Traumatol Arthrosc 17(3):270–276. doi:10.1007/s00167-008-0680-1

42. Amano H, Toritsuka Y, Uchida R, Mae T, Ohzono K, Shino K (2015) Outcome of anatomical double-bundle ACL reconstruction using hamstring tendons via an outside-in approach. Knee Surg Sports Traumatol Arthrosc 23(4):1222–1230. doi:10.1007/s00167-014-2950-4
43. Hensler D, Working ZM, Illingworth KD, Thorhauer ED, Tashman S, Fu FH (2011) Medial portal drilling: effects on the femoral tunnel aperture morphology during anterior cruciate ligament reconstruction. J Bone Joint Surg Am 93(22):2063–2071. doi:10.2106/JBJS.J.01705
44. Lubowitz JH, Akhavan S, Waterman BR, Aalami-Harandi A, Konicek J (2013) Technique for creating the anterior cruciate ligament femoral socket: optimizing femoral footprint anatomic restoration using outside-in drilling. Arthroscopy 29(3):522–528. doi:10.1016/j.arthro.2012.10.007
45. Matsubara H, Okazaki K, Osaki K, Tashiro Y, Mizu-Uchi H, Hamai S, Iwamoto Y (2014) Optimal entry position on the lateral femoral surface for outside-in drilling technique to restore the anatomical footprint of anterior cruciate ligament. Knee Surg Sports Traumatol Arthrosc. doi:10.1007/s00167-014-3460-0
46. Okazaki K, Matsubara H, Osaki K, Tashiro Y, Mizu-Uchi H, Hamai S, Doi T, Iwamoto Y (2014) Femoral tunnel apertures on the lateral cortex in anterior cruciate ligament reconstruction: an analysis of cortical button fixation. Arthroscopy 30(7):841–848. doi:10.1016/j.arthro.2014.03.004
47. Osaki K, Okazaki K, Matsubara H, Kuwashima U, Murakami K, Iwamoto Y (2015) Asymmetry in femoral tunnel socket length during anterior cruciate ligament reconstruction with transportal, outside-in, and modified transtibial techniques. Arthroscopy 31:2365–2370
48. Shino K, Nakata K, Nakamura N, Toritsuka Y, Nakagawa S, Horibe S (2005) Anatomically oriented anterior cruciate ligament reconstruction with a bone-patellar tendon-bone graft via rectangular socket and tunnel: a snug-fit and impingement-free grafting technique. Arthroscopy 21(11):1402. doi:10.1016/j.arthro.2005.08.017
49. Shino K, Nakata K, Nakamura N, Toritsuka Y, Horibe S, Nakagawa S, Suzuki T (2008) Rectangular tunnel double-bundle anterior cruciate ligament reconstruction with bone-patellar tendon-bone graft to mimic natural fiber arrangement. Arthroscopy 24(10):1178–1183. doi:10.1016/j.arthro.2008.06.010
50. Shino K, Mae T, Tachibana Y (2015) Anatomic ACL reconstruction: rectangular tunnel/bone-patellar tendon-bone or triple-bundle/semitendinosus tendon grafting. J Orthop Sci 20 (3):457–468. doi:10.1007/s00776-015-0705-9
51. Suzuki T, Shino K, Nakagawa S, Nakata K, Iwahashi T, Kinugasa K, Otsubo H, Yamashita T (2011) Early integration of a bone plug in the femoral tunnel in rectangular tunnel ACL reconstruction with a bone-patellar tendon-bone graft: a prospective computed tomography analysis. Knee Surg Sports Traumatol Arthrosc 19(Suppl 1):S29–S35. doi:10.1007/s00167-011-1481-5
52. Araki D, Kuroda R, Matsumoto T, Nagamune K, Matsushita T, Hoshino Y, Oka S, Nishizawa Y, Kurosaka M (2014) Three-dimensional analysis of bone tunnel changes after anatomic double-bundle anterior cruciate ligament reconstruction using multidetector-row computed tomography. Am J Sports Med 42(9):2234–2241. doi:10.1177/0363546514540274
53. Tachibana Y, Mae T, Shino K, Kanamoto T, Sugamoto K, Yoshikawa H, Nakata K (2014) Morphological changes in femoral tunnels after anatomic anterior cruciate ligament reconstruction. Knee Surg Sports Traumatol Arthrosc. doi:10.1007/s00167-014-3252-6
54. Kawaguchi Y, Kondo E, Kitamura N, Kai S, Inoue M, Yasuda K (2011) Comparisons of femoral tunnel enlargement in 169 patients between single-bundle and anatomic double-bundle anterior cruciate ligament reconstructions with hamstring tendon grafts. Knee Surg Sports Traumatol Arthrosc 19(8):1249–1257. doi:10.1007/s00167-011-1455-7

55. Taketomi S, Inui H, Sanada T, Yamagami R, Tanaka S, Nakagawa T (2014) Eccentric femoral tunnel widening in anatomic anterior cruciate ligament reconstruction. Arthroscopy 30 (6):701–709. doi:10.1016/j.arthro.2014.02.016

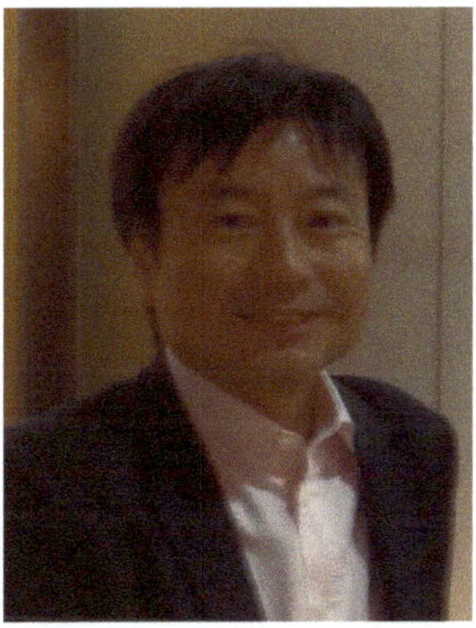

Ken Okazaki, M.D., PhD, Department of Orthopaedic Surgery, Graduate School of Medical Sciences, Kyushu University, Fukuoka, Japan.

Chapter 17
Tibial Bone Tunnel Placement in Double-Bundle Anterior Cruciate Ligament Reconstruction Using Hamstring Tendons

Takashi Ohsawa, Kenji Takagishi, and Masashi Kimura

Abstract There have been many discussions about the femoral tunnel positions during double-bundle anterior cruciate ligament (ACL) reconstruction, and several authors have reported that the femoral ACL attachment was behind the "resident's ridge" and that femoral tunnels should be created behind that ridge. On the other hand, the tibial ACL attachment is variable. Bedi et al. reported that the over-the-top and anterior tibial tunnel positions provided good control in the Lachman test and the pivot shift test compared with posterior tibial tunnel positions. However, the over-the-top tibial tunnel position may cause roof impingement, so a landmark for the anterior border of the tibial tunnels is needed. We reported that the transverse ligament and Parsons' knob are useful as anterior landmarks for tibial sagittal insertions of anteromedial (AM) tunnels. The tibial intertubercular ridge is useful as a posterior landmark for tibial sagittal insertions of posterolateral (PL) tunnels. Furthermore, the medial intercondylar ridge is useful as a medial landmark for insertions of both tunnels. In this chapter, we introduce the technique of arthroscopic anatomical double-bundle ACL reconstruction, focusing on tibial tunnel creation in particular.

Keyword Tibial tunnel • Transverse ligament • Parsons' knob • Tibial intertubercular ridge • Medial intercondylar ridge

T. Ohsawa, M.D., PhD (✉) • K. Takagishi
Department of Orthopaedic Surgery, Gunma University, 3-39-15 Showa-machi, Maebashi, Gunma 371-8511, Japan
e-mail: tk.ohsawa@gmail.com

M. Kimura
Gunma Sports Medicine Research Center, Zenshukai Hospital, Gunma, Japan

M. Ochi et al. (eds.), *ACL Injury and Its Treatment*,
DOI 10.1007/978-4-431-55858-3_17

17.1 Introduction

Anterior cruciate ligament (ACL) reconstruction is performed widely all over the world. Recently, the femoral tunnel position has been well described in the literature [1–3]. Several authors reported that the femoral ACL attachment was behind the "resident's ridge" and that femoral tunnels should be created behind that ridge [4–6]. In association with the discussions about femoral tunnel positions, the discussions about tibial tunnel positions have thrived. Howell et al. reported that the tibial tunnels should be posterior because of roof impingement [7], but the femoral and tibial tunnel placements were not anatomical. Iriuchishima et al. proved that roof impingement does not occur if the femoral and tibial tunnels are created anatomically [8]. Bedi et al. reported that the over-the-top and anterior tibial tunnel positions provided good control in the Lachman test and the pivot shift test compared with posterior tibial tunnel positions [9]. However, an anterior tibial tunnel position increased the risk of roof impingement in extension. Thus, a landmark for the anterior border of the tibial tunnels is needed. Kongcharoensombat et al. reported that a transverse ligament that connects the anterior margin of the lateral meniscus to the anterior horn of the medial meniscus is useful as a landmark for tibial sagittal insertions during arthroscopic surgery [10]. However, the position of the transverse ligament changes with knee flexion angle and has some variations [11]. Berg reported that a bony prominence called Parsons' knob (tuberculum intercondylare tertium), located anterior to the anterior horn of the medial meniscus and the ACL, is useful as a landmark for the anterior edge of the anteromedial (AM) tunnel on sagittal X-ray [12]. However, it is difficult to clarify the position of Parsons' knob during arthroscopy. Therefore, using both the transverse ligament and Parsons' knob is useful for checking the anterior edge of the AM tunnel. We reported the clinical results comparing two tibial tunnel positions during double-bundle ACL reconstruction [13]. We concluded that patients in the anterior tunnel position group showed better knee stability and range of motion for flexion than those in the posterior tibial tunnel group and that the transverse ligament and Parsons' knob are useful as landmarks for the anterior edge of the AM tunnel. Purnell et al. reported that the medial intercondylar ridge can be used as the medial edge of the ACL tunnel [14]. Recently, Siebold et al. reported the ACL tibial "C"-shaped insertion site and the relationship of the ACL tibial attachment and the bony insertion of the anterior root of the lateral meniscus [15]. They concluded that no posterolateral inserting ACL fibers were found, but posteromedial inserting ACL fibers were found. The anterior root attachment of the lateral meniscus was found posterolateral to the ACL fibers. We usually create the PL tunnel just lateral to the medial intercondylar ridge to avoid injuring the anterior root attachment of the lateral meniscus. Tensho et al. reported the three bony landmarks, Parson's knob as an anterior landmark, the medial intercondylar ridge as a medial landmark, the lateral groove as a lateral landmark, and the intertubercular fossa as a posterior landmark on 3D CT [16]. In this chapter, we introduce the technique of arthroscopic anatomical double-bundle ACL reconstruction, focusing particularly on tibial tunnel creation.

17.2 Methods

17.2.1 Surgical Procedure

17.2.1.1 Graft Harvesting and Preparation

Only the semitendinosus tendon or the semitendinosus and gracilis tendons are harvested with a tendon harvester after an approximately 4-cm longitudinal incision is made. If double-looped grafts for the AM and posterolateral (PL) bundles are smaller than 6 mm in diameter and 60 mm in length, we add gracilis tendons. An EndoButton CL (Smith & Nephew Endoscopy, Andover, MA) is connected to the loop end, and a Telos artificial ligament (Telos, Marburg, Germany) is tied to the free end of the graft.

17.2.1.2 Tibial Tunnel Creation

Double-bundle ACL reconstruction is performed with a tibial insertion site length of 14 mm or more [17]. An anteromedial portal is usually used for arthroscopic viewing of the ACL tibial attachment. We make an AM tunnel lateral to the medial intercondylar ridge and posterior to the transverse ligament or Parsons' knob at 90° of knee flexion (Figs. 17.1 and 17.2). It is important to carefully check the medial intercondylar ridge and the transverse ligament. The border of the medial intercondylar ridge and ACL remnant can be checked by the anteromedial portal. We do not usually use the anterior root attachment of the lateral meniscus as a landmark because the attachment is variable [18] and not visible during tibial remnant-preserved technique. The 2.4-mm guide wires are inserted into the tibial cortical surface 1–2 cm proximal from the tibial attachment of the hamstrings using outside-in technique with an acufex director ACL aimer (Smith & Nephew Endoscopy) via a far anteromedial portal. We always check that the 2.4-mm guide wire has been inserted just behind Parsons' knob by a sagittal X-ray and just lateral to the medial intercondylar ridge by a coronal X-ray (Fig. 17.3). If the guide wire goes through Parsons' knob, the guide wire should be inserted more posterior. A 5.0- to 7.0-mm tunnel is then drilled over the guide wire for the AM tunnel. The 2.4-mm guide wires are inserted into the tibial cortical surface about one finger medial to the AM tunnel. The PL tunnel is also created just lateral to the medial intercondylar ridge. If the PL tunnel position is too lateral, impingement to the intercondylar notch may occur. The PL tunnel's position in front of the tibial intertubercular ridge and the 8–9-mm distance between it and the guide wire for the AM tunnel are also checked by a sagittal X-ray. The two tunnels have no direct line of communication.

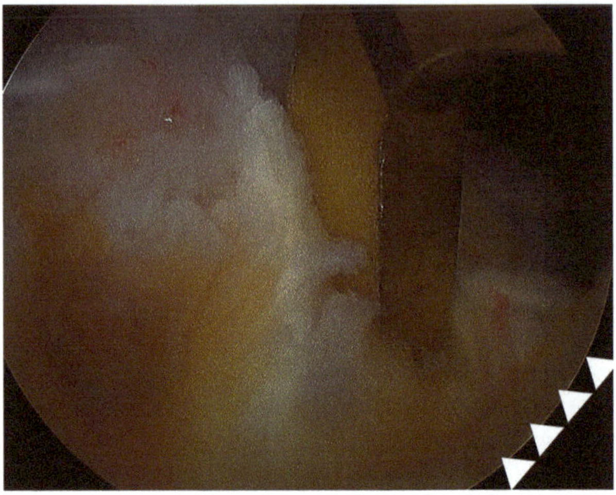

Fig. 17.1 Intraoperative arthroscopic view from the anterolateral portal
▽ shows the transverse ligament. The 2.4-mm guide wire for the AM tunnel should be inserted just posterior to the transverse ligament at 90° knee flexion. The AM tunnel position must not be too anterior to the ACL tibial attachment. It is important to maintain 90° knee flexion to avoid misplacement caused by changing the position of the transverse ligament

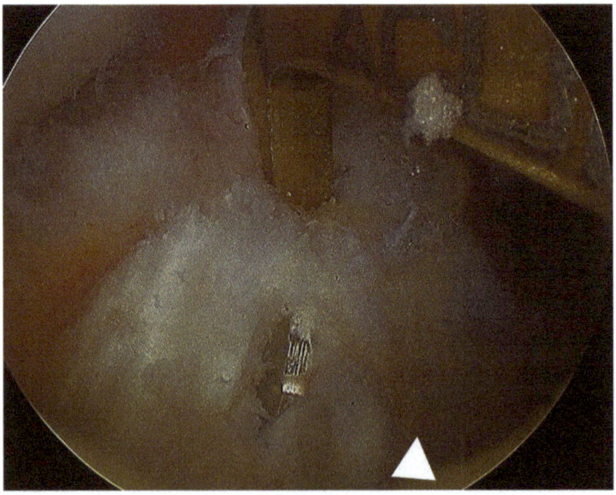

Fig. 17.2 Intraoperative arthroscopic view from the anteromedial portal
△ shows the medial intercondylar ridge. The guide wire for the AM tunnel is inserted just posterior to the transverse ligament and lateral to the medial intercondylar ridge. The guide wire for the PL tunnel is inserted lateral to the medial intercondylar ridge and anterior to the tibial intertubercular ridge. The anteromedial portal is useful for checking the position of the medial intercondylar ridge, the tibial intertubercular ridge, and the relationships of the AM and PL tunnels

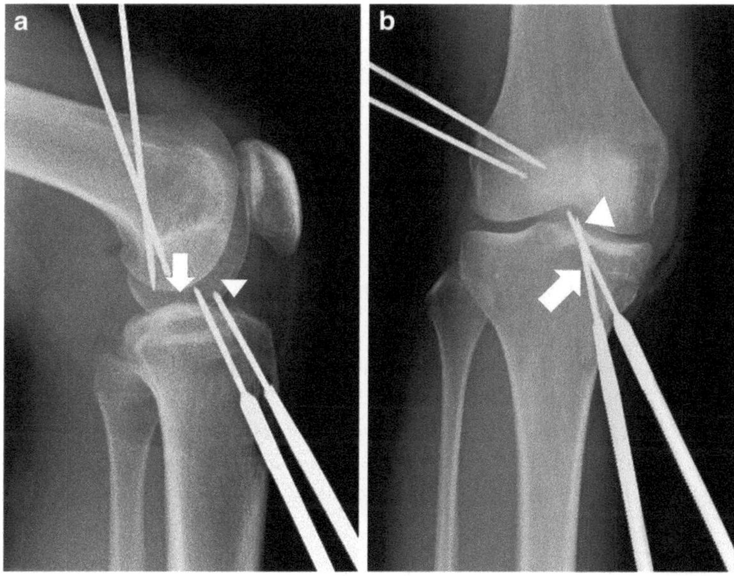

Fig. 17.3 Intraoperative X-rays.
(a) Intraoperative sagittal X-ray
▽ shows Parsons' knob, and ⇩ shows the tibial intertubercular ridge. An intraoperative sagittal X-ray is always taken to check the relationship of the position of the 2.4-mm guide wire with the AM tunnel and Parsons' knob. If the 2.4-mm guide wire for the AM tunnel is positioned through Parsons' knob, the guide wire is reinserted just posterior to Parsons' knob.
(b) Intraoperative coronal X-ray
⇩ shows the guide wire for the AM and PL tunnels. We usually check that both guide wires are positioned just lateral to the medial intercondylar ridge (▽ shows the medial intercondylar ridge) and do not go through too close to the medial tibial plateau

17.2.1.3 Femoral Tunnel Creation

We usually check the "resident's ridge" on the lateral wall after cleaning up the ACL remnant. The "resident's ridge" is defined as a vertical-to-transverse cortical thickening of the lateral femoral condyle at 90° of knee flexion. We make femoral tunnels behind the "resident's ridge," using a far anteromedial portal technique or the outside-in technique for making the AM and PL tunnels. Far anteromedial portal viewing is useful for checking the relationships between the "resident's ridge" and the AM and PL tunnels. A 2.4-mm guide wire is inserted in the footprint behind the ridge. Then, a 5.0- to 7.0-mm tunnel is drilled over the guide wire for the AM and PL grafts.

17.2.1.4 Graft Fixation

The graft for the PL bundle is first introduced through the joint to the femoral drill hole using a passing pin (Smith & Nephew Endoscopy). The EndButton is flipped and fixed on the femoral cortical surface. Then, the graft for the AM bundle is introduced and fixed in the same manner. Staples are used for the graft fixation on the tibial side at 20° of knee flexion, and both grafts are fixed together. The tibial fixation of the AM and PL grafts is carried out with 30 N of traction applied to each bundle. Postoperatively, a knee brace is used to immobilize the knee at 20° of flexion.

17.2.2 Postoperative Management

Continuous passive motion is started 2 days postoperatively. Two weeks postoperatively, weight-bearing is initiated, and full weight-bearing is started at 4 weeks. Jogging is encouraged after 3 months postoperatively. Sprinting and various competitive exercises are allowed 6 months postoperatively, and return to full sports activities is allowed at 8 months postoperatively.

17.3 Postoperative Evaluations

A case at 1 year after surgery is shown.

17.3.1 Postoperative CT

Postoperative CT is shown in Fig. 17.4. The AM tunnel was created just behind Parsons' knob, and the PL tunnel was just in front of the tibial intertubercular ridge. Both tunnels were positioned just lateral to the medial intercondylar ridge.

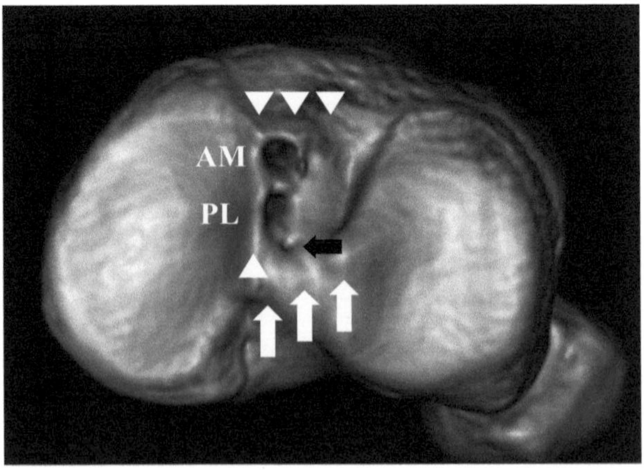

Fig. 17.4 3D CT at 1-year postoperative
▽ shows Parsons' knob, and ⇩ shows the tibial intertubercular ridge. The AM and PL tunnels are positioned just lateral to the medial intercondylar ridge (△ shows the medial intercondylar ridge). ➡ shows the intertubercular fossa; the PL tunnel is just anterior to the fossa. Both tunnels have no direct line of communication

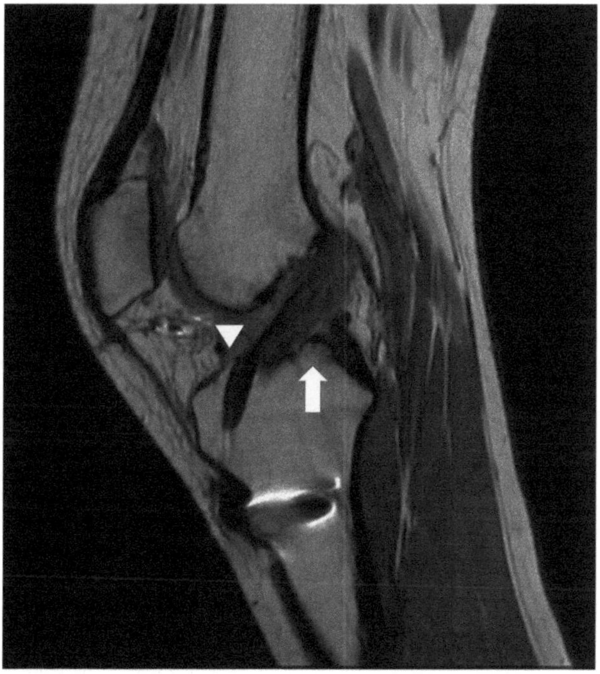

Fig. 17.5 Sagittal MRI at 1-year postoperative Roof impingement and cyclops regions were not suspected in this case. The AM tunnel is positioned just posterior to Parsons' knob. The PL tunnel is positioned just anterior to the tibial intertubercular ridge. ▽ shows Parsons' knob, and ⇩ shows the tibial intertubercular ridge

17.3.2 Postoperative MRI

Roof impingement and cyclops regions were not suspected on MRI (Fig. 17.5).

17.3.3 Second-Look Arthroscopy

Figure 17.6 shows the view at second-look arthroscopy at 1-year postoperative in a case in which the technique mentioned above was performed. The approach to second-look arthroscopy was reported previously [13]. There were no tears and impingement, the synovial cover was evaluated as excellent, and the tension of the graft was evaluated as being taut.

17.4 Conclusion

The relationship between femoral and tibial tunnel positions is important to avoid causing impingement. During ACL reconstruction, the transverse ligament and Parsons' knob are useful as anterior landmarks, the medial intercondylar ridge is

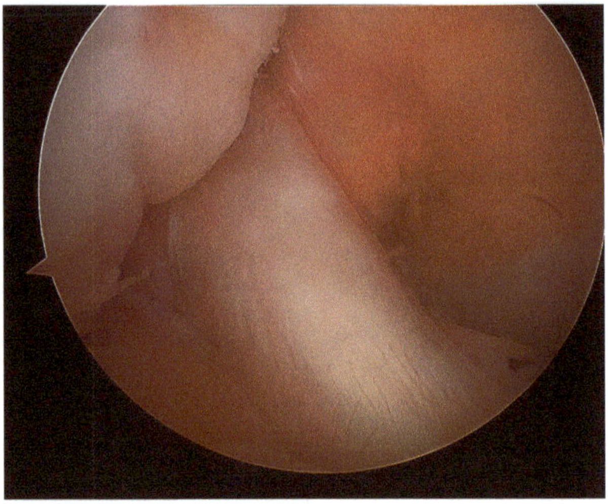

Fig. 17.6 Second-look arthroscopy at 1-year postoperative
This is a reconstructed AM graft of the ACL from the anterolateral portal. The synovial cover is evaluated as excellent, tension is evaluated as taut, and there is no tear of the AM graft. This view of second-look arthroscopy shows that this tunnel position does not cause roof impingement

useful as a medial landmark, and the tibial intertubercular ridge is useful as a posterior landmark.

References

1. Yasuda K, Kondo E, Ichiyama H, Tanabe Y, Tohyama H (2006) Clinical evaluation of anatomic double-bundle anterior cruciate ligament reconstruction procedure using hamstring tendon grafts: comparisons among 3 different procedures. Arthroscopy 22:240–251
2. Muneta T, Koga H, Mochizuki T et al (2007) A prospective randomized study of 4-strand semitendinosus tendon anterior cruciate ligament reconstruction comparing single-bundle and double-bundle techniques. Arthroscopy 23:618–628
3. Zantop T, Diermann N, Schumacher T, Schanz S, Fu FH, Petersen W (2008) Anatomical and nonanatomical double-bundle anterior cruciate ligament reconstruction: importance of femoral tunnel location on knee kinematics. Am J Sports Med 36(4):678–685. doi:10.1177/0363546508314414
4. Hutchinson MR, Ash SA (2003) Resident's ridge: assessing the cortical thickness of the lateral wall and roof of the intercondylar notch. Arthroscopy 19:931–935
5. Ferretti M, Ekdahl M, Shen W, Fu FH (2007) Osseous landmarks of the femoral attachment of the anterior cruciate ligament: an anatomic study. Arthroscopy 23:1218–1225
6. Shino K, Suzuki T, Iwahashi T et al (2010) The resident's ridge as an arthroscopic landmark for anatomical femoral tunnel drilling in ACL reconstruction. Knee Surg Sports Traumatol Arthrosc 18(9):1164–1168
7. Howell SM, Wallace MP, Hull ML, Deutsch ML (1999) Evaluation of the single-incision arthroscopic technique for anterior cruciate ligament replacement: a study of tibial tunnel placement, intraoperative graft tension, and stability. Am J Sports Med 27(3):284–293
8. Iriuchishima T, Tajima G, Ingham SJ, Shen W, Smolinski P, Fu FH (2010) Impingement pressure in the anatomical and nonanatomical anterior cruciate ligament reconstruction: a cadaver study. Am J Sports Med 38(8):1611–1617. doi:10.1177/0363546510363461

9. Bedi A, Maak T, Musahl V, Citak M, O'Loughlin PF, Choi D, Pearle AD (2011) Effect of tibial tunnel position on stability of the knee after anterior cruciate ligament reconstruction: is the tibial tunnel position most important? Am J Sports Med 39(2):366–373. doi:10.1177/0363546510388157
10. Kongcharoensombat W, Ochi M, Abouheif M, Adachi N, Ohkawa S, Kamei G, Okuhara A, Shibuya H, Niimoto T, Nakasa T, Nakamae A, Deie M (2011) The transverse ligament as a landmark for tibial sagittal insertions of the anterior cruciate ligament: a cadaveric study. Arthroscopy 27(10):1395–1399. doi:10.1016/j.arthro.2011.05.019
11. Nelson EW, LaPrade RF (2000) The anterior intermeniscal ligament of the knee. An anatomic study. Am J Sports Med 28(1):74–76
12. Berg EE (1993) Parsons' knob (tuberculum intercondylare tertium): a guide to tibial anterior cruciate ligament insertion. Clin Orthop Relat Res 292:229–231
13. Ohsawa T, Kimura M, Hagiwara K, Yorifuji H, Takagishi K (2012) Clinical and second-look arthroscopic study comparing 2 tibial landmarks for tunnel insertions during double-bundle ACL reconstruction with a minimum 2-year follow-up. Am J Sports Med 40(11):2479–2486. doi:10.1177/0363546512458257
14. Purnell ML, Larson AI, Clancy W (2008) Anterior cruciate ligament insertions on the tibia and femur and their relationships to critical bony landmarks using high-resolution volume-rendering computed tomography. Am J Sports Med 36(11):2083–2090. doi:10.1177/0363546508319896
15. Siebold R, Schuhmacher P, Fernandez F, Smigielski R, Fink C, Brehmer A, Kirsch J (2015) Flat midsubstance of the anterior cruciate ligament with tibial "C"-shaped insertion site. Knee Surg Sports Traumatol Arthrosc 23(11):3136–42. doi:10.1007/s00167-014-3058-6
16. Tensho K, Shimodaira H, Aoki T, Narita N, Kato H, Kakegawa A, Fukushima N, Moriizumi T, Fujii M, Fujinaga Y, Saito N (2014) Bony landmarks of the anterior cruciate ligament tibial footprint: a detailed analysis comparing 3-dimensional computed tomography images to visual and histological evaluations. Am J Sports Med 42(6):1433–1440
17. Van Eck CF, Lesniak BP, Schreiber VM, Fu FH (2010) Anatomic single- and double-bundle anterior cruciate ligament reconstruction flowchart. Arthroscopy 26(2):258–268. doi:10.1016/j.arthro.2009.07.027
18. Ferretti M, Doca D, Ingham SM, Cohen M, Fu FH (2012) Bony and soft tissue landmarks of the ACL tibial insertion site: an anatomical study. Knee Surg Sports Traumatol Arthrosc 20(1):62–68. doi:10.1007/s00167-011-1592-z

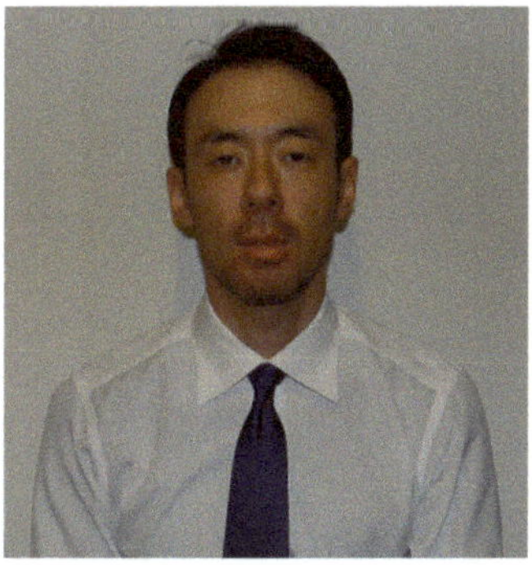

Takashi Ohsawa, M.D., PhD., Department of Orthopaedic Surgery, Gunma University, Gunma, Japan.

Chapter 18
Tensioning and Fixation of the Graft

Tatsuo Mae and Konsei Shino

Abstract Initial tension at graft fixation in ACL reconstruction is one of the important factors for successful outcomes. Excessive low tension leads to lax knee, which resulted in an unsatisfied outcome, while too much tension may bring the abnormal tibial position relative to femur and the deleterious effects of articular cartilage, which resulted in graft tear or cartilage degeneration. However, there is still no clear consensus on the optimal initial tension in clinical situation, though the initial tension must be within the safety range. Laxity match pretension (LMP), which is the graft tension to obtain the normal anterior-posterior laxity in ACL reconstruction, can be the standard of graft tension, whereas that depends on the graft materials and the surgical procedures. Thus, a safe range of initial tension based on the LMP should be taken into account in ACL reconstruction. Additionally, the tensioning boot system is quite useful to apply the intended tension to the graft, because this system makes it possible to give tension to graft on the basis of the tibia at graft fixation.

Keywords ACL • Graft • Tension • Laxity match pretension • Tensioning boot system

18.1 Introduction

Initial tension at graft fixation is one of the key factors for satisfactory outcomes after ACL reconstruction. There were some studies to investigate the effect of initial tension on the outcomes after ACL reconstruction, while the optimal initial tension at graft fixation still has room for discussion. Excessive low tension leads to lax knee immediately after fixation, which resulted in an unsatisfied outcome. Fleming et al. reported that anterior tibial displacement decreased with increase

T. Mae, M.D., PhD (✉)
Department of Orthopaedic Surgery, Osaka University Graduate School of Medicine, 2-2 Yamada-oka, Suita, Osaka 565-0871, Japan
e-mail: ta-mae@umin.ac.jp

K. Shino, M.D., PhD
Sports Orthopaedic Center, Yukioka Hospital, 2-2-3 Ukita, Kita-ku, Osaka 530-0021, Japan

M. Ochi et al. (eds.), *ACL Injury and Its Treatment*,
DOI 10.1007/978-4-431-55858-3_18

of initial tension in response to anterior tibial load in cadaveric ACL reconstruction and showed that larger initial tension at graft fixation had advantage for anterior knee stability [1]. It could be reasonably assumed indispensable to apply greater initial tension than the physiological tension of the normal ACL for restoration of knee stability after ACL reconstruction, as the stress relaxation and the remodeling of graft must be taken into account after graft fixation. On the other hand, some investigators warned that excessive great initial tension might lead to loss of extension, graft failure, abnormal femur-tibial relationship, and cartilage degeneration [2–7]. Yoshiya et al. reconstructed ACL with 1 or 39 N of initial tension for medial one third of patellar tendon graft in canine model and suggested that minimal tension should be applied to the graft, as poor vascularity and focal myxoid degeneration was found at 3 months within the grafts which had been pretensioned at 39 N [7]. These studies suggest excessive low and high initial tension should be avoided. Therefore, it is necessary to determine the optimal initial tension at graft fixation in ACL reconstruction.

18.2 Effect of Initial Tension

ACL graft runs from the supero-posterior margin of the lateral wall of the intercondylar notch to anteromedial portion of the tibial plateau. Once graft fixes on the femoral side in ACL reconstruction, tibia can move on the basis of femur in pulling graft with tension. Melby III et al. described increase of graft tensioning in ACL reconstruction which resulted in posterior subluxation of the tibia and lateral/external rotation tibial subluxations [2]. Brady et al. clarified the effects of initial graft tension on the tibiofemoral compressive force and joint position after ACL reconstruction and mentioned an increase in initial graft tension which increased the tibiofemoral compressive force and produced a posterior neutral shift and external rotation of the tibia relative to the femur in the quasi-static, passively flexed human cadaveric knee [8]. They concluded that a low initial tension on the patellar tendon graft (1–15 N) best simulated the normal tibiofemoral compressive force and neutral position. We also investigated the effect of initial tension on the tibial position and mentioned that the tibia moved posterolaterally with external and valgus rotation and that the proximal movement of the tibia consequently brought the increase of the contact force in both compartments of femorotibial joint with an increase of initial tension [9] (Fig. 18.1). Thus, excessive large initial tension at graft fixation may bring deleterious effects to the articular surface, leading to cartilage degeneration and graft tear.

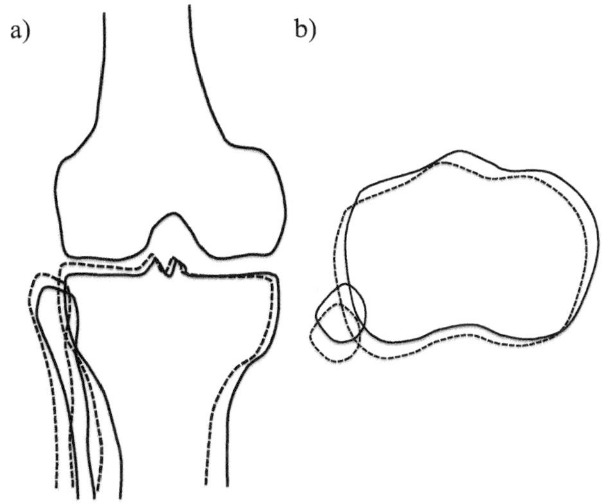

Fig. 18.1 Effect of initial tension on tibiofemoral relationship. Tibia moves posterolaterally with external and valgus rotation with an increase of initial tension. (**a**) Coronal plane, (**b**) axial plane. *Solid line*, previous tibial position; *dot line*, tibial position after graft fixation with some amount of tension

18.3 Clinical study

There are some studies regarding the effect of initial tension on the clinical outcomes after ACL reconstruction. Yasuda et al. compared among 20, 40, and 80 N of three different initial tensions at graft fixation in conventional single-bundle ACL reconstruction with autogenous hamstring tendon graft and described the postoperative side-to-side difference in anterior laxity was significantly less in 80 N group than that in 20 N group 2 years or more after surgery [10]. Thus, they concluded that relatively high tension reduced the postoperative anterior laxity after ACL reconstruction. On the other hand, Yoshiya et al. investigated the effect of the initial tension on the clinical outcome after ACL reconstruction with two different initial tensions of 25 N and 50 N and followed up their patients up to 2 years after ACL reconstruction with autogenous bone-patellar tendon-bone graft [11]. They found no significant difference in the clinical outcomes throughout the follow-up. Van Kampen et al. compared clinical outcomes 2 years after ACL reconstruction using autogenous bone-patellar tendon-bone graft between 20 N and 40 N of initial tension [12]. They described that there were no significant differences on outcomes after ACL reconstruction with two different initial tensions and that graft tension of 20 N seemed to be sufficient without the risk of over-constraining the knee joint. Thus, there is still no clear consensus on the optimal initial tension in clinical situation, though the initial tension must be within the safety range. We preliminarily performed isometric Rosenberg bi-socket ACL reconstruction with three different amounts of initial tension of 60, 80, and 100 N and measured the side-to-side difference with KT knee arthrometer at 2-year follow-up. Then the dispersion in 100 N group was largest among three groups, though there was no significant difference in the average side-to-side difference (Fig. 18.2). Therefore, excessive large tension is unnecessary for steady ACL outcomes.

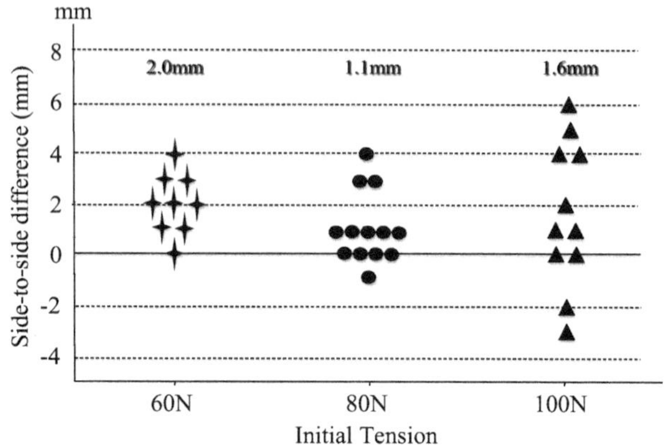

Fig. 18.2 Distribution of KT side-to-side difference after ACL reconstruction at 2 years

18.4 Laxity Match Pretension

The standard of tension is required to determine the optimal initial tension. Laxity match pretension (LMP), which is the graft tension to obtain the normal anterior-posterior laxity in ACL reconstruction, is quite useful as the standard of graft tension. Burks et al. measured the LMP for several graft materials in the isometric single-bundle ACL reconstruction and reported that the LMP value was 3.6 lb (16 N) for BTB graft, 8.5 lb (37.8 N) for doubled semitendinosus graft, and 13.6 lb (60.5 N) for iliotibial band graft, showing the required tension varied among the graft materials [13]. We also reported that the LMP in ACL reconstruction with hamstring tendon graft was 44 N for isometric single-socket technique, 25 N for isometric bi-socket one, and 7.3 N for anatomic double-bundle one and elucidated that the initial tension was different depending on the surgical procedure [14, 15]. Therefore, the optimal graft initial tension should be determined, based on the graft materials and the operative techniques.

18.5 Optimal Initial Tension

It is our belief that the initial graft tension should be slightly larger than the LMP to achieve good clinical outcomes, as the graft tension decreases after fixation because of stress relaxation or creep of the construct. We performed the anatomic double-bundle ACL reconstruction with hamstring tendon graft with 20 N of total initial tension, based on 7.3 N of LMP value (range from 2.2 to 14 N) in this technique, and reported good clinical outcomes including KT side-to-side difference and second-look arthroscopic findings at 2 years postoperatively [16]. Thus, 20 N of initial tension is minimally required tension within safety range for the anatomic double-bundle technique. Shino et al. recently developed the anatomic triple-bundle ACL reconstruction with two femoral and three tibial tunnels within the

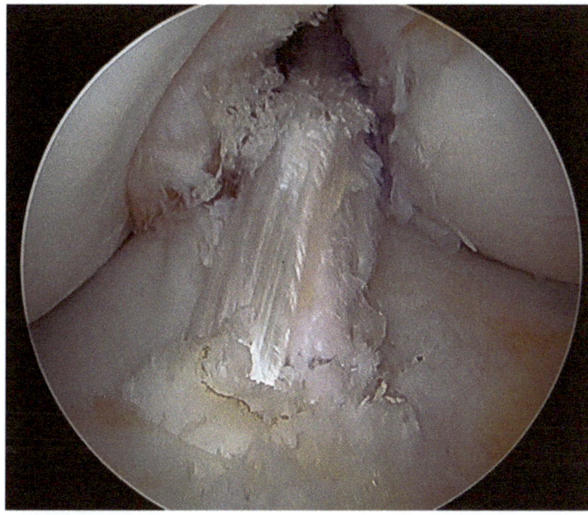

Fig. 18.3 ACL graft in anatomic triple-bundle reconstruction

ACL attachment, while this procedure more closely mimics the morphology of the normal ACL [17] (Fig. 18.3). We then compared the anterior knee laxity with KT knee arthrometer immediately after anatomic ACL reconstruction between the double-bundle and the triple-bundle techniques with initial tension of 20 N and found that the mean anterior laxity was smaller in the triple-bundle technique than that in the double-bundle technique. This suggests that greater contact area between the tibial tunnel wall and the graft in the triple-bundle technique contributed to better knee stability [18]. Thus, less than 20 N for initial tension can be enough for good outcomes in this triple-bundle technique.

Markolf et al. measured the tension to normal ACL on cadaveric knees and reported that the ACL tension at 20° was nearly 0 N [19]. Thus, we believe that the initial graft tension at 20° should be minimized to mimic the tension pattern of the native ACL. Moreover, the smaller the initial tension is applied, the less stress is imposed to the graft, its fixation sites, or articular cartilage. In this point of view, the triple-bundle technique can more closely mimic the normal ACL.

18.6 Femoral Fixation

A lot of devices for graft fixation at femoral side are available. Those included absorbable or nonabsorbable devices with cortical, intra-tunnel, or aperture fixations [20–24]. For hamstring tendon graft, suspensory fixation devices including suture loop and titanium button settled on the lateral femoral cortex are widely used. They have advantages such as easy fixation, while they have disadvantages of longer inter-fixation distance, which resulted in more bungee cord motion

[25]. Recently, adjustable-length loop devices became available to adjust the length of graft in the tunnel, but had a risk of loosening during range of motion or walking in the early phase [26–29]. Petre et al. suggested that adjustable-length loop devices need to be retensioned after cycling the knee and fixing the tibial side to account for the increased initial displacement seen with these devices, as the fixed-length loop devices displaced significantly less than the adjustable-length loop devices [27]. Intra-tunnel fixation like cross pin for hamstring tendons can shorten the inter-fixation distance, but had the difficulty to make two tunnels in the anatomical ACL attachment. Interference screw is common for fixation of BTB graft that could shorten the inter-fixation distance but show a large variation of fixation strength depending on the bone quality and the screw position [30, 31]. Therefore, we must take into account the advantages and the disadvantages of each device at the time of graft fixation to the femur.

18.7 Tibial Fixation

At graft fixation to tibia, sutures tied to the graft are generally fixed to the post screw with manually maximum tension. Yoshihara et al. compared the pretensioned graft load and the residual load in the implanted graft among three different fixation techniques: interference screw, suture-post, and suture-button techniques [32]. They described that the interference screw fixation technique obtained the highest graft tension in spite of overload beyond the intended set force and that the applied load was well maintained during fixation in the suture-post technique, while the graft load in the suture-button technique was reduced probably due to slippage of the button. On the other hand, the suture-post method includes some indefinite factors: (1) difficulty to give the consistent tension to graft as the manually maximum tension is different among the surgeons, (2) risk of loosening or break of suture at the time of knot tying, and (3) stress relaxation of the construct after fixation. Double-staple technique combined with polyester tape and spike washer with a screw for soft tissue graft is also available to control tension with a tensioner. But these fixation techniques could not escape from the risk of slippage of graft under devices, resulting in loss of tension. Shino et al. developed double-spike plate/DSP (Meira Co., Nagoya, Japan), which could allow us to fix graft with any intended tension for tibial fixation [33] (Fig. 18.4). They reported that the graft tension temporarily increased, while the base spikes were being hammered, but the intended tension was maintained even 5 min after fixation. They showed high reliability in initial fixation using DSP.

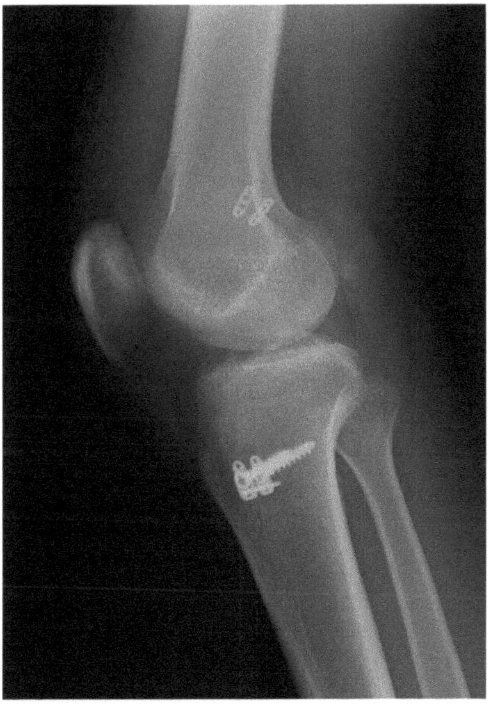

Fig. 18.4 Tibial graft fixation with DSP (double-spike plate) and screw

18.8 Tensioning Technique

In case of graft fixation at the tibia with a tensioner, quantitative tension is usually applied by manual pulls. This technique is quite simple, but the graft tension after fixation could be assumed to change, because the measured tension was based on the surgeon's hand holding the tensioner, not the tibia itself. Then the tension to the graft fixed between the femur and the tibia immediately decreases after fixation according to posterior and proximal translation of tibia. Shino developed a tensioning boot system made of metal (Fig. 18.5). This metal shell boot has tensioners connected to grafts and is fixed to the calf with a bandage. This system makes it possible to give tension to the grafts on the basis of the tibia, as the boot is connected to the tibia. During tensioning of the graft with this boot system, the measured tension based on the tibia or the exact tension of the graft to be fixed between the femur and the tibia is monitored. The tensioner could show the decrease in tension, while the tibia gradually moves posteriorly. Thus, further tightening of the graft could be accomplished monitoring the graft tension based on the tibia. Then the decrease in tension to the graft could be assumed little after fixation between the femur and the tibia, leaving the intended amount of tension to the graft.

We believe the initial tension at graft fixation should be as low as possible, because the tension in the normal ACL is nearly zero around 20 ° of flexion where

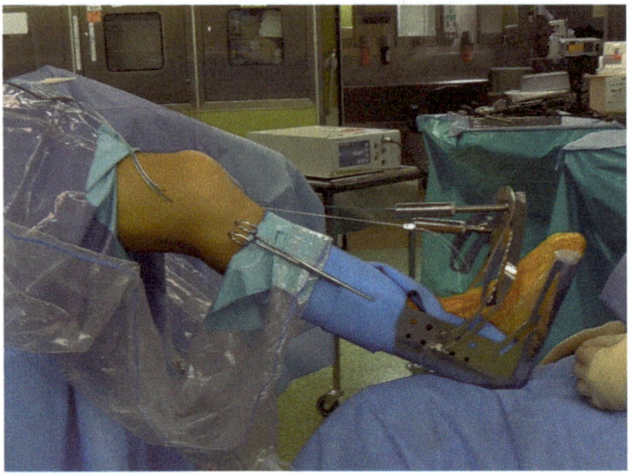

Fig. 18.5 Pretensioning with the tensioning boot

the graft is fixed [19]. However it is not recommendable to apply such small amount of tension manually with a tensioner without the boot system, as the tension loaded to the graft will decrease soon after fixation. Therefore, it is our recommendation to use the tensioning boot system to apply such low initial tension to the graft at the time of fixation in ACL reconstruction.

18.9 Summary

Excessively great amount of tension to the graft potentially makes cartilage degeneration or is harmful to graft healing, while too low tension leads to lax knee. Thus, a safe range of initial tension based on the laxity match pretension should be taken into account in ACL reconstruction. Thus, the tensioning boot system should be utilized at the time of graft fixation in ACL reconstruction to apply the intended tension to the graft.

References

1. Fleming B, Beynnon B, Howe J, McLeod W, Pope M (1992) Effect of tension and placement of a prosthetic anterior cruciate ligament on the anteroposterior laxity of the knee. J Orthop Res 10:177–186
2. Melby A III, Noble JS, Askew MJ, Boom AA, Hurst FW (1991) The effects of graft tensioning on the laxity and kinematics of the anterior cruciate ligament reconstructed knee. Arthroscopy 7:257–266
3. Nabors ED, Richmond JC, Vannah WM, McConville OR (1995) Anterior cruciate ligament graft tensioning in full extension. Am J Sports Med 23:488–492
4. O'Donoghue DH, Rockwood CCA Jr, Frank GR, Jack SC, Kenyon R (1966) Repair of the anterior cruciate ligament in dogs. J Bone Joint Surg Am 48:503–519

5. Bylski-Austrow DI, Grood ES, Hefzy MS, Holden P, Butler DL (1990) Anterior cruciate ligament replacements: a mechanical study of femoral attachment location, flexion angle at tensioning, and initial tension. J Orthop Res 8(4):522–531
6. Eagar P, Hull ML, Howell SM (2004) How the fixation technique stiffness and initial tension affect anterior load–displacement of the knee and tension in anterior cruciate ligament grafts: a study in cadaveric knees using a double-loop hamstrings graft. J Orthop Res 22(3):613–624
7. Yoshiya S, Andrish JT, Manley MT, Bauer TW (1987) Graft tension in anterior cruciate ligament reconstruction. An in vivo study in dogs. Am J Sports Med 15:464–470
8. Brady MF, Bradley MP, Fleming BC, Fadale PD, Hulstyn MJ, Banerjee R (2007) Effects of initial graft tension on the tibiofemoral compressive forces and joint position after anterior cruciate ligament reconstruction. Am J Sports Med 35:395–403
9. Mae T, Shino K, Nakata K, Toritsuka Y, Otsubo H, Fujie H (2008) Optimization of graft fixation at the time of anterior cruciate ligament reconstruction: part I. Effect of initial tension. Am J Sports Med 36:1087–1093. doi:10.1177/0363546508314433
10. Yasuda K, Tsujino J, Tanabe Y, Kaneda K (1997) Effects of initial graft tension on clinical outcome after anterior cruciate ligament reconstruction. Autogenous doubled hamstring tendons connected in series with polyester tapes. Am J Sports Med 25:99–106
11. Yoshiya S, Kurosaka M, Ouchi K, Kuroda R, Mizuno K (2002) Graft tension and knee stability after anterior cruciate ligament reconstruction. Clin Orthop Relat Res 394:154–160
12. van Kampen A, Wymenga AB, van der Heide HJL, Bakens HJAM (1998) The effect of different graft tensioning in anterior cruciate ligament reconstruction: a prospective randomized study. Arthroscopy 14:845–850
13. Burks RT, Leland R (1988) Determination of graft tension before fixation in anterior cruciate ligament reconstruction. Arthroscopy 4:260–266
14. Mae T, Shino K, Miyama T, Shinjo H, Ochi T, Yoshikawa H, Fujie H (2001) Single- versus two-femoral socket anterior cruciate ligament reconstruction technique: biomechanics analysis using a robotic simulator. Arthroscopy 17:708–716
15. Mae T, Shino K, Matsumoto N, Hamada M, Yoneda M, Nakata K (2007) Two-bundle ACL reconstructions using autogenous hamstring tendons – anatomical two-bundle vs. Rosenberg's isometric bi-socket procedure: a biomechanical comparison in laxity match pretension. Knee Surg Sports Traumatol Arthrosc 15:328–334
16. Mae T, Shino K, Matsumoto N, Natsu-ume T, Yoneda K, Yoshikawa H, Yoneda M (2010) Anatomic double-bundle anterior cruciate ligament reconstruction using hamstring tendons with minimally-required initial tension. Arthroscopy 26:1289–1295. doi:10.1016/j.arthro.2010.02.017
17. Shino K, Nakata K, Nakamura N, Mae T, Otsubo H, Iwahashi T, Nakagawa S (2005) Anatomic anterior cruciate ligament reconstruction using two double-looped hamstring tendon grafts via twin femoral and triple tibial tunnels. Oper Tech Orthop Surg 15:130–134. doi:10.1053/j.oto.2004.10.012
18. Mae T, Shino K, Matsumoto N, Yoneda K, Yoshikawa H, Nakata K (2013) Immediately postoperative anterior knee stability: double- versus triple-bundle anterior cruciate ligament reconstructions. Arthroscopy 29:213–219. doi:10.1016/j.arthro.2012.08.012
19. Markolf KL, Gorek JF, Kabo M, Shapiro MS (1990) Direct measurement of resultant forces in the anterior cruciate ligament. An in vitro study performed with a new experimental technique. J Bone Joint Surg Am 72:557–567
20. Kousa P, Jarvinen TTL, Kannus P, Jarvinen M (2001) Initial fixation strength of bioabsorbable and titanium interference screws in anterior cruciate ligament reconstruction. Biomechanical evaluation by single cycle and cycling loading. Am J Sports Med 29:420–425
21. Kousa P, Jarvinen TL, Vihavainen M, Kannus P, Jarvinen M (2003) The fixation strength of six hamstring tendon graft fixation devices in anterior cruciate ligament reconstruction. Part I: femoral site. Am J Sports Med 31:174–181

22. Milano G, Mulas PD, Ziranu F, Piras S, Manunta A, Fabbriciani C (2006) Comparison between different femoral fixation devices for ACL reconstruction with doubled hamstring tendon graft: a biomechanical analysis. Arthroscopy 22:660–668
23. Hammond KE, Dierckman BD, Potini VC, Xerogeanes JW, Labib SA, Hutton WC (2012) Lateral femoral cortical breach during anterior cruciate ligament reconstruction: a biomechanical analysis. Arthroscopy 28:365–371. doi:10.1016/j.arthro.2011.08.309
24. Kamelger FS, Onder U, Schmoei W, Tecklenburg K, Arora R, Fink C (2009) Suspensory fixation of grafts in anterior cruciate ligament reconstruction: a biomechanical comparison of 3 implants. Arthroscopy 25:767–776. doi:10.1016/j.arthro.2009.01.021
25. Hoher J, Moller HD, Fu FH (1998) Bone tunnel enlargement after anterior cruciate ligament reconstruction: fact or fiction ? Knee Surg Sports Traumatol Arthrosc 6:231–240
26. Conner CS, Perez BA, Morris RP, Buckner JW, Buford WL Jr, Ivey FM (2010) Three femoral fixation devices for anterior cruciate ligament reconstruction: comparison of fixation on the lateral cortex versus the anterior cortex. Arthroscopy 26:796–807. doi:10.1016/j.arthro.2009.10.015
27. Petre BM, Smith SD, Jansson KS, de Meijer PP, Hackett TR, LaPrade RF, Wijdicks CA (2013) Femoral cortical suspensory devices for soft tissue anterior cruciate ligament reconstruction: a comparative biomechanical study. Am J Sports Med 41:416–422. doi:10.1177/0363546512469875
28. Barrow AE, Pilia M, Guda T, Kadrmas WR, Burns TC (2013) Femoral suspension devices for anterior cruciate ligament reconstruction. do adjustable loop lengthen ? Am J Sports Med 42:343–349. doi:10.1177/0363546513507769
29. Eguchi A, Ochi M, Adachi N, Deie M, Nakamae A, Usman MA (2014) Mechanical properties of suspensory fixation devices for anterior cruciate ligament reconstruction: comparison of the fixed-length loop device versus the adjustable-length loop device. Knee 21:743–748. doi:10.1016/j.knee.2014.02.009
30. Paschal SO, Seemann MD, Ashman RB, Allard RN, Montgomery JB (1994) Interference fixation versus postfixation of bone-patellar tendon-bone grafts for anterior cruciate ligament reconstruction. Clin Orthop Relat Res 300:281–287
31. Matthews LS, Soffer SR (1989) Pitfalls in the use of interference screws for anterior cruciate ligament reconstruction: brief report. Arthroscopy 5:225–226
32. Yoshihara Y, Yoshiya S, Kurosaka M, Yamamoto T, Kuroada R, Muratsu H (2005) The load of an implanted graft during and after fixation in anterior cruciate ligament reconstruction. Knee Surg Sports Traumatol Arthrosc 13:101–106
33. Shino K, Mae T, Maeda A, Miyama T, Shinjo H, Kawakami H (2002) Graft fixation with predetermined tension using a new device, the double spike plate. Arthroscopy 18:908–911

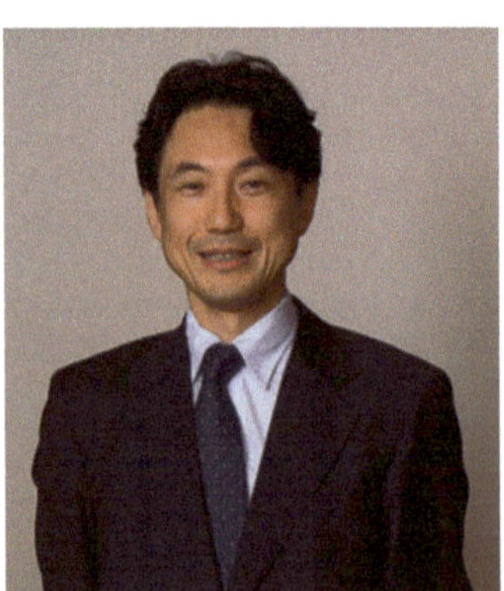

Tatsuo Mae, M.D., PhD, Department of Orthopaedic Surgery, Osaka University Graduate School of Medicine, Osaka, Japan.

Chapter 19
Tendon Regeneration After Harvest for ACL Reconstruction

Shinichi Yoshiya

Abstract It has been reported that tissue regeneration at the graft harvest site takes place following harvest of autogenous tendon grafts, such as bone-patellar tendon-bone (B-PT-B) or hamstring tendon grafts, in ligament reconstructive surgery. In addition, it has also been shown that the regenerated tissue is gradually remodeled to regain properties resembling normal tendons through the subsequent remodeling process. Previous imaging studies using MRI, CT, and ultrasonographic examinations reported a considerably high tendon regeneration rate of more than 70 %; however, the morphology of the whole muscle-tendon unit does not regain its original topography. Moreover, when the biological, biochemical, and biomechanical properties of the regenerated tissue is compared to those of the original tendon, distinct differences are identified between the original and the regenerated tissues. Consequently, postoperative functional deficits, such as muscle weakness, caused by the harvest of the graft cannot be fully discovered even years after surgery, and a caution should be exercised for use of the reharvested tendon graft in revision surgeries.

Keywords Tendon regeneration • Graft harvest • ACL reconstruction • Revision reconstruction

19.1 Introduction

Use of autogenous tendon graft is generally a primary option for graft selection in anterior cruciate ligament (ACL) reconstruction. Among the tendon tissues used as graft materials, a bone-patellar tendon-bone graft and a hamstring tendon graft are the most popular options in our current practice. Harvest of autogenous tissue is inevitably associated with potential loss of the functionality originally provided by the harvested tissue. Moreover, incomplete healing at the graft harvest site may result in undesirable symptoms such as pain and discomfort. These potential

S. Yoshiya, M.D. (✉)
Department of Orthopaedic Surgery, Hyogo College of Medicine, 1-1 Mukogawa-cho, Nishinomiya, Hyogo 663-8501, Japan
e-mail: yoshiya@hyo-med.ac.jp

M. Ochi et al. (eds.), *ACL Injury and Its Treatment*,
DOI 10.1007/978-4-431-55858-3_19

problems associated with graft harvest are called "graft donor-site morbidities." In order to manage and minimize the donor-site morbidities, an understanding of tissue regeneration after graft harvest is critical.

This chapter deals with this issue of clinical importance based on the review of previous relevant studies. The content focuses on the extent and time course of tissue healing and regeneration following graft harvest, its effect on the clinical outcome, and potential factors that may influence the tissue regeneration/ healing process at the donor site.

19.2 Bone-Patellar Tendon-Bone Graft

The bone-patellar tendon-bone graft has been one of the most popularly used graft materials, and a number of studies have been performed to investigate tissue regeneration at the graft harvest site [1–10].

19.2.1 Tendon Regeneration

19.2.1.1 Animal Studies

Cabaud et al. [11] examined the healing following harvest of the medial third of the patellar tendon in dogs and reported that the operated patellar tendon regained its original strength as well as normal microscopic appearance with oriented collagen fibers. Following this study, Laprade et al. [12] performed a canine study examining the histological and biomechanical properties of the regenerated tissue after harvest of the central third of the patellar tendon. Based on the study results, they concluded that the regenerated tendon did not have the same properties as the native patellar tendon for up to 1 year. Burks et al. [13] examined the biomechanical properties of canine patellar tendons after removal of their central third and showed that the operated patellar tendon had significantly decreased its strength and stiffness at 6 months. By contrast, Linder et al. [14] investigated the histological and biomechanical properties of patellar tendons at 3 and 6 months after removal of their medial third in a canine model and showed an increased cross-sectional area and comparable strength compared to those of control tendons. Proctor et al. [15] examined the mechanical, histological, and ultrastructural properties of the repair tissue 21 months after removal of the central third of the patellar tendon in a goat model and showed that the repair tissue exhibited inferior properties compared to the control tissue. Tohyama et al. [16] and Maeda et al. [17] conducted detailed biomechanical analyses of the regenerated tissue in the patellar tendon after removal of its central portion in a rabbit model. They showed that the mechanical properties of the regenerated tissue remained inferior to those of the normal control tendon.

In addition to the studies examining the healing process after graft harvest, potential measures to enhance the tissue healing at the graft harvest site have also been investigated in some animal studies. Karaoglu et al. [18] showed that implantation of a bioscaffold (porcine small intestinal submucosa) at the defect could induce improved tissue healing in a rabbit model. Atkinson et al. [19] used an augmentation device (a nylon monofilament with a metal plate and clips) to fill the defect in a rabbit model and showed better healing with less adhesion and fibrosis in the augmented tendons.

19.2.1.2 Clinical Studies

There have been clinical studies that investigated the healing status at the graft harvest site after removal of the central one third of the patellar tendon. In 1992, Coupens et al. [2] conducted an MRI study for tissue regeneration after graft harvest and showed gradual morphologic return to normal MRI appearances up to 18 months. Bemicker et al. [4] conducted a serial MRI evaluation of the regenerated tissue after harvest. They reported that the width of the defect had reduced with time up to 1 year after surgery, while complete closure of the defect was attained only in two of the 12 patients. Kartus et al. [6] performed a serial MRI examination with a mean follow-up period of 26 months and reported a gradual reduction in width and an increase in thickness. The histological examination in that study showed a significant increase in cellularity and vascularity as compared to normal control tendons, and they concluded that the graft donor site did not regain normal properties for at least up to 2 years.

There were some studies that the investigated long-term sequence of the tissue healing at the donor site based on MRI results. Koseoglu et al. [9] compared the gap width between patients with a short time interval (2–12 months) and those with a long time interval (12–96 months). MRI evaluation at various postoperative time periods revealed gradual gap filling with closure of the graft donor site observed for 6 of the 14 patients in the long time interval group. By contrast, Svensson et al. [10] conducted serial MRI examinations up to 6 years after surgery and reported persistent thinning of the central part of the graft harvest site up to 6 years after surgery. Serial ultrasonographic imaging studies showed similar results to those of MRI studies. Jävelä et al. [7] examined sonographic morphologic changes at the graft harvest site 10 years after patellar tendon ACL reconstruction and reported that normal sonographic appearance was observed in only three of the 31 patients. Those imaging studies have shown that the gap at the graft harvest site is gradually filled with time, while the regenerative tissue cannot regain the original properties of a normal tendon.

Regarding the factors potentially influencing tissue healing at the graft harvest site, closing the defect has not been shown to induce any clinical advantages over the condition with the defect left open [20–22]. The effect of platelet-rich plasma (PRP) on the healing at the graft donor site was investigated in three studies [23–25], and those studies showed improved tissue healing in the PRP group compared to the control group.

19.2.2 Reharvest of the Regenerated Patellar Tendon in Revision Reconstruction

Karns et al. [26] presented a case of a patient who underwent revision ACL reconstruction using a reharvested central third patellar tendon. They reported the microscopic appearance of the reharvested tendon with well-oriented collagen fibers resembling a normal tendon. O'Shea et al. [27] reported satisfactory outcomes for revision ACL reconstruction using a graft consisting of 7 to 8 mm of the regenerated tendon and 2 to 3 mm of previously untouched tendon, while Kartus et al. [28] found inferior clinical results for a revision reconstruction using the reharvested patellar tendon compared to that with the use of the contralateral patellar tendon graft. In addition, Linden et al. [29] reported unsatisfactory clinical results after revision reconstruction using the reharvested graft with abnormal MRI appearance at the harvest site even at 10 years after surgery.

19.3 Hamstring Tendon Graft

Tendon regeneration after hamstring tendon harvest was first reported by Cross et al. in 1992 [30]. Since then, there have been a number of clinical studies that examined the rate and status of tendon regeneration after hamstring autograft harvest in ACL reconstruction. Those studies were recently summarized by Suijkerbuijk et al. [31] and Papalia et al. [32].

19.3.1 Review of Previous Clinical Studies on Tendon Regeneration

We carried out a literature search for articles published up to September 2015 using the PubMed database. In addition, a hand search for relevant articles was also performed. Consequently, 20 articles were selected for review. The design and contents of those studies are summarized in Table 19.1.

19.3.1.1 Regeneration Rate

Cross et al. [30] first reported tendon regeneration following harvest for ACL reconstruction in 1992. Subsequent to this paper, Eriksson et al. reported the results of an MRI study showing regeneration of the semitendinosus (ST) tendon with normal topography to the level of the tibial plateau in eight of 11 patients [33]. There have been a number of studies that examined tissue regeneration after graft harvest [30, 33–52]; however, healing rates reported in those previous studies are variable. In the majority of the studies, regeneration rates ranging from 70 to 100 % were reported.

Table 19.1 Previous studies investigating hamstring tendon regeneration following harvest

Authors (year)	Level of evidence	Number of patients	Mean (median) follow-up period, months	Imaging methods	Regeneration rate (%)	Morphology of muscle, muscle-tendon junction, insertion
Eriksson et al. (1999) [33]	III	11	6–12	MRI	ST 73 %	Fusion of the ST and G tendon in 3/8
						Muscle: smaller area with high signal
Papandrea et al. (2000) [34]	III	40	24 (Serial: 0.5, 1, 2, 3, 6, 12, 18, and 24)	US	ST 100 % (40/40)	
Eriksson et al. (2001) [35]	IV	16	7	MRI	ST 75 % (12/16)	Histology of the regenerative tendon resembled that of the normal tendon
Rispoli et al. (2001) [36]	IV	20	32	MRI	ST, G 100 % (20/20)	More proximal insertion of the regenerated ST tendon
Tadokoro et al. (2004) [37]	III	28	67	MRI	ST 79 %	
					G 46 %	
Williams et al. (2004) [38]	IV	8	6	MRI	100 %	A significant reduction in volume and length was noted for both ST and G muscles
Nakamura et al. (2004) [39]	IV	8	37	3D-CT, MRI	ST 63 % (5/8)	The distal part of the regenerated tendon attached into the medial surface of the popliteal fascia
Nakamae et al. (2005) [40]	III	28	12	3D-CT	ST 100 %	
Nishino et al. (2006) [41]	III	23	23	MRI	ST 91 % (21/23)	Shortening of muscle length and proximal shift of the musculotendinous junction were noted

(continued)

Table 19.1 (continued)

Authors (year)	Level of evidence	Number of patients	Mean (median) follow-up period, months	Imaging methods	Regeneration rate (%)	Morphology of muscle, muscle-tendon junction, insertion
Okahashi et al. (2006) [42]	IV	11	12	Histological examination of the biopsied tissue	ST 82 % (9/11)	Histologic evaluation of the regenerated tissue showed similar properties to the normal tendons.
Takeda et al. (2006) [43]	IV	11	12.7	MRI	ST 100 % (11/11)	Recovery of muscle activation was observed by increased T2 relaxation time after knee flexion exercise
Åhlén et al. (2012) [44]	IV	19	102 (range, 6–11 years)	MRI	ST 89 % (17/19)	The regenerated tendon had a cross-sectional area similar to that on the contralateral side
					G 95 % (18/19)	
Bedi et al. (2013) [45]	IV	15 (18 knees)	12	US	ST 50 % (9/18)	Proximal retraction of the amputated stump was observed. Neither normal excursion nor physiological function similar to the native muscle-tendon unit was reproduced
Choi et al. (2012) [46]	IV	45	36.4	MRI	ST 80 % (36/45)	Distal shift of the distal tendon insertion and proximal shift of the musculotendinous junction were observed
					G 76 % (34/45)	
Janssen et al. (2013) [47]	II	22	12	MRI	ST 64 % (14/22)	Significant reductions in the surface area of the ST and G muscle were noted. Retraction of the ST muscle was increased in cases without tendon regeneration
					G 100 % (22/22)	
Murakami et al. (2012) [48]	III	20	15	MRI	ST 100 % (20/20)	A branch of the ST tendon was retained and sutured to the pes anserinus to induce regeneration

Nakamae et al. (2012) [49]	III	39	12	3D-CT	ST 97 % (38/39)	Proximal shift of the muscle-tendon junction was observed
Snow et al. (2012) [50]	IV	10	129 (9–11 years)	MRI	ST 80 % (8/10)	Reduction in muscle volume was observed for both ST and G muscles
Stevanovic et al. (2013) [51]	II	50	24	US	ST 72 % (36/50)	The regenerated ST tendon fused with the G tendon. Histological finding of the regenerated tendon resembled to that of the normal tendon
Nomura et al. (2014) [52]	IV	24	28	MRI	ST 88 % (21/24)	Reduction in the muscle volume as well as length was noted

ST semitendinosus; *G* gracilis; *US* ultrasonography

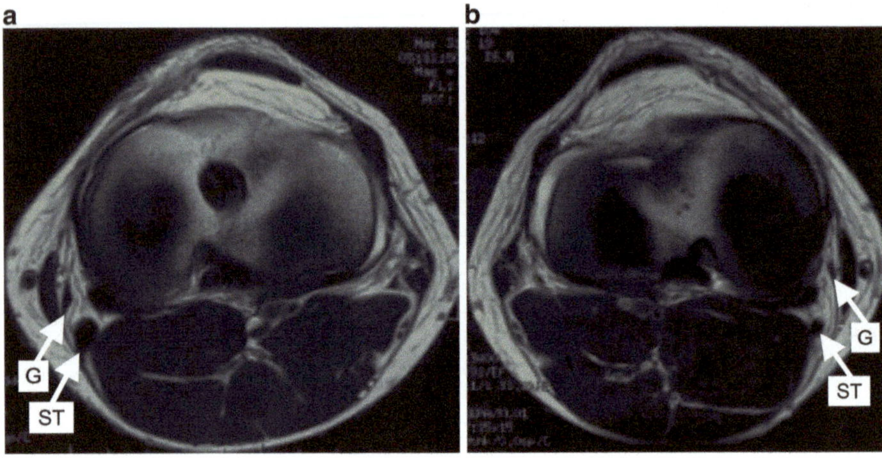

Fig. 19.1 Axial MRI images demonstrating tendon regeneration following graft harvest (*ST*: semitendinosus tendon, *G*: gracilis tendon).
(**a**) Regenerated tendons on the MRI image at 2 years after surgery.
(**b**) Comparative MRI image on the contralateral nonoperated side

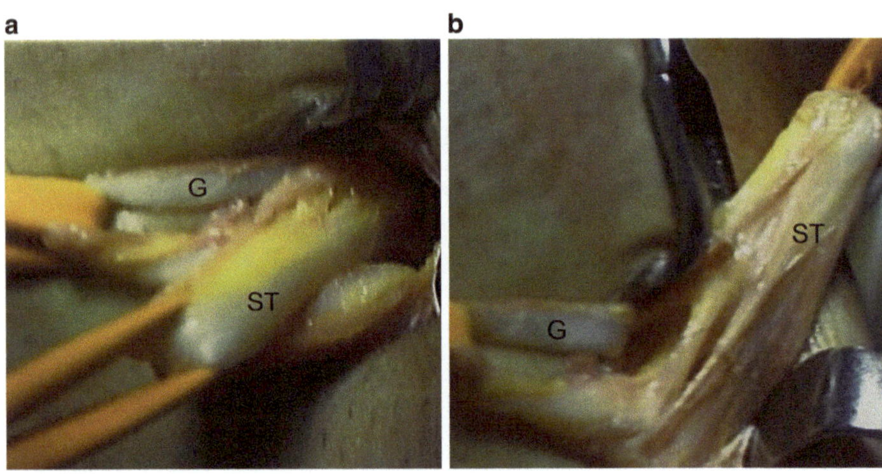

Fig. 19.2 Regeneration of the semitendinosus tendon (ST) observed during the revision reconstructive procedure (at 8 months after the initial ACL reconstruction).
(**a**) The regenerated semitendinosus tendon (ST) adjacent to the gracilis tendon (G).
(**b**) The insertion of the regenerated tendon is scarred and adherent to the surrounding tissue (*white arrow*)

In general, the regeneration rate was not different between the ST and the gracilis (G) tendons (Figs. 19.1 and 19.2). When the regeneration rate was compared between the short-term and long-term studies, no apparent difference (increased regeneration rate with time course) was noted.

19.3.1.2 Morphologic Features of Regenerated Tendon

One of the morphologic changes observed for the regenerated tendon is alteration of the distal tendon insertion. Although a high regeneration rate has been reported in previous imaging studies, it has also been shown that anatomic tendon insertion at the proximal tibia is not reestablished [38, 39, 45, 51]. Another change noted is the proximal shift of the muscle-tendon junction with retraction of muscle belly [38, 41, 45–47, 49, 52]. These morphologic changes are thought to be associated with functional deficit as manifested by a reduction of knee flexor strength.

19.3.1.3 Biological Observation of Regenerated Tendon

Eriksson et al. examined the histologic appearance of regenerated ST tendons in six patients with the postoperative period ranging from 7 to 28 months after surgery [53]. It was shown that the collagen fibers in the regenerated tissue were randomly oriented in the specimen taken at 7 months, while well-oriented fibers were noted in the patient examined at 27 months. Ferreti et al. [54] similarly reported a progressive remodeling based on the histological examination of the specimens obtained at the time of revision surgery. Okahashi et al. [42] conducted histological and immunohistochemical examinations for the biopsied samples at 1 year and reported that the findings of the regenerated tendons closely resembled those of the control tendons. Yoshiya et al. [55] examined the ultrastructure of the regenerated tendon taken at 8 months after surgery. The electron microscopic examination of the biopsied sample revealed a smaller collagen fibril diameter compared to that in the control tendons. Gill et al. [56] extensively examined the biological and biomechanical properties of the regenerated tendon in a rabbit model. At 9 to 12 months after the tendon harvest, regenerated tendons could be identified in 26 of the 35 knees (74 %), and the histological and immunohistochemical examinations of the regenerated tissue showed normal tendon-like findings. However, the ultrastructural and biochemical analyses revealed a smaller collagen fibril diameter and lower glycosaminoglycan and collagen levels in the neo-tendon tissues.

19.3.2 Analysis of Factors That Potentially Influence Tendon Regeneration

Nakamae et al. [49] conducted a comparative clinical study examining whether postoperative immobilization up to 2 weeks could induce better tendon regeneration. A comparison was made between the groups with 3-day immobilization and immobilization for a longer period (10 to 14 days). At 12 months after surgery, tendon regeneration was observed in almost all cases (38 of the 39 knees), while no significant differences in the regeneration rate and the morphologic features were demonstrated between the groups. Murakami et al. [48] reported their technique of "inducer grafting" in which a branch of the ST graft toward the gastrocnemius muscle was retained during the graft harvest and sutured to the pes anserinus. They reported that this technique could successfully promote the hypertrophy of the regenerated tendon.

19.3.3 Reharvest of the Regenerated Tendon in Revision Reconstruction

Yoshiya et al. [55] reported a case of a patient who underwent revision ACL reconstruction using a reharvested ST tendon combined with an initially untouched G tendon. Stevanovic et al. [51] addressed the feasibility of regenerated tendon use in revision reconstructive surgery and reported a case with medial patellofemoral ligament reconstruction using the reharvested ST tendon. Considering the difference in tissue properties between the regenerated and the native tendons, however, it is still recommended to be cautious about using the reharvested tendon alone for revision surgeries.

References

1. Berg EE (1992) Intrinsic healing of a patellar tendon donor site defect after anterior cruciate ligament reconstruction. Clin Orthop Relat Res 278:160–163
2. Coupens SD, Yates CK, Sheldon C et al (1992) Magnetic resonance imaging evaluation of the patellar tendon after use of its central one-third for anterior cruciate ligament reconstruction. Am J Sports Med 20(3):332–335
3. Wiley JP, Bray RC, Wiseman DA et al (1997) Serial ultrasonographic imaging evaluation of the patellar tendon after harvesting its central one third for anterior cruciate ligament reconstruction. J Ultrasound Med 16(4):251–255
4. Bernicker JP, Haddad JL, Lintner DM et al (1998) Patellar tendon defect during the first year after anterior cruciate ligament reconstruction: appearance on serial magnetic resonance imaging. Arthroscopy 14(8):804–809
5. Kiss ZS, Kellaway DP, Cook JL et al (1998) Postoperative patellar tendon healing: an ultrasound study. VIS tendon study group. Australas Radiol 42(1):28–32
6. Kartus J, Movin T, Papadogiannakis N et al (2000) A radiographic and histologic evaluation of the patellar tendon after harvesting its central third. Am J Sports Med 28(2):218–226
7. Järvelä T, Paakkala T, Kannus P et al (2004) Ultrasonographic and power Doppler evaluation of the patellar tendon ten years after harvesting its central third for reconstruction of the anterior cruciate ligament: comparison of patients without or with anterior knee pain. Am J Sports Med 32(1):39–46
8. Svensson M, Kartus J, Ejerhed L et al (2004) Does the patellar tendon normalize after harvesting its central third?: a prospective long-term MRI study. Am J Sports Med 32(1): 34–38
9. Koseoglu K, Memis A, Argin M et al (2004) MRI evaluation of patellar tendon defect after harvesting its central third. Eur J Radiol 50(3):292–295

10. Svensson M, Kartus J, Christensen LR et al (2005) A long-term serial histological evaluation of the patellar tendon in humans after harvesting its central third. Knee Surg Sports Traumatol Arthorosc 13(5):398–404
11. Cabaud HE, Feagin JA, Rodkey WG (1980) Acute anterior cruciate ligament injury and augmented repair. Experimental studies. Am J Sports Med 8(6):395–401
12. LaPrade RF, Hamilton CD, Montgomery RD et al (1997) The reharvested central third of the patellar tendon. A histologic and biomechanical analysis. Am J Sports Med 25(6):779–785
13. Burks RT, Haut RC, Lancaster RL (1990) Biomechanical and histological observations of the dog patellar tendon after removal of its central one-third. Am J Sports Med 18(2):146–153
14. Linder LH, Sukin DL, Burks RT et al (1994) Biomechanical and histological properties of the canine patellar tendon after removal of its medial third. Am J Sports Med 22(1):136–142
15. Proctor CS, Jackson DW, Simon TM (1997) Characterization of the repair tissue after removal of the central one-third of the patellar ligament. An experimental study in a goat model. J Bone Joint Surg Am 79(7):997–1006
16. Tohyama H, Yasuda K, Kitamura Y et al (2003) The changes in mechanical properties of regenerated and residual tissues in the patellar tendon after removal of its central portion. Clin Biomech (Bristol, Avon) 18(8):765–772
17. Maeda E, Noguchi H, Tohyama H et al (2007) The tensile properties of collagen fascicles harvested from regenerated and residual tissues in the patellar tendon after removal of the central third. Biomed Mater Eng 17(2):77–85
18. Karaoglu S, B Fisher M, Woo SL et al (2008) Use of a bioscaffold to improve healing of a patellar tendon defect after graft harvest for ACL reconstruction: a study in rabbits. J Orthop Res 26(2):255–263
19. Atkinson PJ, Oyen-Tiesma M, Zukosky DK et al (1999) Patellar tendon augmentation after removal of its central third limits joints tissue changes. J Orthop Res 17(1):28–36
20. Brandsson S, Faxén E, Eriksson BI et al (1998) Closing patellar tendon defects after anterior cruciate ligament reconstruction: absence of any benefit. Knee Surg Sports Traumatol Arthrosc 6(2):82–87
21. Adriani E, Mariani PP, Maresca G et al (1995) Healing of the patellar tendon after harvesting of its mid-third for anterior cruciate ligament reconstruction and evolution of the unclosed donor site defect. Knee Surg Sports Traumatol Arthrosc 3(3):138–143
22. Cerullo G, Puddu G, Gianní E et al (1995) Anterior cruciate ligament patellar tendon reconstruction: it is probably better to leave the tendon defect open. Knee Surg Sports Traumatol Arthrosc 3(1):14–17
23. Cervellin M, De Girolamo L, Bait C et al (2012) Autologous platelet-rich plasma gel to reduce donor-site morbidity after patellar tendon graft harvesting for anterior cruciate ligament reconstruction: a randomized, controlled clinical study. Knee Surg Sports Traumatol Arthrosc 20(1):114–120
24. De Almeida AM, Demange MK, Sobrado MF et al (2012) Patellar tendon healing with platelet-rich plasma: a prospective randomized controlled trial. Am J Sports Med 40(6): 1282–1288
25. Seijas R, Rius M, Ares O et al (2015) Healing of donor site in bone-tendon-bone ACL reconstruction accelerated with plasma rich in growth factors: a randomized clinical trial. Knee Surg Sports Traumatol Arthrosc 23(4):991–997
26. Karns DJ, Heidt RS Jr, Holladay BR et al (1994) Case report: revision anterior cruciate ligament reconstruction. Arthroscopy 10(2):148–151
27. O'Shea JJ, Shelbourne KD (2002) Anterior cruciate ligament reconstruction with a reharvested bone-patellar tendon-bone graft. Am J Sports Med 30(2):208–213
28. Kartus J, Stener S, Lindahl S et al (1998) Ipsi- or contralateral patellar tendon graft in anterior cruciate ligament revision surgery. A comparison of two methods. Am J Sports Med 26: 499–504

29. Lidén M, Ejerhed L, Sernert N et al (2006) The course of the patellar tendon after reharvesting its central third for ACL revision surgery: a long-term clinical and radiographic study. Knee Surg Sports Traumatol Arthrosc 14(11):1130–1138
30. Cross MJ, Roger G, Kujawa P et al (1992) Regeneration of the semitendinosus and gracilis tendons following their transection for repair of the anterior cruciate ligament. Am J Sports Med 20(2):221–223
31. Suijkerbuijk MA, Reijman M, Lodewijks SJ et al (2015) Hamstring tendon regeneration after harvesting: a systematic review. Am J Sports Med 43:2591–2598
32. Papalia R, Franceschi F, D'Adamio S et al (2015) Hamstring tendon regeneration after harvest for anterior cruciate ligament reconstruction: a systematic review. Arthroscopy 31(6): 1169–1183
33. Eriksson K, Larsson H, Wredmark T et al (1999) Semitendinosus tendon regeneration after harvesting for ACL reconstruction. A prospective MRI study. Knee Surg Sports Traumatol Arthrosc 7(4):220–225
34. Papandrea P, Vulpiani MC, Ferretti A et al (2000) Regeneration of the semitendinosus tendon harvested for anterior cruciate ligament reconstruction. Evaluation using ultrasonography. Am J Sports Med 28(4):556–561
35. Eriksson K, Hamberg P, Jansson E et al (2001) Semitendinosus muscle in anterior cruciate ligament surgery: morphology and function. Arthroscopy 17(8):808–817
36. Rispoli DM, Sanders TG, Miller MD et al (2001) Magnetic resonance imaging at different time periods following hamstring harvest for anterior cruciate ligament reconstruction. Arthroscopy 17(1):2–8
37. Tadokoro K, Matsui N, Yagi M et al (2004) Evaluation of hamstring strength and tendon regrowth after harvesting for anterior cruciate ligament reconstruction. Am J Sports Med 32(7):1644–1650
38. Williams GN, Snyder-Mackler L, Barrance PJ et al (2004) Muscle and tendon morphology after reconstruction of the anterior cruciate ligament with autologous semitendinosus-gracilis graft. J Bone Joint Surg Am 86(9):1936–1946
39. Nakamura E, Mizuta H, Kadota M et al (2004) Three-dimensional computed tomography evaluation of semitendinosus harvest after anterior cruciate ligament reconstruction. Arthroscopy 20(4):360–365
40. Nakamae A, Deie M, Yasumoto M et al (2005) Three-dimensional computed tomography imaging evidence of regeneration of the semitendinosus tendon harvested for anterior cruciate ligament reconstruction: a comparison with hamstring muscle strength. J Comput Assist Tomogr 29(2):241–245
41. Nishino A, Sanada A, Kanehisa H et al (2006) Knee-flexion torque and morphology of the semitendinosus after ACL reconstruction. Med Sci Sports Exerc 38(11):1895–1900
42. Okahashi K, Sugimoto K, Iwai M et al (2006) Regeneration of the hamstring tendons after harvesting for arthroscopic anterior cruciate ligament reconstruction: a histological study in 11 patients. Knee Surg Traumatol Arthrosc 14(6):542–545
43. Takeda Y, Kashiwaguchi S, Matsuura T et al (2006) Hamstring muscle function after tendon harvest for anterior cruciate ligament reconstruction: evaluation with T2 relaxation time of magnetic resonance imaging. Am J Sports Med 34(2):281–288
44. Åhlén M, Lidén M, Bovaller Å et al (2012) Bilateral magnetic resonance imaging and functional assessment of the semitendinosus and gracilis tendons a minimum of 6 years after ipsilateral harvest for anterior cruciate ligament reconstruction. Am J Sports Med 40(8): 1735–1741
45. Bedi A, Srinivasan RC, Salata MJ et al (2013) Structural and functional analysis of the semitendinosus tendon after harvest for soft tissue reconstructive procedures: a dynamic ultrasonographic study. Knee Surg Sports Traumatol Arthrosc 21(3):606–614
46. Choi JY, Ha JK, Kim YW et al (2012) Relationship among tendon regeneration on MRI, flexor strength, and functional performance after anterior cruciate ligament reconstruction with hamstring autograft. Am J Sports Med 40(1):152–162

47. Janssen RP, van der Velden MJ, Pasmans HL et al (2013) Regeneration of hamstring tendons after anterior cruciate ligament reconstruction. Knee Surg Sports Traumatol Arthrosc 21(4): 898–905
48. Murakami H, Soejima T, Inoue T et al (2012) Inducement of semitendinosus tendon regeneration to the pes anserinus after its harvest for anterior cruciate ligament reconstruction-A new inducer grafting technique. Sports Med Arthrosc Rehabil Ther Technol 4(1):17
49. Nakamae A, Deie M, Adachi N et al (2012) Effects of knee immobilization on morphological changes in the semitendinosus muscle-tendon complex after hamstring harvesting for anterior cruciate ligament reconstruction: evaluation using three-dimensional computed tomography. J Orthop Sci 17(1):39–45
50. Snow BJ, Wilcox JJ, Burks RT et al (2012) Evaluation of muscle size and fatty infiltration with MRI nine to eleven years following hamstring harvest for ACL reconstruction. J Bone Joint Surg Am 94(14):1274–1282
51. Stevanović V, Blagojević Z, Petković A et al (2013) Semitendinosus tendon regeneration after anterior cruciate ligament reconstruction: can we use it twice? Int Orthop 37(12):2475–2481
52. Nomura Y, Kuramochi R, Fukubayashi T (2015) Evaluation of hamstring muscle strength and morphology after anterior cruciate ligament reconstruction. Scand J Med Sci Sports 25(3): 301–307
53. Eriksson K, Kindblom LG, Hamberg P et al (2001) The semitendinosus tendon regenerates after resection: a morphologic and MRI analysis in 6 patients after resection for anterior cruciate ligament reconstruction. Acta Orthop Scand 72(4):379–384
54. Ferretti A, Conteduca F, Morelli F et al (2002) Regeneration of the semitendinosus tendon after its use in anterior cruciate ligament reconstruction: a histologic study of three cases. Am J Sports Med 30(2):204–207
55. Yoshiya S, Matsui N, Matsumoto A et al (2004) Revision anterior cruciate ligament reconstruction using the regenerated semitendinosus tendon: analysis of ultrastructure of the regenerated tendon. Arthroscopy 20(5):532–535
56. Gill SS, Turner MA, Battaglia TC et al (2004) Semitendinosus regrowth: biochemical, ultrastructural, and physiological characterization of the regenerate tendon. Am J Sports Med 32(5):1173–1181

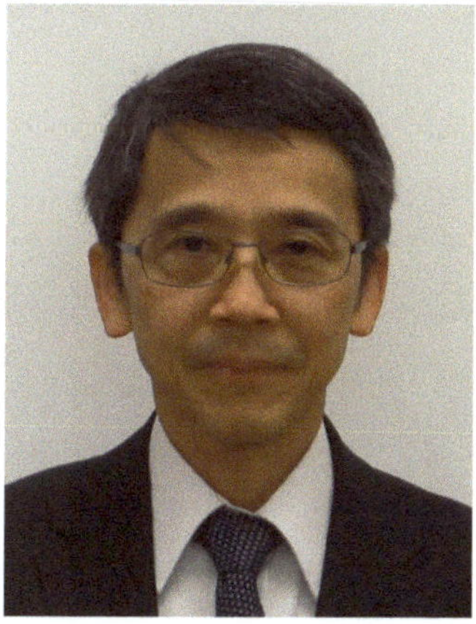

Shinichi Yoshiya, M.D., Department of Orthopaedic Surgery, Hyogo College of Medicine, Hyogo, Japan.

Chapter 20
Second-Look Arthroscopic Evaluation After ACL Reconstruction

Atsuo Nakamae and Mitsuo Ochi

Abstract Second-look arthroscopy after ACL reconstruction is one of the most reliable types of examination to provide valuable prognostic information on a graft such as synovial coverage and damage of the graft. Second-look arthroscopy shows that synovial coverage of the grafts differs substantially between cases and that graft loosening or partial tear can occur even in clinically successful knees. Second-look arthroscopy is also the most dependable procedure to evaluate the postoperative status of meniscal repairs. Moreover, this examination is the most precise way to determine the condition of the articular cartilage. Osteoarthritis is typically diagnosed using radiography. However, by using arthroscopy, even minimal articular cartilage damage consistent with incipient osteoarthritis can be detected long before the classic criteria of osteoarthritis are fulfilled. Arthroscopy demonstrates that although proper ACL reconstruction is clearly important, meniscal repair should be performed, where possible, to limit the progression of articular cartilage damage. This chapter describes the procedure and advantages of second-look arthroscopy and also reviews the literature on second-look arthroscopic findings after ACL reconstruction.

Keywords Anterior cruciate ligament (ACL) • Augmentation technique • Second-look arthroscopy • Knee • Cartilage injury

20.1 Advantages of Second-Look Arthroscopy

Second-look arthroscopy is one of the most reliable examination strategies after knee surgery. After ACL reconstruction, second-look arthroscopy is useful in providing valuable prognostic information on the graft, such as synovial coverage,

A. Nakamae, M.D., Ph.D. (✉)
Department of Orthopaedic Surgery, Integrated Health Sciences, Institute of Biomedical & Health Sciences, Hiroshima University, 1-2-3 Kasumi, Minami-ku, Hiroshima 734-8551, Japan
e-mail: nakamae@hiroshima-u.ac.jp

M. Ochi, M.D., Ph.D.
President of Hiroshima University, 1-3-2 Kagamiyama, Higashi-Hiroshima 739-8511, Japan

M. Ochi et al. (eds.), *ACL Injury and Its Treatment*,
DOI 10.1007/978-4-431-55858-3_20

tension, and damage of the graft, as well as on synovial coverage of the space between the opening of the femoral bone tunnel and the graft [1–13]. This examination is also the most dependable procedure to evaluate the postoperative status of meniscal repairs [14–19]. Moreover, second-look arthroscopy is the most precise way to determine the condition of the articular cartilage [20, 21]. Osteoarthritis is typically diagnosed using radiography. However, by using arthroscopy, even small articular cartilage damage consistent with incipient osteoarthritis can be found long before the classic criteria of osteoarthritis are fulfilled [22].

20.2 Evaluation of the Graft by Second-Look Arthroscopy

20.2.1 Procedure of Second-Look Arthroscopy

Arthroscopic intra-articular inspections are performed through lateral and medial infrapatellar portals with a 30° oblique arthroscope. A thorough arthroscopic probing is needed to assess the reconstructed ACL, meniscus and articular cartilage precisely. For the arthroscopic evaluation of the graft, arthroscopic examination should be performed in various knee flexion angles to ensure good visualization of the graft and femoral bone tunnel. The status of the posterolateral bundle of the ACL can be evaluated with the knee in a figure-of-4 position for good visualization of the femoral attachment of the posterolateral bundle [23].

20.2.2 Tension and Damage of the Graft

To evaluate the tension of the graft, arthroscopic examination should be performed with the knee in various angles of flexion to allow observation of the different tension patterns of the fibers. Initial tension applied to the graft at the time of graft fixation may influence the tension and damage of the graft at the time of second-look arthroscopy. Position of the femoral bone tunnel may also influence the tension pattern of the graft. Excessive tension to the graft at the time of primary ACL reconstruction may cause abnormal knee kinematics, hinder flexion–extension, and lead to graft failure or articular cartilage degeneration [7]. Therefore, evaluating graft tension and damage by second-look arthroscopy is meaningful not only for patients but also for improvement of the surgical procedure.

In 2004, Toritsuka and Shino et al. [10] evaluated the tension and thickness of the grafts by second-look arthroscopy after ACL reconstruction with multistranded autogenous hamstring tendon grafts. The patients were all clinically evaluated as experiencing successful outcomes. In their series, 96 knees were surgically treated with the single-socket procedure, and the remaining 60 were treated with the bi-socket procedure. As a result, 11 % of the hamstring ACL grafts showed looseness, and 34 % had a partial tear in the clinically successful knees. No statistically significant difference was seen between the two surgical procedures in any of the findings.

Otsubo and Shino et al. [9] performed second-look arthroscopic evaluation of the transplanted graft after anatomic double-bundle ACL reconstruction, with emphasis on graft tension and the presence of graft damage. An initial tension to the graft of 20–30 N was applied to each tensioning suture, based on the diameter of the graft. The grafts were secured onto the tibia with two double-spike plates at 20° of knee flexion. The authors reported that none of the anteromedial grafts showed rupture, while 11 % of the posterolateral grafts showed substantial damage around the femoral tunnel aperture. Both the anteromedial and posterolateral grafts were evaluated as lax in 9 % of the knees. They concluded that their double-bundle ACL reconstruction and postoperative regimen required improvement, in order to achieve better postoperative graft morphology.

In response to the results of the above-cited study, Mae et al. [7] investigated the clinical results and second-look arthroscopic findings after anatomic double-bundle ACL reconstruction with a total of 20 N of low initial tension (10 N to each graft). They reported that their ACL reconstruction yielded good clinical outcomes at 2 years postoperatively, and second-look arthroscopy showed that most grafts were evaluated as being taut in tension and free of tear damage. They concluded that low initial tension applied to grafts was enough to restore normal stability in ACL reconstruction. This study is informative for the further development of ACL reconstruction.

20.2.3 Synovial Coverage of the Grafts

The extent of synovial coverage over the grafts is also one of the most important findings in second-look arthroscopic evaluation. Good synovial coverage over the graft may accelerate cellular proliferation and revascularization of the grafted tendon. In addition, good synovial coverage may improve proprioceptive function of the knee after ACL reconstruction. It is accepted that the normal ACL is extensively innervated by mechanoreceptors and has an important proprioceptive role. Many mechanoreceptors in the synovia may play an important afferent role in proprioception.

An augmentation technique for the treatment of ACL injury has recently received attention from orthopedic surgeons, because preservation of the ACL remnant may have several potential advantages. One of the proposed advantages is preservation of the mechanoreceptors within the ACL remnant. We investigated 216 patients who underwent ACL reconstruction or augmentation to evaluate the clinical outcomes and second-look arthroscopic findings of single-bundle ACL augmentation in comparison with those of central anatomic single- or double-bundle ACL reconstruction [1]. In 94 of the 216 patients, proprioceptive function of the knees was evaluated using the threshold to detect passive motion test (TTDPM) before and 12 months after surgery. Second-look arthroscopy showed

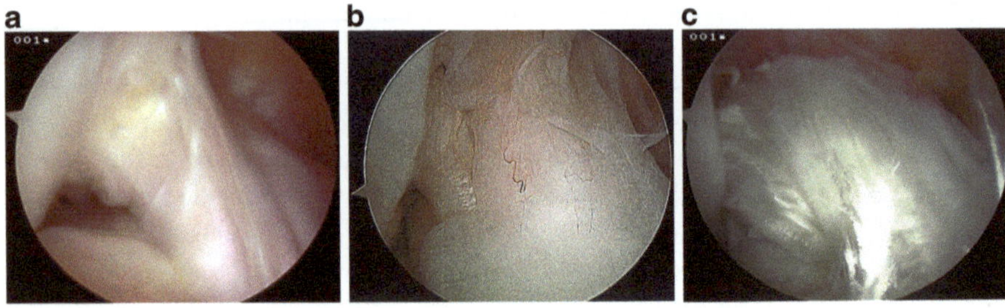

Fig. 20.1 Second-look arthroscopic view of the reconstructed anterior cruciate ligament. The synovial coverage of the grafts was classified as follows: (**a**) good (synovial coverage of >80 % of the graft), (**b**) fair (50–80 % coverage), and (**c**) poor (<50 % coverage)

significantly better synovial coverage of the graft in the augmentation group (good, 82 %; fair, 14 %; poor, 4 %) [Fig. 20.1] than in the other groups. The mean side-to-side difference measured with a KT-2000 arthrometer was 0.4 mm in the augmentation group, 0.9 mm in the double-bundle group, and 1.3 mm in the single-bundle group. Hence, the result differed significantly between the augmentation and single-bundle groups. No significant difference in the Lysholm score or pivot-shift test was seen between the three groups. In patients with good synovial coverage, three of the four measurements used revealed significant improvement in proprioceptive function. In conclusion, patients in the ACL augmentation group exhibited better knee stability than those in the standard single-bundle reconstruction group and better synovial coverage of the graft upon second-look arthroscopy than those in the standard single- and double-bundle reconstruction groups. Improvement in proprioceptive function was observed in patients with good synovial coverage of the graft. Therefore, ACL augmentation may be a reasonable treatment option for patients with favorable ACL remnants.

20.3 Evaluation of Articular Cartilage and Meniscus After ACL Reconstruction by Second-Look Arthroscopy

20.3.1 Importance of Articular Cartilage in the Knee

It is well known that articular cartilage injury often occurs in conjunction with ACL injury. Although the incidence of articular cartilage injury under arthroscopy varies among the literature, the incidence of severe articular cartilage injury in acute ACL tears is estimated to be between 16 % and 46 % [24]. Several studies support an increasing incidence of cartilage injury with increasing time from injury [24].

Damage to the articular cartilage is typically described as the most important predictor of poor clinical outcomes after ACL reconstruction. In addition, the damage is also a significant predictor of failure to return to sporting activities following ACL reconstruction. Proper anatomic ACL reconstruction is of course important to obtain normal knee stability and function. However, even when knee stability and function have been achieved using anatomic ACL reconstruction, the long-term results of successful ACL reconstruction are affected by the condition of the articular cartilage [24, 25]. Shelbourne et al. [25] concluded that patients with articular cartilage damage at the time of their ACL reconstruction had more subjective symptoms at follow-up. Potter et al. [26] reported that each increase in the Outerbridge score for the medial femoral condyle resulted in a 13-point decrease in the International Knee Documentation Committee subjective knee score.

20.3.2 Classification of the Articular Cartilage Injury Under Arthroscopy

The incidence of articular cartilage injury depends on the definition of cartilage injury. Classification of cartilage lesions is important to evaluate the condition of the articular cartilage. The International Cartilage Repair Society Classification scale is one of the leading classification systems for cartilage lesions [27].

Grade 0 – Normal
Grade 1 – Nearly normal: Superficial lesions. Soft indentation (A) and/or superficial fissures and cracks (B)
Grade 2 – Abnormal: Lesions extending down to <50 % of cartilage depth
Grade 3 – Severely abnormal: Cartilage defects extending down >50 % of cartilage depth (A) as well as down to the calcified layer (B) and down to, but not through, the subchondral bone (C). Blisters are included in this Grade (D)
Grade 4 – Severely abnormal

The Outerbridge classification scale is another leading classification system for cartilage lesions [28].

Grade 0 – Normal
Grade I – Cartilage with softening and swelling
Grade II – A partial-thickness defect with fissures on the surface that do not reach subchondral bone or exceed 1.5 cm in diameter
Grade III – Fissuring to the level of subchondral bone in an area with a diameter more than 1.5 cm.
Grade IV – Exposed subchondral bone

20.3.3 ACL Injury and Osteoarthritis

Osteoarthritis is a degenerative disease that affects the hyaline cartilage on the articular surface. ACL injuries have been implicated in the progression of osteoarthritis of the knee. The incidence of osteoarthritis following an ACL injury varies among the literature, ranging from 10 to 100 % between 10 and 30 years post-injury [22, 29–31]. In cases of osteoarthritis, both joint changes and symptoms progress slowly over the years, and there is limited association between osteoarthritis changes on X-rays and symptoms. The joint changes in osteoarthritis in the ACL-deficient knee are caused by multifactors, including presence of meniscal or cartilage injury, age at time of injury, time from injury to reconstruction, changes in gait mechanism, instability of the knee joint, certain work or leisure activities, muscle weakness, and obesity [26, 30, 32]. Among the proposed mechanisms for osteoarthritis after ACL injury, the condition of meniscus and articular cartilage at the time of surgery is considered particularly important [25, 26].

20.3.4 ACL Reconstruction and Articular Cartilage Injury

ACL reconstruction is expected not only to restore knee stability but also to protect the knee from further damage to articular cartilage and meniscus. A majority of American orthopedic surgeons believed that ACL reconstruction reduced the rate of osteoarthritis [33]. To date, however, no study has yet conclusively indicated that conventional ACL reconstruction protects the knee from the development of osteoarthritis [22, 34–41]. The reported prevalence of radiological osteoarthritis after ACL reconstruction varies from 10 to 90 %. Fithian et al. [36] tested their treatment algorithm on patients with acute ACL tears. Early ACL reconstruction with a patellar tendon autograft was recommended to high-risk patients and conservative care to low-risk patients. They found that there were more cases of degenerative change on radiographs in the early reconstructed group and that more additional meniscus surgeries were performed in the conservative management group. This was backed up by a previous report, in 1994: "the literature does not lend support to the efficacy of cruciate ligament repair or reconstruction in retarding the progression of osteoarthritis after knee injury" [42].

Current ACL reconstruction is directed toward restoring the normal structure and function of the knee. The normal ACL consists of two major functional bundles: the anteromedial (AM) and the posterolateral (PL). Double-bundle ACL reconstruction aims to reconstruct both the AM and PL bundles of the ACL. Interest in double-bundle ACL reconstruction has increased over the last 10 years, because several studies have shown that double-bundle ACL reconstruction can closely mimic the structure and function of the native ACL [43–48]. Anatomic double-bundle reconstruction may protect the knee from long-term joint damage. Second-look arthroscopy is one of the most reliable examination methods for assessing cartilage damage. Gong et al. [2] compared single- and double-bundle ACL reconstruction in terms of the prevalence of cartilage damage using second-look arthroscopic evaluation. In this study, they excluded patients who had any meniscus or cartilage injury. The authors concluded that chondral lesions were found postoperatively in both single- and double-bundle ACL reconstruction groups and also that double-bundle ACL reconstruction was more likely than single-bundle reconstruction to reduce patellofemoral cartilage damage.

However, several biomechanical studies have shown that central anatomic single-bundle ACL reconstruction can also restore normal anterior translation for simulated pivot shift or anterior tibial loading [49–51]. In this method, the openings of the femoral and tibial bone tunnels are placed in the centers of their respective ACL footprints. Therefore, when performing single-bundle ACL reconstruction, orthopedic surgeons prefer central anatomic single-bundle reconstruction rather than conventional nonanatomic single-bundle reconstruction. Song et al. [52] compared anatomic single- and double-bundle ACL reconstruction in terms of the prevalence of osteoarthritis and clinical outcomes with a minimum 4-year follow-up. Although the authors did not use second-look arthroscopic evaluation, their study showed that five patients (9.6 %) in the double-bundle group and six patients (10 %) in the single-bundle group had more degenerative change on radiographs. The authors concluded that double-bundle reconstruction was not more effective than central anatomic single-bundle reconstruction in protecting against long-term cartilage damage. We compared single-bundle ACL reconstruction, double-bundle reconstruction, and the ACL augmentation procedure in terms of the prevalence of cartilage damage, using second-look arthroscopic evaluation. This study also suggested that the surgical technique used for ACL reconstruction did not significantly influence the progression of the cartilage damage (ongoing study).

20.3.5 Meniscus Injury and Articular Cartilage Injury

Normal meniscus of the knee is involved in load transmission, lubrication, and nutrition of the articular cartilage. In addition, the menisci themselves are also known to contribute to knee stability. Several long-term follow-up studies have identified preoperative meniscal injury and meniscectomy as posing a high risk of cartilage loss, and unacceptable long-term clinical results after meniscectomy have been reported by many surgeons [22, 53, 54]. In a 10-year follow-up, Nakata et al. [53] reported that radiographic degenerative changes were present in 87 % of knees that had undergone meniscectomy compared with 26 % of knees with intact menisci. Even partial meniscectomy for meniscus lesion has been linked to an increased incidence of osteoarthritis [37, 55, 56]. A systematic review found the patients with partial meniscectomy to be five times more likely to exhibit radiographic osteoarthritis than those with intact menisci [57]. Nevertheless, a recent study has reported that meniscectomy is performed two to three times more frequently than meniscus repair during ACL reconstruction [58].

In cases of isolated meniscus lesion, there is a lack of evidence to support the theory that repair of the meniscus prevents progression of osteoarthritis [22, 59]. However, concomitant ACL reconstruction is usually described as one of the most favorable factors of successful meniscal repair. Several studies [15, 60, 61] showed a high success rate of meniscal repair with concurrent ACL reconstruction. Well-repaired meniscus may provide protection against long-term joint damage. In fact, some studies showed that patients with meniscectomy and ACL reconstruction had more pain and degenerative change in the knee compared with meniscal repair and ACL reconstruction, even though the procedure of ACL reconstruction was a conventional method [54, 62, 63]. In 1991, Ferretti et al. [62] found that ACL reconstruction had a chondroprotective effect in cases of knees with ACL injuries without meniscal tear or meniscal repair but not in cases where irreparable meniscal tears or meniscectomy occurred. Recently, Barenius et al. [54] performed a randomized controlled trial to investigate the prevalence of radiographic osteoarthritis after conventional ACL reconstruction and compared the osteoarthritis prevalence between quadrupled semitendinosus tendon (65 cases) and bone–patellar tendon–bone grafts (69 cases). They concluded that there was no difference in the prevalence of osteoarthritis between the two surgical procedures and also that patients with a resected medial meniscus had an increased risk of osteoarthritis of the medial compartment compared with patients with a repaired medial meniscus. Brophy et al. [64] used arthroscopy to evaluate the condition of articular cartilage at the time of ACL revision surgery. The authors demonstrated that previous meniscal repair was associated with a lower incidence of chondral changes in knees undergoing revision ACL reconstruction compared with previous partial meniscectomy. Although their study included only cases of ACL revision surgeries and the results may reflect underlying differences in the knee at the time of prior surgery, they concluded that meniscal repair is preferable when possible at the time of ACL reconstruction.

We also investigated the relationship between the progression of articular cartilage damage and meniscal surgery (normal, repair, or partial meniscectomy) in conjunction with anatomic ACL reconstruction, using second-look arthroscopy. The results indicate that although partial meniscectomy was associated with progression of articular cartilage damage, meniscal repair was not associated with the progression (ongoing study). Several studies reported that ACL reconstruction may provide protection against later meniscus surgery [15, 22, 36, 65]. Although proper anatomic ACL reconstruction is clearly important, meniscal repair should be performed, where possible, to limit the progression of articular cartilage damage.

References

1. Nakamae A, Ochi M, Deie M, Adachi N, Shibuya H, Ohkawa S, Hirata K (2014) Clinical outcomes of second-look arthroscopic evaluation after anterior cruciate ligament augmentation: comparison with single- and double-bundle reconstruction. Bone Joint J 96-B:1325–1332
2. Gong X, Jiang D, Wang YJ, Wang J, Ao YF, Yu JK (2013) Second-look arthroscopic evaluation of chondral lesions after isolated anterior cruciate ligament reconstruction: single-versus double-bundle reconstruction. Am J Sports Med 41:2362–2367
3. Ohsawa T, Kimura M, Hagiwara K, Yorifuji H, Takagishi K (2012) Clinical and second-look arthroscopic study comparing 2 tibial landmarks for tunnel insertions during double-bundle ACL reconstruction with a minimum 2-year follow-up. Am J Sports Med 40:2479–2486

4. Ohsawa T, Kimura M, Kobayashi Y, Hagiwara K, Yorifuji H, Takagishi K (2012) Arthroscopic evaluation of preserved ligament remnant after selective anteromedial or posterolateral bundle anterior cruciate ligament reconstruction. Arthroscopy 28:807–817
5. Tanaka Y, Shino K, Horibe S, Nakamura N, Nakagawa S, Mae T, Otsubo H, Suzuki T, Nakata K (2012) Triple-bundle ACL grafts evaluated by second-look arthroscopy. Knee Surg Sports Traumatol Arthrosc 20:95–101
6. Kinugasa K, Mae T, Matsumoto N, Nakagawa S, Yoneda M, Shino K (2011) Effect of patient age on morphology of anterior cruciate ligament grafts at second-look arthroscopy. Arthroscopy 27:38–45
7. Mae T, Shino K, Matsumoto N, Natsu-Ume T, Yoneda K, Yoshikawa H, Yoneda M (2010) Anatomic double-bundle anterior cruciate ligament reconstruction using hamstring tendons with minimally required initial tension. Arthroscopy 26:1289–1295
8. Kondo E, Yasuda K (2007) Second-look arthroscopic evaluations of anatomic double-bundle anterior cruciate ligament reconstruction: relation with postoperative knee stability. Arthroscopy 23:1198–1209
9. Otsubo H, Shino K, Nakamura N, Nakata K, Nakagawa S, Koyanagi M (2007) Arthroscopic evaluation of ACL grafts reconstructed with the anatomical two-bundle technique using hamstring tendon autograft. Knee Surg Sports Traumatol Arthrosc 15:720–728
10. Toritsuka Y, Shino K, Horibe S, Mitsuoka T, Hamada M, Nakata K, Nakamura N, Yoshikawa H (2004) Second-look arthroscopy of anterior cruciate ligament grafts with multistranded hamstring tendons. Arthroscopy 20:287–293
11. Shino K, Oakes BW, Horibe S, Nakata K, Nakamura N (1995) Collagen fibril populations in human anterior cruciate ligament allografts. Electron microscopic analysis. Am J Sports Med 23:203–208
12. Ochi M, Yamanaka T, Sumen Y, Ikuta Y (1993) Arthroscopic and histologic evaluation of anterior cruciate ligaments reconstructed with the Leeds-Keio ligament. Arthroscopy 9:387–393
13. Shino K, Inoue M, Horibe S, Nakata K, Maeda A, Ono K (1991) Surface blood flow and histology of human anterior cruciate ligament allografts. Arthroscopy 7:171–176
14. Tachibana Y, Sakaguchi K, Goto T, Oda H, Yamazaki K, Iida S (2010) Repair integrity evaluated by second-look arthroscopy after arthroscopic meniscal repair with the FasT-Fix during anterior cruciate ligament reconstruction. Am J Sports Med 38:965–971
15. Feng H, Hong L, Geng XS, Zhang H, Wang XS, Jiang XY (2008) Second-look arthroscopic evaluation of bucket-handle meniscus tear repairs with anterior cruciate ligament reconstruction: 67 consecutive cases. Arthroscopy 24:1358–1366
16. Horibe S, Shino K, Nakata K, Maeda A, Nakamura N, Matsumoto N (1995) Second-look arthroscopy after meniscal repair. Review of 132 menisci repaired by an arthroscopic inside-out technique. J Bone Joint Surg (Br) 77:245–249
17. Ihara H, Miwa M, Takayanagi K, Nakayama A (1994) Acute torn meniscus combined with acute cruciate ligament injury. Second look arthroscopy after 3-month conservative treatment. Clin Orthop Relat Res 307:146–154
18. Uchio Y, Ochi M, Adachi N, Kawasaki K, Iwasa J (2003) Results of rasping of meniscal tears with and without anterior cruciate ligament injury as evaluated by second-look arthroscopy. Arthroscopy 19:463–469
19. Asahina S, Muneta T, Yamamoto H (1996) Arthroscopic meniscal repair in conjunction with anterior cruciate ligament reconstruction: factors affecting the healing rate. Arthroscopy 12:541–545
20. Asano H, Muneta T, Ikeda H, Yagishita K, Kurihara Y, Sekiya I (2004) Arthroscopic evaluation of the articular cartilage after anterior cruciate ligament reconstruction: a short-term prospective study of 105 patients. Arthroscopy 20:474–481
21. Shino K, Nakagawa S, Inoue M, Horibe S, Yoneda M (1993) Deterioration of patellofemoral articular surfaces after anterior cruciate ligament reconstruction. Am J Sports Med 21:206–211

22. Lohmander LS, Englund PM, Dahl LL, Roos EM (2007) The long-term consequence of anterior cruciate ligament and meniscus injuries: osteoarthritis. Am J Sports Med 35:1756–1769
23. Sonnery-Cottet B, Chambat P (2007) Arthroscopic identification of the anterior cruciate ligament posterolateral bundle: the figure-of-four position. Arthroscopy 23:1128.e1–1128.e3
24. Brophy RH, Zeltser D, Wright RW, Flanigan D (2010) Anterior cruciate ligament reconstruction and concomitant articular cartilage injury: incidence and treatment. Arthroscopy 26:112–120
25. Shelbourne KD, Gray T (2000) Results of anterior cruciate ligament reconstruction based on meniscus and articular cartilage status at the time of surgery. Five- to fifteen-year evaluations. Am J Sports Med 28:446–452
26. Potter HG, Jain SK, Ma Y, Black BR, Fung S, Lyman S (2012) Cartilage injury after acute, isolated anterior cruciate ligament tear: immediate and longitudinal effect with clinical/MRI follow-up. Am J Sports Med 40:276–285
27. ICRS Cartilage Injury Evaluation Package. http://www.cartilage.org/_files/contentmanagement/ICRS_evaluation.pdf#search='ICRS+classification+cartilage'
28. Outerbridge RE (1961) The etiology of chondromalacia patellae. J Bone Joint Surg (Br) 43-B:752–757
29. Louboutin H, Debarge R, Richou J, Selmi TA, Donell ST, Neyret P, Dubrana F (2009) Osteoarthritis in patients with anterior cruciate ligament rupture: a review of risk factors. Knee 16:239–244
30. Neuman P, Englund M, Kostogiannis I, Fridén T, Roos H, Dahlberg LE (2008) Prevalence of tibiofemoral osteoarthritis 15 years after nonoperative treatment of anterior cruciate ligament injury: a prospective cohort study. Am J Sports Med 36:1717–1725
31. Neyret P, Donell ST, DeJour D, DeJour H (1993) Partial meniscectomy and anterior cruciate ligament rupture in soccer players. A study with a minimum 20-year followup. Am J Sports Med 21:455–460
32. Irie K, Uchiyama E, Iwaso H (2003) Intraarticular inflammatory cytokines in acute anterior cruciate ligament injured knee. Knee 10(1):93–96
33. Marx RG, Jones EC, Angel M, Wickiewicz TL, Warren RF (2003) Beliefs and attitudes of members of the American Academy of Orthopaedic Surgeons regarding the treatment of anterior cruciate ligament injury. Arthroscopy 19:762–770
34. Daniel DM, Stone ML, Dobson BE, Fithian DC, Rossman DJ, Kaufman KR (1994) Fate of the ACL-injured patient. A prospective outcome study. Am J Sports Med 22:632–644
35. Myklebust G, Holm I, Maehlum S, Engebretsen L, Bahr R (2003) Clinical, functional, and radiologic outcome in team handball players 6 to 11 years after anterior cruciate ligament injury: a follow-up study. Am J Sports Med 31:981–989
36. Fithian DC, Paxton EW, Stone ML, Luetzow WF, Csintalan RP, Phelan D, Daniel DM (2005) Prospective trial of a treatment algorithm for the management of the anterior cruciate ligament-injured knee. Am J Sports Med 33:335–346
37. Salmon LJ, Russell VJ, Refshauge K, Kader D, Connolly C, Linklater J, Pinczewski LA (2006) Long-term outcome of endoscopic anterior cruciate ligament reconstruction with patellar tendon autograft: minimum 13-year review. Am J Sports Med 34:721–732
38. von Porat A, Roos EM, Roos H (2004) High prevalence of osteoarthritis 14 years after an anterior cruciate ligament tear in male soccer players: a study of radiographic and patient relevant outcomes. Ann Rheum Dis 63:269–273
39. Hertel P, Behrend H, Cierpinski T, Musahl V, Widjaja G (2005) ACL reconstruction using bone-patellar tendon-bone press-fit fixation: 10-year clinical results. Knee Surg Sports Traumatol Arthrosc 13:248–255
40. Oiestad BE, Holm I, Aune AK, Gunderson R, Myklebust G, Engebretsen L, Fosdahl MA, Risberg MA (2010) Knee function and prevalence of knee osteoarthritis after anterior cruciate ligament reconstruction: a prospective study with 10 to 15 years of follow-up. Am J Sports Med 38:2201–2210

41. Kessler MA, Behrend H, Henz S, Stutz G, Rukavina A, Kuster MS (2008) Function, osteoarthritis and activity after ACL-rupture: 11 years follow-up results of conservative versus reconstructive treatment. Knee Surg Sports Traumatol Arthrosc 16:442–448
42. Lohmander LS, Roos H (1994) Knee ligament injury, surgery and osteoarthrosis. Truth or consequences? Acta Orthop Scand 65:605–609
43. Kondo E, Merican AM, Yasuda K, Amis AA (2010) Biomechanical comparisons of knee stability after anterior cruciate ligament reconstruction between 2 clinically available transtibial procedures: anatomic double bundle versus single bundle. Am J Sports Med 38:1349–1358
44. Yasuda K, Kondo E, Ichiyama H, Tanabe Y, Tohyama H (2006) Clinical evaluation of anatomic double-bundle anterior cruciate ligament reconstruction procedure using hamstring tendon grafts: comparisons among 3 different procedures. Arthroscopy 22:240–251
45. Yasuda K, Kondo E, Ichiyama H, Kitamura N, Tanabe Y, Tohyama H, Minami A (2004) Anatomic reconstruction of the anteromedial and posterolateral bundles of the anterior cruciate ligament using hamstring tendon grafts. Arthroscopy 20:1015–1025
46. Yasuda K, Ichiyama H, Kondo E, Miyatake S, Inoue M, Tanabe Y (2008) An in vivo biomechanical study on the tension-versus-knee flexion angle curves of 2 grafts in anatomic double-bundle anterior cruciate ligament reconstruction: effects of initial tension and internal tibial rotation. Arthroscopy 24:276–284
47. Muneta T, Koga H, Mochizuki T, Ju YJ, Hara K, Nimura A, Yagishita K, Sekiya I (2007) A prospective randomized study of 4-strand semitendinosus tendon anterior cruciate ligament reconstruction comparing single-bundle and double-bundle techniques. Arthroscopy 23:618–628
48. Muneta T, Koga H, Morito T, Yagishita K, Sekiya I (2006) A retrospective study of the midterm outcome of two-bundle anterior cruciate ligament reconstruction using quadrupled semitendinosus tendon in comparison with one-bundle reconstruction. Arthroscopy 22:252–258
49. Ho JY, Gardiner A, Shah V, Steiner ME (2009) Equal kinematics between central anatomic single-bundle and double-bundle anterior cruciate ligament reconstructions. Arthroscopy 25:464–472
50. Kondo E, Merican AM, Yasuda K, Amis AA (2011) Biomechanical comparison of anatomic double-bundle, anatomic single-bundle, and nonanatomic single-bundle anterior cruciate ligament reconstructions. Am J Sports Med 39:279–288
51. Goldsmith MT, Jansson KS, Smith SD, Engebretsen L, LaPrade RF, Wijdicks CA (2013) Biomechanical comparison of anatomic single- and double-bundle anterior cruciate ligament reconstructions: an in vitro study. Am J Sports Med 41:1595–1604
52. Song EK, Seon JK, Yim JH, Woo SH, Seo HY, Lee KB (2013) Progression of osteoarthritis after double- and single-bundle anterior cruciate ligament reconstruction. Am J Sports Med 41:2340–2346
53. Nakata K, Shino K, Horibe S, Tanaka Y, Toritsuka Y, Nakamura N, Koyanagi M, Yoshikawa H (2008) Arthroscopic anterior cruciate ligament reconstruction using fresh-frozen bone plug-free allogeneic tendons: 10-year follow-up. Arthroscopy 24:285–291
54. Barenius B, Ponzer S, Shalabi A, Bujak R, Norlén L, Eriksson K (2014) Increased risk of osteoarthritis after anterior cruciate ligament reconstruction: a 14-year follow-up study of a randomized controlled trial. Am J Sports Med 42:1049–1057
55. Macnicol MF, Thomas NP (2000) The knee after meniscectomy. J Bone Joint Surg (Br) 82:157–159
56. Pernin J, Verdonk P, Si Selmi TA, Massin P, Neyret P (2010) Long-term follow-up of 24.5 years after intra-articular anterior cruciate ligament reconstruction with lateral extra-articular augmentation. Am J Sports Med 38:1094–1102
57. Magnussen RA, Mansour AA, Carey JL, Spindler KP (2009) Meniscus status at anterior cruciate ligament reconstruction associated with radiographic signs of osteoarthritis at 5- to 10-year follow-up: a systematic review. J Knee Surg 22:347–357

58. Noyes FR, Barber-Westin SD (2012) Treatment of meniscus tears during anterior cruciate ligament reconstruction. Arthroscopy 28:123–130
59. Hunter DJ, Zhang YQ, Niu JB, Tu X, Amin S, Clancy M, Guermazi A, Grigorian M, Gale D, Felson DT (2006) The association of meniscal pathologic changes with cartilage loss in symptomatic knee osteoarthritis. Arthritis Rheum 54:795–801
60. Pujol N, Beaufils P (2009) Healing results of meniscal tears left in situ during anterior cruciate ligament reconstruction: a review of clinical studies. Knee Surg Sports Traumatol Arthrosc 17:396–401
61. O'Shea JJ, Shelbourne KD (2003) Repair of locked bucket-handle meniscal tears in knees with chronic anterior cruciate ligament deficiency. Am J Sports Med 31:216–220
62. Ferretti A, Conteduca F, De Carli A, Fontana M, Mariani PP (1991) Osteoarthritis of the knee after ACL reconstruction. Int Orthop 15:367–371
63. Aglietti P, Zaccherotti G, De Biase P, Taddei I (1994) A comparison between medial meniscus repair, partial meniscectomy, and normal meniscus in anterior cruciate ligament reconstructed knees. Clin Orthop Relat Res 307:165–173
64. Brophy RH, Wright RW, David TS, McCormack RG, Sekiya JK, Svoboda SJ, Huston LJ, Haas AK, Steger-May K, Multicenter ACL Revision Study (MARS) Group (2012) Association between previous meniscal surgery and the incidence of chondral lesions at revision anterior cruciate ligament reconstruction. Am J Sports Med 40:808–814
65. Dunn WR, Lyman S, Lincoln AE, Amoroso PJ, Wickiewicz T, Marx RG (2004) The effect of anterior cruciate ligament reconstruction on the risk of knee reinjury. Am J Sports Med 32:1906–1914

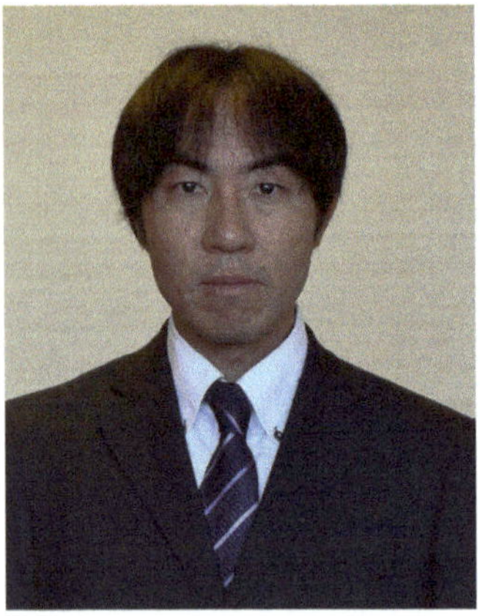

Atsuo Nakamae M.D., Ph.D., Department of Orthopaedic Surgery, Integrated Health Sciences, Institute of Biomedical & Health Sciences, Hiroshima University, Hiroshima, JAPAN.

Chapter 21
Bone Tunnel Changes After ACL Reconstruction

Daisuke Araki, Takehiko Matsushita, and Ryosuke Kuroda

Abstract Femoral and tibial bone tunnel enlargement has been reported after anterior cruciate ligament (ACL) reconstruction. Although the exact etiology of bone tunnel enlargement after ACL reconstruction remains unknown, a complex interplay between mechanical and biological factors has been proposed to explain this phenomenon. The mechanical factors include motion of the graft within the bone tunnel, fixation methods or devices, stress shielding of the graft, improper graft placement, and rehabilitation protocols. The biological factors include the infiltration of inflammatory cytokines or synovial fluid into the bone tunnel, the use of allograft tissue, and the bioabsorbable fixation device. These factors are thought to induce osteolysis and bone tunnel enlargement after ACL reconstruction. Several studies reported that bone tunnel enlargement did not affect the clinical results; however, enlarged bone tunnel often complicates revision ACL reconstruction. This chapter describes the multiple causes of bone tunnel enlargement after ACL reconstruction. Future research and improvement of surgical technique are aimed at prevention of bone tunnel enlargement.

Keywords Anterior cruciate ligament • Bone tunnel enlargement • Tunnel changes • Mechanical factor • Biological factor

21.1 Introduction

Anterior cruciate ligament (ACL) reconstruction has been the established surgical technique for patients with anterior knee instability. As the number of ACL reconstructions is increasing, femoral and tibial bone tunnel enlargement has been increasingly reported after surgery over time [3]. Several studies investigated bone tunnel enlargement using radiography (Fig. 21.1) [14, 28, 30, 52, 63], computed tomography (CT) scans (Fig. 21.2) [3, 22, 24], and magnetic resonance imaging (MRI) (Fig. 21.3) [27, 62]. Classically, bone tunnel enlargement was

D. Araki, M.D., Ph.D. (✉) • T. Matsushita • R. Kuroda
Department of Orthopedic Surgery, Kobe University Graduate School of Medicine, 7-5-2 Kusunoki-cho, Chuo-ku, Kobe, Hyogo 650-0017, Japan
e-mail: isuke@pop21.odn.ne.jp

M. Ochi et al. (eds.), *ACL Injury and Its Treatment*,
DOI 10.1007/978-4-431-55858-3_21

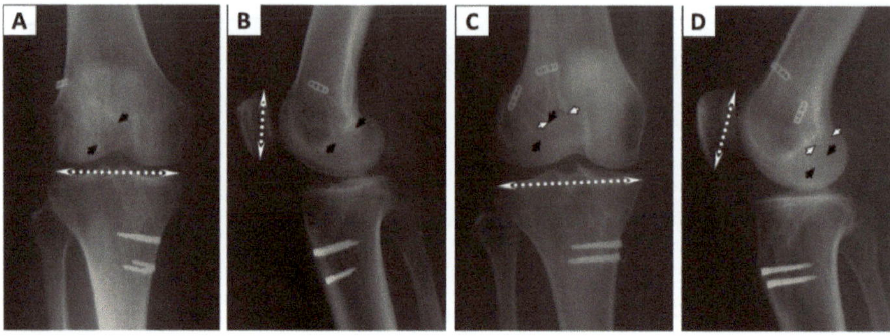

Fig. 21.1 The radiographic measurement method of bone tunnel width. Bone tunnel enlargements were observed in two-dimensional plane. (**a**) Anterior/posterior view on single-bundle ACL reconstruction. (**b**) Lateral view on single-bundle ACL reconstruction. (**c**) Anterior/posterior view on double-bundle ACL reconstruction. (**d**) Lateral view on double-bundle ACL reconstruction (Figure from "Kawaguchi Y, Kondo E, Kitamura N, Kai S, Inoue M, Yasuda K (2011) Comparisons of femoral tunnel enlargement in 169 patients between single-bundle and anatomic double-bundle anterior cruciate ligament reconstructions with hamstring tendon grafts. Knee Surg Sports Traumatol Arthrosc 19 (8):1249–1257")

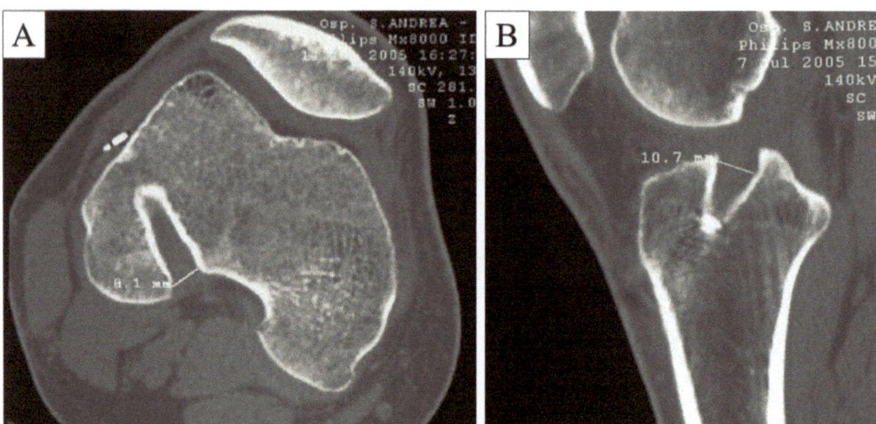

Fig. 21.2 The CT measurement method of bone tunnel width. (**a**) Axial view, (**b**) sagittal view (Figure from "Iorio R, Vadala A, Argento G, Di Sanzo V, Ferretti A (2007) Bone tunnel enlargement after ACL reconstruction using autologous hamstring tendons: a CT study. Int Orthop 31 (1):49–55")

assessed in two-dimensional view measuring the tunnel diameter using anterior/posterior and lateral views. However, recent studies demonstrated imaging in three-dimensional view in order to evaluate this phenomenon more accurately [3].

The exact etiology of bone tunnel enlargement remains unknown. However, many factors have been postulated to explain this phenomenon represented including mechanical and biological factors [64]. The mechanical factors include motion

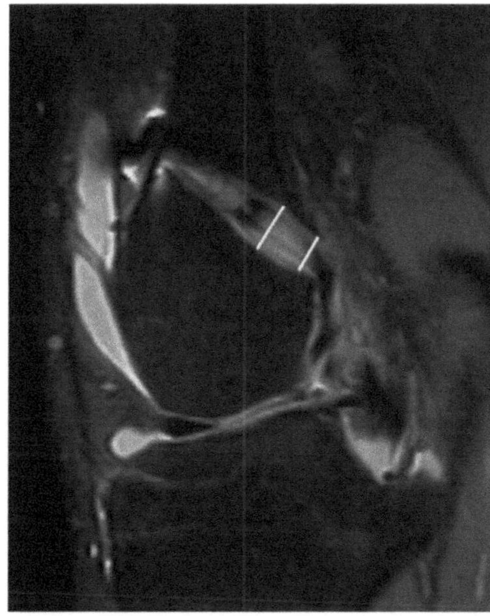

Fig. 21.3 The MRI measurement method of bone tunnel width (Figure from "Silva A, Sampaio R, Pinto E (2010) Femoral tunnel enlargement after anatomic ACL reconstruction: a biological problem? Knee Surg Sports Traumatol Arthrosc 18 (9):1189–1194")

of the graft within the bone tunnel, fixation methods or devices, stress shielding of the graft, improper graft placement, and rehabilitation protocols. The biological factors include infiltration of inflammatory cytokines or synovial fluid into the bone tunnel, the use of allograft tissue, and bioabsorbable fixation device. These factors are thought to induce osteolysis and bone tunnel enlargement after ACL reconstruction.

Although many studies have examined bone tunnel enlargement after ACL reconstruction, most of them reported no significant difference in clinical score with respect to laxity of the graft or increased failure rates [1, 3, 7, 8, 11, 13, 15, 19, 48, 63, 68]. Even though bone tunnel enlargement does not affect the clinical results, enlarged bone tunnel often complicates revision ACL reconstruction [1, 3, 7, 11, 13, 15, 21, 26, 33, 34, 48, 57, 63]. In addition, enlarged bone tunnel increases the risks of stress reactions, tibial plateau fracture, and tibial tunnel-associated cysts. For these cases, bone grafting should be considered in patients with severe bone tunnel enlargement in order to prevent future stress fracture, cyst formation, or consistent pain. For the cases of ACL revision, enlarged femoral and tibial bone tunnels interfere with the anatomical placement and size of the new bone tunnel [64]. Tunnel enlargement in the revision cases poses a technically difficult challenge with possible compromise of graft placement, fixation, and ultimately graft healing within the tunnels. These factors have a significant effect on the final outcome of the revision surgery. Therefore, bone tunnel grafting renders necessary to provide proper placement and fixation of the revision graft.

In this chapter, the etiology of bone tunnel enlargement after ACL reconstruction will be described based on both mechanical and biological factors. Surgeons should consider these factors in order to prevent bone tunnel enlargement and to improve surgical techniques.

21.2 Mechanical Factors

21.2.1 Graft–Bone Tunnel Micromotion

The current standard technique of ACL reconstruction is to create bone tunnel for the ACL graft placement. Although bone-patellar tendon–bone graft or hamstring tendon graft is commonly used, reproducing the anatomical ACL attachment morphology is difficult. Rodeo et al. reported in a cadaveric study that the graft–tunnel motion was highest at the tunnel aperture and lowest at the distal end of the tunnel within the femur, when using suspensory fixation [49]. When bone-patellar tendon–bone graft is used and the bone plug is properly placed at the position of articular aperture, direct bone-to-bone healing is expected. However, mimicking the anatomical insertion site remains difficult, and a gap between the bone tunnel and bone plug is produced. In addition, filling the bone tunnel aperture on the other side is difficult. In contrast, hamstring tendon graft is usually fixed by the suspensory fixation device, with the mismatch between bone tunnel and soft tissue graft consequently producing a gap. The resulting gap between the bone tunnel and the ACL graft may cause graft–bone tunnel micromotion. The predominant theory for tunnel enlargement after ACL reconstruction has been motion at the graft–tunnel interface [64]. Current graft substitutes and fixation techniques have been unable to recreate the normal attachment sites of the ACL.

This phenomenon may induce the "windshield wiper effect" [47, 52] which is caused by the sliding movement of the knee and the "bungee cord effect" [11, 20, 21] which is produced by the longitudinal movement of the graft. The windshield wiper effect is the reported transverse motion of ACL graft in the articular tunnel apertures, producing increased influx of synovial fluid into the bone tunnels [21]. In contrast, the bungee cord effect is the longitudinal graft–tunnel motion within the bone tunnels. These effects combined lead to bone tunnel enlargement. As a result, tunnel enlargement continues to be seen with all types of grafts and fixation methods [1, 11, 13, 15, 21, 26, 33, 48, 57, 58, 63].

Hamstring tendon autografts exhibit higher rates of bone tunnel enlargement than bone-patellar tendon–bone autografts [11, 31, 33, 63]. Clatworthy et al. compared the incidence of bone tunnel widening between bone-patellar tendon–bone and hamstring tendon grafts [11]. They showed a significant increase in tunnel widening both in the femur and in the tibia in the hamstring tendon group at a minimum of 12 months after surgery. This study suggested that the bone-to-bone interface might play an important role in decreasing micromotion of the graft once incorporation occurs. L'Insalata et al. reported that mean percentage increases in tunnel size were 30.2 % for femoral tunnel and 25. 5 % for tibial tunnel when hamstring tendon autograft was used with the suspensory fixation device for the femur and with the post-screw fixation for the tibia [33]. These values were greater when the bone-patellar tendon–bone graft was used. In addition, a statistically significant difference with respect to tunnel enlargement was found in both the femur and tibia. The authors concluded that the distant points of fixation for the hamstring grafts created a larger force moment during graft cycling, potentially leading to tunnel widening. Webster et al. also stated that bone tunnel widening stabilized after the first few months, possibly indicating graft–tunnel incorporation [63]. The longer time required for graft incorporation resulted in more time available for graft–tunnel micromotion. Thus, Morgan et al. claimed that aperture fixation of the femoral and tibial tunnels may prevent bone tunnel enlargement [40].

However, although rapid biologic bone-to-bone healing is expected using bone-patellar tendon–bone graft with interference screw fixation, a small gap is still produced between the bone plug and tunnel. Fink et al. and Höher et al. reported that synovial fluid may contribute to the bone tunnel enlargement through the gap between the graft and bone tunnel and may delay bone graft incorporation [15, 20]. Therefore, Wilson et al. claimed that the fixation of the graft was important [64]. The recent technique of rectangular anatomic ACL reconstruction matches the bone plug and tunnel aperture [53, 54] and may reduce bone tunnel enlargement, if dead space around the graft is filled with a bone plug. Mutsuzaki et al. reported that the calcium phosphate (CaP)-hybridized tendon graft improved anterior knee stability and Lysholm scores at the 2-year follow-up and reduced the percentage of bone tunnel enlargement in both tunnels at the 1-year follow-up compared with the conventional method for single-bundle ACL reconstruction [43]. Zhai et al. reported that the platelet-rich gel + deproteinized bone compound could effectively trigger tendon–bone healing by promoting maturation and ossification of the tendon–bone tissue and might improve tensile strength of the healing interface and reduce bone tunnel enlargement [67]. This new technique may enhance bone tunnel incorporation rapidly. Besides, Silva et al. compared the enlargement of the femoral tunnels at their aperture and in the middle and found that the enlargement was fusiform [56]. They concluded that biological factors might affect bone tunnel enlargement more than the mechanical factors, although response of tunnels to mechanical stress can be modified by the cortical bone at their entrance. Further studies are needed to describe the effect of micromotion at the articular bone tunnel aperture.

21.2.2 Graft Selection

ACL graft selection is also a factor for bone tunnel enlargement. Typically, bone-patellar tendon–bone auto- and allografts, Achilles tendon allografts, and hamstring tendon auto- and allografts are used for ACL graft [31, 38]. Wilson et al. claimed that the proposed mechanism in the attainment of large tunnels may be quite different for each graft source [64]. Among these grafts, hamstring tendon autograft is used increasingly because of easy harvesting technique, less donor site morbidity, reduced pain, and easier rehabilitation [33]. However, hamstring autografts had exhibited higher rates of tunnel enlargement than bone-patellar tendon–bone autografts in many previous studies [64]. One rationale is that more rapid bone-to-bone integration is expected by using bone-patellar tendon–bone graft than by using hamstring tendon graft [38]. Another rationale is that most of the fixation for the hamstring tendon graft is performed by using a suspensory fixation device. Fujii et al. demonstrated that the semitendinosus tendon graft shifted at the tunnel aperture with graft bending using a simulated femoral bone tunnel [16]. The authors reported that although the femoral tunnel was created in the center of the ACL insertion site, the graft shifted within the tunnel in the direction of the tension applied to the graft during knee movement. Therefore, a small gap between the graft and bone tunnel must be produced when a suspensory fixation device is used. In addition, distant fixation point from the joint line may lead to further graft elongation occurring with knee flexion and extension [20, 60]. Therefore, the "bungee cord effect" and the "windshield wiper effect" induced bone tunnel enlargement more than that induced by a bone-patellar tendon–bone graft, which is often fixed by aperture fixation [63]. Clatworthy et al. compared the incidence of tunnel widening between bone-patellar tendon–bone and hamstring grafts [11]. They showed a significant increase in tunnel enlargement in both the femur and tibia in the hamstring graft group at a minimum of 1 year after surgery. This study suggested that the bone-to-bone interface might play an important role in decreasing micromotion of the graft once incorporation occurs. Thus, for bone tunnel enlargement, graft fixation method is closely related to graft selection.

21.2.3 Graft Fixation Method

As explained earlier, graft fixation methods strongly affect bone tunnel enlargement. In ACL reconstruction, several fixation devices, represented by cortical suspensory fixation and aperture intra-tunnel fixation, are used for the femur and tibia. Theoretically, each technique has several advantages. For suspensory fixation, the femoral and tibial insertions of the ACL have been shown to cover the footprint, which may be reproduced to a greater extent using suspensory fixation. In contrast, as mentioned above, the "bungee cord effect" and the "windshield wiper effect" allow the graft to move back and forth between the tunnel margins during knee flexion and extension. Meanwhile, aperture fixation results in a shorter total length of the graft construct, which increases stiffness of the knee, if the elastic modulus of the graft is assumed to be constant over its length, due to mitigation of the "bungee cord effect." Lubowitz et al. compared ACL soft tissue allograft reconstruction using suspensory versus aperture fixation [35]. They showed no significant differences in knee anterior-posterior stability or clinical outcomes comparing all-inside ACL allograft reconstruction using aperture fixation to all-inside ACL allograft reconstruction using suspensory fixation. However, Buelow et al. reported that the immediately postoperative bone tunnel area was 75 % larger than the initial tunnel area in hamstring graft fixation with bioabsorbable interference screws [8]. The insertion of an interference screw apparently not only compresses the graft in the tunnel but also leads to an enlargement of the bone tunnel itself. Therefore, the compressive stiffness of the screw and graft is thought to be often greater than that of the cancellous bone of the proximal tibial metaphysis leading to tunnel enlargement. Thus, compressive stiffness of the fixation device graft construct versus cancellous bone may be an additional factor for tunnel enlargement.

Besides, the recent report by Saygi et al. investigated in different femoral fixation devices, whether tight (undersize drilled) fit technique decreased the tunnel widening and improved the clinical outcome compared to conventional technique in ACL reconstruction using hamstring tendon autograft [50]. They concluded that undersize drilling might be preferred in suspensory button fixation in order to reduce tunnel enlargement. Therefore, the utilized surgical technique may reduce bone tunnel enlargement.

21.2.4 Surgical Technique

Mechanical factors contributing to tunnel enlargement include the "windshield wiper effect" of a graft within the tunnel wall and the graft–tunnel motion and the "bungee cord effect," which results from the elastic property of the graft construct. These increased graft forces may be distributed at the tunnel entrances, resulting in tunnel wall lysis. Segawa et al. reported that one of the main factors associated with tunnel enlargement is the location of tunnels and the angle of the femoral tunnel [51]. An acute femoral tunnel angle may increase the mechanical stress on the anterior margin of the femoral tunnel. The "windshield wiper effect" of the graft may be enhanced by the changing tension in the graft due to tunnel malposition.

Furthermore, graft bending angle on the bone tunnel aperture strongly affects stress distribution to the bone tunnel wall. Fujii et al. experiment examined soft tissue graft shift at the tunnel aperture with graft bending using a simulated femoral bone tunnel [16]. Their results revealed that during knee movement, the graft shifted within the tunnel in the direction of the applied tension, enhancing stress distribution to the bone tunnel wall. In order to reduce this stress distribution to the wall, several investigators focused on the graft bending angle [44, 45]. Nishimoto et al. compared the three-dimensional bending angle of the graft at the femoral tunnel aperture in the transtibial and the transportal technique and suggested that the use of the transportal technique might result in lower stress on the graft at the femoral tunnel aperture [45]. Niki et al. assessed graft bending angle and three-dimensional characteristics of femoral bone tunnels and compared them between outside-in and transportal techniques. Their results claimed that surgeons should create the femoral tunnel considering not only the anatomic positioning of the bone tunnel aperture but also the bone tunnel direction and subsequent graft bending angle. These technical points should be taken into consideration to reduce stress contribution to the bone tunnel aperture.

Besides, in order to enhance the pullout strength of ACL graft, bone tunnel dilation technique using serial dilator was used [9, 12]. Whether bone tunnel dilation enhances the pullout strength remains controversial [46]. However, Maeda et al. investigated the time-course influence of dilation of the bone tunnel wall in ligament reconstruction on the tissue around the bone tunnel and histologically examined the mechanism of preventing the complication of bone tunnel enlargement, using rabbit tibia [36]. Their histological results suggested that the dilation promoted callus formation in the bone tunnel wall and prevented the complication of bone tunnel enlargement after ligament reconstruction. Therefore, bone tunnel dilation technique may also prevent subsequent bone tunnel enlargement.

21.2.5 Rehabilitation Protocol

Some authors claimed that aggressive rehabilitation protocols might promote tunnel enlargement, especially in hamstring tendon graft [18, 42, 61, 66]. Since Shelbourne started “accelerated rehabilitation” protocol in 1990, the incidences of arthrofibrosis, loss of motion, and anterior knee pain were reported to significantly reduce. Their postoperative rehabilitation protocol allows full weight bearing, immediate unlimited range of motion, and strengthening exercises emphasizing full extension of the knee just after surgery. Some authors investigated the relationship between postoperative rehabilitation protocol and bone tunnel enlargement. Murty et al. reported that immobilization for 2 weeks after surgery was associated with an increased bone tunnel enlargement [42]. In contrast, Hantes et al. and Yu et al. reported that a nonaggressive rehabilitation procedure resulted in a lower increase in tunnel widening [18, 66]. They suggested that less aggressive rehabilitation could reduce longitudinal micromotion of the graft in the early postoperative days. Vadalà et al. evaluated the effect of a brace-free rehabilitation on the tunnel enlargement after ACL reconstruction using hamstring tendon grafts [61]. They enrolled 45 consecutive patients undergoing ACL reconstruction who were randomly assigned to enter the standard postoperative rehabilitation group or the brace-free accelerated rehabilitation group. A CT scan was used to exactly determine the diameters of both femoral and tibial tunnels at various levels of lateral femoral condyle and proximal tibia. Their results suggested significantly higher increase in femoral and tunnel diameters in the accelerated rehabilitation group than in the standard rehabilitation group. These results may be attributed to the accelerated rehabilitation protocol, influencing ligamentization after ACL reconstruction. Thus, graft-to-tunnel healing could possibly be compromised by motion occurring between these interfaces during cycling of the knee [5]. As a result, graft–tunnel motion such as the “windshield wiper effect” or the “bungee cord effect” may delay this process. However, how these accelerated rehabilitation protocols affect bone tunnel enlargement remains unclear. Many studies have reported that tunnel enlargement is an early phenomenon occurring within 3 months after ACL reconstruction. Further studies are needed to investigate the relationship between accelerated rehabilitation and bone tunnel enlargement.

21.3 Biological Factors

21.3.1 Inflammatory Cytokines

Biological factors have been claimed to play an important role in the pathogenesis of bone tunnel enlargement after ACL reconstruction. Cameron et al. showed that the concentrations of inflammatory cytokines, such as tumor necrosis factor alpha (TNF-α), interleukin (IL)-1β, and IL-6, are elevated in the synovial fluid both immediately and several weeks after ACL injury [10]. These cytokines are released by macrophages, act as intercellular messengers, and are synthesized during inflammatory or antigenic stimulation. In addition, they are known to stimulate osteoclastic activity and contribute to bone resorption [23]. "Synovial bathing effect" has been proposed that postulates synovial fluid leakage into the bone tunnel after ACL reconstruction, exposing the bone to the inflammatory cytokines [15, 20, 33, 64]. This phenomenon was reported in total joint arthroplasty, where high levels of macrophages and cytokines were induced around loose implants [4]. Berg et al. examined intra-articular bone tunnel healing in a rabbit animal model after ACL reconstruction [6]. They found that bone tunnel healing was slower and less complete in the articular part of the tunnel than in the tunnel parts that were farther from the synovial environment. Zysk et al. investigated the synovial fluid concentrations of TNF-α, IL-1β, and IL-6 immediately before and 7 days after ACL reconstruction [69]. IL-6 levels increased significantly from the pre- to the postoperative measurements, while TNF-α concentrations were lower postoperatively. IL-1β concentrations remained unchanged throughout the course of ACL surgery. These data suggested that ACL reconstruction has a greater impact on IL-6 than on TNF-α or IL-1β synovial fluid levels in the time period assessed.

Synovial fluid tracking along the graft–bone tunnel interface after ACL reconstruction has been reported [11]. The bone tunnel is subsequently exposed to the increased levels of cytokines within the synovial fluid, which induces osteolysis. In normal synovial fluid, a high concentration of IL-1 receptor antagonist protein exists, while other cytokines are present in lower levels. However, after ACL injury, large increases of the IL family and TNF occur acutely. Associated injuries such as bone bruises and meniscus tears may affect the cytokine profile. These cytokines may decrease and stabilize over time or continue to be elevated [10, 20]. Moreover, IL-1 receptor antagonist protein apparently becomes depleted over time and is somewhat undetectable in chronic ACL situations [64]. Therefore, aperture fixation and rapid graft–bone tunnel healing may prevent these biological reactions along ACL graft and subsequent bone tunnel enlargement.

21.3.2 Graft Type (Autograft Versus Allograft)

The tendon–bone healing process is generally divided into the following four stages: (1) inflammation, (2) proliferation, (3) matrix synthesis, and (4) matrix remodeling [17]. For ACL reconstruction, both autograft and allograft tendons are widely used. Allograft can be easily used without any donor site morbidity. Meanwhile, allograft tendons have the risk of a foreign-body immune response compared to autograft tendons. Therefore, bone tunnel enlargement has been reported in association with the use of allograft tissue for ACL reconstruction.

The incidence of tunnel enlargement with the use of allografts compared to autografts was reported. Fahey et al. examined a radiography study comparing patellar tendon autografts and patellar tendon allografts at 1-year follow-up [13]. They showed significantly increased incidence of tunnel enlargement in the allograft group than in the autograft group. Although they hypothesized that a subclinical immune response caused the difference, their clinical outcomes were not adversely affected. Linn et al. reported on fresh-frozen Achilles tendons without a calcaneal bone block fixed using screws and washers on both the femur and tibia. This study reported that most patients had evidence of tunnel enlargement; however, the grafts were clinically stable [34]. The recent study by Ge et al. compared tendon–bone healing between autograft and allograft tendons after ACL reconstruction using 3.0 T MRI [17]. They compared MRI scans of 18 patients with autograft and 18 with allograft obtained at least 2 years after ACL reconstruction. They found that the allograft tendons had inferior remodeling in the bone tunnel compared to the autograft tendons. However, no significant difference was found between the allograft group and autograft group for the femoral and tibial tunnel aperture areas. The graft remodeling condition in the bone tunnel appeared to have has no direct relationship with the bone tunnel area enlargement. They concluded that the biomechanical effect of graft motion might have played a significant role in the tunnel aperture for both the autograft and allograft group. Based on the literature, further studies are needed to prove an increased risk of tunnel enlargement with allograft tissue as compared with autograft.

21.3.3 Bioabsorbable Interference Screw

Traditionally, ACL graft fixation method was often performed with metal interference screws [32]. Although good fixation by metal interference screws has been reported, there are concerns regarding the distortion on MRI evaluation as well as the requirement for implant removal for revision surgery. To avoid these potential problems, bioabsorbable screws have been proposed for graft fixation. However, since Martinek et al. reported a case of osteolytic tibial bone tunnel enlargement in association with pretibial cyst formation 8 months after ACL graft fixation with a poly-D, -L-lactide interference screw [37], bioabsorbable interference screws in the graft incorporation area are postulated to cause a local inflammatory response that induces cell necrosis and associated bone tunnel enlargement [21].

In contrast, Stähelin et al. examined six tibial biopsy specimens after ACL reconstructions performed by using interference screws made of polylactic acid, polyglycolic acid, or a polylactic acid–polyglycolic acid copolymer. They observed the presence of foreign-body giant cells in only one case, with no clinical inflammatory reaction [59]. However, the recent study by Kim et al. compared an autogenous bone plug and a bioabsorbable interference screw for tibial fixation with respect to bone tunnel enlargement as assessed with MRI [29]. They found that autogenous bone plugs reduced the tibial tunnel enlargement without inducing instability compared with bioabsorbable interference screws. Therefore, the influence of bioabsorbable interference screw on bone tunnel enlargement remains unclear. Further comparative studies are required.

21.3.4 New Biological Approach to Minimize Bone Tunnel Enlargement

As described above, firm tendon–bone tunnel healing near the joint may prevent bone tunnel enlargement after ACL reconstruction. Therefore, several researchers have tried to improve tendon–bone healing using new biological approaches. Mutsuzaki et al. examined the tendon–bone healing by hybridizing CaP with a tendon graft using an alternating soaking process [43]. They applied this method to human ACL reconstruction and compared the clinical results with those of conventional single-bundle ACL reconstruction with hamstring tendon. The tendon grafts were soaked in a calcium solution for 30 s and then soaked in a $NaHPO_4$ solution for 30 s. They repeated this cycle ten times. They found that CaP-hybridized tendon graft reduced the percentage of bone tunnel enlargement in both tunnels at the 1 year follow-up compared with the conventional method for single-bundle ACL reconstruction. Matsumoto et al. investigated an effect of autologous ruptured ACL tissue on the maturation of bone–tendon integration in ACL reconstruction using a canine model [39]. Twenty healthy adult beagle dogs underwent bilateral ACL reconstruction using the ipsilateral flexor digitorum superficialis tendon and were divided into two groups: right knee (a tissue-treated group) and left knee (a control group). The tissue-treated group received autologous ruptured ACL tissue, which was obtained 2 days after resection and sutured to the tibial side of the graft. Histological, radiographic, and biomechanical assessments were performed. In addition, immunohistochemical staining was performed to assess angiogenesis and osteogenesis. Histological assessment and staining for osteoblasts and endothelial cells at week 2 demonstrated early healing, inducing endochondral ossification-like integration with enhanced angiogenesis and osteogenesis in the tissue-treated group's grafts. Computed tomography at week 4 showed a significantly smaller tibial bone tunnel in the tissue-treated group.

Furthermore, biomechanical testing of force during loading to ultimate failure at week 4 demonstrated a significantly higher strength in the tissue-treated group. They elucidated that transplantation of ACL-ruptured tissue, which was sutured to the tibial side of the graft, contributed to early tendon–bone healing in a canine model of ACL reconstruction. Therefore, ACL-ruptured tissue may have a therapeutic potential in promoting an appropriate environment for tendon-to-bone healing in bone tunnels of ACL reconstruction. Jang et al. investigated whether non-autologous transplantation of human umbilical cord blood-derived mesenchymal stem cells (hUCB-MSCs) could be integrated safely at the bone–tendon junction without immune rejection and whether it could enhance bone–tendon healing effectively during ACL reconstruction in an animal model [25]. They found enhanced tendon–bone tunnel healing through broad fibrocartilage formation with higher histologic scores and decreased femoral and tibial tunnel enlargement compared with the control group. Therefore, they indicated that non-autologous transplantation of hUCB-MSCs had therapeutic potential in promoting tendon-to-bone tunnel healing after ACL reconstruction.

In contrast, Vadalà et al. tried to apply platelet-rich plasma (PRP) for reducing femoral and tibial tunnel enlargement in patients after ACL reconstruction [61]. They compared 20 patients after ACL reconstruction with PRP with 20 controls. For the PRP group, 5 ml of PRP was added between the peripheral part of the graft and the tunnel wall before passing the graft through the femoral tunnel. Next, another 5 ml of semisolid PRP was added above the graft before it was pulled down into the femoral tunnel. Similarly, on the tibial side, 5 ml of liquid and semisolid PRP were added before fixing the graft with the metallic screw. However, no significant differences were found in bone tunnel diameter between these two groups. They concluded that the use of PRP did not seem to be effective in preventing femoral and tibial tunnel enlargement in patients after ACL reconstruction with hamstrings.

The application of these techniques is quite new, and several new therapies of regenerative medicine have been introduced. These new techniques may enhance graft–bone tunnel healing and subsequently prevent bone tunnel enlargement. However, further studies are definitely needed to prove the efficacy of these new techniques for preventing bone tunnel enlargement.

21.4 Bone Tunnel Changes After Double-Bundle ACL Reconstruction

Recently, on the basis of several biomechanical studies [41, 65], double-bundle ACL reconstruction, which is designed to reproduce both the anteromedial bundle (AMB) and the posterolateral bundle (PLB), became increasingly popular over the past decade, because this procedure was able to more closely restore the rotational stability compared with the conventional single-bundle technique [2]. Siebold et al. first investigated the amount of tibial and femoral bone tunnel enlargement after double-bundle ACL reconstruction [55]. They found significant bone tunnel enlargement for both tibial and femoral bone tunnels at a mean follow-up period of 1 year postoperatively on MRI. The mean enlargement was 43 % for each individual tibial bone tunnel and 35 % and 48 % for the AMB and PLB femoral bone tunnels, respectively. Järvela compared tunnel enlargement in patients with double-bundle and single-bundle ACL reconstruction [27]. They showed that double-bundle ACL reconstruction resulted in less tunnel enlargement in each tunnel on the tibial side than the single-bundle technique. In addition, no tunnel communication was observed in the patients undergoing double-bundle ACL reconstruction. Thus, even though bone tunnel enlargement is observed in double-bundle ACL reconstruction, less tunnel enlargement was reported in double-bundle ACL reconstruction than in single-bundle technique.

Most of the previous reports that evaluated bone tunnel enlargement were by two-dimensional analysis, and no previous reports have assessed the direction of bone tunnel volume change and that of the transposition after anatomic double-bundle ACL reconstruction. Therefore, authors tried to extract the bone tunnel region to compare site-specific (articular one-third and outer one-third) volume changes and to assess the direction of transposition of the bone tunnel by the use of three-dimensional multidetector-row computed tomography (MDCT) data [3]. Eleven patients who underwent unilateral double-bundle ACL reconstruction with hamstring tendon autografts were included, and MDCT scanning of their knees was performed at 3 weeks and 1 year after surgery. The bone tunnel regions were extracted from the MDCT images, and the longitudinal axis of each bone tunnel was divided into three equal sections. The centroids of the outside and the articular thirds were then extracted from the bone tunnel position. Changes in the bone tunnel volume and the transposition of the articular third were calculated and compared. At 1 year postoperatively, as compared with the 3-week postoperative value (set at 100 %), the femoral bone tunnel volume of the AMB and PLB changed to 77.4 ± 15.3 % and 102.3 ± 19.2 % in the outside third and 122.3 ± 31.8 % and 112.5 ± 34.4 % in the articular third, respectively. The tibial bone tunnel volume of the AMB and the PLB changed to 108.6 ± 28.7 % and 105.4 ± 22.6 % in the tibial articular third and 54.9 ± 25.8 % and 52.5 ± 26.9 % in the outside third, respectively. The femoral outside third of the AMB and the tibial outside third of both the AMB and PLB were significantly reduced in bone tunnel volume. The centroid of the femoral articular third of the AMB moved 13°, 1.1 ± 0.6 mm posterodistally, and that of the PLB moved 35°, 0.8 ± 0.4 mm anterodistally. Furthermore, the centroid of the tibial articular third of the AMB moved 14°, 2.0 ± 1.6 mm posterolaterally, and that of the PLB moved 72°, 1.0 ± 1.3 mm posterolaterally. Compared with 3 weeks postoperatively, the articular side outlets of the femoral and tibial bone tunnels at 1 year postoperatively had enlarged slightly, but their volume was maintained, and they had moved a little in the direction in which the grafts were pulled (Fig. 21.4). From the result of this study, within ACL insertion site, surgeons should consider the direction in which the bone tunnels move.

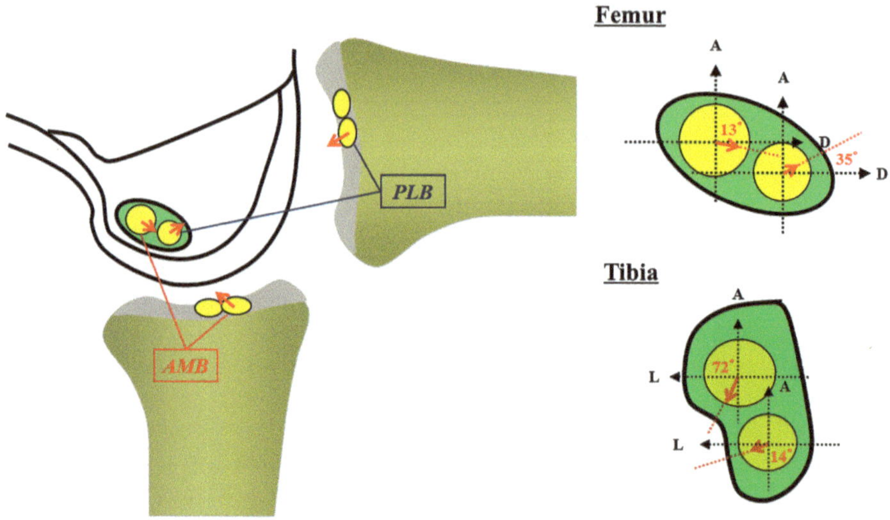

Fig. 21.4 The direction of bone tunnel enlargement. The centroid of the bone tunnel in articular sides moved in the direction that the grafts were pulled

Therefore, surgeons should consider this direction of bone tunnel change proposed by the new three-dimensional analysis.

21.5 Summary

The exact etiology of bone tunnel enlargement after ACL reconstruction remains unclear and seems to be multifactorial. As described above, a complex interplay between mechanical and biological factors has been proposed to describe bone tunnel enlargement. The mechanical factors identified include local stress deprivation of the bone tunnels in the early postoperative period or excessive graft–tunnel motion in the coronal or sagittal planes. The mechanical environment is affected by the surgical technique such as graft position, graft tension, graft fixation, and aggressive rehabilitation. The biologic factors involved may include synovial fluid-derived cytokines and inflammatory mediators, the graft choice, and bioabsorbable fixation devices. In addition, allograft-specific factors that may contribute include the immune response to allograft and potential toxicity of chemicals used during allograft processing.

A recent study by Weber et al. examined the predictive value of demographic data and preoperative bone quality on functional outcome scores, manual and instrumented laxity measurements, and changes in bone tunnel area over time using logistic regression modeling [62]. They investigated 18 patients after ACL reconstruction and found that younger age (<30 years), male sex, and time from injury to ACL reconstruction (>1 year) may be potential risks for enlargement. To

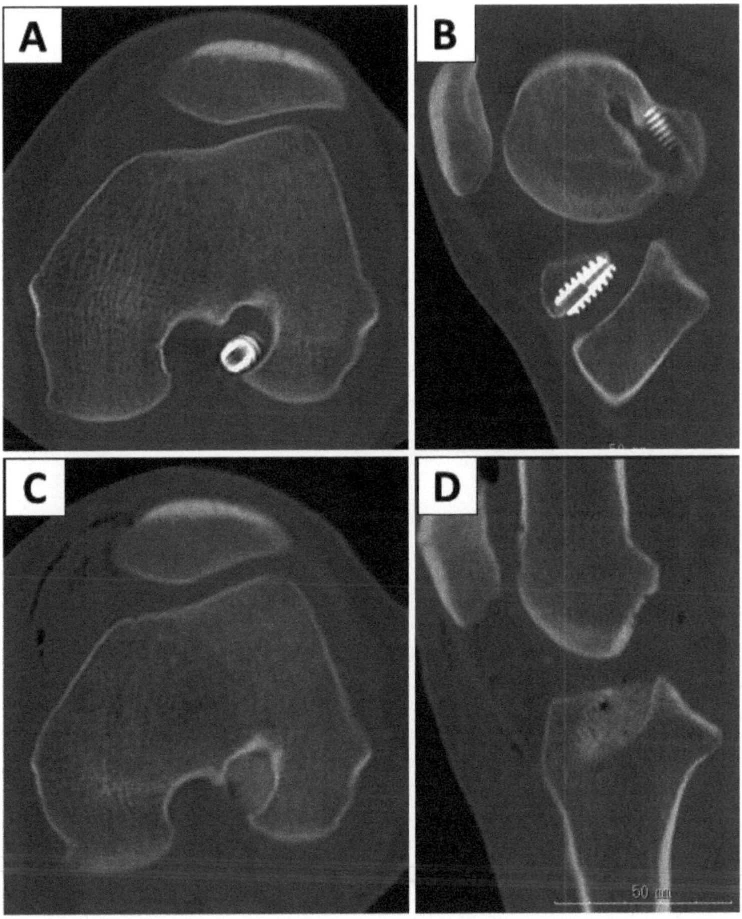

Fig. 21.5 Two-staged surgery case with bone grafting of the tunnels. Twenty-seven years old female. Preoperative CT images; (**a**) axial view and (**b**) sagittal view. Postoperative CT images (after autologous bone grafting); (**c**) axial view and (**d**) sagittal view

our knowledge, this study, despite its small sample size, is the first to predict the effect of demographic factors on bone tunnel enlargement. Further studies are required to examine the relationship between younger age, male sex, and time from injury to ACL reconstruction as potential risk factors for postoperative bone tunnel enlargement.

The etiology of tunnel widening remains unknown, but is most likely multifactorial. Concluding from the several studies on bone tunnel enlargement and aperture fixation in the femoral and tibial tunnels may decrease tunnel enlargement. Autografts may cause less tunnel enlargement than allografts due to a proposed cellular reaction to allograft tissue. Postoperative rehabilitation methods need to allow for sufficient graft incorporation. Tunnel placement may affect the direction of bone tunnel enlargement. Although bone tunnel enlargement does not appear to adversely affect clinical outcome in the short term, the long-term relationship with potential knee laxity or increased traumatic failure rate is unknown. However, tunnel enlargement may definitely complicate revision surgery. In addition, the results of revision surgery show increased laxity compared to primary surgery. Large tunnels create complications for graft fixation and graft placement. Patients with large bone tunnel enlargement may need a two-staged surgery with bone grafting of the tunnels followed by delayed ACL reconstruction (Fig. 21.5). Therefore, it is important to prevent bone tunnel enlargement after ACL reconstruction. The surgeon must consider these potential causes of bone tunnel enlargement and attempt to minimize these risks. Techniques that enhance graft fixation or avoid mechanical stress should be developed, and further research should be pursued aiming at the prevention of bone tunnel enlargement after ACL reconstruction.

References

1. Aglietti P, Zaccherotti G, Simeone AJ, Buzzi R (1998) Anatomic versus non-anatomic tibial fixation in anterior cruciate ligament reconstruction with bone-patellar tendon-bone graft. Knee Surg Sports Traumatol Arthrosc 6(Suppl 1):S43–S48
2. Araki D, Kuroda R, Kubo S, Fujita N, Tei K, Nishimoto K, Hoshino Y, Matsushita T, Matsumoto T, Nagamune K, Kurosaka M (2011) A prospective randomised study of anatomical single-bundle versus double-bundle anterior cruciate ligament reconstruction: quantitative evaluation using an electromagnetic measurement system. Int Orthop 35(3):439–446
3. Araki D, Kuroda R, Matsumoto T, Nagamune K, Matsushita T, Hoshino Y, Oka S, Nishizawa Y, Kurosaka M (2014) Three-dimensional analysis of bone tunnel changes after anatomic double-bundle anterior cruciate ligament reconstruction using multidetector-row computed tomography. Am J Sports Med 42(9):2234–2241
4. Archibeck MJ, Jacobs JJ, Roebuck KA, Glant TT (2001) The basic science of periprosthetic osteolysis. Instr Course Lect 50:185–195
5. Aune AK, Ekeland A, Cawley PW (1998) Interference screw fixation of hamstring vs patellar tendon grafts for anterior cruciate ligament reconstruction. Knee Surg Sports Traumatol Arthrosc 6(2):99–102
6. Berg EE, Pollard ME, Kang Q (2001) Interarticular bone tunnel healing. Arthroscopy 17 (2):189–195
7. Buelow JU, Siebold R, Ellermann A (2000) A new bicortical tibial fixation technique in anterior cruciate ligament reconstruction with quadruple hamstring graft. Knee Surg Sports Traumatol Arthrosc 8(4):218–225
8. Buelow JU, Siebold R, Ellermann A (2002) A prospective evaluation of tunnel enlargement in anterior cruciate ligament reconstruction with hamstrings: extracortical versus anatomical fixation. Knee Surg Sports Traumatol Arthrosc 10(2):80–85
9. Cain EL, Phillips BB, Charlebois SJ, Azar FM (2005) Effect of tibial tunnel dilation on pullout strength of semitendinosus-gracilis graft in anterior cruciate ligament reconstruction. Orthopedics 28(8):779–783
10. Cameron M, Buchgraber A, Passler H, Vogt M, Thonar E, Fu F, Evans CH (1997) The natural history of the anterior cruciate ligament-deficient knee. Changes in synovial fluid cytokine and keratan sulfate concentrations. Am J Sports Med 25(6):751–754

11. Clatworthy MG, Annear P, Bulow JU, Bartlett RJ (1999) Tunnel widening in anterior cruciate ligament reconstruction: a prospective evaluation of hamstring and patella tendon grafts. Knee Surg Sports Traumatol Arthrosc 7(3):138–145
12. Dargel J, Schmidt-Wiethoff R, Bruggemann GP, Koebke J (2007) The effect of bone tunnel dilation versus extraction drilling on the initial fixation strength of press-fit anterior cruciate ligament reconstruction. Arch Orthop Trauma Surg 127(9):801–807
13. Fahey M, Indelicato PA (1994) Bone tunnel enlargement after anterior cruciate ligament replacement. Am J Sports Med 22(3):410–414
14. Fauno P, Kaalund S (2005) Tunnel widening after hamstring anterior cruciate ligament reconstruction is influenced by the type of graft fixation used: a prospective randomized study. Arthroscopy 21(11):1337–1341
15. Fink C, Zapp M, Benedetto KP, Hackl W, Hoser C, Rieger M (2001) Tibial tunnel enlargement following anterior cruciate ligament reconstruction with patellar tendon autograft. Arthroscopy 17(2):138–143
16. Fujii M, Sasaki Y, Araki D, Furumatsu T, Miyazawa S, Ozaki T, Linde-Rosen M, Smolinski P, Fu FH (2014) Evaluation of the semitendinosus tendon graft shift in the bone tunnel: an experimental study. Knee Surg Sports Traumatol Arthrosc [Epub ahead of print]
17. Ge Y, Li H, Tao H, Hua Y, Chen J, Chen S (2015) Comparison of tendon-bone healing between autografts and allografts after anterior cruciate ligament reconstruction using magnetic resonance imaging. Knee Surg Sports Traumatol Arthrosc 23(4):954–960
18. Hantes ME, Mastrokalos DS, Yu J, Paessler HH (2004) The effect of early motion on tibial tunnel widening after anterior cruciate ligament replacement using hamstring tendon grafts. Arthroscopy 20(6):572–580
19. Hogervorst T, van der Hart CP, Pels Rijcken TH, Taconis WK (2000) Abnormal bone scans of the tibial tunnel 2 years after patella ligament anterior cruciate ligament reconstruction: correlation with tunnel enlargement and tibial graft length. Knee Surg Sports Traumatol Arthrosc 8(6):322–328
20. Hoher J, Livesay GA, Ma CB, Withrow JD, Fu FH, Woo SL (1999) Hamstring graft motion in the femoral bone tunnel when using titanium button/polyester tape fixation. Knee Surg Sports Traumatol Arthrosc 7(4):215–219
21. Hoher J, Moller HD, Fu FH (1998) Bone tunnel enlargement after anterior cruciate ligament reconstruction: fact or fiction? Knee Surg Sports Traumatol Arthrosc 6(4):231–240
22. Iorio R, Vadala A, Argento G, Di Sanzo V, Ferretti A (2007) Bone tunnel enlargement after ACL reconstruction using autologous hamstring tendons: a CT study. Int Orthop 31(1):49–55
23. Jacobs JJ, Roebuck KA, Archibeck M, Hallab NJ, Glant TT (2001) Osteolysis: basic science. Clin Orthop Relat Res 393:71–77
24. Jagodzinski M, Geiges B, von Falck C, Knobloch K, Haasper C, Brand J, Hankemeier S, Krettek C, Meller R (2010) Biodegradable screw versus a press-fit bone plug fixation for hamstring anterior cruciate ligament reconstruction: a prospective randomized study. Am J Sports Med 38(3):501–508
25. Jang KM, Lim HC, Jung WY, Moon SW, Wang JH (2015) Efficacy and safety of human umbilical cord blood-derived mesenchymal stem cells in anterior cruciate ligament reconstruction of a rabbit model: new strategy to enhance tendon graft healing. Arthroscopy 31 (8):1530–1539
26. Jansson KA, Harilainen A, Sandelin J, Karjalainen PT, Aronen HJ, Tallroth K (1999) Bone tunnel enlargement after anterior cruciate ligament reconstruction with the hamstring autograft and endobutton fixation technique. A clinical, radiographic and magnetic resonance imaging study with 2 years follow-up. Knee Surg Sports Traumatol Arthrosc 7(5):290–295
27. Jarvela T, Moisala AS, Paakkala T, Paakkala A (2008) Tunnel enlargement after double-bundle anterior cruciate ligament reconstruction: a prospective, randomized study. Arthroscopy 24(12):1349–1357
28. Kawaguchi Y, Kondo E, Kitamura N, Kai S, Inoue M, Yasuda K (2011) Comparisons of femoral tunnel enlargement in 169 patients between single-bundle and anatomic double-

bundle anterior cruciate ligament reconstructions with hamstring tendon grafts. Knee Surg Sports Traumatol Arthrosc 19(8):1249–1257
29. Kim SJ, Bae JH, Song SH, Lim HC (2013) Bone tunnel widening with autogenous bone plugs versus bioabsorbable interference screws for secondary fixation in ACL reconstruction. J Bone Joint Surg Am 95(2):103–108
30. Klein JP, Lintner DM, Downs D, Vavrenka K (2003) The incidence and significance of femoral tunnel widening after quadrupled hamstring anterior cruciate ligament reconstruction using femoral cross pin fixation. Arthroscopy 19(5):470–476
31. Kobayashi M, Nakagawa Y, Suzuki T, Okudaira S, Nakamura T (2006) A retrospective review of bone tunnel enlargement after anterior cruciate ligament reconstruction with hamstring tendons fixed with a metal round cannulated interference screw in the femur. Arthroscopy 22 (10):1093–1099
32. Kurosaka M, Yoshiya S, Andrish JT (1987) A biomechanical comparison of different surgical techniques of graft fixation in anterior cruciate ligament reconstruction. Am J Sports Med 15 (3):225–229
33. L'Insalata JC, Klatt B, Fu FH, Harner CD (1997) Tunnel expansion following anterior cruciate ligament reconstruction: a comparison of hamstring and patellar tendon autografts. Knee Surg Sports Traumatol Arthrosc 5(4):234–238
34. Linn RM, Fischer DA, Smith JP, Burstein DB, Quick DC (1993) Achilles tendon allograft reconstruction of the anterior cruciate ligament-deficient knee. Am J Sports Med 21 (6):825–831
35. Lubowitz JH, Schwartzberg R, Smith P (2015) Cortical suspensory button versus aperture interference screw fixation for knee anterior cruciate ligament soft-tissue allograft: a prospective, randomized controlled trial. Arthroscopy 31(9):1733–1739
36. Maeda S, Ishikawa H, Tanigawa N, Miyazaki K, Shioda S (2012) Histological observation of regions around bone tunnels after compression of the bone tunnel wall in ligament reconstruction. Acta Histochem Cytochem 45(2):107–112
37. Martinek V, Friederich NF (1999) Tibial and pretibial cyst formation after anterior cruciate ligament reconstruction with bioabsorbable interference screw fixation. Arthroscopy 15 (3):317–320
38. Matsumoto A, Yoshiya S, Muratsu H, Yagi M, Iwasaki Y, Kurosaka M, Kuroda R (2006) A comparison of bone-patellar tendon-bone and bone-hamstring tendon-bone autografts for anterior cruciate ligament reconstruction. Am J Sports Med 34(2):213–219
39. Matsumoto T, Kubo S, Sasaki K, Kawakami Y, Oka S, Sasaki H, Takayama K, Tei K, Matsushita T, Mifune Y, Kurosaka M, Kuroda R (2012) Acceleration of tendon-bone healing of anterior cruciate ligament graft using autologous ruptured tissue. Am J Sports Med 40 (6):1296–1302
40. Morgan CD, Stein DA, Leitman EH, Kalman VR (2002) Anatomic tibial graft fixation using a retrograde bio-interference screw for endoscopic anterior cruciate ligament reconstruction. Arthroscopy 18(7), E38
41. Muneta T (2015) Twenty-year experience of a double-bundle anterior cruciate ligament reconstruction. Clin Orthop Surg 7(2):143–151
42. Murty AN, el Zebdeh MY, Ireland J (2001) Tibial tunnel enlargement following anterior cruciate reconstruction: does post-operative immobilisation make a difference? Knee 8 (1):39–43
43. Mutsuzaki H, Kanamori A, Ikeda K, Hioki S, Kinugasa T, Sakane M (2012) Effect of calcium phosphate-hybridized tendon graft in anterior cruciate ligament reconstruction: a randomized controlled trial. Am J Sports Med 40(8):1772–1780
44. Niki Y, Nagai K, Harato K, Suda Y, Nakamura M, Matsumoto M (2015) Effects of femoral bone tunnel characteristics on graft-bending angle in double-bundle anterior cruciate ligament reconstruction: a comparison of the outside-in andtransportal techniques. Knee Surg Sports Traumatol Arthrosc [Epub ahead of print]

45. Nishimoto K, Kuroda R, Mizuno K, Hoshino Y, Nagamune K, Kubo S, Yagi M, Yamaguchi M, Yoshiya S, Kurosaka M (2009) Analysis of the graft bending angle at the femoral tunnel aperture in anatomic double bundle anterior cruciate ligament reconstruction: a comparison of the transtibial and the far anteromedial portal technique. Knee Surg Sports Traumatol Arthrosc 17(3):270–276
46. Nurmi JT, Kannus P, Sievanen H, Jarvela T, Jarvinen M, Jarvinen TL (2004) Interference screw fixation of soft tissue grafts in anterior cruciate ligament reconstruction: part 2: effect of preconditioning on graft tension during and after screw insertion. Am J Sports Med 32 (2):418–424
47. Pederzini L, Adriani E, Botticella C, Tosi M (2000) Technical note: double tibial tunnel using quadriceps tendon in anterior cruciate ligament reconstruction. Arthroscopy 16(5), E9
48. Peyrache MD, Djian P, Christel P, Witvoet J (1996) Tibial tunnel enlargement after anterior cruciate ligament reconstruction by autogenous bone-patellar tendon-bone graft. Knee Surg Sports Traumatol Arthrosc 4(1):2–8
49. Rodeo SA, Kawamura S, Kim HJ, Dynybil C, Ying L (2006) Tendon healing in a bone tunnel differs at the tunnel entrance versus the tunnel exit: an effect of graft-tunnel motion? Am J Sports Med 34(11):1790–1800
50. Saygi B, Karaman O, Sirin E, Arslan I, Demir AI, Oztermeli A (2015) Comparison of different femoral fixation implants and fit techniques for tunnel widening and clinical outcome in ACL reconstruction using hamstring autograft. Arch Orthop Trauma Surg [Epub ahead of print]
51. Segawa H, Koga Y, Omori G, Sakamoto M, Hara T (2003) Influence of the femoral tunnel location and angle on the contact pressure in the femoral tunnel in anterior cruciate ligament reconstruction. Am J Sports Med 31(3):444–448
52. Segawa H, Omori G, Tomita S, Koga Y (2001) Bone tunnel enlargement after anterior cruciate ligament reconstruction using hamstring tendons. Knee Surg Sports Traumatol Arthrosc 9 (4):206–210
53. Shino K, Nakata K, Nakamura N, Toritsuka Y, Horibe S, Nakagawa S, Suzuki T (2008) Rectangular tunnel double-bundle anterior cruciate ligament reconstruction with bone-patellar tendon-bone graft to mimic natural fiber arrangement. Arthroscopy 24(10):1178–1183
54. Shino K, Nakata K, Nakamura N, Toritsuka Y, Nakagawa S, Horibe S (2005) Anatomically oriented anterior cruciate ligament reconstruction with a bone-patellar tendon-bone graft via rectangular socket and tunnel: a snug-fit and impingement-free grafting technique. Arthroscopy 21(11):1402
55. Siebold R (2007) Observations on bone tunnel enlargement after double-bundle anterior cruciate ligament reconstruction. Arthroscopy 23(3):291–298
56. Silva A, Sampaio R, Pinto E (2010) Femoral tunnel enlargement after anatomic ACL reconstruction: a biological problem? Knee Surg Sports Traumatol Arthrosc 18(9):1189–1194
57. Simonian PT, Erickson MS, Larson RV, O'Kane JW (2000) Tunnel expansion after hamstring anterior cruciate ligament reconstruction with 1-incision EndoButton femoral fixation. Arthroscopy 16(7):707–714
58. Simonian PT, Monson JT, Larson RV (2001) Biodegradable interference screw augmentation reduces tunnel expansion after ACL reconstruction. Am J Knee Surg 14(2):104–108
59. Stahelin AC, Weiler A, Rufenacht H, Hoffmann R, Geissmann A, Feinstein R (1997) Clinical degradation and biocompatibility of different bioabsorbable interference screws: a report of six cases. Arthroscopy 13(2):238–244
60. Steiner ME, Hecker AT, Brown CH Jr, Hayes WC (1994) Anterior cruciate ligament graft fixation. Comparison of hamstring and patellar tendon grafts. Am J Sports Med 22 (2):240–246; discussion 246–247
61. Vadala A, Iorio R, De Carli A, Argento G, Di Sanzo V, Conteduca F, Ferretti A (2007) The effect of accelerated, brace free, rehabilitation on bone tunnel enlargement after ACL reconstruction using hamstring tendons: a CT study. Knee Surg Sports Traumatol Arthrosc 15 (4):365–371

62. Weber AE, Delos D, Oltean HN, Vadasdi K, Cavanaugh J, Potter HG, Rodeo SA (2015) Tibial and femoral tunnel changes after ACL reconstruction: a prospective 2-year longitudinal MRI study. Am J Sports Med 43(5):1147–1156
63. Webster KE, Feller JA, Hameister KA (2001) Bone tunnel enlargement following anterior cruciate ligament reconstruction: a randomised comparison of hamstring and patellar tendon grafts with 2-year follow-up. Knee Surg Sports Traumatol Arthrosc 9(2):86–91
64. Wilson TC, Kantaras A, Atay A, Johnson DL (2004) Tunnel enlargement after anterior cruciate ligament surgery. Am J Sports Med 32(2):543–549
65. Yagi M, Wong EK, Kanamori A, Debski RE, Fu FH, Woo SL (2002) Biomechanical analysis of an anatomic anterior cruciate ligament reconstruction. Am J Sports Med 30(5):660–666
66. Yu JK, Paessler HH (2005) Relationship between tunnel widening and different rehabilitation procedures after anterior cruciate ligament reconstruction with quadrupled hamstring tendons. Chin Med J (Engl) 118(4):320–326
67. Zhai W, Lv C, Zheng Y, Gao Y, Ding Z, Chen Z (2013) Weak link of tendon-bone healing and a control experiment to promote healing. Arch Orthop Trauma Surg 133(11):1533–1541
68. Zijl JA, Kleipool AE, Willems WJ (2000) Comparison of tibial tunnel enlargement after anterior cruciate ligament reconstruction using patellar tendon autograft or allograft. Am J Sports Med 28(4):547–551
69. Zysk SP, Gebhard H, Plitz W, Buchhorn GH, Sprecher CM, Jansson V, Messmer K, Veihelmann A (2004) Influence of orthopedic particulate biomaterials on inflammation and synovial microcirculation in the murine knee joint. J Biomed Mater Res B Appl Biomater 71 (1):108–115

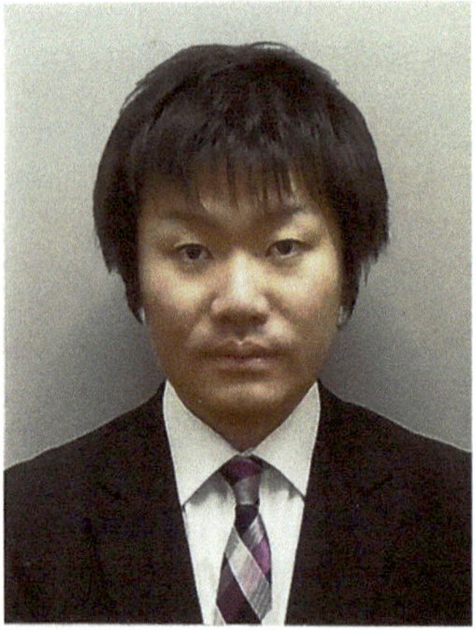

Daisuke Araki M.D. Ph.D., Department of Orthopaedic Surgery, Kobe University Graduate School of Medicine, Hyogo, Japan.

Chapter 22
Graft Impingement

Hideyuki Koga and Takeshi Muneta

Abstract When performing anterior cruciate ligament (ACL) reconstruction, graft impingement is one of the major concerns surgeons have to take into account. When the reconstructed graft was placed in a wrong position, it would be impinged to surrounding structures such as the intercondylar roof of the femur and posterior cruciate ligament (PCL) during knee range of motion. It has been reported that graft impingement could cause anterior knee pain and loss of knee range of motion. In addition, continuous graft impingement could lead to graft failure, resulting in residual knee instability. Therefore, avoiding graft impingement during ACL reconstruction is critical for successful clinical results. In traditional nonanatomic single-bundle ACL reconstruction where femoral tunnel was placed "high noon," posterior tibial tunnel placement and notchplasty had been recommended to avoid graft impingement. The recent strategy of anatomic ACL reconstruction reduced the risk of graft impingement. Anatomic double-bundle ACL reconstruction without notchplasty did not increase the incidence of loss of extension and graft failure; rather notchplasty likely caused over-constrained knees. Therefore, except in cases with spur formation on the intercondylar notch or narrow notch, routine notchplasty is not recommended in anatomic double-bundle ACL reconstruction.

Keywords Anterior cruciate ligament reconstruction • Graft impingement • Notchplasty

22.1 Introduction

When performing anterior cruciate ligament (ACL) reconstruction, graft impingement is one of the major concerns surgeons have to take into account. When the reconstructed graft was placed in a wrong position, it would be impinged to surrounding structures such as the intercondylar roof of the femur and posterior cruciate ligament (PCL) during knee range of motion. It has been reported that graft

H. Koga (✉) • T. Muneta
Department of Joint Surgery and Sports Medicine, Graduate School of Medicine, Tokyo Medical and Dental University, 1-5-45 Yushima, Bunkyo-ku, Tokyo 113-8519, Japan
e-mail: koga.orj@tmd.ac.jp

M. Ochi et al. (eds.), *ACL Injury and Its Treatment*,
DOI 10.1007/978-4-431-55858-3_22

impingement could cause anterior knee pain and loss of knee range of motion. In addition, continuous graft impingement could lead to graft failure, resulting in residual knee instability [1, 2]. Therefore, avoiding graft impingement during ACL reconstruction is critical for successful clinical results.

ACL reconstruction was performed as a single-bundle reconstruction until the 1990s [3], and in the traditional transtibial technique, the femoral tunnel was made at the isometric point on the lateral wall of the intercondylar notch, which was placed at a higher position than the anatomic ACL footprint on the femur [4]. In this isometric "nonanatomic" technique, anterior placement of the tibial tunnel causes intercondylar roof impingement of the ACL graft; therefore, posterior tibial tunnel placement and notchplasty had been recommended to avoid graft impingement [1, 2, 5, 6]. However, normal restoration of the knee kinematics and stability would be impaired in the nonanatomic single-bundle technique with such a "vertical graft placement" [7].

Recently, the strategy of ACL reconstruction has been shifting toward anatomic reconstruction, in which the ACL graft is placed within the native ACL footprint at both the femoral and tibial sides. It has been reported that anatomic femoral tunnels are located more posterior to the traditional position [8], and making the femoral tunnels accurately in the femoral ACL foot print would prevent the intercondylar roof impingement [9]. With regard to the tibial tunnels, the tibial tunnel of the anteromedial bundle (AMB) in the anatomic reconstruction is placed more anterior to the tibial tunnel in the traditional transtibial single-bundle technique [10]. It is also reported that native ACL made contact with the intercondylar roof in hyper-extension of the knee [11]; it may be that anatomic ACL causes physiologic roof impingement [12, 13].

In this chapter, significances of graft impingement are described both in nonanatomic single-bundle reconstruction and anatomic reconstruction.

22.2 Graft Impingement in Nonanatomic Single-Bundle Reconstruction

As mentioned, in traditional single-bundle reconstruction using the transtibial technique, the femoral tunnel was made at the isometric point on the lateral wall of the intercondylar notch. This "traditional" femoral tunnel position was higher and more anterior to the anatomic ACL footprint; therefore, various types of ACL graft impingement have been reported in this technique.

22.2.1 Intercondylar Roof Impingement in Nonanatomic Single-Bundle Reconstruction

Intercondylar roof impingement has been reported most commonly among the various types of ACL graft impingement. Roof impingement occurs when an ACL graft contacts the intercondylar roof before the knee reaches terminal

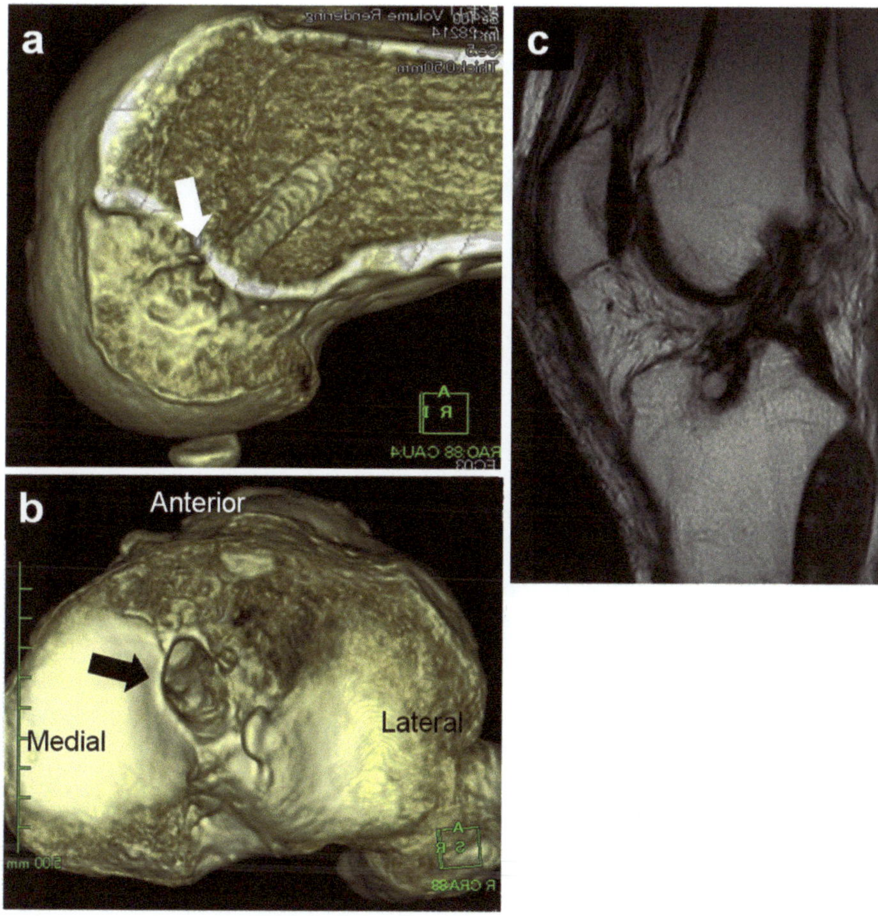

Fig. 22.1 A case with residual instability after nonanatomic single-bundle ACL reconstruction, without graft tear by obvious reinjury. (**a, b**) Femoral tunnel position (**a**, *white arrow*) and tibial tunnel position (**b**, *black arrow*) in three-dimensional computed tomography. (**c**) Magnetic resonance imaging (sagittal view). The femoral tunnel was made at the "high noon" position on the lateral wall of the intercondylar notch. Tibial tunnel was placed posteriorly to avoid graft impingement. However, normal restoration of the knee kinematics and stability would be impaired with such a "vertical graft placement"

extension [10]. In the early 1990s, Howell et al. reported several studies regarding intercondylar roof impingement [1, 2, 5, 6, 14]. They showed that, in the isometric single-bundle reconstruction technique, tibial tunnel placement was correlated with roof impingement pressure on the ACL graft, and anterior placement of the tibial tunnel induced roof impingement. The graft impingement could cause anterior knee pain and loss of knee range of motion (loss of extension), and eventually, continuous graft impingement could lead to graft failure, resulting in residual knee instability. Their conclusion from those studies was that posterior tibial tunnel placement and notchplasty were necessary to avoid roof impingement (Figs. 22.1 and 22.2).

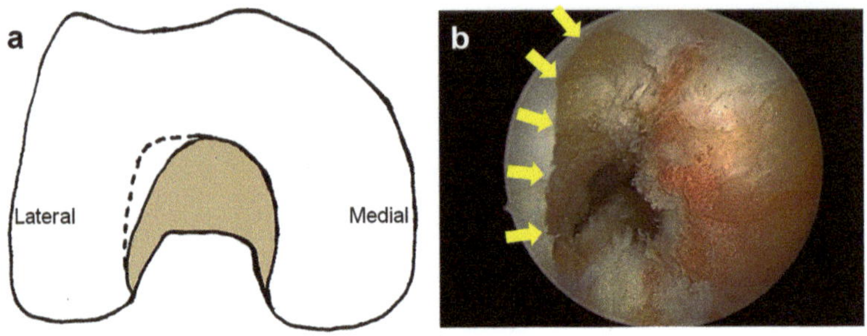

Fig. 22.2 (**a**) Scheme of notchplasty. Notchplasty is performed by removing a certain amount of the roof and lateral femoral wall to avoid graft impingement. (**b**) Arthroscopic view of notchplasty (*yellow arrows*) from the anterolateral portal

22.2.2 Notchplasty in Nonanatomic Single-Bundle Reconstruction

Therefore, notchplasty had been widely performed in nonanatomic single-bundle reconstruction, in order to avoid roof impingement (Fig. 22.2). Another concept of notchplasty was that because narrow intercondylar notch dimensions have been reported to be associated with the risk of noncontact ACL injuries [15–17]; this anatomic variation needed to be corrected by notchplasty to maximize the success rate of the reconstruction surgery. It has been reported that roof impingement pressure decreased after a 3-mm notchplasty [18]. It has also been reported, in an in vivo rabbit study, that notchplasty increases the cross-sectional area of the regenerated ACL [19], suggesting that providing space for graft healing by notchplasty might improve the healing process, although the mechanical strength of the reconstructed ACL with notchplasty was identical to that without notchplasty.

However, it has been warned that notchplasty has a potentially harmful effect on the patellar articular cartilage, because of the contact area of the intercondylar cartilage of the femur [20]. Aggressive notchplasty had detrimental effects on the histopathological characteristics of articular cartilage consistent with early degenerative disease [19, 21], whereas the minimum extent of notchplasty had no harmful effect [19]. Moreover, notch regrowth after notchplasty is not uncommon, which could potentially result in late graft demise in the ACL-reconstructed knee [21, 22].

22.2.3 PCL Impingement in Nonanatomic Single-Bundle Reconstruction

ACL graft-PCL impingement was first hypothesized by Strobel et al.[23], who reported a case of extension loss after ACL reconstruction in which the graft was placed on the femoral site in the "high noon" position. Simmons et al. also reported in the cadaveric study that high graft tension in flexion might be caused by PCL impingement, which resulted from placing the femoral tunnel medially at the apex of the notch in the coronal plane [24]. Fujimoto et al. first detected ACL graft impingement against PCL in nonanatomic single-bundle reconstruction using MRI and reported that ACL grafts with positive PCL impingement were more vertical than those with negative PCL impingement, and PCL impingement affected anteroposterior knee stability [25]. Iriuchishima et al. also reported that in nonanatomic reconstruction, high femoral tunnel position made it closer to the femoral PCL insertion site, leading to high ACL-PCL impingement pressure [26].

22.3 Graft Impingement in Anatomic Reconstruction

As mentioned above, posterior tibial tunnel placement and notchplasty had been recommended to avoid graft impingement [1, 2, 5, 6]. However, normal restoration of the knee kinematics and stability would be impaired in the traditional nonanatomic single-bundle technique with such a "vertical graft placement" [7]. Therefore, the strategy of ACL reconstruction has been shifting toward anatomic reconstruction in the past 10 years, in which the ACL graft is placed within the native ACL footprint at both the femoral and tibial sides (Fig. 22.3). This also has changed the concept of graft impingement.

22.3.1 Intercondylar Roof Impingement in Anatomic Reconstruction

It has been reported that in anatomic reconstruction, femoral tunnels are located more posterior to the traditional position [8], and making the femoral tunnels accurately in the femoral ACL footprint would prevent the intercondylar roof impingement [9]. Maak et al. reported in their cadaveric study that in single-bundle reconstruction with the tibial tunnel created at the AMB footprint, the risk of roof impingement was higher when the femoral tunnel was created at the AMB footprint compared to the center of the ACL footprint [27]. Iriuchishima et al. reported that there was no difference in roof impingement pressure between native ACL and the ACL graft after anatomic double-bundle reconstruction [10]. They also showed in a clinical study using MRI that no positive graft-roof impingement was observed after anatomic double-bundle reconstruction [12]. Based on these results, it is likely that as long as the ACL graft is accurately positioned in the native femoral ACL footprint, the risk of roof impingement would be reduced.

When it comes to the tibial tunnel position, the risk of roof impingement might be higher in anatomic reconstruction, as the tibial tunnel of the AMB in anatomic

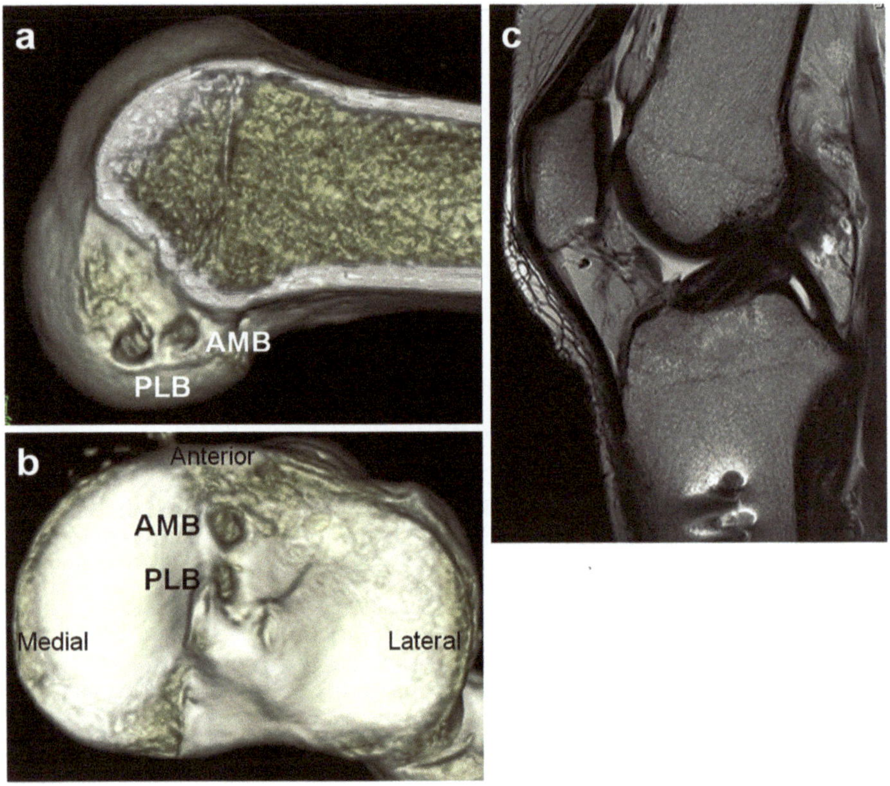

Fig. 22.3 A representative case after anatomic double-bundle ACL reconstruction. (**a, b**) Femoral tunnel positions (**a**) and tibial tunnel positions (**b**) in three-dimensional computed tomography. (**c**) Magnetic resonance imaging (*sagittal view*). Both femoral and tibial tunnels were created within native ACL footprints

reconstruction is placed more anterior to the tibial tunnel in the traditional transtibial single-bundle technique [10]. Bedi et al. evaluated the effect of tibial tunnel position on restoration of knee kinematics and stability after ACL reconstruction and showed that the anterior placement of the tibial tunnel resulted in significantly reduced anterior tibial translation compared with the posterior placement of the tibial tunnel [7]. On the other hand, Matsubara et al. reported in a MRI simulation study that roof impingement was observed in hyperextended knees greater than 10° after anatomic double-bundle reconstruction [28]. It is reported that native ACL made contact with the intercondylar roof in hyperextension of the knee [11, 28]; it may be that anatomic ACL causes physiologic roof impingement [12, 13]. Hatayama et al. reported that anterior placement of the tibial tunnel led to better anterior knee stability and did not increase the incidence of loss of extension and graft failure in anatomic double-bundle reconstruction [29]. However, it still remained unclear whether the physiologic roof impingement is tolerated or how much impingement is tolerated after anatomic double-bundle reconstruction.

22.3.2 Effect of Notchplasty in Anatomic Reconstruction

Therefore, the effects of notchplasty on the clinical outcome after anatomic double-bundle ACL reconstruction were evaluated in a cohort study [30]. One hundred and thirty-seven patients who underwent anatomic double-bundle ACL reconstruction were included in this study. Seventy-three patients without notchplasty were classified as the control group, and 64 patients with two-millimeter notchplasty were classified as the notchplasty group. The following evaluation methods were used: loss of extension, patient's subjective feeling of limited extension and pain at passive full extension, muscle strength, manual laxity tests, KT-1000 measurement, patellofemoral joint findings, Tegner score, Lysholm score, subjective scores, and time to return to sports. Tear of the reconstructed ACL and additional synovectomy was recorded. Both tibial and femoral tunnel positions were also measured using two-view radiographs, a Rosenberg view, and a lateral view.

Loss of extension and the number of cases with feeling of limited extension were larger in the notchplasty group. Six cases required additional synovectomy because of the prolonged loss of extension in the notchplasty group, whereas no case required additional synovectomy in the control group. There were no differences regarding muscle strength, patellofemoral findings, Lysholm score, Tegner score, subjective scores, and time to return to sports. KT measurement was better in the notchplasty group (1.2 mm vs. 0.4 mm, $p = 0.002$). However, six cases showed over-constrained knees (KT measurement ≤ -2 mm) in the notchplasty group, whereas only one case did in the control group. There were no differences in other manual laxity tests. There were no differences in the tunnel positions.

It was unexpected that loss of extension, as well as the number of cases with subjective feeling of limited extension, was significantly larger in the notchplasty group, as notchplasty is supposed to avoid intercondylar roof impingement of the ACL graft, which is the cause of loss of extension. However, it has been reported that regrowth after notchplasty is not uncommon [21, 22]. Moreover, six cases required additional arthroscopic synovectomy because of the prolonged loss of extension, supposedly caused by the fibrosis of the infrapatellar fat pad, in the notchplasty group (Fig. 22.4). These results suggest that bleeding from the notchplasty site caused the fibrosis of the infrapatellar fat pad, resulting in loss of extension in some cases. On the other hand, it seems that tibial tunnel placement allowing physiologic roof impingement did not increase the incidence of loss of extension without notchplasty.

The result of KT measurement was significantly better in the notchplasty group. However, it seems to be due to the fact that there were more cases with over-constrained knees in the notchplasty group, probably caused by the same reason as larger loss of extension in the notchplasty group. Rather, there was no case with graft failure in the control group, and there were no differences in other manual laxity tests. Therefore, the results regarding knee stability in the current study should be interpreted with caution.

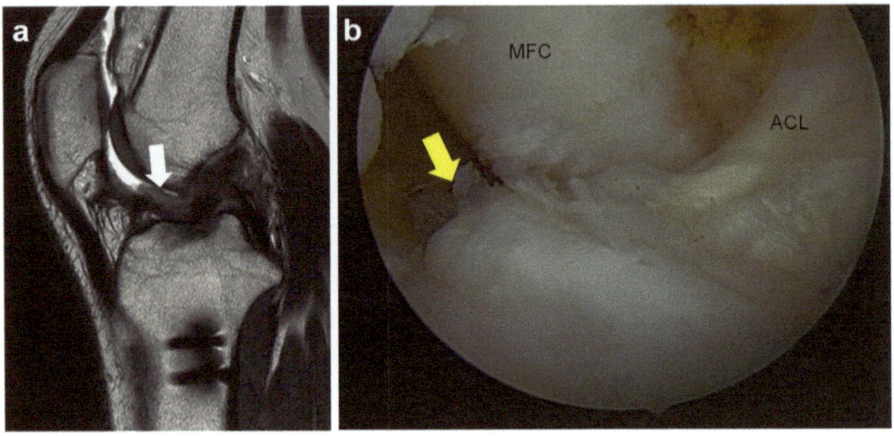

Fig. 22.4 A case that required additional synovectomy because of the prolonged loss of extension after anatomic double-bundle ACL reconstruction with notchplasty. (**a**) MRI (*sagittal view*) taken 3 months after surgery showed fibrosis of the infrapatellar fat pad (*white arrow*) adhered to the reconstructed ACL. (**b**) Arthroscopic view from the anterolateral portal. Fibrosis of the infrapatellar fat pad (*yellow arrow*) adhered to the reconstructed ACL

The conclusions of this study are that, in anatomic double-bundle ACL reconstruction, anterior stability was improved and there were no harmful effects on patellofemoral joint findings by 2-mm notchplasty; however, notchplasty likely caused over-constrained knees, leading to a need for additional synovectomy in some cases. On the other hand, anatomic double-bundle ACL reconstruction without notchplasty did not increase the incidence of loss of extension and graft failure. Therefore, except in cases with spur formation on the intercondylar notch or narrow notch, routine notchplasty is not recommended in anatomic double-bundle ACL reconstruction.

22.3.3 PCL Impingement in Anatomic Reconstruction

As already mentioned, vertical graft placement by high femoral tunnel position increased the risk of ACL-PCL impingement in nonanatomic single-bundle reconstruction. On the other hand, in anatomic reconstruction where the grafts were placed more laterally, the risk of PCL impingement would be lower. Simmons et al. reported in the cadaveric study that in single-bundle reconstruction, lateral femoral tunnel placement lowered ACL graft tension caused by PCL impingement [24]. Iriuchishima et al. also reported that there were no significant differences in the PCL impingement pressure between anatomic single-bundle reconstruction and native ACL [26].

The advantage of double-bundle reconstruction over single-bundle reconstruction in PCL impingement should also be noted. Fujimoto et al. described that a normal oblique ACL axial MR image was not round but spindle shaped, whereas most single-bundle reconstructed ACL grafts were rounder and wider than the normal ACL, which might be one reason for the PCL impingement. They suggested that double-bundle reconstruction might resolve this morphological problem [25]. Iriuchishima et al. also reported that anatomic double-bundle reconstruction showed no ACL-PCL impingement [10].

22.4 Summary

In nonanatomic single-bundle ACL reconstruction where the femoral tunnel was placed "high noon," posterior tibial tunnel placement and notchplasty had been recommended to avoid graft impingement. The recent strategy of anatomic ACL reconstruction reduces the risk of graft impingement. Anatomic double-bundle ACL reconstruction without notchplasty did not increase the incidence of loss of extension and graft failure; rather notchplasty likely caused over-constrained knees. Therefore, except in cases with spur formation on the intercondylar notch or narrow notch, routine notchplasty is not recommended in anatomic double-bundle ACL reconstruction.

References

1. Howell SM, Taylor MA (1993) Failure of reconstruction of the anterior cruciate ligament due to impingement by the intercondylar roof. J Bone Joint Surg Am 75(7):1044–1055
2. Howell SM, Barad SJ (1995) Knee extension and its relationship to the slope of the intercondylar roof. Implications for positioning the tibial tunnel in anterior cruciate ligament reconstructions. Am J Sports Med 23(3):288–294
3. Harner CD, Vogrin TM (2002) What's new in sports medicine. J Bone Joint Surg Am 84-A (6):1095–1099
4. Schindler OS (2012) Surgery for anterior cruciate ligament deficiency: a historical perspective. Knee Surg Sports Traumatol Arthrosc 20(1):5–47
5. Howell SM (1992) Arthroscopic roofplasty: a method for correcting an extension deficit caused by roof impingement of an anterior cruciate ligament graft. Arthroscopy 8(3):375–379
6. Howell SM, Clark JA, Farley TE (1991) A rationale for predicting anterior cruciate graft impingement by the intercondylar roof. A magnetic resonance imaging study. Am J Sports Med 19(3):276–282
7. Bedi A, Maak T, Musahl V, Citak M, O'Loughlin PF, Choi D, Pearle AD (2011) Effect of tibial tunnel position on stability of the knee after anterior cruciate ligament reconstruction: is the tibial tunnel position most important? Am J Sports Med 39(2):366–373
8. Kopf S, Forsythe B, Wong AK, Tashman S, Anderst W, Irrgang JJ, Fu FH (2010) Nonanatomic tunnel position in traditional transtibial single-bundle anterior cruciate ligament reconstruction evaluated by three-dimensional computed tomography. J Bone Joint Surg Am 92 (6):1427–1431
9. Iriuchishima T, Shirakura K, Fu FH (2013) Graft impingement in anterior cruciate ligament reconstruction. Knee Surg Sports Traumatol Arthrosc 21(3):664–670
10. Iriuchishima T, Tajima G, Ingham SJ, Shen W, Smolinski P, Fu FH (2010) Impingement pressure in the anatomical and nonanatomical anterior cruciate ligament reconstruction: a cadaver study. Am J Sports Med 38(8):1611–1617

11. Jagodzinski M, Richter GM, Passler HH (2000) Biomechanical analysis of knee hyperextension and of the impingement of the anterior cruciate ligament: a cinematographic MRI study with impact on tibial tunnel positioning in anterior cruciate ligament reconstruction. Knee Surg Sports Traumatol Arthrosc 8(1):11–19
12. Iriuchishima T, Shirakura K, Horaguchi T, Morimoto Y, Fu FH (2011) Full knee extension magnetic resonance imaging for the evaluation of intercondylar roof impingement after anatomical double-bundle anterior cruciate ligament reconstruction. Knee Surg Sports Traumatol Arthrosc 19(Suppl 1):S22–S28
13. Zantop T, Wellmann M, Fu FH, Petersen W (2008) Tunnel positioning of anteromedial and posterolateral bundles in anatomic anterior cruciate ligament reconstruction: anatomic and radiographic findings. Am J Sports Med 36(1):65–72
14. Howell SM, Berns GS, Farley TE (1991) Unimpinged and impinged anterior cruciate ligament grafts: MR signal intensity measurements. Radiology 179(3):639–643
15. Al-Saeed O, Brown M, Athyal R, Sheikh M (2013) Association of femoral intercondylar notch morphology, width index and the risk of anterior cruciate ligament injury. Knee Surg Sports Traumatol Arthrosc 21(3):678–682
16. Swami VG, Mabee M, Hui C, Jaremko JL (2013) Three-dimensional intercondylar notch volumes in a skeletally immature pediatric population: a magnetic resonance imaging-based anatomic comparison of knees with torn and intact anterior cruciate ligaments. Arthroscopy 29 (12):1954–1962
17. Zeng C, Gao SG, Wei J, Yang TB, Cheng L, Luo W, Tu M, Xie Q, Hu Z, Liu PF, Li H, Yang T, Zhou B, Lei GH (2013) The influence of the intercondylar notch dimensions on injury of the anterior cruciate ligament: a meta-analysis. Knee Surg Sports Traumatol Arthrosc 21 (4):804–815
18. Jagodzinski M, Leis A, Iselborn KW, Mall G, Nerlich M, Bosch U (2003) Impingement pressure and tension forces of the anterior cruciate ligament. Knee Surg Sports Traumatol Arthrosc 11(2):85–90
19. Asahina S, Muneta T, Ezura Y (2000) Notchplasty in anterior cruciate ligament reconstruction: an experimental animal study. Arthroscopy 16(2):165–172
20. Shino K, Nakagawa S, Inoue M, Horibe S, Yoneda M (1993) Deterioration of patellofemoral articular surfaces after anterior cruciate ligament reconstruction. Am J Sports Med 21 (2):206–211
21. LaPrade RF, Terry GC, Montgomery RD, Curd D, Simmons DJ (1998) Winner of the Albert Trillat young investigator award. The effects of aggressive notchplasty on the normal knee in dogs. Am J Sports Med 26(2):193–200
22. Bents RT, Jones RC, May DA, Snearly WS (1998) Intercondylar notch encroachment following anterior cruciate ligament reconstruction: a prospective study. Am J Knee Surg 11 (2):81–88
23. Strobel MJ, Castillo RJ, Weiler A (2001) Reflex extension loss after anterior cruciate ligament reconstruction due to femoral "high noon" graft placement. Arthroscopy 17(4):408–411
24. Simmons R, Howell SM, Hull ML (2003) Effect of the angle of the femoral and tibial tunnels in the coronal plane and incremental excision of the posterior cruciate ligament on tension of an anterior cruciate ligament graft: an in vitro study. J Bone Joint Surg Am 85-A (6):1018–1029
25. Fujimoto E, Sumen Y, Deie M, Yasumoto M, Kobayashi K, Ochi M (2004) Anterior cruciate ligament graft impingement against the posterior cruciate ligament: diagnosis using MRI plus three-dimensional reconstruction software. Magn Reson Imaging 22(8):1125–1129
26. Iriuchishima T, Tajima G, Ingham SJ, Shirakura K, Fu FH (2012) PCL to graft impingement pressure after anatomical or non-anatomical single-bundle ACL reconstruction. Knee Surg Sports Traumatol Arthrosc 20(5):964–969
27. Maak TG, Bedi A, Raphael BS, Citak M, Suero EM, Wickiewicz T, Pearle AD (2011) Effect of femoral socket position on graft impingement after anterior cruciate ligament reconstruction. Am J Sports Med 39(5):1018–1023

28. Matsubara H, Okazaki K, Tashiro Y, Toyoda K, Uemura M, Hashizume M, Iwamoto Y (2013) Intercondylar roof impingement after anatomic double-bundle anterior cruciate ligament reconstruction in patients with knee hyperextension. Am J Sports Med 41(12):2819–2827
29. Hatayama K, Terauchi M, Saito K, Higuchi H, Yanagisawa S, Takagishi K (2013) The importance of tibial tunnel placement in anatomic double-bundle anterior cruciate ligament reconstruction. Arthroscopy 29(6):1072–1078
30. Koga H, Muneta T, Yagishita K, Watanabe T, Mochizuki T, Horie M, Nakamura T, Sekiya I (2014) Effect of notchplasty in anatomic double-bundle anterior cruciate ligament reconstruction. Am J Sports Med 42(8):1813–1821

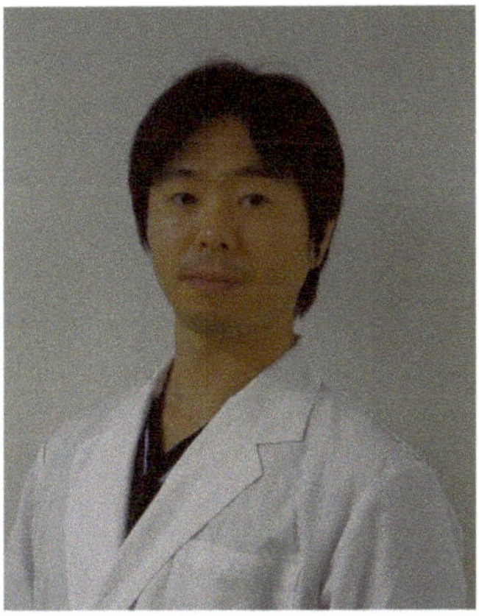

Hideyuki Koga, M.D., Ph.D., Department of Joint Surgery and Sports Medicine, Tokyo Medical and Dental University, Tokyo, Japan.

Chapter 23
Fixation Procedure

Akio Eguchi

Abstract The fixation of the graft in anterior cruciate ligament (ACL) reconstruction is considered as the factor most influential on its mechanical property at the timing before the graft is fixed biologically within the bone tunnel especially immediately after surgery. Nowadays, various fixation devices are available for the soft tissue graft and the bone-patella tendon-bone graft, and there are many studies that compared them. Despite biomechanical differences, clinical results seem to be acceptable with most fixation procedures. The best fixation method has not yet been defined. We summarized the mechanisms of the ACL graft fixation procedures and the main properties of the ACL graft fixation devices.

Keywords Anterior cruciate ligament • Reconstruction • Graft • Fixation

23.1 Introduction

Anterior cruciate ligament (ACL) reconstruction surgery is one of the most advanced procedures in the field of sports medicine. Given, however, that the key to success of ACL reconstruction surgery depends on several elements such as mechanical property of each graft, remodeling process, the position of the bone tunnel, the complicated damage in the meniscus or cartilage, and postoperative rehabilitation, it still remains unclear and unpredictable. Above all, the fixation of the graft is considered as the factor most influential on its mechanical property at the time before the graft is fixed biologically within the bone tunnel especially immediately after surgery. In this context, with the increasing needs for the introduction of an accelerated rehabilitation program and for early functional recovery, a secure mechanical fixation of the graft is required especially at a time immediately after surgery [1]. For graft in ACL reconstruction surgery, however, there are several fixation devices such as cortical suspension devices, transfixation

A. Eguchi, M.D., Ph.D. (✉)
Department of Orthopaedic Surgery, Matsuyama Red Cross Hospital, 1 Bunkyo-cho, Matsuyama, Ehime 790-8524, Japan
e-mail: eguchi.ak@matsuyama.jrc.or.jp

M. Ochi et al. (eds.), *ACL Injury and Its Treatment*,
DOI 10.1007/978-4-431-55858-3_23

devices, interference screws, staple, and buttons, resulting in no clear consensus yet as to which one is most appropriate [2].

In 1984, Noyes et al. [3] conducted a high strain-rate failure test to experiment the strength and the elongation property of various ligament grafts and compared the results with the normal ACL mechanical property of young adults. They reported that the structural property of the bone-patellar tendon-bone (BPTB) graft was superior to the soft tissue graft such as a single hamstring tendon, multiple hamstring tendons, or iliotibial band. They also provided the estimation of the in vivo loading on ACL during normal activity (mean: 454 N). In 1987, Kurosaka et al. [4] conducted a biomechanical study to investigate the fixation method of ACL graft. They described the better mechanical strength of the BPTB graft fixed with titanium interference screws than staples or sutures tied over buttons, and on the other hand, they concluded that the fixation site was the weakest link of ACL reconstruction. Later, Hamner et al. [5] reported that compound graft made of twofold semitendinosus tendon and the gracilis tendon that were fixed by adding tension equally was superior to the previously reported BPTB graft in strength and stiffness. Nowadays, various fixation devices are available for the soft tissue graft and the BPTB graft, and there are many studies that compared them [6–9]. Some studies experimentally found a significant difference using various fixation methods, all of which reported excellent clinical results [10–13]. In recent years, therefore, the area of interest has shifted from the fixation method of the ACL graft to the anatomical reconstruction and the appropriate tunnel placement, which account for most of the factors that contribute to the poor results of ACL reconstruction.

23.2 Graft Fixation Mechanisms

The major factors of the fixation of the graft are strength and stiffness. For fixation of the graft to the bone, the following elements are required: (1) enough strength to prevent failure, (2) stiffness to restore load displacement response and allow biological incorporation of the graft into the bone tunnels, and (3) secure enough to resist slippage or stretch under cyclic loading [14]. The factors that define the magnitude and the direction of the graft include the graft selection (soft tissue or BPTB graft), the design of the fixation device, and the bone mineral density (BMD).

ACL fixation method can be categorized into two types regardless of the kinds of the graft. One is the fixation at the opening of the bone tunnel or within the bone tunnel (e.g., interference screws or cross pins), and the other is the extra-articular fixation (e.g., cortical fixation device or staples). Some fixation devices can be used regardless of the graft being the soft tissue or the BPTB. Biomechanical examinations are being carried out for the ideal fixation method of the graft. The strength and stiffness of the fixation method that are close to those of a human normal anterior cruciate ligament are required. In many cases, actually, the threshold of the physiological load is over 450 N proposed by Noyes et al.

Biomechanical examination is usually performed using an animal model (porcine or bovine knee) in vitro or ex vivo or a human cadaver. Usually, two types of biomechanical examinations, i.e., the single cycle load-to-failure test and the cyclic loading test, are carried out as the test of the mechanical behavior regarding the graft fixation method of ACL reconstruction [15]. The load-to-failure test to examine the ultimate failure load, yield load, linear stiffness, and displacement at failure can measure the structural properties of the bone-graft-fixation device complex. The benefit of these kinds of tests is to be able to discern the weaknesses of the method of fixation of the graft, i.e., the state/site of destruction and the upper limit of the strength. The cycle loading test can evaluate the quality of the bone-graft-fixation device complex against elongation and projection under the maximum load repeated over time [16]. It is actually very difficult to simply compare the mechanical properties of various fixation devices. One of the reasons is that using study models and mechanical tests that are different with each other makes the comparison among them difficult. In addition, it is usually difficult to conduct a study using human cadaveric specimens of younger generations for whom ACL reconstruction is generally performed, and instead, studies using specimens of elder donors are being conducted. Under the circumstances, the strength of the fixation devices is underestimated and presented as it is [17]. Moreover, animal models such as porcine bones are still used for a study of ACL graft fixation method, though they are described as inappropriate for these study purposes [18]. Lastly, in an in vivo biomechanical study, parameters such as ultimate failure load, yield point, breakage state, stiffness, and quantity of displacement at time zero point are evaluated. When the weakness of the strength shifts from the ACL graft fixation-bone tunnel interface to the intra-articular part of ACL graft during the course of biologic adherence of the ACL graft, little information is provided regarding as to how much those parameters would shift [19].

23.3 Graft Selection

Soft tissue grafts that are most commonly used among autologous tendon graft are the semitendinosus tendon and the gracilis tendon. Biological fixation between the soft tissue graft and the bone tunnel is generally considered to take longer than that of the BPTB graft. It starts within 4–12 weeks after surgery in an animal experiment [20]. That is why the fixation of the soft tissue graft in early stage has long been considered to have an important role.

The patellar tendon with bone plug and the quadriceps muscle tendon with bone plug are also reconstruction materials used commonly. It is reported that healing of the bone block would complete within 6–12 weeks after surgery in the ACL reconstruction using the BPTB graft. Therefore, powerful fixation strength is required within 4–12 weeks after surgery until biological healing is established [21].

Several fixation methods for each transplanted tendon have been advocated in the past 10 years.

23.4 Graft Fixation Procedures

23.4.1 Cortical Suspension Device

Cortical suspension device is widely used as a fixation method of the soft tissue graft. Cortical suspension devices such as EndoButton® (Smith & Nephew, Andover, Massachusetts), TightRope® (Arthrex, Naples, Florida), ToggleLoc® (Biomet, Warsaw, Indiana), Rigidloop® (Depuy Synthes Mitek, Raynham, Massachusetts), and XO Button® (Conmed Linvatec, Largo, Florida) are constructed by metal plates with suture loops (Fig. 23.1). The fixation principle of these methods relies on the structure in which hardware is set to the lateral cortex of the distal femur to suspend the graft into the femoral tunnel. In this type of fixation methods, the directions of the resistance vectors are parallel, and the pullout force is converged to the cortical bone of the distal femur, which is the contact point of the bone and the hardware. Therefore, a smaller contact surface of the fixation device allows a greater stress concentration, which depends on the design of the fixation device. In addition, the mechanical properties of the artificial ligaments to suspend the graft are factors involved in the fixation strength.

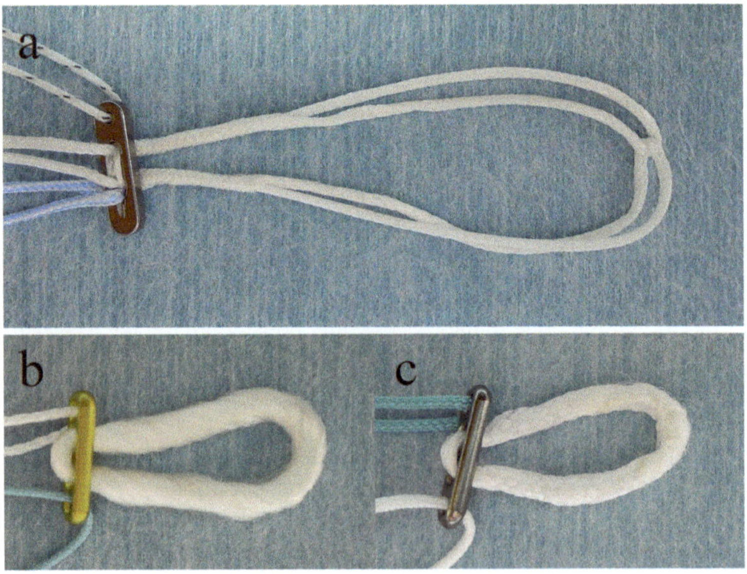

Fig. 23.1 Cortical suspension devices. (**a**) TightRope® (Arthrex), (**b**) EndoButton® (Smith & Nephew), (**c**) Rigidloop® (Depuy Synthes Mitek)

Compared with the fixation method within the bone tunnel, the following elements are considered as the benefits of this method: (1) the powerful strength owing to the cortical bone that is stronger than the cancellous bone, (2) the wide contact of the tendon and the bone within the tunnel that is beneficial for healing, and (3) the circumstantial healing that is obtained from the tunnel filled with the tendon. On the other hand, the disadvantage is that a phenomenon that could lead to the tunnel expansion such as the bungee-cord effect and the windshield-wiper effect might occur because the graft is not fixed on the anatomical ACL insertion site.

Ochi [22] developed a looped artificial ligament without a mechanical weak point such as a knot and reported its excellent mechanical strength. It is suggested that it can minimize the bungee-cord effect and the elongation of the device because it is superior to the suture and the existing artificial ligaments in its strength and stiffness and because the amount of elongation was found to be small in the cyclic loading test. Even now, the fixation devices that reflect these concepts are widely used.

Recently, on the other hand, adjustable-length loop devices such as TightRope® and ToggleLoc® have been developed. One of the features is that there is no need to overdrill the tunnel to flip the button, which is considered as beneficial from the viewpoint of bone preservation and dead space. However, there are doubts as to whether the loop adjusted in vivo after fixation could come loose [23–25]. The authors comparatively examined the mechanical properties of these kinds of devices and found that the adjustable-length loop device might elongate until it is pulled back with a certain level of strength and reported that it wouldn't elongate any further if a certain level of strength is applied [26]. In other words, it is suggested that postoperative loosening might be caused when the loop is not tightened up enough or is stuck at a certain site in the bone tunnel, indicating a need to know the mechanical properties of these devices when using them.

23.4.2 Interference Screw

Interference screw fixation of the BPTB graft is most commonly used and considered as the gold standard. The properties of the interference screw fixation for BPTB graft are specified as the frictional force among the bone plugs and the bone tunnel wall as well as the engagement of the thread grooves with the bone plugs and the bone tunnel wall. The fixation strength of the interference screw is subject to various factors such as the screw diameter and size of the gap, deviation of the screw, the screw length, and the BMD [27]. Currently, different types of interference screws such as metal screws, biodegradable screws, and biosynthetic screws are available. Metal interference screw used to be a classic fixation method for ACL reconstruction for a long time (Fig. 23.2a). This fixation method will bring about powerful primary fixation strength at an early stage until the bone invasion occurs. Although excellent results of metal interference screws have been reported, there exist concerns such as damage of the transplanted tendon when setting a screw,

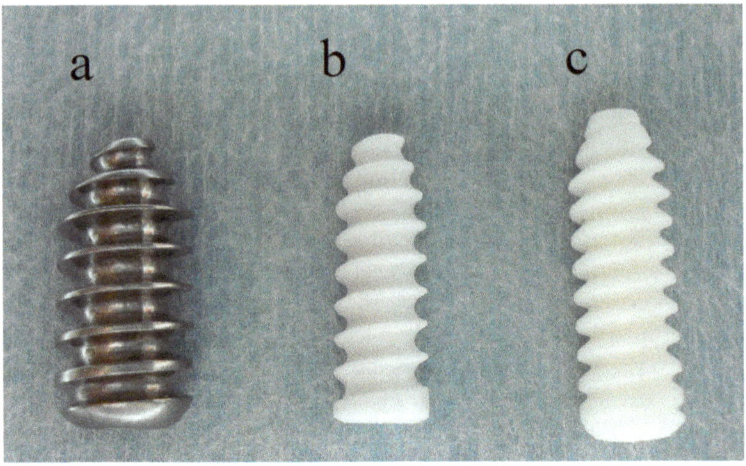

Fig. 23.2 Interference screws. (**a**) Metal interference screw, Softsilk® (Smith & Nephew), (**b**) biocomposite interference screw (PLLA and HA), BioRCI-HA® (Smith & Nephew), (**c**) biocomposite interference screw (PLA and β-TCP), Milagro-BR® (Depuy Synthes Mitek)

destruction of the posterior wall, projection of the fixation device into the joint, distortion of the MRI images after surgery, and the need to pull out the fixation device at revision surgery [28]. Consequently, along with the development of bioengineering and biomaterial science, it has long been considered that an ideal implant should be biocompatible, biosimilar, and biodegradable. Under the circumstances, a biodegradable screw was invented. Biodegradable interference screws can be classified into those with early biodegradability and those with late biodegradability. Screws with early biodegradability might be highly prone to soft tissue response [29]. Generally, biodegradable screws are composed of several stereoisomers of lactic acid molecules such as polyglycolic acid (PGA), poly-l-lactic acid (PLLA), and poly-d-lactic acid (PDLA) as well as copolymers such as polyglycolic acid/polylactic acid (PGA/PLA). Each polymer has material-specific characteristics, and implants made of one kind of polymer can be defined by its nature. Therefore, copolymers can combine and mix the characteristics needed for different polymers and can exceed the limit of the polymer of one kind.

In recent years, biocomposite materials are also being developed (Fig. 23.2b–c). These materials are composed of a combination of the previously listed polymers and osteoconductive materials, such as beta-tricalcium phosphate (β-TCP) or hydroxyapatite (HA). In particular, β-TCP that can be used as synthetic implant material has appropriate ultrastructural properties for cell adhesion [30].

Compared with metal interference screws, these biodegradable interference screws are expected to dissolve concerns such as the need to pull out the fixation device, the adverse effect on MRI images, and injury risks of the transplanted tendon. Some other biomechanical studies indicated that the primary fixation property of biodegradable screws and biosynthetic screws has a similar strength and stiffness as the metal screws.

On the other hand, complications associated with the use of biodegradable interference screws involve damage during early stage of surgery, inflammatory reaction originated from a large quantity of oxides produced during the course of resolution implants, aberrant screw implantation due to additional damage, and a risk of tunnel expansion.

Some clinical studies investigated the biodegradable interference screws and metal interference screws and compared the residual anterior laxity evaluated by manual examination or a KT arthrometer as well as subjective/objective functional evaluation end points such as the Lysholm Knee scoring scale and the IKDC score. However, none of them showed a clinically significant difference.

23.4.3 Tibial Fixation

Fixation on the tibial side is considered as generally difficult compared with that on the femoral side at least mainly due to following two reasons: (1) BMD is obviously low compared with the distal femur; (2) the fixation device on the tibial side needs to be able to resist the tension exerted parallel on the axis of the tibial tunnel. The potential bifurcation in the fixation method on the tibial side may lead to the loosening and the tunnel expansion that can cause residual disability including the disconnection of the graft and micromotion. For these reasons, fixation on the tibial side can become the weakness of the femur-graft-tibial complex immediately after ACL reconstruction. Fixation method on the tibial side includes interference screws, staples, spiked washers, and post screws (Fig. 23.3). Ishibashi et al. [31] investigated the fixation method of BPTB graft on the tibial side and reported that the primary fixation strength of the more proximal fixation using interference screws was superior to that of the distal fixation using staples. To improve the fixation power of the transplanted tendon and decrease the risk of displacement, the following combinations were tested as hybrid fixation methods: screws and washers and bone nails, screws and washers and interference screws, interference screws

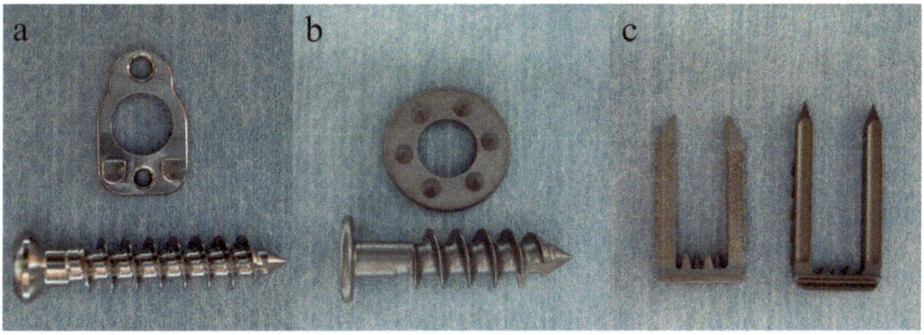

Fig. 23.3 Tibial Fixation Devices. (**a**) Double-spike plate (smith & Nephew), (**b**) screw & washer (Arthrex), (**c**) staples

and staples, interference screws and double-spike plates, interference screws and autologous transplanted tendon/bone reinforcement, and interference screws and Bio-Tenodesis screws, all of which were reported to have a good mechanical property compared with a conventional, unreinforced fixation method [32, 33]. However, a clinically significant difference was not observed in any of these cases [34].

References

1. Harvey A, Thomas NP, Amis AA (2005) Fixation of the graft in reconstruction of the anterior cruciate ligament. J Bone Joint Surg (Br) 87:593–603
2. Miyata K, Yasuda K, Kondo E et al (2000) Biomechanical comparisons of anterior cruciate ligament: reconstruction procedures with flexor tendon graft. J Orthop Sci 5:585–592
3. Noyes FR, Butler DL, Grood ES et al (1984) Biomechanical analysis of human ligament grafts used in knee-ligament repairs and reconstructions. J Bone Joint Surg Am 66:344–352
4. Kurosaka M, Yoshiya S, Andrish JT et al (1987) A biomechanical comparison of different surgical techniques of graft fixation in anterior cruciate ligament reconstruction. Am J Sports Med 15:225–229
5. Hamner DL, Brown CH, Steiner ME et al (1999) Hamstring tendon grafts for reconstruction of the anterior cruciate ligament: biomechanical evaluation of the use of multiple strands and tensioning techniques. J Bone Joint Surg Am 81:549–557
6. Ahmad CS, Gardner TR, Groh M et al (2004) Mechanical properties of soft tissue femoral fixation devices for anterior cruciate ligament reconstruction. Am J Sports Med 32:635–640
7. Milano G, Mulas PD, Ziranu F et al (2006) Comparison between different femoral fixation devices for ACL reconstruction with doubled hamstring tendon graft: a biomechanical analysis. Arthroscopy 22:660–668
8. Zantop T, Ruemmler M, Welbers B et al (2005) Cyclic loading comparison between biodegradable interference screw fixation and biodegradable double cross-pin fixation of human bone-patellar tendon-bone grafts. Arthroscopy 21:934–941
9. Milano G, Mulas PD, Ziranu F et al (2007) Comparison of femoral fixation methods for anterior cruciate ligament reconstruction with patellar tendon graft: a mechanical analysis in porcine knees. Knee Surg Sports Traumatol Arthrosc 15:733–738
10. Shen C, Jiang SD, Jiang LS et al (2010) Bioabsorbable versus metallic interference screw fixation in anterior cruciate ligament reconstruction: a meta-analysis of randomized controlled trials. Arthroscopy 26:705–713
11. Emond CE, Woelber EB, Kurd SK (2011) A comparison of the results of anterior cruciate ligament reconstruction using bioabsorbable versus metal interference screws: a meta-analysis. J Bone Joint Surg Am 93:572–580
12. Colvin A, Sharma C, Parides M et al (2011) What is the best femoral fixation of hamstring autografts in anterior cruciate ligament reconstruction?: a meta-analysis. Clin Orthop Relat Res 469:1075–1081
13. Han DL, Nyland J, Kendzior M et al (2012) Intratunnel versus extratunnel fixation of hamstrung autograft for anterior cruciate ligament reconstruction. Arthroscopy 28:1555–1566
14. Milano G, Petersen W, Hoeher J et al (2014) Fixation. In: Siebold R, Dejour D, Zaffagnini S (eds) Anterior cruciate ligament reconstruction: a practical surgery guide. ESSKA ASBL, Luxembourg

15. Beynnon BD, Amis AA (1998) In vitro testing protocols for the cruciate ligaments and ligament reconstructions. Knee Surg Sports Traumatol Arthrosc 6:S70–S76
16. Yamanaka M, Yasuda K, Tohyama H et al (1999) The effect of cyclic displacement on the biomechanical characteristics of anterior cruciate ligament reconstructions. Am J Sports Med 27:772–777
17. Brown GA, Peña F, Grøntvedt T et al (1996) Fixation strength of interference screw fixation in bovine, young human, and elderly human cadaver knees: influence of insertion torque, tunnel-bone block gap, and interference. Knee Surg Sports Traumatol Arthrosc 3:238–244
18. Nurmi JT, Sievänen H, Kannus P et al (2004) Porcine tibia is a poor substitute for human cadaver tibia for evaluating interference screw fixation. Am J Sports Med 32:765–771
19. Milano G, Mulas PD, Sanna-Passino E et al (2005) Evaluation of bone plug and soft tissue anterior cruciate ligament graft fixation over time using transverse femoral fixation in a sheep model. Arthroscopy 21:532–539
20. Rodeo SA, Arnoczky SP, Torzilli PA et al (1993) Tendon-healing in a bone tunnel. A biomechanical and histological study in the dog. J Bone Joint Surg Am 75:1795–1803
21. Yoshiya S, Nagano M, Kurosaka M et al (2000) Graft healing in the bone tunnel in anterior cruciate ligament reconstruction. Clin Orthop Relat Res 376:278–286
22. Uchio Y, Ochi M, Sumen Y et al (2002) Mechanical properties of newly developed loop ligament for connection between the EndoButton and hamstring tendons: comparison with ethibond sutures and EndoButton Tape. J Biomed Mater Res 63:173–181
23. Petre BM, Smith SD, Jansson KS et al (2013) Femoral cortical suspension devices for soft tissue anterior cruciate ligament reconstruction: a comparative biomechanical study. Am J Sports Med 41:416–422
24. Barrow AE, Pilia M, Guda T et al (2014) Femoral suspension devices for anterior cruciate ligament reconstruction: do adjustable loops lengthen? Am J Sports Med 42:343–349
25. Johnson JS, Smith SD, LaPrade CM et al (2015) A biomechanical comparison of femoral cortical suspension devices for soft tissue anterior cruciate ligament reconstruction under high loads. Am J Sports Med 43:154–160
26. Eguchi A, Ochi M, Adachi N et al (2014) Mechanical properties of suspensory fixation devices for anterior cruciate ligament reconstruction: comparison of the fixed-length loop device versus the adjustable-length loop device. Knee 21:743–748
27. Shino K, Pflaster DS (2000) Comparison of eccentric and concentric screw placement for hamstring graft fixation in the tibial tunnel. Knee Surg Sports Traumatol Arthrosc 8:73–75
28. Marti C, Imhoff AB, Bahrs C et al (1997) Metallic versus bioabsorbable interference screw for fixation of bone-patellar tendon-bone autograft in arthroscopic anterior cruciate ligament reconstruction: a preliminary report. Knee Surg Sports Traumatol Arthrosc 5:217–221
29. Konan S, Haddad FS (2009) The unpredictable material properties of bioabsorbable PLC interference screws and their adverse effects in ACL reconstruction surgery. Knee Surg Sports Traumatol Arthrosc 17:293–297
30. Bernstein A, Techlenburg K, Südkamp P et al (2012) Adhesion and proliferation of human osteoblast-like cells on different biodegradable implant materials used for graft fixation in ACL-reconstruction. Arch Orthop Trauma Surg 132:1637–1645
31. Ishibashi Y, Rudy TW, Livesay GA et al (1997) The effect of anterior cruciate ligament graft fixation site at the tibia on knee stability: evaluation using a robotic testing system. Arthroscopy 13:177–182
32. Tesumura S, Fujita A, Nakajima M et al (2006) Biomechanical comparison of different fixation methods on the tibial side in anterior cruciate ligament reconstruction: a biomechanical study in porcine tibial bone. J Orthop Sci 11:278–282
33. Yoo JC, Ahn JH, Kim JH et al (2006) Biomechanical testing of hybrid hamstring graft tibial fixation in anterior cruciate ligament reconstruction. Knee 13:455–459

34. Hoh JH, Yang BG, Yi SR et al (2012) Hybrid tibial fixation for anterior cruciate ligament reconstruction with achilles tendon allograft. Arthroscopy 28:1540–1546

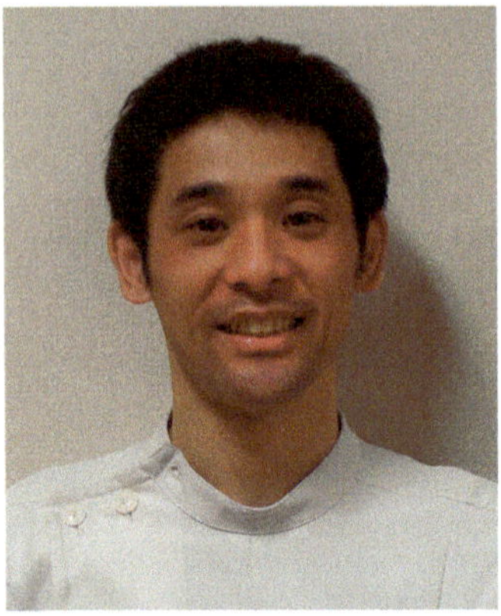

Akio Eguchi M.D., Ph.D., Department of Orthopaedic Surgery, Matsuyama Red Cross Hospital, Ehime, Japan.

Part V
Multiple Bundle ACL Reconstruction

Chapter 24
Single- Vs. Double-Bundle ACL Reconstruction

Masahiro Kurosaka, Ryosuke Kuroda, and Kanto Nagai

Abstract Multiple bundle ACL reconstruction, especially focused on double-bundle ACL reconstruction was discussed in this article. Although crucial factors and denominators that influence the outcome of ACL reconstruction are not elucidated, we believe that anatomically oriented graft replacement in reconstruction of the ruptured ACL structure will be certainly the future direction of this surgery. The study of anatomy of the ACL insertion site and intra-articular graft orientation in the young and normal population would be mandatory for the better understanding of future ACL reconstruction. Also better evaluation system that includes both subjective and objective approach should be refined in the future. As the technology advancement is seen in many fields of surgical technique, navigation system or some other types of newer technique will surely be introduced in ACL reconstruction technique field. Biological intervention of ACL surgery is surely one of the challenging issues for future ACL reconstruction. Since ACL is the tissue that has blood supply, biological application to facilitate the implanted graft to heal to normal ACL tissue may be one of the attainable possibilities and may be easier than healing of nonvascularized tissue like an articular cartilage damage or torn meniscus. We are still on the way to get the normal ACL tissue back to the torn ACL knee; however, anatomic approach of the double-bundle ACL reconstruction of the ACL tissue may be one of the possible solutions to this currently unsolved problem for the athletic population.

Keywords Single-bundle • Double-bundle • ACL reconstruction

24.1 Historical Background

First anatomic reconstruction concept was reported by Mott in 1983 by using the semitendinosus tendon [1]. Since then much attention has not been paid to double-bundle ACL reconstruction until Muneta et al. reported their technique of

M. Kurosaka, M.D., Ph.D. (✉) • R. Kuroda, M.D., Ph.D. • K. Nagai, M.D.
Department of Orthopaedic Surgery, Kobe University Graduate School of Medicine, 7-5-1 Kusunoki-cho, Chuo-ku, Kobe, Hyogo 650-0017, Japan
e-mail: kurosaka@med.kobe-u.ac.jp

M. Ochi et al. (eds.), *ACL Injury and Its Treatment*,
DOI 10.1007/978-4-431-55858-3_24

double-bundle ACL reconstruction in 2007 [2]. This report was a prospective randomized study of 4-strand semitendinosus tendon ACL reconstruction comparing single-bundle and double-bundle techniques. There were several studies published from Japan regarding the double-bundle ACL reconstructions [3–12]; however, most of the studies reported the theoretical advantages of double-bundle ACL reconstruction. Toritsuka et al. reported double-bundle ACL reconstruction in satisfactory outcome after short-term follow-up [7]. Also Yagi et al. showed the superiority of double-bundle ACL reconstruction [13] and especially emphasized the importance of posterolateral (PL) bundle that predominantly controlled tibial internal rotation when the tibia was internally rotated as pivot shift test-like force applied to the tibia by using robotic universal force-moment sensor (UFS) device [14]. Our personal experience of anatomic double-bundle reconstruction started in 2002. During those days Yasuda et al. [15] reported the femoral anatomical insertion site of PL bundle located distal and more posterior than usually perceived by most of the double-bundle ACL reconstruction surgeons. Our general understanding of importance of the isometricity of the ACL fibers led us to create two anteromedial (AM) bundle femoral tunnels instead of truly anatomically located insertion sites. Dr. Yasuda's report influenced quite a few surgeons to create the PL new femoral drill tunnels positioning. There are still controversial issues whether the double-bundle ACL reconstruction brings better outcome comparing to single-bundle reconstruction [16]. Meta-analysis has shown that there was not significant difference between single- and double-bundle ACL reconstruction [17]. However, this result may be due to the evaluation modality that was available for us to judge the outcome of ACL surgery at the time the analysis was conducted. Recent first class review guidelines [18] have shown that both double-bundle and single-bundle ACL reconstruction confirmed the similarity of both techniques that can be recommended for the patients. With the currently available evaluation technique, there might be a limit to clearly define the difference of both techniques. That really indicates the necessity to develop the better and more accurate evaluation modality developed in the future. Recently, we have developed a three-dimensional electromagnetic measurement system (EMS) to evaluate the knee stability and reported the accuracy of this measurement system [19, 20], and several outcomes and comparisons between single- and double-bundle ACL reconstruction were also reported [11, 21]. There are other evaluation systems reported recently using accelerometer [22, 23] and image analysis by using the iPad [24], etc. These newer techniques along with better patients' subjective evaluation also with better imaging system will make our evaluation more precise and objective in the future.

24.2 Insertion Site Evaluation

Until now there have been quite a few literatures existing regarding the insertion site of ACL. As to the femoral insertion, historically, it is known that the insertion site is relatively broad extending from the bone cartilage junction to the what is called resident ridge that usually exist on the lateral femoral condylar wall. We were taught that the creation of the femoral tunnel above the resident ridge is the nonanatomical malpositioned poor technique. Fu and his group reported that there is a ridge in between AM and PL bundle (bifurcate ridge) that separates both bundles posterior to the resident ridge [25]. Shino et al. reported similar findings with the more detailed histological study [26, 27]. However, a recently new concept of the anatomy of the femoral insertion was published by several authors [28, 29]. They found by anatomical dissection that the predominantly functioning femoral insertion of ACL existed more anteriorly than was reported [28]. Their finding shows that the functioning femoral insertion site existed on the resident ridge area that is far anterior than most of the surgeon believed. This new concept is totally different than what we have understood in the past, and this new concept of femoral insertion site can change the currently practiced surgical technique. Similar dispute on the insertion of the tibial insertion recently came into the attention among ACL reconstruction surgeons. Tibial ACL insertion was believed to be quite wide anteriorly and PL bundle insertion was known to be located posterolaterally to AM bundle insertion. The anatomical landmark that can be referenced at the time of surgery can be the anterior horn of both medial and lateral meniscus and the ridge of the tibial spines. The new concept of the anatomical tibial insertion of the ACL exhibits that tibial insertion site is J or C shaped and that it extends from the very anterior portion of the ACL fibers to the very medial that is next to the medial ridge of the tibial spine [30]. This indicates that tibial insertion of PL bundle is quite medial, so this structure could be called as posteromedial bundle rather than posterolateral bundle according to their report [28]. This concept is quite new and may influence our daily surgical procedures in the future. However, the criticism to these new studies can be that they only examined old degenerated specimens and there should be the difference between young and athletic population knee anatomy and old degenerated specimens. I personally believe this criticism should be cleared by more high-resolution imaging techniques available to precisely analyze the insertion site of native ACLs in the young and active population in the future.

24.3 Our Surgical Technique

Our surgical technique to ACL deficiency is what is called anatomic ACL reconstruction for most of the cases. The exception is the patients with wide open epiphysis and multiple-ligament reconstruction cases. For the patients with wide open epiphysis, we try to avoid the epiphyseal plate injury by approaching from outside-in technique for the femoral side that makes double-bundle reconstruction difficult (Fig. 24.1). For the cases with multiple-ligament reconstruction, we try to

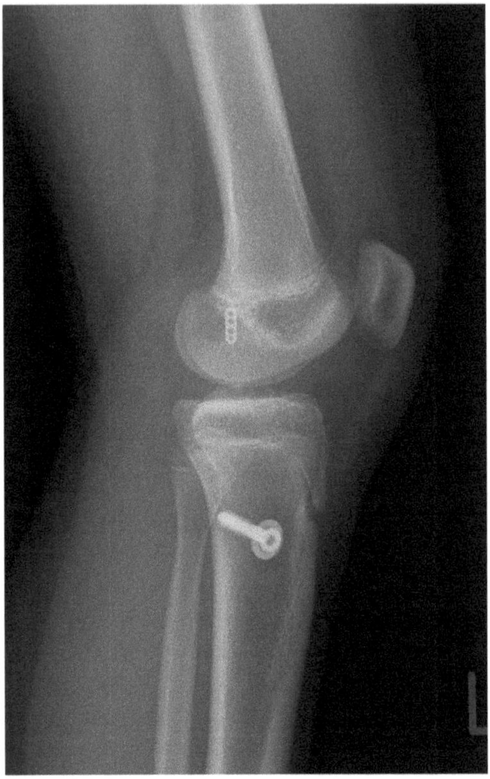

Fig. 24.1 The postoperative lateral radiograph after ACL reconstruction of the *left knee*. The ACL injured patient was 13 y.o. female with open epiphysis. For the femoral side, outside-in technique was used to avoid the injury of epiphyseal plate, and fixed with a suspensory button. For the tibial side, the transphyseal technique was used and fixed with a post screw

do anatomic double-bundle reconstruction as much as possible because we believe anatomical reconstruction will be better than single-bundle reconstruction to mimic normal knee structure. However, for the cases of ACL, posterior cruciate ligament (PCL), plus other ligaments, it is difficult to do it in a single tourniquet time, and so we stay in the single-bundle technique. For the other cases like the small patients or elderly patients, we basically do anatomic double-bundle technique because we believe that double-bundle reconstruction is more anatomical and natural for their knees. Fu et al. reported that even in the fetus, double-bundle ACL exists [31]. We use semitendinosus tendon for the double-bundle ACL reconstruction. So, the first part of this procedure is the harvest of semitendinosus tendon (Fig. 24.2). We make the 5 cm oblique skin incision in the medial side of the anterior part of the knee. After the sharp dissection on the top of pes anserinus soft tissue, we can separate the semitendinosus and gracilis from the pes anserinus. The semitendinosus tendon can be separated from the rest of the pes anserinus tendon and this can be harvested by open tendon stripper. The length of the tendon needs to be a minimum of 24 cm. Two doubled semitendinosus tendon is prepared for AM and PL bundle reconstruction in the back table by a graft master assistant while the surgeon prepares the bony

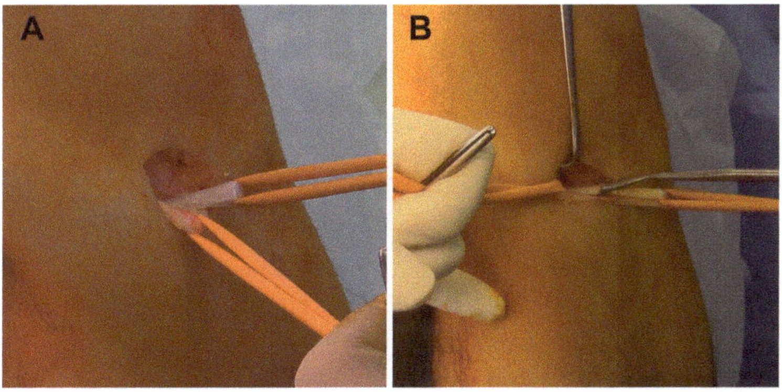

Fig. 24.2 Harvesting of hamstring tendon graft. The semitendinosus tendon was identified from the surface of pes anserinus tissue. Then, the semitendinosus tendon was isolated from the underneath of the gracilis tendon and harvested with tendon stripper (*left knee*)

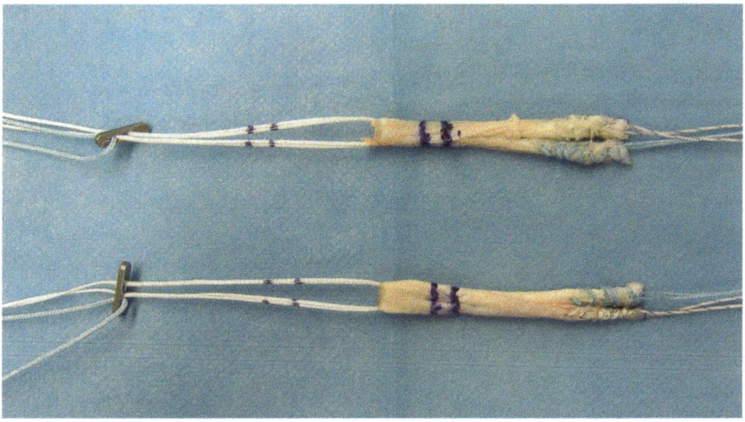

Fig. 24.3 Graft preparation for double-bundle ACL reconstruction. The doubled semitendinosus tendons were prepared with suspensory buttons

tunnels for both AM and PL bundles (Fig. 24.3). The first step for intra-articular tunnel preparation is identification of the drilling hole sites. We use regular 30° angle arthroscopy with anterior lateral, medial, and far anterior medial accessory portals. Viewing the insertion site both from lateral and medial is extremely important especially for the femoral insertion site identification. We try to use the remnant tissue for both the femoral and tibial side to identify the insertion site and mark the point for drilling by a thermal instrument (Fig. 24.4a, b). For the femoral tunnel creation, we have reported that the femoral tunnels shift anteriorly and distally during the follow-up after the surgery [32]. Thus our tunnel location is in the posterior and proximal margin underneath the resident ridge for AM bundle. PL bundle insertion is marked just distal and slightly posterior to the AM bundle

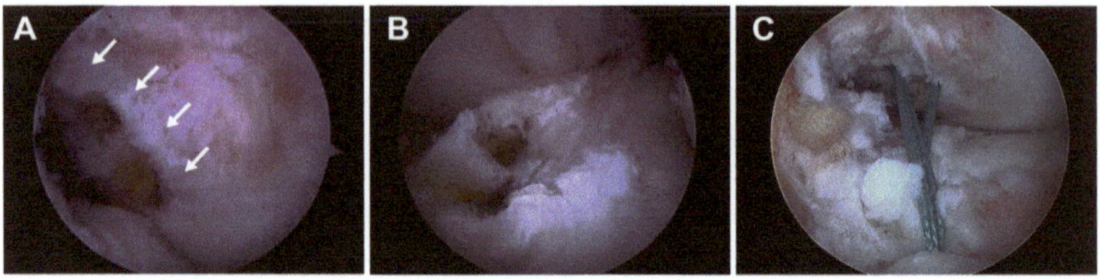

Fig. 24.4 Intraoperative arthroscopic images of double-bundle ACL reconstruction for the *left knee*. (**a**) Marking of femoral ACL insertion site of AM and PL bundles by using the thermal device. Arrows indicate the resident ridge. (**b**) Marking of tibial insertion site of AM and PL bundles by using the thermal device. (**c**) Graft passage leading sutures were placed through AM and PL bone tunnels

insertion. We usually create the drilling holes of both AM and PL bundles from the far anterior medial portal. We make sure that tunnel coalition in both does not happen. We use the suspensory type of fixation for the femoral side; thus we create the femoral drill hole as the graft is tightly fit in diameter and get the minimum length of 1.5 cm graft incorporation in both AM and PL bundles. After the creation of the femoral tunnels, tibial drill holes are prepared and drilled. AM tibial tunnels are near to the anterior horn of the medial meniscus; thus it is the anterior that we used to create AM bundle. PL tibial tunnel can be created toward more lateral and near to the posterior edge of the anterior horn of the lateral meniscus and just medial to the medial tibial spine. Both AM and PL tibial tunnels are created by outside-in drilling fashion. By the time you create these four tunnels in the femur and the tibia (Fig. 24.4c), the grafts for both tunnels are manipulated and be ready for implantation in the back table. PL bundle insertion is done first and followed by AM graft insertion. After the graft insertion and femoral side suspensory type graft fixation is completed, isometricity of the graft can be checked by the knee in full extension to full flexion. In our experience, graft isometricity is nearly isometric or slightly tight in extension in the AM bundle, and in the PL bundle, it gets tighter in extension and usually minimal change occurs in flexion. Our fixation technique is the suture tied to the fixation post screw with a washer in the tibia. Since the isometricity of the graft is tight in extension in most of the cases, we fix the graft near to the extension position. We believe that graft will undergo load relaxation phenomenon and they will stay in the certain tension in 24 h after the surgery because we have the several points where the load relaxation occurs after implantation such as soft tissue between femoral suspensory device to the bone, suture, and graft material junction and sutures tied to the fixation post screw. We carefully examine the intra-articular graft seating, notch impingement, and other structures such as cartilage and meniscus. Additional procedure necessary at this stage is extremely rare.

24.4 Future Directions

Obviously, our technique has changed in the past 10 years and tunnel positioning has become more standardized. But in the future, insertion site study should be more refined and more standardized technique will be developed. Possible technology change may take surgery to a more computer-navigated direction. So some technology will be developed and preoperative and intraoperative identification of the insertion sites may become more precise. In some areas of the surgery like urology, da Vinci telerobotic surgery [33] became very standard. We are not sure if we have the tendency toward that direction, but for sure some computer-navigated surgery will be incorporated to ACL reconstruction. From the biological standpoint, significant advancement of tissue regeneration has been made in the past as represented in the creation of induced pluripotent stem (iPS) cells by the Nobel Prize laureate Professor Shinya Yamanaka [34, 35]. There is certainly a possibility that some kind of biological manipulation on the process of ligamentization may be available and change the story of ligament-healing process. Although the facilitation of the maturation process of implanted ligament graft might be difficult, facilitation of the muscular recovery may be more easily attained. We have found the possibility to use the carbon dioxide gas (CO_2) with the special gel applied from the skin that facilitates the absorption of CO_2 gas to the muscular tissue which in turn resulted in high concentration of oxygen in the muscular tissue [36] (Figs. 24.5 and, 24.6). In fact, in the animal model, a positive effect of muscular strength recovery was found, and this result was reported in several journals [36, 37]. Not only the muscular strength but also muscle-to-nerve coordination and proprioception recovery could be the possible solution of earlier return to sports after ACL reconstruction in the future.

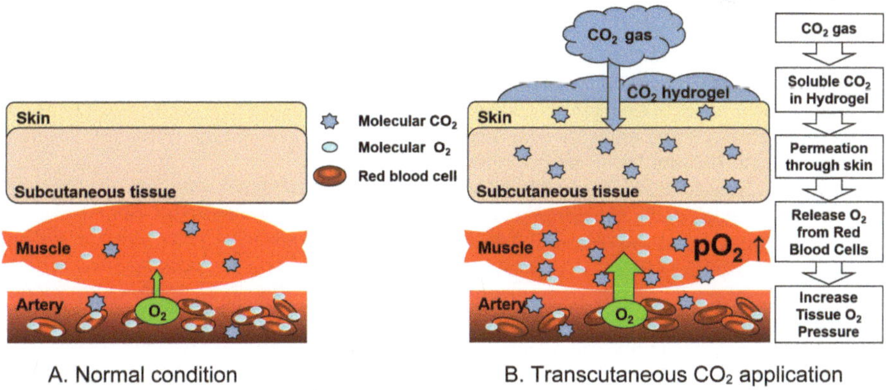

Fig. 24.5 The mechanism of transcutaneous carbon dioxide (CO_2) gas application. (**a**). In normal condition, the use of the muscles creates CO_2 in muscular tissue that is replaced by oxygen (O_2). (**b**). By applying excessive CO_2 though the skin to the muscular tissues. CO_2 concentration in the muscular tissues becomes abnormally high. After this phenomenon, CO_2 is replaced by the O_2 from the artery, and eventually O_2 concentration in the muscular tissue becomes extremely high

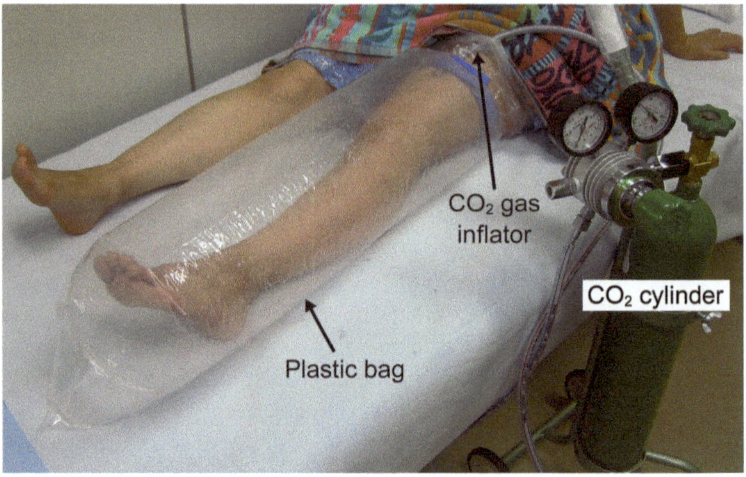

Fig. 24.6 The application of carbon dioxide (CO_2) gas for the lower limb. The lower limb is covered by CO_2 absorption-enhancing hydrogel and placed into the plastic bag. Then CO_2 gas is fulfilled through the tube in the plastic bag

References

1. Mott HW (1983) Semitendinosus anatomic reconstruction for cruciate ligament insufficiency. Clin Orthop Relat Res 172:90–92
2. Muneta T, Koga H, Mochizuki T, Ju YJ, Hara K, Nimura A, Yagishita K, Sekiya I (2007) A prospective randomized study of 4-strand semitendinosus tendon anterior cruciate ligament reconstruction comparing single-bundle and double-bundle techniques. Arthroscopy 23 (6):618–628. doi:10.1016/j.arthro.2007.04.010
3. Adachi N, Ochi M, Uchio Y, Iwasa J, Kuriwaka M, Ito Y (2004) Reconstruction of the anterior cruciate ligament. Single- versus double-bundle multistranded hamstring tendons. J Bone Joint Surg Br Vol 86(4):515–520
4. Shino K, Nakata K, Nakamura N, Toritsuka Y, Nakagawa S, Horibe S (2005) Anatomically oriented anterior cruciate ligament reconstruction with a bone-patellar tendon-bone graft via rectangular socket and tunnel: a snug-fit and impingement-free grafting technique. Arthroscopy 21(11):1402. doi:10.1016/j.arthro.2005.08.017
5. Yasuda K, Kondo E, Ichiyama H, Tanabe Y, Tohyama H (2006) Clinical evaluation of anatomic double-bundle anterior cruciate ligament reconstruction procedure using hamstring tendon grafts: comparisons among 3 different procedures. Arthroscopy 22(3):240–251. doi:10.1016/j.arthro.2005.12.017
6. Shino K, Nakata K, Nakamura N, Toritsuka Y, Horibe S, Nakagawa S, Suzuki T (2008) Rectangular tunnel double-bundle anterior cruciate ligament reconstruction with bone-patellar tendon-bone graft to mimic natural fiber arrangement. Arthroscopy 24(10):1178–1183. doi:10.1016/j.arthro.2008.06.010
7. Toritsuka Y, Amano H, Kuwano M, Iwai T, Mae T, Ohzono K, Shino K (2009) Outcome of double-bundle ACL reconstruction using hamstring tendons. Knee Surg Sports Traumatol Arthrosc 17(5):456–463. doi:10.1007/s00167-008-0707-7

8. Kanaya A, Ochi M, Deie M, Adachi N, Nishimori M, Nakamae A (2009) Intraoperative evaluation of anteroposterior and rotational stabilities in anterior cruciate ligament reconstruction: lower femoral tunnel placed single-bundle versus double-bundle reconstruction. Knee Surg Sports Traumatol Arthrosc 17(8):907–913. doi:10.1007/s00167-009-0757-5
9. Yasuda K, Tanabe Y, Kondo E, Kitamura N, Tohyama H (2010) Anatomic double-bundle anterior cruciate ligament reconstruction. Arthroscopy 26(9 Suppl):S21–S34. doi:10.1016/j.arthro.2010.03.014
10. Yasuda K, van Eck CF, Hoshino Y, Fu FH, Tashman S (2011) Anatomic single- and double-bundle anterior cruciate ligament reconstruction, part 1: basic science. Am J Sports Med 39 (8):1789–1799. doi:10.1177/0363546511402659
11. Araki D, Kuroda R, Kubo S, Fujita N, Tei K, Nishimoto K, Hoshino Y, Matsushita T, Matsumoto T, Nagamune K, Kurosaka M (2011) A prospective randomised study of anatomical single-bundle versus double-bundle anterior cruciate ligament reconstruction: quantitative evaluation using an electromagnetic measurement system. Int Orthop 35(3):439–446. doi:10.1007/s00264-010-1110-9
12. Nakamae A, Ochi M, Adachi N, Deie M, Nakasa T (2012) Clinical comparisons between the transtibial technique and the far anteromedial portal technique for posterolateral femoral tunnel drilling in anatomic double-bundle anterior cruciate ligament reconstruction. Arthroscopy 28(5):658–666. doi:10.1016/j.arthro.2011.10.025
13. Yagi M, Kuroda R, Nagamune K, Yoshiya S, Kurosaka M (2007) Double-bundle ACL reconstruction can improve rotational stability. Clin Orthop Relat Res 454:100–107. doi:10.1097/BLO.0b013e31802ba45c
14. Yagi M, Wong EK, Kanamori A, Debski RE, Fu FH, Woo SL (2002) Biomechanical analysis of an anatomic anterior cruciate ligament reconstruction. Am J Sports Med 30(5):660–666
15. Yasuda K, Kondo E, Ichiyama H, Kitamura N, Tanabe Y, Tohyama H, Minami A (2004) Anatomic reconstruction of the anteromedial and posterolateral bundles of the anterior cruciate ligament using hamstring tendon grafts. Arthroscopy 20(10):1015–1025. doi:10.1016/j.arthro.2004.08.010
16. Kondo E, Merican AM, Yasuda K, Amis AA (2011) Biomechanical comparison of anatomic double-bundle, anatomic single-bundle, and nonanatomic single-bundle anterior cruciate ligament reconstructions. Am J Sports Med 39(2):279–288. doi:10.1177/0363546510392350
17. Meredick RB, Vance KJ, Appleby D, Lubowitz JH (2008) Outcome of single-bundle versus double-bundle reconstruction of the anterior cruciate ligament: a meta-analysis. Am J Sports Med 36(7):1414–1421. doi:10.1177/0363546508317964
18. Shea KG, Carey JL, Richmond J, Sandmeier R, Pitts RT, Polousky JD, Chu C, Shultz SJ, Ellen M, Smith A, LaBella CR, Anderson AF, Musahl V, Meyer GD, Jevsevar D, Bozic KJ, Shaffer W, Cummins D, Murray JN, Patel N, Shores P, Woznica A, Martinez Y, Gross L, Sevarino K, American Academy of Orthopaedic S (2015) The American Academy of Orthopaedic Surgeons evidence-based guideline on management of anterior cruciate ligament injuries. J Bone Joint Surg Am Vol 97(8):672–674
19. Hoshino Y, Kuroda R, Nagamune K, Yagi M, Mizuno K, Yamaguchi M, Muratsu H, Yoshiya S, Kurosaka M (2007) In vivo measurement of the pivot-shift test in the anterior cruciate ligament-deficient knee using an electromagnetic device. Am J Sports Med 35 (7):1098–1104. doi:10.1177/0363546507299447
20. Araki D, Kuroda R, Kubo S, Nagamune K, Hoshino Y, Nishimoto K, Takayama K, Matsushita T, Tei K, Yamaguchi M, Kurosaka M (2011) The use of an electromagnetic measurement system for anterior tibial displacement during the Lachman test. Arthroscopy 27(6):792–802. doi:10.1016/j.arthro.2011.01.012
21. Fujita N, Kuroda R, Matsumoto T, Yamaguchi M, Yagi M, Matsumoto A, Kubo S, Matsushita T, Hoshino Y, Nishimoto K, Araki D, Kurosaka M (2011) Comparison of the clinical outcome of double-bundle, anteromedial single-bundle, and posterolateral single-

bundle anterior cruciate ligament reconstruction using hamstring tendon graft with minimum 2-year follow-up. Arthroscopy 27(7):906–913. doi:10.1016/j.arthro.2011.02.015
22. Lopomo N, Zaffagnini S, Signorelli C, Bignozzi S, Giordano G, Marcheggiani Muccioli GM, Visani A (2012) An original clinical methodology for non-invasive assessment of pivot-shift test. Comput Meth Biomech Biomed Eng 15(12):1323–1328. doi:10.1080/10255842.2011.591788
23. Lopomo N, Signorelli C, Bonanzinga T, Marcheggiani Muccioli GM, Visani A, Zaffagnini S (2012) Quantitative assessment of pivot-shift using inertial sensors. Knee Surg Sports Traumatol Arthrosc 20(4):713–717. doi:10.1007/s00167-011-1865-6
24. Hoshino Y, Araujo P, Ahlden M, Samuelsson K, Muller B, Hofbauer M, Wolf MR, Irrgang JJ, Fu FH, Musahl V (2013) Quantitative evaluation of the pivot shift by image analysis using the iPad. Knee Surg Sports Traumatol Arthrosc 21(4):975–980. doi:10.1007/s00167-013-2396-0
25. Ferretti M, Ekdahl M, Shen W, Fu FH (2007) Osseous landmarks of the femoral attachment of the anterior cruciate ligament: an anatomic study. Arthroscopy 23(11):1218–1225. doi:10.1016/j.arthro.2007.09.008
26. Otsubo H, Shino K, Suzuki D, Kamiya T, Suzuki T, Watanabe K, Fujimiya M, Iwahashi T, Yamashita T (2012) The arrangement and the attachment areas of three ACL bundles. Knee Surg Sports Traumatol Arthrosc 20(1):127–134. doi:10.1007/s00167-011-1576-z
27. Shino K, Suzuki T, Iwahashi T, Mae T, Nakamura N, Nakata K, Nakagawa S (2010) The resident's ridge as an arthroscopic landmark for anatomical femoral tunnel drilling in ACL reconstruction. Knee Surg Sports Traumatol Arthrosc 18(9):1164–1168. doi:10.1007/s00167-009-0979-6
28. Smigielski R, Zdanowicz U, Drwiega M, Ciszek B, Ciszkowska-Lyson B, Siebold R (2014) Ribbon like appearance of the midsubstance fibres of the anterior cruciate ligament close to its femoral insertion site: a cadaveric study including 111 knees. Knee Surg Sports Traumatol Arthrosc. doi:10.1007/s00167-014-3146-7
29. Mochizuki T, Fujishiro H, Nimura A, Mahakkanukrauh P, Yasuda K, Muneta T, Akita K (2014) Anatomic and histologic analysis of the mid-substance and fan-like extension fibres of the anterior cruciate ligament during knee motion, with special reference to the femoral attachment. Knee Surg Sports Traumatol Arthrosc 22(2):336–344. doi:10.1007/s00167-013-2404-4
30. Siebold R, Schuhmacher P, Fernandez F, Smigielski R, Fink C, Brehmer A, Kirsch J (2014) Flat midsubstance of the anterior cruciate ligament with tibial "C"-shaped insertion site. Knee Surg Sports Traumatol Arthrosc. doi:10.1007/s00167-014-3058-6
31. Ferretti M, Levicoff EA, Macpherson TA, Moreland MS, Cohen M, Fu FH (2007) The fetal anterior cruciate ligament: an anatomic and histologic study. Arthroscopy 23(3):278–283. doi:10.1016/j.arthro.2006.11.006
32. Araki D, Kuroda R, Matsumoto T, Nagamune K, Matsushita T, Hoshino Y, Oka S, Nishizawa Y, Kurosaka M (2014) Three-dimensional analysis of bone tunnel changes after anatomic double-bundle anterior cruciate ligament reconstruction using multidetector-row computed tomography. Am J Sports Med. doi:10.1177/0363546514540274
33. Ballantyne GH, Moll F (2003) The da Vinci telerobotic surgical system: the virtual operative field and telepresence surgery. Surg Clin N Am 83(6):1293–1304. doi:10.1016/S0039-6109(03)00164-6, vii
34. Takahashi K, Tanabe K, Ohnuki M, Narita M, Ichisaka T, Tomoda K, Yamanaka S (2007) Induction of pluripotent stem cells from adult human fibroblasts by defined factors. Cell 131(5):861–872. doi:10.1016/j.cell.2007.11.019
35. Takahashi K, Yamanaka S (2006) Induction of pluripotent stem cells from mouse embryonic and adult fibroblast cultures by defined factors. Cell 126(4):663–676. doi:10.1016/j.cell.2006.07.024

36. Sakai Y, Miwa M, Oe K, Ueha T, Koh A, Niikura T, Iwakura T, Lee SY, Tanaka M, Kurosaka M (2011) A novel system for transcutaneous application of carbon dioxide causing an "artificial Bohr effect" in the human body. PLoS ONE 6(9), e24137. doi:10.1371/journal.pone.0024137
37. Oe K, Ueha T, Sakai Y, Niikura T, Lee SY, Koh A, Hasegawa T, Tanaka M, Miwa M, Kurosaka M (2011) The effect of transcutaneous application of carbon dioxide (CO(2)) on skeletal muscle. Biochem Biophys Res Commun 407(1):148–152. doi:10.1016/j.bbrc.2011.02.128

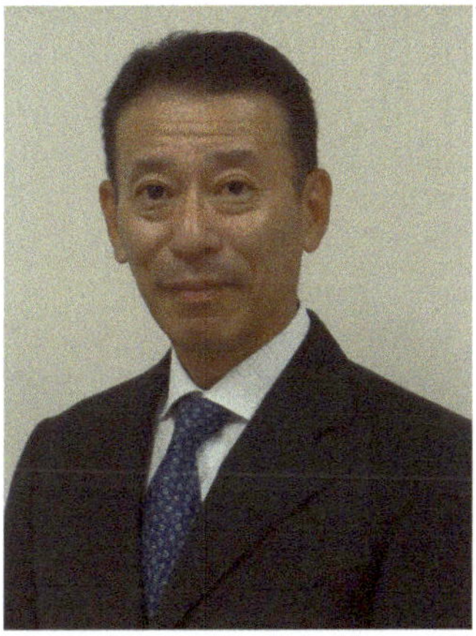

Masahiro Kurosaka, M.D., Ph.D., Department of Orthopaedic Surgery, Kobe University Graduate School of Medicine, Hyogo, Japan.

Chapter 25
Anatomic Double-Bundle Reconstruction Procedure

Kazunori Yasuda, Eiji Kondo, and Nobuto Kitamura

Abstract The anterior cruciate ligament (ACL) is composed of the anteromedial (AM) and posterolateral (PL) bundles, each with a different function. Based on our basic studies, the authors established the theory and the practical procedure to anatomically reconstruct the two bundles using hamstring tendon grafts. In the anatomic double-bundle bundle procedure, four ends of two tendon grafts should be grafted at the center of the direct attachment of the AM or PL mid-substance fibers, respectively, not only on the tibia but on the femur. In biomechanical evaluations, the knee stability after the anatomic double-bundle procedure was almost equal to that in the normal knee and significantly superior to that after the conventional single-bundle reconstruction procedure. Our comparative clinical studies demonstrated that the anatomic double-bundle procedure significantly improved the postoperative knee stability in comparison with the conventional single-bundle procedure, without providing any adverse clinical effects. Recently, we developed the remnant-preserving procedure for anatomic double-bundle reconstruction. Our clinical study indicated that preservation of the ACL remnant tissue was significantly effective to improve knee stability after anatomic double-bundle ACL reconstruction without any adverse effects in functional evaluations. Thus, we believe that the anatomic double-bundle ACL reconstruction with preservation of a sufficient amount of remnant tissue can bring the clinical results of ACL reconstruction closer to the ideal goal.

Keywords Anatomic reconstruction • Double-bundle reconstruction • Transtibial technique • Remnant preservation

---

K. Yasuda (✉) • E. Kondo • N. Kitamura
Department of Sports Medicine, Hokkaido University Graduate School of Medicine, Kita-15, Nishi-7, 060-8638 Kita-ku, Sapporo, Hokkaido, Japan
e-mail: kazu-yasuda@rouge.plala.or.jp

M. Ochi et al. (eds.), *ACL Injury and Its Treatment*,
DOI 10.1007/978-4-431-55858-3_25

25.1 Introduction

The anterior cruciate ligament (ACL) is functionally composed of the anteromedial (AM) and posterolateral (PL) bundles. The authors reported the first practical double-bundle procedure to anatomically reconstruct both the AM and PL bundles using the hamstring tendon in 2004 [1]. The greatest feature of this procedure was that all four ends of two tendon grafts are grafted at the center of the anatomical attachment of the AM bundle or the PL bundle, not only on the tibia but also on the femur. Then, we reported the first clinical results compared with a conventional single-bundle procedure in 2006 [2] and 2008 [3]. These studies demonstrated that the postoperative anterior and rotational stability after the anatomic double-bundle ACL reconstruction was significantly better than that after the conventional single-bundle reconstruction. In addition, our biomechanical study using cadaver knees showed advantages of this double-bundle procedure in terms of restoration of knee stability in comparison with a conventional single-bundle procedure [4]. In this chapter, the authors explain the surgical theory, the practical procedure, and the evaluations of our anatomical double-bundle ACL reconstruction procedure. In addition, we introduce our recent studies to further improve the clinical results after this procedure by preserving the ACL remnant tissue.

25.2 History of Double-Bundle ACL Reconstruction Procedures

In 1983, Mott [5] showed the first idea to reconstruct the ACL with two bundles, although he did not show where he created the intra-articular outlets of the two tunnels in the femur or the tibia. In 1994, a technical manual produced under the advice of Rosenberg and Graf [6] displayed a few important drawings on an arthroscopically assisted double-bundle procedure using two femoral and one tibial tunnels, although this manual was not regarded as a scientific paper. According to these drawings, the two femoral tunnels were created between the 11:00 and 12:00 o'clock point. In 1999, Muneta et al. [7] improved upon this procedure by creating two tunnels in the tibia. They described that the two femoral tunnels were created at the 10:30 and 11:30 (or 12:30 and 1:30) o'clock orientations, respectively. Hereafter, several technical papers for double-bundle ACL reconstruction procedures were published [8]. These procedures, however, did not include the concept of anatomic reconstruction of the PL bundle but rather meant to reconstruct the AM bundle with two bundles. In 2004, Yasuda et al. [1] reported the first anatomic reconstruction procedure of the AM and PL bundles with two-year follow-up results, in which the two bundles were reconstructed with four independent tunnels created at the center of the four normal attachments. Hereafter, a number of prospective comparative clinical trials were conducted to compare the anatomic double-bundle reconstruction with the conventional single-bundle reconstruction [8].

25.3 Theory of the Anatomic Double-Bundle ACL Reconstruction Procedure

25.3.1 Where Should Surgeons Create Femoral Tunnels in the Anatomic DB ACL Reconstruction?

It is critical to understand functional anatomy and biomechanics of the AM and PL bundles of the ACL in order to understand the theory of the anatomic double-bundle ACL reconstruction. It has been well known that the mid-substance fibers of the AM and PL bundles have different functions: The AM bundle mid-substance is stretched in the full extension position, relaxed at 20–60 ° of knee flexion, and again stretched in a flexion position of more than 90° [9]. The PL bundle mid-substance is stretched in the full extension position, whereas it becomes slack in a flexion position [9]. In response to an anterior tibial load, the magnitude of the in situ force in the PL bundle mid-substance was larger than that in the AM bundle mid-substance at knee flexion angles between 0 ° and 45 ° [10]. Under a combined rotatory load, the PL bundle mid-substance is as important as the AM bundle mid-substance, especially when the knee is in the near extension position [11].

Concerning the ACL attachment on the femur, Mochizuki et al. [12] described that the broad attachment of the ACL is composed of the attachment of the mid-substance fibers and the fanlike extension fibers. Recently, the authors have clarified functional anatomy of the ACL attachment in detail: In the whole attachment, the mid-substance fiber attachment is relatively narrow and long, with its long axis inclined toward the posterior direction by 30 ° to the long axis of the femur [1, 13]. The fanlike extension fibers extend from the mid-substance fibers and broadly spread out like a fan on the posterior condyle. The authors discovered that a deep fold is formed at the border between the mid-substance and the fanlike extension fibers during knee flexion [14] (Fig. 25.1). This fact suggested that a force from the ACL mid-substance might not be distributed to the fanlike extension fibers over this fold. Most recently, our biomechanical study demonstrated that, in

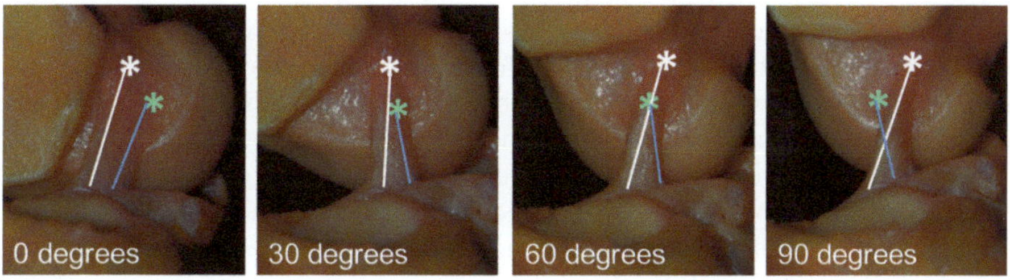

Fig. 25.1 A deep fold is formed at the border between the mid-substance and the fanlike extension fibers during knee flexion. Therefore, it is meaningless to reconstruct the fanlike extension fibers in ACL reconstruction. However, the mid-substance fibers of the AM and PL bundles can be reconstructed by creating two tunnels at the center of the femoral direct attachment of the AM or PL mid-substance fibers, respectively

anterior tibial displacement, the attachment of the mid-substance fibers resisted 82–90 % of the anterior drawer force, while the fanlike extension fibers contributed very little [15].

The above-described anatomical and biomechanical facts suggest that it is not of value to reconstruct the fanlike extension fibers in ACL reconstruction and that what should be anatomically reconstructed in the anatomic DB ACL reconstruction are the mid-substance fibers of the AM and PL bundles including the direct attachment on the femur and the tibia [1, 14, 15]. To reconstruct such bundles, four ends of two tendon grafts should be grafted at the center of the direct attachment of the AM or PL mid-substance fibers, respectively, not only on the tibia but on the femur (Fig. 25.1).

25.3.2 How to Determine the Center of the Femoral Attachment of the AM and PL Mid-Substance Fiber Bundles

In the anatomic double-bundle ACL reconstruction, two femoral tunnel positions are particularly critical to obtain better clinical results [2]. Nevertheless, no studies have shown a quantitative method available in arthroscopic surgery. For example, the quadrant grid method cannot be applied to actual arthroscopic surgery. The resident's ridge cannot be quantitatively used as a reference in ACL reconstruction surgery, as shown in our anatomical study [16]. How should we create two femoral tunnels at the center of the direct attachment of the AM and PL mid-substance fibers, respectively? The authors developed a clinically available quantitative method to precisely insert a guidewire at the averaged center of the direct attachment of the AM and PL mid-substance fibers [1, 17].

Concerning the AM bundle reconstruction, the anatomic study reported that the averaged center of the direct attachment of the AM bundle mid-substance fibers was located on the cylindrical surface of the femoral intercondylar notch at "10:37" (or "1:23") o'clock orientation in the distal view and at 5.0-mm from the proximal outlet of the intercondylar notch (POIN) in the lateral view (Fig. 25.2) [17]. Based on this fact, the authors developed the following quantitative method to insert a guidewire into this point: Through the tibial tunnel, we introduced a 5-mm offset guide (Twisted Offset Guide, Smith and Nephew Endoscopy Japan Inc, Tokyo, Japan) into the joint cavity and set the hook-shaped tip of this guide at the POIN at 90–100 ° of knee flexion. Keeping the hook at this point, we aimed a guide wire at the "1:30" or "10:30" o'clock orientation, an eighth of a circle, in the arthroscopic visual field (Fig. 25.3) [17]. In the postoperative evaluation of the accuracy of this technique, the average location of the AM tunnel actually created in ACL reconstruction was at "10:41" (or "1:19") o'clock orientation and at 5.0 mm from the POIN. There was no significant difference between the averaged center location of the native AMB attachment and that of the actually created tunnels [17]. The results

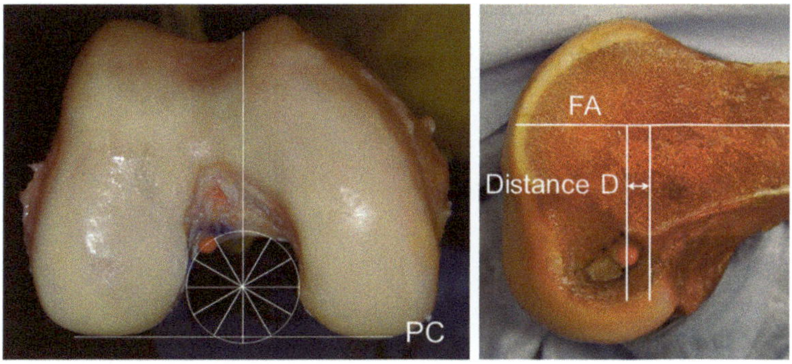

Fig. 25.2 The averaged center (*red marker*) of the direct attachment of the AM bundle mid-substance fibers was located on the cylindrical surface of the femoral intercondylar notch at "10:37" (or "1:23") o'clock orientation in the distal view and at 5.0 mm (Distance D) from the proximal outlet of the intercondylar notch (POIN) in the lateral view. *PC*: posterior condylar line. *FA*: femoral axis. (From ref. 17 with permission)

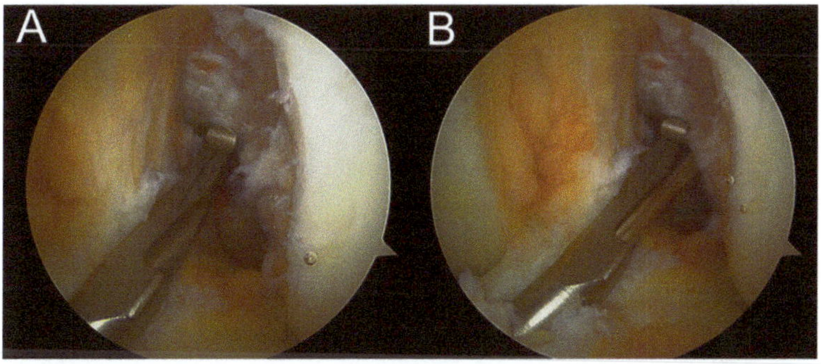

Fig. 25.3 Through the tibial tunnel, we introduced a 5-mm "twisted" offset guide into the joint cavity and set the *hook*-shaped tip of this guide at the POIN at 90 to 100 ° of knee flexion (**a**). Keeping the hook at this point, we inserted a guide wire at the "1:30" or "10:30" o'clock orientation (**b**)

suggest that the above-described quantitative technique is useful to insert a guidewire into the averaged center of the native AM bundle attachment.

Regarding PL bundle reconstruction, the authors reported a geometric method to estimate the averaged center of the direct attachment of the PL bundle mid-substance in the original procedure [1]. In an arthroscopic visual field, we could draw an imaginary vertical line through the contact point between the lateral femoral condyle and the tibial plateau at 90 ° of knee flexion (Fig. 25.4). This line and the long axis of the ACL remnant were crossed at the point 5–8 mm anterior to the edge of the joint cartilage. The averaged center of the normal attachment of the PL bundle was located approximately at this crossing point. The surgeon manually held a guidewire and aimed it at the crossing point on the femur through the tibial tunnel. Then, the surgeon hammered the wire into the femur and then drilled it. The

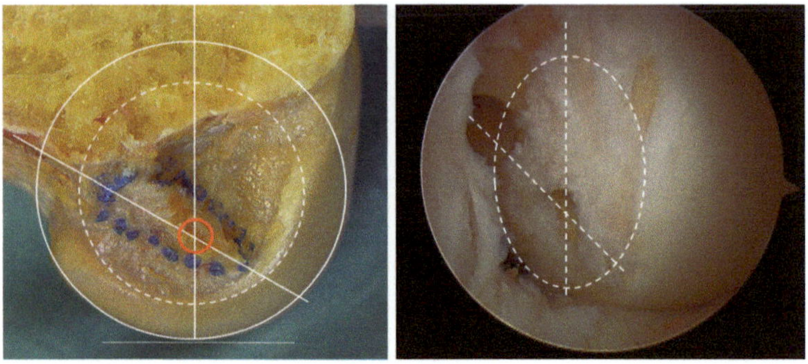

Fig. 25.4 In an arthroscopic visual field, we can draw an imaginary vertical line through the contact point between the lateral femoral condyle and the tibial plateau at 90 ° of knee flexion. The averaged center of the normal attachment of the PL bundle was located approximately at a crossing point of this line and the long axis of the ACL remnant

accuracy of this geometric method was evaluated to be sufficient for clinical use in our radiological study [18].

25.4 Practical Procedure to Reconstruct the Mid-Substance Fibers of the AM and PL Bundles

25.4.1 Preparation

Surgery is performed with an air tourniquet in the standard supine position. Preoperative setup is critical to accurately perform the transtibial tunnel technique, which is one of the features of our procedure, keeping a sterile condition. A surgeon attaches an edge of a sterile drape to his lumbar portion and then sits beside the knee joint of the patient. The surgeon puts the patient's leg hanging beside the table on his knee covered by the drape (Fig. 25.5). This setup allows the surgeon to control the patient's knee position using the surgeon's own knee in a sterile condition.

25.4.2 Essence of the Transtibial Tunnel Technique

We use the transtibial tunnel technique to perform this procedure. This technique is not a simple technique which is defined as a femoral tunnel creation through a tibial tunnel, which has been created independently to the femoral tunnel. There are two greatest keys to the success of the transtibial tunnel technique [19]: One is to create a tibial tunnel with an appropriate three-dimensional direction. In other words, a tibial tunnel should be created so that a guidewire for femoral tunnel creation can be

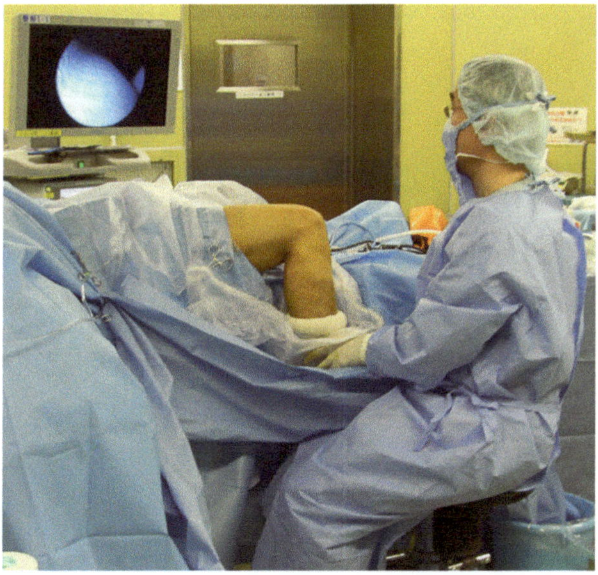

Fig. 25.5 Preoperative setup is critical to successfully perform the transtibial tunnel technique. A surgeon attaches an edge of a sterile drape to his lumbar portion and then sits beside the knee joint of the patient. The surgeon puts the patient's leg hanging beside the table on his knee covered by the drape

easily inserted at a targeted point on the lateral condyle through the tibial tunnel. The other key is to utilize the physiological knee laxity in order to insert a guidewire at the most appropriate point on the femur. Namely, the "leg-hanging" position (Fig. 25.5), in which a distraction force is applied to the knee, is essentially needed for the transtibial tunnel technique. If it is difficult to insert the wire at this point in this knee position, we recommend to change the "leg-hanging" position to the "figure-4" position, in which varus and internal rotatory forces are applied to the tibia. This position enables a surgeon to easily insert the wire at the appropriate point.

25.4.3 Creation of Tibial Tunnels

The practical procedure has been reported in detail in the original papers [1]. To create such tibial tunnels for the PL and AM bundles, we use a previously developed guidewire navigator device (Guidewire navigator III, Smith and Nephew Endoscopy Japan, Tokyo, Japan). This device is composed of a navi-tip and a wire sleeve. The navi-tip consists of sharp tibial and femoral indicators. The axis of the wire sleeve passes through the tip of the tibial indicator (Fig. 25.6). The navi-tip is introduced into the joint cavity through the medial infrapatellar portal. The surgeon holds the tibia at 90 ° of knee flexion, keeping the femur horizontal. The tibial indicator of the navi-tip is placed at the center of each bundle footprint on the tibia. Then, we aim the femoral indicator at the center of each footprint on the femur (Fig. 25.6), and the proximal end of the extra-articularly located wire sleeve is fixed

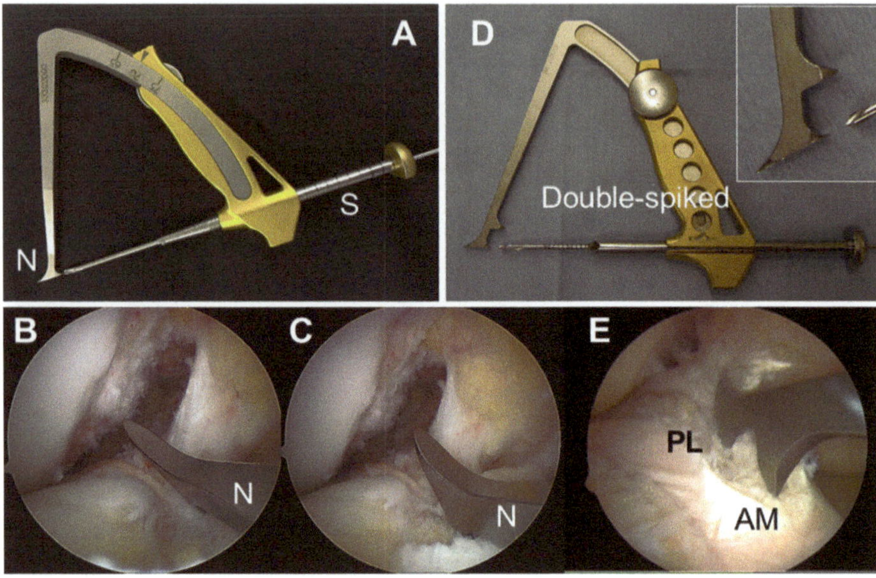

Fig. 25.6 (**a**) The guidewire navigator device is composed of a navi-tip (*N*) and a wire sleeve (*S*). The axis of the wire sleeve passes through the tip of the tibial indicator. The tibial indicator of the device is placed at the center of bundle footprint on the tibia, and the femoral indicator is aimed at the center of each bundle footprint on the femur (**b**): PL tunnel creation. (**c**): AM tunnel creation. (**d**) Recently, we developed a "double-spiked" navigator-modified device for PL tunnel creation. (**e**) When the AM indicator (AM) was set at the AM center, the PL indicator (PL) was automatically set at the PL center

on the anteromedial aspect of the tibia through the skin incision made for the graft harvest. Namely, the proximal end and the direction of the wire sleeve are automatically determined on the anteromedial aspect of the tibia, depending on the direction of the intra-articular navi-tip. A Kirschner wire of 2 mm in diameter is drilled through the sleeve in the tibia. The first tunnel is made for the PL bundle reconstruction with a cannulated drill which corresponds to the measured diameter of the prepared substitute (commonly 6 mm). Then, the second tunnel is drilled for the AM bundle reconstruction in the same manner (commonly 7 mm).

25.4.4 Creation of Femoral Tunnels

First, through the second tibial tunnel, we insert a Kirschner wire in the average center of the femoral footprint of the AM bundle mid-substance, according to the above-described method using a 5-mm offset guide (Fig. 25.3). Using this wire as a guide, a tunnel is made with a 4.5-mm cannulated drill. The length of the tunnel is measured with a scaled probe. A socket is created for the AM bundle reconstruction with a cannulated drill in the Endobutton fixation system (Acufex Microsurgical,

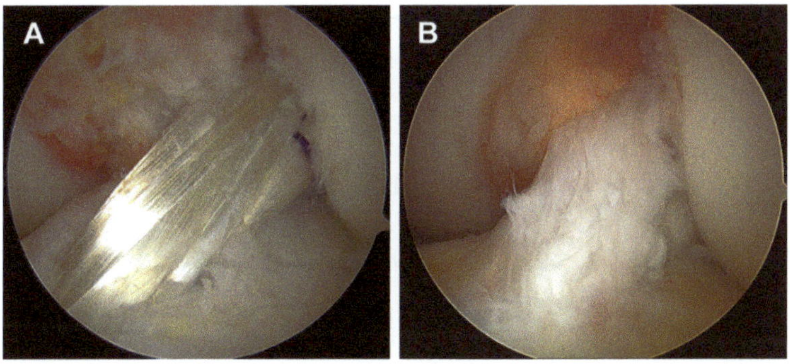

Fig. 25.7 Two tendon grafts having different directions are placed intra-articularly (**a**). In the remnant tissue-preserving procedure, the same two tendon grafts were placed, penetrating the remnant tissue (**b**)

Mansfield, MA), the diameter of which is matched to the prepared graft. Then, keeping the femur horizontal at 90 ° of knee flexion, the lateral condyle is observed with a 30 ° arthroscope inserted through the medial infrapatellar portal. The center point of the PL bundle footprint is identified using the above-described method (Fig. 25.4). The femoral tunnel, which has been created already for the AM bundle reconstruction using the above-described quantitative technique, can be used as a good landmark to use this method (Fig. 25.4). After inserting a guide wire at this point, a 4.5-mm diameter tunnel is drilled using this wire as a guide. The tunnel length is measured in the same manner. A socket is created for the PL bundle reconstruction with a cannulated drill in the same manner (Fig. 25.4).

25.4.5 Graft Fashioning, Placement, and Fixation

The semitendinosus tendon is harvested using a tendon stripper. When it is too thin or short, the gracilis tendon is harvested. Using these tendon materials, the hybrid grafts are then fashioned. Namely, a commercially available polyester tape (Leeds-Keio Artificial Ligament, Neoligament, Leeds, United Kingdom) is mechanically connected in series with the other end of the doubled tendons, using the original technique [1]. At the looped end of each doubled tendon graft, an Endobutton-CL (Acufex Microsurgical, Mansfield, MA) is attached. The length of the Endobutton-CL is determined such that a 15–20-mm long tendon portion can be placed within the bone tunnel. The PLB graft is first introduced through the tibial tunnel to the femoral tunnel using a passing pin and is fixed on the femur by an Endobutton. Then the graft for the AM bundle is placed in the same manner. Thus, the two bundles having different directions are grafted in the intercondylar space (Fig. 25.7a). An assistant surgeon simultaneously applies tension of 30 N to each graft for 2 min at 10 ° of knee flexion, using a spring tensiometer. A surgeon simultaneously secures the two tape portions onto the anteromedial aspect of the tibia using two spiked staples in the turnbuckle fashion.

25.5 Evaluations of this Procedure

25.5.1 Biomechanical Evaluations of this Procedure

Yasuda et al. [20] evaluated the function of the two grafts placed in the two femoral tunnels, which were created with the above-described quantitative technique. Namely, they intraoperatively measured the tension of the AM and PL bundle grafts during flexion-extension motion of the knee, using a strain gauge-type tensiometer. The averaged tension-versus-flexion curves were significantly different between the AM and PL grafts under each initial tension condition, and each curve was similar to that of the normal AM or PL bundle, which was reported in previous biomechanical studies with cadaver knees [9–11]. The maximal internal rotation of the tibia significantly increased the tension on both the AM and PL suture grafts at knee flexion angles of less than 60°. This study implied that the two femoral tunnel locations determined with the above-described quantitative technique were appropriate to reconstruct the anatomical location and orientation of the mid-substance fibers of the AM and PL bundles.

Kondo et al. [4] reported a unique laboratory study to verify biomechanical effects of this ACL reconstruction procedure. Namely, they arthroscopically performed this anatomic double-bundle reconstruction procedure and the conventional single-bundle reconstruction procedure with cadaver knees and biomechanically compared the knee stability among the two procedures and the normal knee, under the following loading conditions: 90-N anterior tibial force, 5-Nm internal and external tibial torques, and a simulated pivot-shift test. In the results, there were significant reductions of anterior laxity of 3.5 mm and internal rotational laxity of 2.5 mm at 20 ° of flexion and anterior translations (2 mm) and internal rotations (5 °) in the simulated pivot-shift test in the anatomic double-bundle reconstruction as compared with the single-bundle reconstruction. In addition, the knee stability after the anatomic double-bundle procedure was almost equal to that in the normal knee. This study demonstrated that our anatomic double-bundle procedure was significantly superior to the conventional single-bundle reconstruction procedure in terms of restoring the knee stability.

25.5.2 Clinical Evaluations of this Procedure

In 2006, Yasuda et al. [2] reported the first prospective comparative study to evaluate this anatomic double-bundle procedure using 72 patients. Concerning the side-to-side anterior laxity and the pivot-shift test, the anatomic double-bundle group was significantly superior to the single-bundle group. There were no significant differences in the IKDC evaluation, the range of knee motion, and the muscle torque. In 2008, Kondo et al. [3] reported on a large prospective comparative study with 328 patients to compare this anatomic double-bundle procedure with the conventional single-bundle procedure. Concerning all background factors, there were no statistical differences between the two groups. Each patient was examined 2 years after surgery. No serious complications were experienced in either group. As for the results, the anterior laxity was significantly less in the double-bundle reconstruction (mean, 1.2 mm) than in the single-bundle reconstruction (mean, 2.5 mm). In the pivot-shift test, the double bundle (+, 16 %; ++, 3 %) was significantly better than the single bundle (+, 37 %; ++, 12 %). There were no significant differences in the other clinical measures between the two groups. Thus, this study showed that the anatomic double-bundle procedure significantly improved the postoperative knee stability in comparison with the conventional single-bundle procedure, without providing any adverse clinical effects. These clinical results were supported by our second-look arthroscopy study using 123 patients [21], which evaluated graft thickness, apparent tension, and synovium coverage of the reconstructed bundles at 1–2 years after surgery. Namely, the anteromedial bundle was evaluated as excellent in 79.5 % of the knees, fair in 16.7 %, and poor in 3.8 % and the posterolateral bundle was evaluated as excellent in 75.8 %, fair in 21.2 %, and poor in 3.0 %. There was a significant correlation between the evaluation score in the second-look observation and the knee stability.

25.6 Recent Challenges to Further Improve the Clinical Results After Anatomic Double-Bundle Procedure

25.6.1 Development of Remnant-Preserving Procedure

In our previous studies, we found some discrepancy in the knee stability between the biomechanical and clinical results. Namely, the clinical results were worse than the biomechanical results. What causes the discrepancy? It is known that the grafted tendon is necrotized after surgery and undergoes a process of matrix remodeling, which is considered to entail cellular repopulation, revascularization, and collagen deposition [22]. During the remodeling phase, the structural properties of the graft deteriorate, and the reduced properties are not completely restored even at 12 months after surgery [23]. Therefore, there is a strong possibility that the discrepancy between the biomechanical and clinical studies is caused by gradual failure or elongation of the graft, which are induced during the remodeling phase of the graft by low or moderate forces in daily activities. Remnant preservation has been expected to have several potential advantages to improve postoperative knee stability, such as enhanced graft coverage with fibrous tissues, accelerated cell repopulation and revascularization, maintenance of the native broad tibial attachment, and reduction of bone tunnel enlargement, although these points are arguable. No clinical studies, however, have been conducted to compare clinical results between the remnant-preserving and remnant-resecting procedures after anatomic double-bundle reconstruction.

Recently, we developed the remnant-preserving procedure for anatomic double-bundle reconstruction [19], based on the original remnant-resecting procedure [1]. Briefly, first, we inserted a guide wire for the tibial PL tunnel with the wire-navigator device. Because the remnant tissue disturbed arthroscopic observation, we confirmed a position of the device using a C-arm fluoroscope. Then, a shallow longitudinal incision was made on the AM bundle remnant along with the fiber orientation. The wire-navigator device was at the center of the AM bundle attachment through the incision. To insert a guide wire for femoral AM tunnel creation, we made a short, deep incision, which was parallel to the remnant fiber orientation, into the femoral attachment of the remnant tissue at the 1:30- or 10:30-o'clock orientation. Through this incision, a tip of a 5-mm offset guide, which was inserted to the joint cavity through the tibial AM tunnel and the remnant tissue, was placed on the posterior part of the lateral condyle with use of the C-arm fluoroscope. For femoral PL tunnel creation, finally, the surgeon manually inserted a guide wire into the joint cavity through the tibial PL tunnel and the remnant tissue and aimed it at the center of the femoral attachment of the PL bundle mid-substance, using the fluoroscopic method [19]. After each guide wire was inserted without detaching the adherent attachment of the remnant from the PCL or the femur, we gently drilled a tunnel by use of a cannulated drill, penetrating the remnant tissue. In this procedure, the same hybrid tendon grafts were easily placed, penetrating the remnant tissue (Fig. 25.7b) and fixed to the femur and tibia in completely the same manner. The transtibial tunnel technique was beneficial to place the two tendon grafts, penetrating the remnant tissue.

25.6.2 Clinical Evaluations of the Remnant-Preserving Procedure

We conducted a prospective comparative study with a total of 179 patients who underwent anatomic double-bundle ACL reconstruction [24]. Based on the Crain classification of ACL remnant tissue, 81 patients underwent the remnant-preserving procedure (group P) and the remaining 98 patients underwent the remnant-resecting procedure (group R). There were no differences between the two groups concerning all background factors, including preoperative knee instability and intraoperative tunnel positions. The patients were followed for 2 years or more. The rate of complications, including Cyclops syndrome, and the subjective and functional clinical results were comparable between the two reconstructions. The side-to-side anterior laxity was significantly less in group P (0.9 mm) than in group R (1.5 mm). The pivot-shift test was negative in 89 % of group P and 78 % of group R patients; the result for group P was significantly better. The degree of initial graft coverage significantly affected postoperative knee stability. In arthroscopic evaluation, the remnant-preserving procedure was significantly better than remnant-resecting procedure concerning postoperative laceration or tear of the grafts as well as the synovial and fibrous tissue coverage of the grafts. These results showed a strong possibility that preservation of the ACL remnant tissue was effective in improving knee stability after anatomic double-bundle ACL reconstruction without any adverse effects in functional evaluations.

25.7 Discussion

In these 15 years, we have made a series of investigations in pursuit of the improvement of the clinical results of ACL reconstruction. In our clinical evaluations, the knee stability has been gradually but significantly improved by development of anatomic double-bundle ACL reconstruction procedure and by preservation of the ACL remnant tissue with this procedure. To each study, there may be a criticism that a mean improvement in knee laxity is small and not clinically meaningful for the patient, even though it is statistically significant. However, this improvement does not mean that the postoperative knee laxity was improved only by the mean improvement value in each knee. The significance in the chi-square test indicates that we should regard the mean improvement as resulting from the finding that each reconstruction procedure could significantly increase the number of the knees with normal knee laxity. In addition, the knees with negative pivot-shift test results were also significantly increased by each development. In our short-term evaluations, the significantly better knee stability in the remnant-preserving group did not result in significantly better results on subjective evaluation. However, this does not mean that the improvement in knee stability was meaningless for the patients with ACL reconstruction. It is clinically important to restore normal knee stability because less than normal knee stability may cause meniscal injuries and osteoarthritic changes in the long term after ACL reconstruction, resulting in reduction of functional results. The significant superiority in knee stability may result in possible superiority in future subjective and functional evaluations. In addition, we should remember that all of the patients who underwent ACL reconstruction simply hoped to achieve the same stability and functionality as in their contralateral knee. We believe that one of the final goals of ACL reconstruction is the complete restoration of normal knee stability in all patients. The anatomic double-bundle ACL reconstruction with preservation of a sufficient amount of remnant tissue can bring the clinical results of ACL reconstruction closer to the ideal goal. In addition, we expect that proprioceptive functions of the reconstructed knees are better in the remnant-preserved knees.

References

1. Yasuda K, Kondo E, Ichiyama H, Kitamura N, Tanabe Y, Tohyama H, Minami A (2004) Anatomic reconstruction of the anteromedial and posterolateral bundles of the anterior cruciate ligament using hamstring tendon grafts. Anatomic and clinical studies. Arthroscopy 20:1015–1025
2. Yasuda K, Kondo E, Ichiyama H, Tanabe Y, Tohyama H (2006) Anatomic double-bundle reconstruction of the anterior cruciate ligament. Comparisons with non-anatomic single- and double-bundle reconstructions. Arthroscopy 22:240–251
3. Kondo E, Yasuda K, Azuma H, Tanabe Y, Yagi T (2008) Prospective clinical comparisons of anatomic double-bundle versus single-bundle anterior cruciate ligament reconstruction procedures in 328 consecutive patients. Am J Sports Med 36:1675–1687
4. Kondo E, Merican AM, Yasuda K, Amis AA (2010) Biomechanical comparisons of knee stability after anterior cruciate ligament reconstruction between 2 clinically available transtibial procedures: anatomic double bundle versus single bundle. Am J Sports Med 38:1349–1358
5. Mott HW (1983) Semitendinosus anatomic reconstruction for cruciate ligament insufficiency. Clin Orthop Relat Res 172:90–92
6. Rosenberg TD, Graf B (1994) Techniques for ACL reconstruction with multi-trac drill guide. Acufex Microsurgical Inc., Mansfield
7. Muneta T, Sekiya I, Yagishita K, Ogiuchi T, Yamamoto H, Shinomiya K (1999) Two-bundle reconstruction of the anterior cruciate ligament using semitendinosus tendon with endobuttons: operative technique and preliminary results. Arthroscopy 15:618–624
8. Yasuda K, Tanabe Y, Kondo E, Kitamura N, Tohyama H (2010) Anatomic double-bundle anterior cruciate ligament reconstruction. Arthroscopy 26:S21–S34
9. Kurosawa H, Yamakoshi K, Yasuda K, Sasaki T (1991) Simultaneous measurement of changes in length of the cruciate ligaments during knee motion. Clin Orthop Relat Res 265:233–240
10. Sakane M, Fox RJ, Woo SL, Livesay GA, Li G, Fu FH (1997) In situ forces in the anterior cruciate ligament and its bundles in response to anterior tibial loads. J Orthop Res 15:285–293
11. Gabriel MT, Wong EK, Woo SL-Y, Yagi M, Debski RE (2004) Distribution of in situ forces in the anterior cruciate ligament in response to rotatory loads. J Orthop Res 22:85–89
12. Mochizuki T, Muneta T, Nagase T, Shirasawa S, Akita KI, Sekiya I (2006) Cadaveric knee observation study for describing anatomic femoral tunnel placement for two-bundle anterior cruciate ligament reconstruction. Arthroscopy 22:356–361
13. Hara K, Mochizuki T, Sekiya I, Yamaguchi K, Akita K, Muneta T (2009) Anatomy of normal human anterior cruciate ligament attachments evaluated by divided small bundles. Am J Sports Med 37:2386–2391
14. Mochizuki T, Fujishiro H, Nimura A, Mahakkanukrauh P, Yasuda K, Muneta T, Akita K (2014) Anatomic and histologic analysis of the mid-substance and fan-like extension fibres of the anterior cruciate ligament during knee motion, with special reference to the femoral attachment. Knee Surg Sports Traumatol Arthrosc 22:336–344
15. Kawaguchi Y, Kondo E, Takeda R, Akita K, Yasuda K, Amis AA (2015) The role of fibers in the femoral attachment of the anterior cruciate ligament in resisting tibial displacement. Arthroscopy 31:435–444
16. Tsukada S, Fujishiro H, Watanabe K, Nimura A, Mochizuki T, Mahakkanukrauh P, Yasuda K, Akita K (2014) Anatomic variations of the lateral intercondylar ridge: relationship to the anterior margin of the anterior cruciate ligament. Am J Sports Med 42:1110–1117
17. Kai S, Kondo E, Kitamura N, Kawaguchi Y, Inoue M, Amis AA, Yasuda K (2013) A quantitative technique to create a femoral tunnel at the averaged center of the anteromedial bundle attachment in anatomic double-bundle anterior cruciate ligament reconstruction. BMC Musculoskelet Disord 14:189. doi:10.1186/1471-2474-14-189

18. Inoue M, Tokuyasu S, Kuwahara S, Yasojima N, Kasahara Y, Kondo E, Onodere S, Yasuda K (2010) Tunnel location in transparent 3-dimensional CT in anatomic double-bundle anterior cruciate ligament reconstruction with the trans-tibial tunnel technique. Knee Surg Sports Traumatol Arthrosc 18:1176–1183
19. Yasuda K, Kondo E, Kitamura N, Kawaguchi Y, Kai S, Tanabe Y (2012) A pilot study of anatomic double-bundle anterior cruciate ligament reconstruction with ligament remnant tissue preservation. Arthroscopy 28:343–353
20. Yasuda K, Ichiyama H, Kondo E, Miyatake S, Inoue M, Tanabe Y (2008) An in vivo biomechanical study on the tension versus-knee flexion angle curves of 2 grafts in anatomic double-bundle anterior cruciate ligament reconstruction: effects of initial tension and internal tibial rotation. Arthroscopy 24:276–284
21. Kondo E, Yasuda K (2007) Second-look arthroscopic evaluations of anatomic double-bundle anterior cruciate ligament reconstruction: relation with postoperative knee stability. Arthroscopy 23:1198–1209
22. Amiel D, Kleiner JB, Akeson WH (1986) The natural history of the anterior cruciate ligament autograft of patellar tendon origin. Am J Sports Med 14:449–462
23. Butler DL, Grood ES, Noyes FR, Olmstead ML, Hohn RB, Arnoczky SP, Siegel MG (1989) Mechanical properties of primate vascularized vs. nonvascularized patellar tendon grafts; changes over time. J Orthop Res 7:68–79
24. Kondo E, Yasuda K, Kawaguchi Y, Onodera J, Kitamura K (2015) Effects of remnant tissue preservation on clinical and arthroscopic results after anatomic double-bundle anterior cruciate ligament reconstruction. Am J Sports Med 43(8):1882–1892

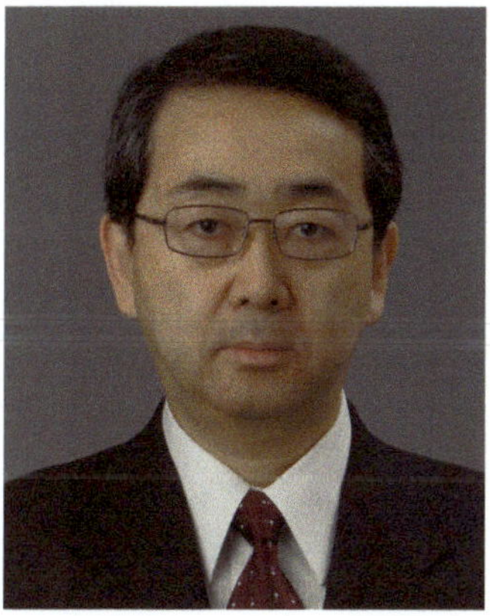

Kazunori Yasuda M.D., PhD, Department of Sports Medicine, Hokkaido University Graduate School of Medicine, Hokkaido, Japan.

Chapter 26
Triple-Bundle ACL Reconstruction with the Semitendinosus Tendon Graft

Yoshinari Tanaka, Konsei Shino, and Tatsuo Mae

Abstract Recent improvement in operative technique and understanding of the normal anatomy have enabled us to perform the anatomic double-bundle ACL reconstruction. According to the previous reports on the functional anatomy and biomechanics of the ACL, however, it could be divided into three bundles. To more precisely mimic the fiber alignment of the normal ACL, the anatomic triple-bundle ACL reconstruction has been developed. Successful results following the triple-bundle ACL reconstruction depend on several points which include tunnel apertures inside the attachment areas, proper graft preparation, and appropriate graft tensioning and fixation. As a result, the triple-bundle procedure has become one of the best techniques to closely mimic the morphology of the native ACL and to restore the stability and the normal tibiofemoral relationship. However, there still remains the problem of graft rupture, and improved preventive training is required to avoid tear of the graft.

Keywords ACL • Triple bundle • Anatomic reconstruction

26.1 Introduction

Anterior cruciate ligament (ACL) reconstruction using hamstring tendon graft has become popular because of improvement in operative technique, which made it possible to perform anatomic double-bundle ACL reconstruction [1, 2]. The double-bundle procedure to mimic the normal anatomy of the ACL showed biomechanically superior performances [3, 4] to the traditional Rosenberg's 1 or 2 femoral sockets ("bi-socket") procedure and could have resulted in more

---

Y. Tanaka
Department of Sports Orthopaedics, Osaka Rosai Hospital, Osaka, Japan

K. Shino, M.D., Ph.D. (✉)
Sports Orthopaedic Center, Yukioka Hospital, 2-2-3 Ukita, Kita-ku, Osaka 530-0021, Japan
e-mail: shinok0220@gmail.com

T. Mae
Department of Orthopaedic Sugery, Osaka University Graduate School of Medicine, Osaka University, Osaka, Japan

M. Ochi et al. (eds.), *ACL Injury and Its Treatment*,
DOI 10.1007/978-4-431-55858-3_26

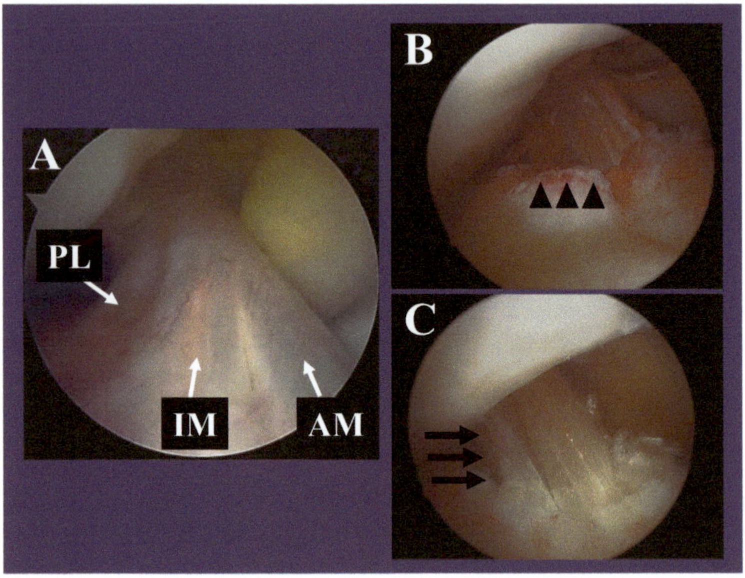

Fig. 26.1 (**a**) Triple bundles of the native ACL of the *right knee*. *AM* anteromedial bundle, *IM* intermediate bundle, *PL* posterolateral bundle. (**b**) Double-bundle reconstruction. Note the graft defect in the anterolateral portion of the tibial footprint (*black arrowheads*). (**c**) Triple-bundle reconstruction. The intermediate graft occupies the anterolateral space (*black arrows*)

favorable clinical results [5]. Although closely mimicking the normal structure is reasonable to restore normal knee function, the authors have found no graft implanted into the anterolateral portion of the tibial footprint in the double-bundle ACL reconstruction (Fig. 26.1).

According to the previous reports on the functional anatomy of the ACL, however, it could be divided into three bundles: the anteromedial (AM), the intermediate (IM), and the posterolateral (PL) [6, 7]. Additionally, it is well-known that the natural ACL forms a crescent-shaped footprint on the femur and a triangular one on the tibia. Furthermore, a recent macroscopic study by Siebold et al. showed that the "C"-shaped tibial insertion runs from along the medial tibial spine to the anterior aspect of the lateral meniscus [8].

Accordingly, one of the authors (KS) developed the triple-bundle ACL reconstruction in 2004, which divided the "anteromedial graft" in the anatomic double-bundle ACL reconstruction into further two bundles (the AM and the IM grafts) to form a triangular shape in the tibial attachment [9]. In this chapter, we describe the concept and the technique of the triple-bundle ACL reconstruction.

26.2 Anatomical and Biomechanical Considerations

26.2.1 Why Triple Bundle?

26.2.1.1 Functional Three Bundles of the Native ACL

According to the previous reports on the functional anatomy of the ACL, it could be divided into three bundles: the anteromedial (AM), the intermediate (IM), and the posterolateral (PL) [6, 7, 10]. Actually, as we could observe these three bundles arthroscopically (Fig. 26.1a), we felt something lacking around the anterolateral portion of the tibial footprint when we performed the double-bundle ACL reconstruction (Fig. 26.1b). Macroscopic investigation of the arrangement of three ACL bundles by Otsubo et al. revealed that all three bundles ran parallel to each other in knee extension, while the bundles became twisted around each other as the knee flexion increased [10], as described in Chap. 2. Additionally, ultrastructure is different among these three bundles: The AM bundle predominantly includes thick, unidirectionally oriented fibrils like tendons, while the PL bundle consists of thinner, multidirectionally oriented fibrils. The IM bundle shows an intermediate structure between the AM and the PL [11]. Furthermore, a biomechanical study by Fujie et al. clarified all three bundles functional, as described in Chap. 6. In brief, the AM bundle is the primary stabilizer to tibial anterior drawer through a wide range of motion, while the IM bundle is the secondary stabilizer in deep flexion angles. The PL bundle is the crucial stabilizer to hyperextension as well as tibial anterior drawer at full extension [12]. These results indicate that the functional three bundles should be reconstructed to restore the stability of the normal knee.

26.2.2 Femoral and Tibial Attachment of the ACL

ACL bundle insertion site anatomy as an implication of multi-bundle reconstruction is precisely described in Chap. 2 and mentioned briefly in this chapter. In terms of the femoral attachment, a microscopic analysis by Iwahashi et al. clarified that the direct insertion of the ACL was located in the fovea between the "resident's ridge" and the articular cartilage margin of the lateral femoral condyle [13, 14] (Fig. 26.3a). The result was ascertained by the other authors [15]. In terms of the location of the femoral tunnels, we usually create the femoral tunnels near the posterior cartilage margin within the footprint (Fig. 26.3b, c) because the femoral tunnels translated anteriorly and distally at the aperture after the anatomic triple-bundle ACL reconstruction [16]. In terms of the tibial attachment, the "Parson's knob" (AIR: the anterior intercondylar ridge of the tibia) is recognized as the anterior border of the ACL [17, 18]. Posteriorly, Girgis et al. described that the most posterior fibers attached to the lower part of the anterior surface of the tibial eminence and the base of the tibial spine is used as the posterior border

[19]. Medially, some reports showed that the ACL was confluent with the apex of the medial intercondylar ridge (MIR) of the tibia [20–22]. Laterally, the fibers of the ACL blend with those of the anterior attachment of the lateral meniscus, and it has been thought to be the landmark for the ACL footprint. Furthermore, recent report by Siebold et al. revealed that the fiber of the attachment of the lateral meniscus was distinguishable from the ACL tibial attachment and it can be thought to be the lateral border [8].

26.3 Operative Technique

26.3.1 Positioning

We recommend the operative leg to be placed in a leg holder to keep the distal thigh horizontal, which enables us to obtain consistent and excellent visualization of the femoral attachment area through the anteromedial portal.

26.3.2 Graft Harvest and Preparation

For autogenous grafting, the entire semitendinosus tendon is harvested through a 4-cm oblique skin incision medial to the tibial tubercle. The tendon is transversely cut in two halves to create two double-looped grafts 55–70 mm in length and 5–6 mm in diameter. According to the difference between the AM and the PL bundle of the native ACL [23], we usually prepared the AM/IM graft is 5–7 mm longer than the PL graft. Next, an ENDOBUTTON CL (Smith & Nephew Endoscopy, MA) is connected to the loop end, and braided polyester or polyester sutures (#3–5) are placed in each free end of the graft using the baseball glove or whip stitches (Fig. 26.2).

26.3.3 Femoral Tunnel Preparation

For consistent creation of the bone tunnels, it has been our policy to directly visualize the anatomical landmarks, which include the resident's ridge and the posterior cartilage margin. While the posterior third of the lateral wall of the intercondylar notch is viewed through the anteromedial portal, the residual fibrous tissue around the femoral footprint is thoroughly removed using a radiofrequency device through the far anteromedial (FAM) portal, which is 2–2.5 cm posterior to the anteromedial portal and just above the medial meniscus [9, 24]. After clearing of the footprint, the anatomical landmarks and the bony attachment area are identified, followed by marking for the AM and the PL tunnels with a chondral

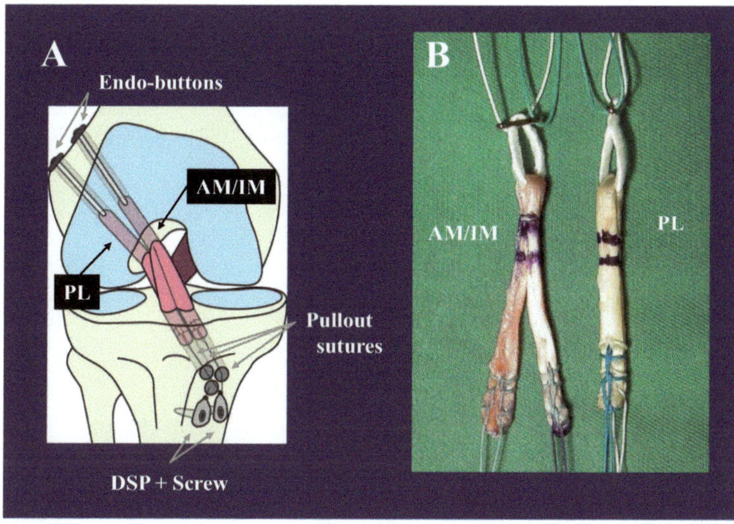

Fig. 26.2 Anatomic triple-bundle ACL reconstruction. (**a**) Schema of the procedure. (**b**) Prepared grafts. A bifurcated AM/IM graft is 5–7 mm longer than a looped PL graft (Modified from Ref. [18])

pick. The mark for the AM is usually created at the level of the superior margin of the articular cartilage, and the PL is anterodistal to the AM. Next, two 2.4-mm guide pins are inserted from the lateral femoral cortex to the marked points using the anterolateral entry femoral aimer (# 6901189 or 7210984, Smith & Nephew, Andover, MA) (Fig. 26.3). Then each wire is over-drilled with a drill bit of appropriate diameter (5–6 mm in diameter) through a 7-mm skin muscle-protective cannula (Smith & Nephew #6901106).

26.3.4 Tibial Tunnel Preparation

While the tibial attachment area is viewed through the anteromedial portal, the remnant of the tibial footprint is removed to expose the slope of the MIR. After identification of the tibial attachment area, a 2.4-mm guide pin is inserted using a tibial drill guide set at an angle of 45° (Smith & Nephew #7205519) from the anterior tibial cortex to the center of the attachment, which is located between the Parson's knob and the posterior margin of the LM attachment. The pin is over-drilled with a 10-mm drill bit to remove the anterior cortex. Then, three parallel guide pins were inserted using the 10-mm offset parallel pin guide (Smith & Nephew #E0014050-7) (Fig. 26.4b, c). According to the recent studies for the tibial footprint [8, 20, 22], we prefer to insert the guide pins of the AM and PL just lateral to the apex of the MIR. Furthermore, we recommend that the position of the guide wires is checked by X-ray, followed by over-drilling with a drill bit of appropriate diameter (5–6 mm in diameter).

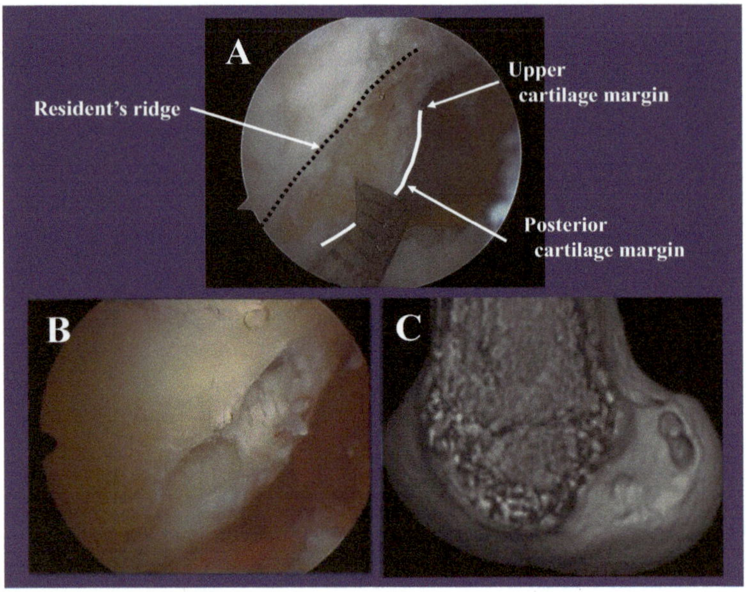

Fig. 26.3 Femoral tunnel creation. (**a**) Femoral attachment area and its three landmarks. (**b**, **c**) The two femoral tunnels are located just anterior to the posterior cartilage margin (Modified from Ref. [18])

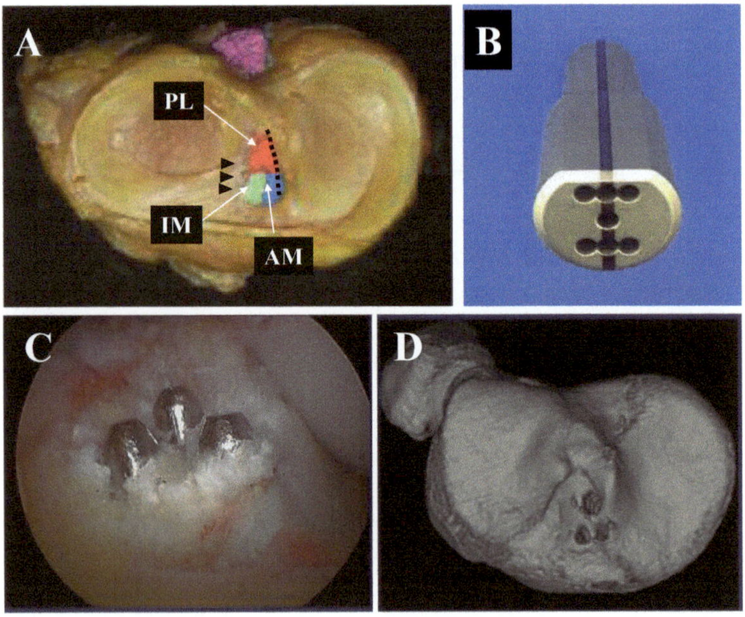

Fig. 26.4 (**a**) Tibial attachment of the three ACL bundles. *Dotted line*: MIR, *Arrowheads*: the anterior horn of the lateral meniscus. (Redrawn from Ref. [10]) (**b**) Parallel pin guide (Smith & Nephew #E0014050-7). (**c**, **d**) Three tibial tunnels. Two tunnels for the AM and PL are created just lateral to the apex of the MIR (Redrawn from Ref. [18])

26.3.5 Graft Passage and Femoral Fixation

The PL looped graft with the ENDOBUTTON CL on the top is introduced through the posterior tibial tunnel to the lower femoral tunnel and fixed to the femur by turning the button. The loop end with the ENDOBUTTON CL for AM/IM graft is passed through the FAM portal to the upper femoral tunnel and fixed with the button. Each free end of the AM/IM graft is introduced into the joint and passed into the anterolateral tibial tunnel as the IM graft and into the anteromedial tunnel as the AM graft in an inside-out fashion.

26.3.6 Tibial Fixation

To control the initial tension of the graft fixation, the authors prefer to use two double spike plates (DSP; Meira Corporation, Aichi, Japan) [25] and a metal tensioning boot (Meira Corporation) (Fig. 26.5). First, the PL graft sutures are manually tensioned and tied to a DSP of small size. Then, the AM and IM graft sutures are also tensioned and tied to the other DSP. These DSPs are tied to the tensioners installed in the tensioning boot, and the creep of each graft is removed by repetitive strong manual pulling for 5 min under a total initial tension of 20 N at 20° of knee flexion. Finally, the grafts are fixed to the tibia with DSPs and two cancellous screws.

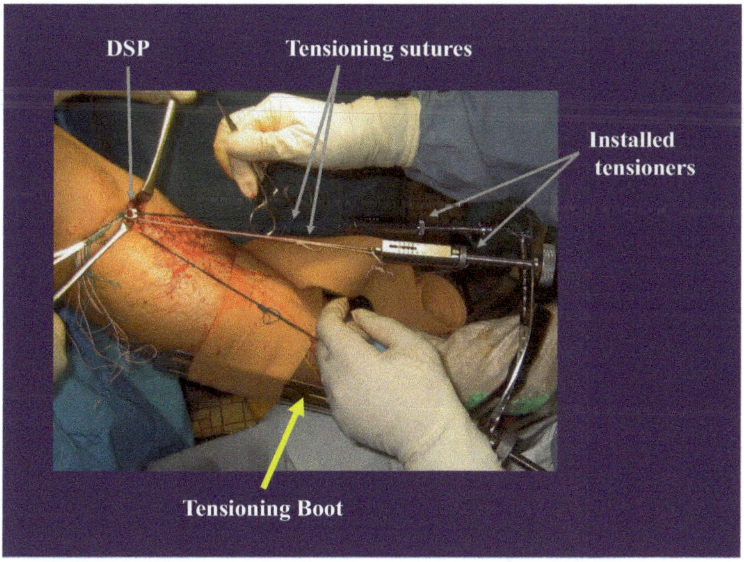

Fig. 26.5 Tibial fixation with tensioning boot system. After removing the creep of the grafts by repetitive manual pulling of tensioning sutures, the grafts are fixed to the tibia with DSPs and two cancellous screws (Courtesy Pr. Shino K)

26.3.7 *Postoperative Rehabilitation*

Postoperatively, the knee *is* immobilized at 10° flexion with a brace for 2 weeks, followed by ROM exercise. Partial weight-bearing was allowed at 3 weeks, followed by full weight-bearing at 4 weeks. Full extension or flexion exceeding 130° is not allowed until 5 weeks. Jogging was allowed at 3 months and running was permitted at 4 months, followed by return to strenuous sports activity at 8–10 months.

26.4 Clinical Studies of the Triple-Bundle Procedure

26.4.1 *Morphology*

The second-look arthroscopy showed that the transplanted triple-bundle grafts had a "fan-out" shape like the native ACL as was ascertained by MRI [26] (Fig. 26.6). An anatomically placed triple-bundle graft revealed no synovial defect in its anterior aspect, which had been seen in the isometric single-bundle reconstruction [27]. However, there were substantial damages in 10 % of the PL grafts as seen in cases of the anatomical double-bundle ACL reconstruction [1]. In addition, poor synovial coverage was observed in 41 % of the PL grafts around the femoral tunnel aperture. As the relatively poor results in the PL graft might be due to its greater length change during extension-flexion movement [23], decrease in the initial tension at the graft fixation and improvement of the rehabilitation program could improve these weak points.

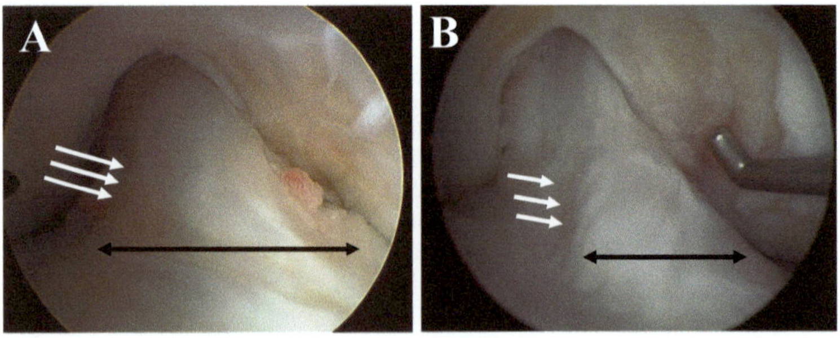

Fig. 26.6 Arthroscopic views of the multi-bundle ACL grafts. (**a**) A triple-bundle graft. Note the "fan-out" morphology approaching to the tibial attachment (*double-headed arrows*). (**b**) A double-bundle graft. Its anterior portion around the tibial attachment looks narrower (*double-headed arrows*). The *white arrows* show boundary between the anterior portion and the posterolateral of the graft (Redrawn from Ref. [26])

26.4.2 Biomechanics

Soft tissue grafts including hamstring tendon graft shift anteriorly in the femoral tunnel and posteriorly in the tibial tunnel in ACL-reconstructed knees, when anterior tibial load is applied. Thus, the more posteriorly the femoral tunnel and the more anteriorly the tibial tunnel are created inside the attachment areas, the closer the graft runs to the native ACL. Consequently, the graft could more efficaciously control instability due to loss of ACL. Moreover, it is important to maximize the contact area between tunnel wall and the graft, as the graft acts efficaciously to resist anterior drawer force. Thus the multiple tunnel reconstruction is advantageous over the single one.

Comparing the triple-bundle technique with the single- or the double-bundle one, the smaller diameter tunnels are created within the precise ACL footprint in the triple-bundle technique. With this technique, two separate smaller femoral tunnels can be created more posterior and superior compared to single-bundle ACLR, and three tibial tunnels can be created more anterior than single- or double-bundle one. We previously compared the anterior laxity immediately after the anatomic triple-bundle (ATB) ACL reconstruction with that after the anatomic double-bundle (ADB) procedure under initial tension of 20 N at 20° at the time of graft fixation [28]. Then the anterior laxity measured with KT knee arthrometer under 89 N of anterior tibial load in the ATB ACL reconstruction was significantly smaller than that in the ADB, and the side-to-side difference of the laxity in ATB (average: −4.2 mm) was greater than that in the ADB (average: −3.2 mm), demonstrating significant difference. Therefore, ATB procedure can achieve better immediate postoperative anterior knee stability compared to the ADB and is more efficacious to control the anterior knee laxity. Thus we could reasonably assume that the graft can be safely fixed with initial tension of 10 N at 20° in ATB procedure; as we reported the minimally required initial tension at graft fixation in the ADB procedure was 20 N [29].

26.4.3 Postoperative Tibiofemoral Relationship

The goal of the ACL reconstruction includes restoration of the normal tibiofemoral relationship, which is expected to prevent the onset of the postoperative degenerative change. Although several previous reports showed that the tibiofemoral relationship was abnormal following the ACL reconstruction [30–32], a few reports on the anatomic double-bundle reconstruction revealed that the procedure could restore the normal knee kinematics in vivo [33–35].

In terms of the tibiofemoral relationship after the triple-bundle reconstruction, Matsuo et al. analyzed the knees with preoperative and postoperative CT images [36]. Preoperatively, the tibia was located anteriorly by 1.4 ± 0.9 mm and rotated internally by $2.1 \pm 1.7°$. Although the tibia was over-constrained posteriorly by

2.0 ± 1.2 mm and rotated externally by $3.4 \pm 3.5°$ at 3 weeks, it regained the normal position at 6 months postoperatively. According to these good clinical results, this procedure may be useful for prevention of osteoarthritis following the ACL reconstruction [37].

26.5 Special Considerations

Although anatomic ACL reconstruction with hamstring tendon graft has made it possible for many young and highly active athletes to return to previous sports without major complications, there still remains a problem of graft rupture which has tended to occur 6–12 months postoperatively [38–40].

Although many physicians allow athletes to return to previous sports in this period, successful return to sports activity is multifactorial [41], and a rational rehabilitation protocol in which multiple factors are taken into account may be required. At the same time, physicians should give the athletes an instruction that remodeling process of the ACL graft is still proceeding in this period [42–45] and advise them to avoid re-injury by risk management measures.

26.6 Summary

Recent improvement in operative technique and understanding of the normal anatomy has enabled us to perform the anatomic double-bundle ACL reconstruction. To more precisely mimic the fiber alignment of the normal ACL, the anatomic triple-bundle ACL reconstruction has been developed. Successful results following the triple-bundle ACL reconstruction depend on several points which include tunnel apertures inside the attachment areas, proper graft preparation, and appropriate graft tensioning and fixation. As a result, the triple-bundle procedure has become one of the best techniques to closely mimic the morphology of the native ACL and to restore the stability and the normal tibiofemoral relationship. However, there still remains a problem of graft rupture and improved preventive training is required to avoid tear of the graft.

References

1. Otsubo H, Shino K, Nakamura N, Nakata K, Nakagawa S, Koyanagi M (2007) Arthroscopic evaluation of ACL grafts reconstructed with the anatomical two-bundle technique using hamstring tendon autograft. Knee Surg Sports Traumatol Arthrosc 15:720–728
2. Toritsuka Y, Amano H, Kuwano M, Iwai T, Mae T, Ohzono K, Shino K (2009) Outcome of double-bundle ACL reconstruction using hamstring tendons. Knee Surg Sports Traumatol Arthrosc 17:456–463. doi:10.1007/s00167-008-0707-7

3. Mae T, Shino K, Matsumoto N, Hamada M, Yoneda M, Nakata K (2007) Anatomical two-bundle versus Rosenberg's isometric bi-socket ACL reconstruction: a biomechanical comparison in laxity match pretension. Knee Surg Sports Traumatol Arthrosc 15:328–334
4. Yagi M, Wong EK, Kanamori A, Debski RE, Fu FH, Woo SL (2002) Biomechanical analysis of an anatomic anterior cruciate ligament reconstruction. Am J Sports Med 30:660–666
5. Muneta T, Koga H, Mochizuki T, Ju YJ, Hara K, Nimura A, Yagishita K, Sekiya I (2007) A prospective randomized study of 4-strand semitendinosus tendon anterior cruciate ligament reconstruction comparing single-bundle and double-bundle techniques. Arthroscopy 23:618–628
6. Norwood LA, Cross MJ (1979) Anterior cruciate ligament: functional anatomy of its bundles in rotatory instabilities. Am J Sports Med 7:23–26
7. Amis AA, Dawkins GP (1991) Functional anatomy of the anterior cruciate ligament. Fibre bundle actions related to ligament replacements and injuries. J Bone Joint Surg (Br) 73:260–267
8. Siebold R, Schuhmacher P, Fernandez F, Smigielski R, Fink C, Brehmer A, Kirsch J (2015) Flat midsubstance of the anterior cruciate ligament with tibial "C"-shaped insertion site. Knee Surg Sports Traumatol Arthrosc 23(11):3136–3142
9. Shino K, Nakata K, Nakamura N, Mae T, Ohtsubo H, Iwahashi T, Nakagawa S (2005) Anatomic anterior cruciate ligament reconstruction using two double-looped hamstring tendon grafts via twin femoral and triple tibial tunnels. Oper Tech Orthop 15:130–134
10. Otsubo H, Shino K, Suzuki D, Kamiya T, Suzuki T, Watanabe K, Fujimiya M, Iwahashi T, Yamashita T (2012) The arrangement and the attachment areas of three ACL bundles. Knee Surg Sports Traumatol Arthrosc 20:127–134. doi:10.1007/s00167-011-1576-z
11. Suzuki D, Otsubo H, Watanabe T, Kamiya T, Nagoya S, Yamashita T, Shino K (2015) Ultrastructure of the three anterior cruciate ligament bundles. Clin Anat 28(7):910–916. doi:10.1002/ca.22586
12. Fujie H, Otsubo H, Fukano S, Suzuki T, Suzuki D, Mae T, Shino K (2011) Mechanical functions of the three bundles consisting of the human anterior cruciate ligament. Knee Surg Sports Traumatol Arthrosc 19:S47–S53. doi:10.1007/s00167-011-1513-1
13. Iwahashi T, Shino K, Nakata K, Otsubo H, Suzuki T, Amano H, Nakamura N (2010) Direct anterior cruciate ligament insertion to the femur assessed by histology and 3-dimensional volume-rendered computed tomography. Arthroscopy 26:S13–S20. doi:10.1016/j.arthro.2010.01.023
14. Shino K, Suzuki T, Iwahashi T, Mae T, Nakamura N, Nakata K, Nakagawa S (2010) The resident's ridge as an arthroscopic landmark for anatomical femoral tunnel drilling in ACL reconstruction. Knee Surg Sports Traumatol Arthrosc 18:1164–1168. doi:10.1007/s00167-009-0979-6
15. Sasaki N, Ishibashi Y, Tsuda E, Yamamoto Y, Maeda S, Mizukami H, Toh S, Yagihashi S, Tonosaki Y (2012) The femoral insertion of the anterior cruciate ligament: discrepancy between macroscopic and histological observations. Arthroscopy 28:1135–1146. doi:10.1016/j.arthro.2011.12.021
16. Tachibana Y, Mae T, Shino K, Kanamoto T, Sugamoto K, Yoshikawa H, Nakata K (2015) Morphological changes in femoral tunnels after anatomic anterior cruciate ligament reconstruction. Knee Surg Sports Traumatol Arthrosc 23(12):3591–3600
17. Berg EE (1993) Parsons' knob (tuberculum intercondylare tertium). A guide to tibial anterior cruciate ligament insertion. Clin Orthop Relat Res 292:229–231
18. Shino K, Mae T, Tachibana Y (2015) Anatomic ACL reconstruction: rectangular tunnel/bone-patellar tendon-bone or triple-bundle/semitendinosus tendon grafting. J Orthop Sci 20:457–468. doi:10.1007/s00776-015-0705-9
19. Girgis FG, Marshall JL, Monajem A (1975) The cruciate ligaments of the knee joint. Anatomical, functional and experimental analysis. Clin Orthop Relat Res 106:216–231
20. Edwards A, Bull AM, Amis AA (2007) The attachments of the anteromedial and posterolateral fibre bundles of the anterior cruciate ligament: part 1: tibial attachment. Knee Surg Sports Traumatol Arthrosc 15:1414–1421

21. Purnell ML, Larson AI, Clancy W (2008) Anterior cruciate ligament insertions on the tibia and femur and their relationships to critical bony landmarks using high-resolution volume-rendering computed tomography. Am J Sports Med 36:2083–2090. doi:10.1177/0363546508319896
22. Tanaka Y, Shiozaki Y, Yonetani Y, Kanamoto T, Tsujii A, Horibe S (2011) MRI analysis of the attachment of the anteromedial and posterolateral bundles of anterior cruciate ligament using coronal oblique images. Knee Surg Sports Traumatol Arthrosc 19:S54–S59. doi:10.1007/s00167-011-1515-z
23. Iwahashi T, Shino K, Nakata K, Nakamura N, Yamada Y, Yoshikawa H, Sugamoto K (2008) Assessment of the "functional length" of the three bundles of the anterior cruciate ligament. Knee Surg Sports Traumatol Arthrosc 16:167–174
24. Shino K, Nakata K, Nakamura N, Toritsuka Y, Horibe S, Nakagawa S, Suzuki T (2008) Rectangular tunnel double-bundle anterior cruciate ligament reconstruction with bone-patellar tendon-bone graft to mimic natural fiber arrangement. Arthroscopy 24:1178–1183. doi:10.1016/j.arthro.2008.06.010
25. Shino K, Mae T, Maeda A, Miyama T, Shinjo H, Kawakami H (2002) Graft fixation with predetermined tension using a new device, the double spike plate. Arthroscopy 18:908–911
26. Tanaka Y, Shino K, Horibe S, Nakamura N, Nakagawa S, Mae T, Otsubo H, Suzuki T, Nakata K (2012) Triple-bundle ACL grafts evaluated by second-look arthroscopy. Knee Surg Sports Traumatol Arthrosc 20:95–101. doi:10.1007/s00167-011-1551-8
27. Toritsuka Y, Shino K, Horibe S, Mitsuoka T, Hamada M, Nakata K, Nakamura N, Yoshikawa H (2004) Second-look arthroscopy of anterior cruciate ligament grafts with multistranded hamstring tendons. Arthroscopy 20:287–293
28. Mae T, Shino K, Matsumoto N, Yoneda K, Yoshikawa H, Nakata K (2013) Immediate postoperative anterior knee stability: double- versus triple-bundle anterior cruciate ligament reconstructions. Arthroscopy 29:213–219. doi:10.1016/j.arthro.2012.08.012
29. Mae T, Shino K, Matsumoto N, Natsu-ume T, Yoneda K, Yoshikawa H, Yoneda M (2010) Anatomic double-bundle anterior cruciate ligament reconstruction using hamstring tendons with minimally-required initial tension. Arthroscopy 26:1289–1295. doi:10.1016/j.arthro.2010.02.017
30. Papannagari R, Gill TJ, Defrate LE, Moses JM, Petruska AJ, Li G (2006) In vivo kinematics of the knee after anterior cruciate ligament reconstruction: a clinical and functional evaluation. Am J Sports Med 34:2006–2012
31. Deneweth JM, Bey MJ, McLean SG, Lock TR, Kolowich PA, Tashman S (2010) Tibiofemoral joint kinematics of the anterior cruciate ligament-reconstructed knee during a single-legged hop landing. Am J Sports Med 38:1820–1828. doi:10.1177/0363546510365531
32. Tashman S, Collon D, Anderson K, Kolowich P, Anderst W (2004) Abnormal rotational knee motion during running after anterior cruciate ligament reconstruction. Am J Sports Med 32:975–983
33. Iriuchishima T, Shirakura K, Horaguchi T, Morimoto Y, Fu FH (2012) Rollback of the femoral condyle in anatomical double-bundle anterior cruciate ligament reconstruction. Knee Surg Sports Traumatol Arthrosc 20:941–946. doi:10.1007/s00167-011-1672-0
34. Kopf S, Moloney G, Freismuth K, Fu FH, Tashman S (2012) Anatomic double bundle anterior cruciate ligament reconstruction restores normal dynamic in vivo knee kinematics. Orth Research Scty 43: Paper No. 0254
35. Zaffagnini S, Marcheggiani Muccioli GM, Lopomo N, Signorelli C, Bonanzinga T, Musiani C, Vassilis P, Nitri M, Marcacci M (2012) Can the pivot-shift be eliminated by anatomic double-bundle anterior cruciate ligament reconstruction? Knee Surg Sports Traumatol Arthrosc 20:743–751. doi:10.1007/s00167-012-1897-6
36. Matsuo T, Mae T, Shino K, Kita K, Tachibana Y, Sugamoto K, Yoshikawa H, Nakata K (2013) Tibiofemoral relationship following anatomic triple-bundle anterior cruciate ligament reconstruction. Knee Surg Sports Traumatol Arthrosc 22:2128–2135. doi:10.1007/s00167-013-2646-1

37. Lohmander LS, Ostenberg A, Englund M, Roos H (2004) High prevalence of knee osteoarthritis, pain, and functional limitations in female soccer players twelve years after anterior cruciate ligament injury. Arthritis Rheum 50:3145–3152
38. Salmon L, Russell V, Musgrove T, Pinczewski L, Refshauge K (2005) Incidence and risk factors for graft rupture and contralateral rupture after anterior cruciate ligament reconstruction. Arthroscopy 21:948–957
39. Tanaka Y, Yonetani Y, Shiozaki Y, Kitaguchi T, Sato N, Takeshita S, Horibe S (2010) Retear of anterior cruciate ligament grafts in female basketball players: a case series. Sports Med Arthrosc Rehabil Ther Technol 2:7. doi:10.1186/1758-2555-2-7
40. Mae T, Shino K, Matsumoto N, Yoneda K, Yoshikawa H, Nakata K (2014) Risk factors for ipsi-lateral graft rupture or contralateral anterior cruciate ligament tear after anatomic double-bundle reconstruction. A-P Smart 1:90–95
41. Zaffagnini S, Grassi A, Serra M, Marcacci M (2015) Return to sport after ACL reconstruction: how, when and why? A narrative review of current evidence. Joints 8:25–30
42. Shino K, Kawasaki T, Hirose H, Gotoh I, Inoue M, Ono K (1984) Replacement of the anterior cruciate ligament by an allogeneic tendon graft. An experimental study in the dog. J Bone Joint Surg (Br) 66:672–681
43. Shino K, Inoue M, Horibe S, Nakata K, Maeda A, Ono K (1991) Surface blood flow and histology of human anterior cruciate ligament allografts. Arthroscopy 7:171–176
44. Weiler A, Peters G, Mäurer J, Unterhauser FN, Südkamp NP (2001) Biomechanical properties and vascularity of an anterior cruciate ligament graft can be predicted by contrast-enhanced magnetic resonance imaging. A two-year study in sheep. Am J Sports Med 29:751–761
45. Arai Y, Hara K, Takahashi T, Urade H, Minami G, Takamiya H, Kubo T (2008) Evaluation of the vascular status of autogenous hamstring tendon grafts after anterior cruciate ligament reconstruction in humans using magnetic resonance angiography. Knee Surg Sports Traumatol Arthrosc 16:342–347. doi:10.1007/s00167-007-0478-6

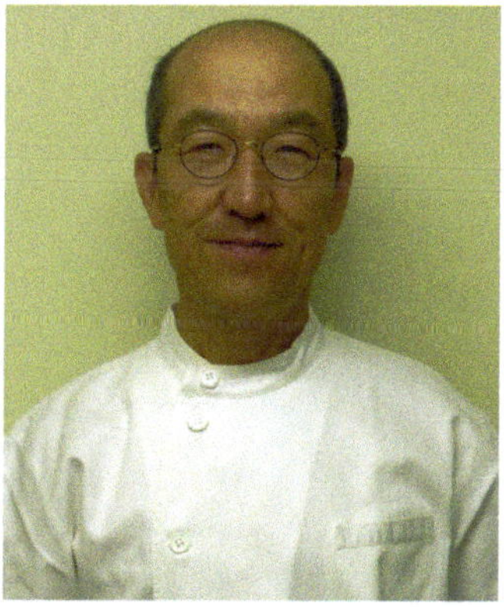

Konsei Shino, M.D., Ph.D, Sports Orthopaedic Center, Yukioka Hospital, Osaka, Japan.

Part VI
ACL Augmentation

Chapter 27
History and Advantages of ACL Augmentation

Mitsuo Ochi and Atsuo Nakamae

Abstract Anterior cruciate ligament (ACL) augmentation (remnant-preserving ACL reconstruction) has attracted much attention in the field of ACL reconstruction, because preservation of the ACL remnant may be beneficial in terms of proprioception, biomechanical functions, and vascularization of the graft. Several ACL augmentation techniques, including selective anteromedial or posterolateral bundle reconstruction and the remnant retensioning technique, have been described. There are five different augmentation procedures for ACL remnant preservation. ACL augmentation is used not only for partial rupture of the ACL but also for complete rupture. It is important to know the history and clinical results of ACL augmentation, in order to precisely understand the current status of this surgery. This chapter shows the potential advantage and history of ACL augmentation. In addition, we reviewed the current evidence to see whether ACL augmentation could obtain better clinical results than the standard single- or double-bundle ACL reconstruction. We believe that the augmentation technique can be a good treatment option for patients whose ACL remnants have certain characteristics.

Keywords Anterior cruciate ligament (ACL) • Augmentation • Remnant preservation • Knee • Review

27.1 ACL Augmentation and Its Potential Advantage

Anatomic anterior cruciate ligament (ACL) reconstruction has received attention from orthopedic surgeons. Restoration of normal biomechanical function is one of the essential factors for successful ACL reconstruction. However, early biological healing of the graft is also vital to obtaining satisfactory clinical results after ACL

M. Ochi, M.D., Ph.D. (✉)
President of Hiroshima University, 1-3-2 Kagamiyama, Higashi-Hiroshima 739-8511, Japan
e-mail: ochim@hiroshima-u.ac.jp

A. Nakamae, M.D., Ph.D.
Department of Orthopaedic Surgery, Integrated Health Sciences, Institute of Biomedical & Health Sciences, Hiroshima University, Hiroshima, Japan

M. Ochi et al. (eds.), *ACL Injury and Its Treatment*,
DOI 10.1007/978-4-431-55858-3_27

reconstruction. Accelerated graft remodeling, ligamentization, and reinnervation of the grafted tendon are necessary, not only for early return to sporting activities but also for reliable remodeling of the graft.

In patients with ACL injury, arthroscopic examination occasionally demonstrates a relatively thick and abundant ACL remnant maintaining a bridge between the tibia and the intercondylar notch. In almost half of these cases, the femoral attachment of the ACL remnant is positioned abnormally. This represents a complete rupture of the ACL. However, sometimes we observe a partial rupture of the ACL. In these cases, although complete rupture of the anteromedial (AM) or posterolateral (PL) bundle can be seen, the other bundle is preserved, if not normally, with an attachment of anatomical femoral origin. In standard single- or double-bundle ACL reconstruction, this ACL remnant is totally debrided, in order to enable clear visualization of the femoral and tibial bone tunnels. However, many orthopedic surgeons are not fully satisfied with the clinical results of standard ACL reconstruction and have searched for better surgical methods. One approach is remnant-preserving ACL reconstruction by means of ACL augmentation [1, 2], which has the following potential advantages:

27.1.1 Proprioceptive Function

It is known that the ACL has an important proprioceptive function for the knee and that human ACL remnants contain several types of mechanoreceptors. When an ACL remnant is preserved during surgery, these mechanoreceptors in the ACL remnant may contribute to the proprioceptive function of the knee [3–6]. Adachi and Ochi et al. [3] showed significantly better results for ACL augmentation than for conventional ACL reconstruction in terms of the knee's proprioceptive function. Recently, Nakamae and Ochi et al. [7] reported that patients in the ACL augmentation group exhibited better synovial coverage of the graft upon second-look arthroscopy than those in the single- and double-bundle reconstruction groups, and improvement in proprioceptive function was observed in patients with good synovial coverage of the graft.

27.1.2 Biomechanical Function

Several studies have shown that the ACL remnant can contribute to biomechanical stability of the knee [8, 9]. Crain et al. [8] investigated the relationship between the ACL remnant's morphological pattern and anterior laxity. The morphological pattern was classified as having one of four types: scarring to the PCL, scarring to the roof of the notch, scarring to the lateral wall of the notch in a position anterior and distal to the anatomic footprint of the ACL, and no identifiable ligament tissue remaining. The greatest increase in anterior laxity following resection of the remnant was observed in knees in which the injured ACL made an aberrant reattachment to the femur. We investigated whether ACL remnants make a biomechanical contribution to anteroposterior and rotational knee stability in patients with complete rupture of the ACL [9]. In this study, we found that ACL remnants contributed to anteroposterior knee stability when evaluated at 30° knee flexion for up to 1 year after injury, beyond which this biomechanical function was lost. However, the ACL remnant made no contribution to rotational knee stability at any stage after injury. Therefore, when the ACL remnant is preserved during surgery, the ACL remnant may contribute to anteroposterior knee stability, thus ensuring mechanical strength in the early postoperative period.

27.1.3 Revascularization and Ligamentization of the Grafted Tendon

Preservation of the ACL remnant may accelerate revascularization and ligamentization of the grafted tendon. An experimental animal study showed greater cellularity and angiogenesis in augmented grafts than in conventionally reconstructed grafts and concluded that selected ACL augmentation promotes tendon graft healing, which appears to result in further mechanical strength of the bone-tendon bone complex [10].

27.2 History and Clinical Results of ACL Augmentation

As outlined above, preservation of the ACL remnant may contribute to knee function from several points of view. Therefore, Ochi considered it beneficial to perform remnant-preserving ACL reconstruction by using ACL augmentation, in terms of its proprioceptive and biomechanical functions. Furthermore, the ACL remnants likely provide more rapid vascularization to the graft. Since 1992, Ochi has been performing ACL augmentation, when indicated, without sacrificing the ACL remnant by using an autogenous semitendinosus tendon under arthroscopy. In 2000, Adachi and Ochi et al. [1] reported that the joint stability and proprioceptive function of 40 patients who underwent arthroscopy-assisted ACL augmentation were superior to those of 40 patients who underwent standard single-bundle ACL reconstruction during the same period. However, the early surgical procedure of ACL augmentation needed two incisions at the medial aspect of the proximal tibia and also at the lateral femoral condyle because the graft was passed through the over-the-top route for the femoral side. In 1996, Ochi started performing ACL augmentation with the one-incision technique using EndoButton-CL and documenting it as a report in 2006 [2]. During this study, the main indication for

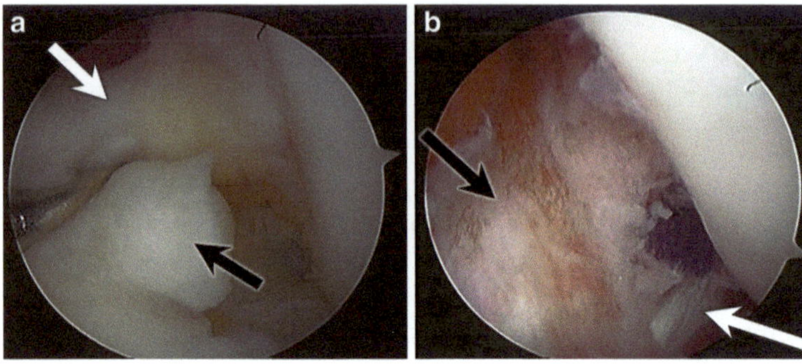

Fig. 27.1 (**a**): Partial rupture of the posterolateral (*PL*) bundle (*black arrow*). The anteromedial (*AM*) bundle (*white arrow*) of the ACL was well preserved although the remaining AM bundle is not completely intact. (**b**): AM bundle preserving ACL augmentation for rupture of the PL bundle (*white arrow*, grafted tendon; *black arrow*, preserved AM bundle)

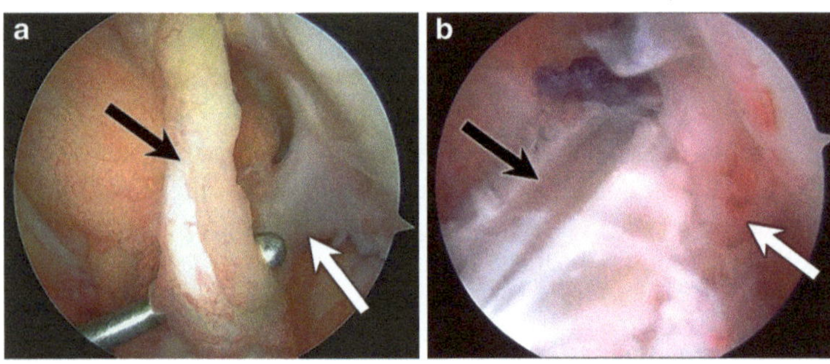

Fig. 27.2 (**a**): Partial rupture of the anteromedial (*AM*) bundle (*black arrow*). The posterolateral (*PL*) bundle (*white arrow*) of the ACL was well preserved although the remaining PL bundle was not completely intact. (**b**): PL bundle preserving ACL augmentation for rupture of the AM bundle (*black arrow*, grafted tendon; *white arrow*, preserved PL bundle)

ACL augmentation was partial rupture of the ACL (Figs. 27.1 and 27.2), with the indication for ACL augmentation comprising 10 % of all ACL reconstruction cases. In cases of partial rupture, although single-bundle reconstruction of the ruptured bundle is desirable to minimize damage to the femoral attachment of the remaining bundle, surgeons should keep in mind that the remaining AM or PL bundle is not completely intact and that the biomechanical function of the remaining bundle probably declines to some extent. In 2008, we started performing ACL augmentation even for patients with continuity of the ACL remnant between the tibia and the femur after complete rupture of the ACL (Fig. 27.3). In this complete rupture group, indication for the procedure comprises cases whose ACL remnant maintains a ligamentous bridge between the tibia and the intercondylar notch. Anatomic central single-bundle ACL augmentation is carried out for patients in this group. We also

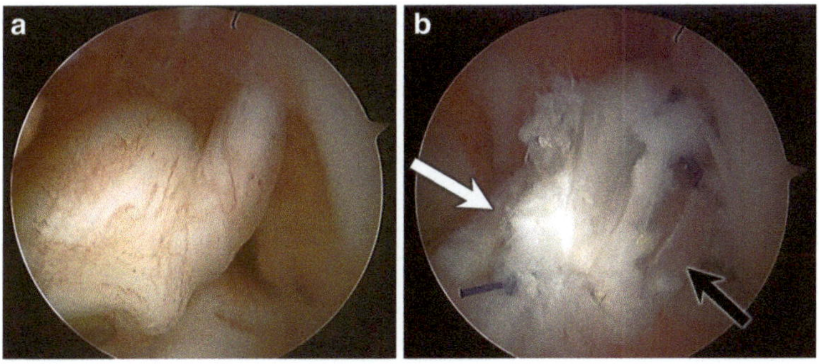

Fig. 27.3 (**a**): Complete rupture of the ACL. The ACL remnant maintained a bridge between the tibia and the intercondylar notch. (**b**): Anatomic central single-bundle ACL augmentation for complete rupture of the ACL (*black arrow*, grafted tendon; *white arrow*, preserved ACL remnant)

perform double-bundle reconstruction with the remnant-preserving technique and single-bundle augmentation using a quadriceps tendon-patellar bone autograft.

27.2.1 Clinical Studies

Since 2006, ACL augmentation has attracted much attention in the field of ACL reconstruction (Table 27.1). Several ACL augmentation techniques, including selective AM or PL bundle reconstruction, the remnant retensioning technique, and preservation of the ACL tibial remnant have been described. It is important to know the history and clinical results of ACL augmentation, in order to precisely understand the current status of this surgery. To summarize the clinical outcomes of patients undergoing ACL augmentation, an online search was performed using a PubMed (1983–2014). The search terms included (anterior cruciate ligament reconstruction AND (augmentation OR preserving OR preservation)). Inclusion criteria are as follows: (1) a clinical study of ACL augmentation, (2) primary ACL reconstruction under arthroscopy, (3) and autograft or allograft used for augmentation. Technical notes were also included. Exclusion criteria are as follows: (1) literature review, current concepts, or case reports and (2) animal study. Table 27.1 shows studies reporting arthroscopic remnant-preserving augmentation in ACL reconstruction. There are five different procedures for ACL remnant preservation: (1) anatomic single-bundle ACL augmentation preserving ACL remnant for complete rupture, (2) anatomic double-bundle ACL augmentation preserving ACL remnant for complete rupture, (3) single-bundle ACL reconstruction with remnant-tensioning technique, (4) selective AM or PL bundle augmentation for partial rupture, and (5) standard ACL reconstruction plus tibial remnant sparing. The ACL remnant in (1) and (2) maintains a bridge between the tibia and the intercondylar notch.

Table 27.1 Studies reporting remnant-preserving augmentation in ACL reconstruction

Study	Study design	Patient number*	Patient's age (years) *	Time from injury to reconstruction (months) *	Mean follow-up (months)*
Adachi and Ochi et al. (2000) [1]	Retrospective comparative study	40	25.8	4.2	38
Ochi et al. (2006) [2]	Technical note	17	31	Not reported	Not reported
Lee BI et al. (2006) [11]	Technical note	Not reported	Not reported	Not reported	Not reported
Buda et al. (2006) [12]	Case series	47	23.3	4.5	(More than 60)
Gohil et al. (2007) [13]	Randomized controlled trial	22	30.5	2	12
Buda et al. (2008) [14]	Case series	28	32.3	Not reported	27
Lee BI et al. (2008) [15]	Case series	16	35.1	5.5	35.1
Ochi et al. (2009) [16]	Case series	45	22	7.9	35
Yoon et al. (2009) [17]	Retrospective comparative study	82	28	7	24
Ahn et al. (2009) [18]	Technical note	65	Not reported	Not reported	Not reported
Kim SJ et al. (2009) [19]	Technical note	21	Not reported	Not reported	12
Ahn et al. (2010) [20]	Cohort study	41	29.2	36.1	6.3
Sonnery-Cottet et al. (2010) [21]	Case series	36	32	6.6	24
Serrano-Fernandez et al. (2010) [22]	Case series	24	25	3	74
Ahn et al. (2011) [23]	Case series	53	32.2	28.2	27.7
Jung et al. (2011) [24]	Retrospective comparative study	76	32	2.5	31
Ochi et al. (2011) [25]	Technical note	Not reported	Not reported	Not reported	Not reported
Pujol et al. (2012) [26]	Randomized controlled trial	29	31.24	5.3	(More than 12)
Hong et al. (2012) [27]	Randomized controlled trial	39	34	10.3	25.8

(continued)

Table 27.1 (continued)

Study	Study design	Patient number*	Patient's age (years) *	Time from injury to reconstruction (months) *	Mean follow-up (months)*
Ohsawa et al. (2012) [28]	Case series	19	(15 to 57)	4.8	40.2
Yasuda et al. (2012) [29]	Case series	44	29	4	16.6
Park et al. (2012) [30]	Retrospective comparative study	55	30.4	7.0	34.1
Demirağ et al. (2012) [31]	Randomized controlled trial	20	28	2.3	24.3
Sonnery-Cottet et al. (2012) [32]	Case series	168	30	3	26
Cha et al. (2012) [33]	Retrospective comparative study	100	31.9	Not reported	Not reported
Muneta et al. (2013) [34]	Cohort study	88	22.1	6.7	(More than 24)
Kazusa and Ochi et al. (2013) [35]	Technical note	Not reported	Not reported	Not reported	Not reported
Maestro et al. (2013) [36]	Retrospective comparative study	39	28.1	1	31.7
Buda et al. (2013) [37]	Case series	52	23.3	4.3	(Up to 60)
Abat et al. (2013) [38]	Case series	28	30.4	2	37.3
Nakamae and Ochi et al. (2014) [7]	Retrospective comparative study	73	26.6	Not reported	28.9
Zhang et al. (2014) [39]	Randomized controlled trial	27	23.5	12.7	24.4
Lee YS et al. (2014) [40]	Retrospective comparative study	16	30.6	Not reported	29.5
Ahn et al. (2014) [41]	Technical note	Not reported	Not reported	Not reported	Not reported
Noh et al. (2014) [42]	Technical note	Not reported	Not reported	Not reported	Not reported
Sonnery-Cottet et al. (2014) [43]	Technical note	Not reported	Not reported	Not reported	Not reported
Muneta et al. (2014) [44]	Cohort study	200	Not reported	Not reported	Not reported

(continued)

Table 27.1 (continued)

Study	Study design	Patient number*	Patient's age (years) *	Time from injury to reconstruction (months) *	Mean follow-up (months)*
Kim MK et al. (2014) [45]	Retrospective comparative study	66	30	3	27
Taketomi et al. (2014) [46]	Technical note	47	31	4	Not reported

*Augmentation group only

27.2.2 Clinical Outcomes

13 clinical studies which compared the outcomes of ACL augmentation techniques with those of the standard ACL reconstruction technique were selected from among studies in Table 27.1 (Tables 27.2 and 27.3). Table 27.2 shows the ACL remnant characteristics and type of graft in each study. Table 27.3 shows clinical outcomes in each study. Ten studies [1, 7, 13, 17, 26, 27, 30, 36, 39, 40] evaluated the side-to-side difference in instrumented knee-laxity testing (anterior displacement of tibia). Three of the studies showed that patients in the ACL augmentation group exhibited better anteroposterior knee stability than those in the single-bundle reconstruction group [1, 7, 26]. The remaining seven studies concluded that there was no significant difference between the groups at final follow-up. Three studies reported similar anteroposterior knee stability between the ACL augmentation group and double-bundle reconstruction group [7, 30, 40]. Ten studies [1, 7, 17, 26, 27, 30, 31, 36, 39, 40] reported data on the clinical scores, and nine studies [1, 7, 17, 26, 27, 30, 31, 36, 40] evaluated results of the pivot shift test. None of the studies indicated that there were significant differences between the groups at final follow-up.

27.3 Conclusions

The ACL augmentation techniques have potential advantages in terms of the proprioceptive function of the knee, biological healing of the graft, and contribution to knee stability. Although appropriately powered randomized controlled trials and a longer follow-up period are necessary before a definitive conclusion can be reached, we believe that ACL augmentation is a valuable procedure.

Table 27.2 Clinical studies which compared the ACL augmentation techniques with the standard ACL reconstruction technique

Study	Conditions of ACL remnant for augmentation	Type of graft
Adachi and Ochi et al. (2000) [1]	ACL remnant bridging the femur and tibia, with a diameter from 1/3 to 1/2 that of the normal ACL	Autogenous hamstring tendons or allogenic fascia lata
Gohil et al. (2007) [13]		Autologous hamstring tendons
Yoonetal.(2009) [17]	ACL remnant bridging the femur and the tibia anatomically, with a thickness of more than 50 % of that of the AM or PL bundle and laxity of less than 5 mm when drawn by a probe	Autologous hamstring tendons
Ahn et al. (2010) [20]	ACL remnant that could be tensioned toward the femoral bone tunnel	Autologous hamstring tendons
Pujol et al. (2012) [26]	Partial ACL tear; a well-inserted PL bundle	Autologous hamstring tendons or bone patellar tendon bone
Hong et al. (2012) [27]	The remnant could be pulled to reach the femoral ACL insertion, and the remnant diameter was more than half of the native ACL	Allogeneic tibialis anterior or hamstring tendon
Park et al. (2012) [30]	Attachment of the remnant bundle between the femur and tibia, the thickness of the ACL exceeding more than 50 % of that of the AM or PL bundle, and laxity of less than 5 mm when drawn by a probe	Autologous hamstring tendons
Demirağ et al. (2012) [31]	ACL remnant with more than one half of its integrity preserved, bridging the tibia and femur, and elongated no more than one half of its length	Autologous hamstring tendons
Cha et al. (2012) [33]	ACL remnant that could be tensioned toward the femoral bone tunnel	Autologous hamstring tendons
Maestro et al. (2013) [36]	Partial ACL tear; a healthy bundle with a diameter equivalent to at least one third of the original ACL was found, which was functional after palpation with a hook probe showing retention of its femoral and tibial insertions	Autologous hamstring tendons
Nakamae and Ochi et al. (2014) [7]	Partial rupture of the ACL; ligamentous fibers were seen to be in continuity from the femur to the tibia, and the femoral attachment of those fibers was within the anatomical femoral insertion of the ACL Complete rupture of the ACL; thick ACL remnant (greater than one third of the original size) maintaining a ligamentous bridge between the tibia and femur and the femoral attachment of the ACL remnant was positioned nonanatomically	Autologous hamstring tendons
Zhang et al. (2014) [39]		Autologous hamstring tendons
Lee YS et al. (2014) [40]	Partial ACL tear; there was a relatively intact bundle during surgery	Autologous hamstring tendons

AM, anteromedial; *PL*, posterolateral

Table 27.3 Outcomes in studies which compared the ACL augmentation techniques with the standard ACL reconstruction technique

Study	The mean side-to-side difference in instrumented knee-laxity testing (anterior displacement of tibia)	Pivot shift test (positive rate)	Other findings	Complications
Adachi and Ochi et al. (2000) [1]	0.7 mm in Group A and 1.8 mm in Group S ($P < .05$)	8 % in Group A and 4 % in Group S (not significant)	Inaccuracy of joint position sense was 0.7° in Group A and 1.7° in Group S ($P < .05$). ACL augmentation technique may contribute to restoring the proprioceptive function of the knee	
Gohil et al. (2007) [13]	3.2 (2 to 5) mm in Group A and 2.75 (2 to 5) mm in Group S		ACL augmentation technique appears to accelerate revascularization, as indicated by increased signal intensity of MRI in the mid-substance of the graft at 2 months	No significant differences were found in incidence of cyclops lesions and ROM
Yoon et al. (2009) [17]	2.2 mm in Group A and 1.9 mm in Group S	12 % in Group A and 12 % in Group S		One case of limited ROM was observed in each group
Ahn et al. (2010) [20]			MRI showed significantly larger ACL grafts in Group A than in Group S, and these preserved remnant bundles showed progressive remodeling in the ACL graft	No significant difference was found in incidence of cyclops lesions
Pujol et al. (2012) [26]	1.24 mm in Group A and 1.87 mm in Group S (P = .03)	17 % in Group A and 28 % in Group S ($P = .4$)	There were no significant differences in subjective IKDC, KOOS, or Lysholm scores between the groups	One patient in Group A developed cyclops lesion
Hong et al. (2012) [27]	1.6 mm in Group A and 1.8 mm in Group S ($P = .69$)	5 % in Group A and 12 % in Group S ($P = .52$)	The passive angle reproduction test for proprioception measurements showed that there was no difference between both groups at final follow-up	In each group, cyclops lesion formation occurred in three patients

Park et al. (2012) [30]	1.5 mm in Group A and 1.7 mm in Group S (double bundle) ($P = .69$)	9 % in Group A and 11 % in Group S (double-bundle) ($P = .74$)	There were no significant differences in the postoperative ROM, visual analog scale score, Lysholm score, Tegner score, and International Knee Documentation Committee knee evaluation form score between the two groups	
Demirağ et al. (2012) [31]		20 % in Group A and 15 % in Group S ($P = .5$)	Tibial and femoral tunnel widening was less in the augmentation group. This difference was more significant on the tibial side	One patient in Group A developed cyclops lesion confirmed by MRI
Cha et al. (2012) [33]			Eight cyclops lesions (3/20 (15.0 %) in Group S and 5/41 (12.2 %) in Group A) were found in the 61 patients who underwent second look (P = .76)	
Maestro et al. (2013) [36]	1.8 mm in Group A and 2.3 mm in Group S	13 % in Group A and 36 % in Group S		No postoperative complications
Nakamae and Ochi et al. (2014) [7]	0.4 mm in Group A, 1.3 mm in single-bundle group, and 0.9 mm in double-bundle group ($P = .013$ between Group A and the single-bundle group)	12 % in Group A, 21 % in single-bundle group, and 15 % in double-bundle group (P = .65)	Second-look arthroscopy showed significantly better synovial coverage of the graft in Group A than in the other groups. Improvement in proprioceptive function (threshold to detect passive motion) was seen in patients with good synovial coverage of the graft	
Zhang et al. (2014) [39]	1.4 mm in Group A and 1.7 mm in Group S (not significant)		The percentage of tibial tunnel enlargement was 25.7 % in Group A and 34.0 % in Group S ($P = .0004$)	
Lee YS et al. (2014) [40]	1.8 mm in Group A and 1.9 mm in Group S (double bundle) (not significant)	6 % in Group A and 6 % in Group S (not significant)	No statistical differences in the Lysholm, Tegner, and International Knee Documentation Committee scores were observed between the two groups	ROM was not statistically different between the groups

Group A, ACL augmentation (remnant-preserving ACL reconstruction) group; Group S, standard ACL reconstruction technique group; ROM, range of motion

References

1. Adachi N, Ochi M, Uchio Y, Sumen Y (2000) Anterior cruciate ligament augmentation under arthroscopy. A minimum 2-year follow-up in 40 patients. Arch Orthop Trauma Surg 120:128–133
2. Ochi M, Adachi N, Deie M, Kanaya A (2006) Anterior cruciate ligament augmentation procedure with a 1-incision technique: anteromedial bundle or posterolateral bundle reconstruction. Arthroscopy 22:463.e1–463.e5
3. Adachi N, Ochi M, Uchio Y, Iwasa J, Ryoke K, Kuriwaka M (2002) Mechanoreceptors in the anterior cruciate ligament contribute to the joint position sense. Acta Orthop Scand 73:330–334
4. Denti M, Monteleone M, Berardi A, Panni AS (1994) Anterior cruciate ligament mechanoreceptors. Histologic studies on lesions and reconstruction. Clin Orthop Relat Res 308:29–32
5. Ochi M, Iwasa J, Uchio Y, Adachi N, Sumen Y (1999) The regeneration of sensory neurones in the reconstruction of the anterior cruciate ligament. J Bone Joint Surg (Br) 81:902–906
6. Ochi M, Iwasa J, Uchio Y, Adachi N, Kawasaki K (2002) Induction of somatosensory evoked potentials by mechanical stimulation in reconstructed anterior cruciate ligaments. J Bone Joint Surg (Br) 84:761–766
7. Nakamae A, Ochi M, Deie M, Adachi N, Shibuya H, Ohkawa S, Hirata K (2014) Clinical outcomes of second-look arthroscopic evaluation after anterior cruciate ligament augmentation: comparison with single- and double-bundle reconstruction. Bone Joint J 96-B:1325–1332
8. Crain EH, Fithian DC, Paxton EW, Luetzow WF (2005) Variation in anterior cruciate ligament scar pattern: does the scar pattern affect anterior laxity in anterior cruciate ligament-deficient knees? Arthroscopy 21:19–24
9. Nakamae A, Ochi M, Deie M, Adachi N, Kanaya A, Nishimori M, Nakasa T (2010) Biomechanical function of anterior cruciate ligament remnants: how long do they contribute to knee stability after injury in patients with complete tears? Arthroscopy 26:1577–1585
10. Mifune Y, Ota S, Takayama K, Hoshino Y, Matsumoto T, Kuroda R, Kurosaka M, Fu FH, Huard J (2013) Therapeutic advantage in selective ligament augmentation for partial tears of the anterior cruciate ligament: results in an animal model. Am J Sports Med 41:365–373
11. Lee BI, Min KD, Choi HS, Kim JB, Kim ST (2006) Arthroscopic anterior cruciate ligament reconstruction with the tibial-remnant preserving technique using a hamstring graft. Arthroscopy 22:340.e1–340.e7
12. Buda R, Ferruzzi A, Vannini F, Zambelli L, Di Caprio F (2006) Augmentation technique with semitendinosus and gracilis tendons in chronic partial lesions of the ACL: clinical and arthrometric analysis. Knee Surg Sports Traumatol Arthrosc 14:1101–1107
13. Gohil S, Annear PO, Breidahl W (2007) Anterior cruciate ligament reconstruction using autologous double hamstrings: a comparison of standard versus minimal debridement techniques using MRI to assess revascularisation. A randomised prospective study with a one-year follow-up. J Bone Joint Surg (Br) 89:1165–1171
14. Buda R, Di Caprio F, Giuriati L, Luciani D, Busacca M, Giannini S (2008) Partial ACL tears augmented with distally inserted hamstring tendons and over-the-top fixation: an MRI evaluation. Knee 15:111–116
15. Lee BI, Kwon SW, Kim JB, Choi HS, Min KD (2008) Comparison of clinical results according to amount of preserved remnant in arthroscopic anterior cruciate ligament reconstruction using quadrupled hamstring graft. Arthroscopy 24:560–568
16. Ochi M, Adachi N, Uchio Y, Deie M, Kumahashi N, Ishikawa M, Sera S (2009) A minimum 2-year follow-up after selective anteromedial or posterolateral bundle anterior cruciate ligament reconstruction. Arthroscopy 25:117–122
17. Yoon KH, Bae DK, Cho SM, Park SY, Lee JH (2009) Standard anterior cruciate ligament reconstruction versus isolated single-bundle augmentation with hamstring autograft. Arthroscopy 25:1265–1274
18. Ahn JH, Lee YS, Ha HC (2009) Anterior cruciate ligament reconstruction with preservation of remnant bundle using hamstring autograft: technical note. Arch Orthop Trauma Surg 129:1011–1015

19. Kim SJ, Jo SB, Kim TW, Chang JH, Choi HS, Oh KS (2009) A modified arthroscopic anterior cruciate ligament double-bundle reconstruction technique with autogenous quadriceps tendon graft: remnant-preserving technique. Arch Orthop Trauma Surg 129:403–407
20. Ahn JH, Lee SH, Choi SH, Lim TK (2010) Magnetic resonance imaging evaluation of anterior cruciate ligament reconstruction using quadrupled hamstring tendon autografts: comparison of remnant bundle preservation and standard technique. Am J Sports Med 38:1768–1777
21. Sonnery-Cottet B, Lavoie F, Ogassawara R, Scussiato RG, Kidder JF, Chambat P (2010) Selective anteromedial bundle reconstruction in partial ACL tears: a series of 36 patients with mean 24 months follow-up. Knee Surg Sports Traumatol Arthrosc 18:47–51
22. Serrano-Fernandez JM, Espejo-Baena A, Martin-Castilla B, De La Torre-Solis F, Mariscal-Lara J, Merino-Ruiz ML (2010) Augmentation technique for partial ACL ruptures using semitendinosus tendon in the over-the-top position. Knee Surg Sports Traumatol Arthrosc 18:1214–1218
23. Ahn JH, Wang JH, Lee YS, Kim JG, Kang JH, Koh KH (2011) Anterior cruciate ligament reconstruction using remnant preservation and a femoral tensioning technique: clinical and magnetic resonance imaging results. Arthroscopy 27:1079–1089
24. Jung YB, Jung HJ, Siti HT, Lee YS, Lee HJ, Lee SH, Cheon HY (2011) Comparison of anterior cruciate ligament reconstruction with preservation only versus remnant tensioning technique. Arthroscopy 27:1252–1258
25. Ochi M, Abouheif MM, Kongcharoensombat W, Nakamae A, Adachi N, Deie M (2011) Double bundle arthroscopic Anterior Cruciate Ligament reconstruction with remnant preserving technique using a hamstring autograft. Sports Med Arthrosc Rehabil Ther Technol 3:30
26. Pujol N, Colombet P, Potel JF, Cucurulo T, Graveleau N, Hulet C, Panisset JC, Servien E, Sonnery-Cottet B, Trojani C, Djian P, French Arthroscopy Society (SFA) (2012) Anterior cruciate ligament reconstruction in partial tear: selective anteromedial bundle reconstruction conserving the posterolateral remnant versus single-bundle anatomic ACL reconstruction: preliminary 1-year results of a prospective randomized study. Orthop Traumatol Surg Res 98(8 Suppl):S171–S177
27. Hong L, Li X, Zhang H, Liu X, Zhang J, Shen JW, Feng H (2012) Anterior cruciate ligament reconstruction with remnant preservation: a prospective, randomized controlled study. Am J Sports Med 40:2747–2755
28. Ohsawa T, Kimura M, Kobayashi Y, Hagiwara K, Yorifuji H, Takagishi K (2012) Arthroscopic evaluation of preserved ligament remnant after selective anteromedial or posterolateral bundle anterior cruciate ligament reconstruction. Arthroscopy 28:807–817
29. Yasuda K, Kondo E, Kitamura N, Kawaguchi Y, Kai S, Tanabe Y (2012) A pilot study of anatomic double-bundle anterior cruciate ligament reconstruction with ligament remnant tissue preservation. Arthroscopy 28:343–353
30. Park SY, Oh H, Park SW, Lee JH, Lee SH, Yoon KH (2012) Clinical outcomes of remnant-preserving augmentation versus double-bundle reconstruction in the anterior cruciate ligament reconstruction. Arthroscopy 28:1833–1841
31. Demirağ B, Ermutlu C, Aydemir F, Durak K (2012) A comparison of clinical outcome of augmentation and standard reconstruction techniques for partial anterior cruciate ligament tears. Eklem Hastalik Cerrahisi 23:140–144
32. Sonnery-Cottet B, Panisset JC, Colombet P, Cucurulo T, Graveleau N, Hulet C, Potel JF, Servien E, Trojani C, Djian P, Pujol N, French Arthroscopy Society (SFA) (2012) Partial ACL reconstruction with preservation of the posterolateral bundle. Orthop Traumatol Surg Res 98 (8 Suppl):S165–S170
33. Cha J, Choi SH, Kwon JW, Lee SH, Ahn JH (2012) Analysis of cyclops lesions after different anterior cruciate ligament reconstructions: a comparison of the single-bundle and remnant bundle preservation techniques. Skeletal Radiol 41:997–1002
34. Muneta T, Koga H, Ju YJ, Horie M, Nakamura T, Sekiya I (2013) Remnant volume of anterior cruciate ligament correlates preoperative patients' status and postoperative outcome. Knee Surg Sports Traumatol Arthrosc 21:906–913
35. Kazusa H, Nakamae A, Ochi M (2013) Augmentation technique for anterior cruciate ligament injury. Clin Sports Med 32:127–140

36. Maestro A, Suárez-Suárez MA, Rodríguez-López L, Villa-Vigil A (2013) Stability evaluation after isolated reconstruction of anteromedial or posterolateral bundle in symptomatic partial tears of anterior cruciate ligament. Eur J Orthop Surg Traumatol 23:471–480
37. Buda R, Ruffilli A, Parma A, Pagliazzi G, Luciani D, Ramponi L, Castagnini F, Giannini S (2013) Partial ACL tears: anatomic reconstruction versus nonanatomic augmentation surgery. Orthopedics 36:e1108–e1113
38. Abat F, Gelber PE, Erquicia JI, Pelfort X, Tey M, Monllau JC (2013) Promising short-term results following selective bundle reconstruction in partial anterior cruciate ligament tears. Knee 20:332–338
39. Zhang Q, Zhang S, Cao X, Liu L, Liu Y, Li R (2014) The effect of remnant preservation on tibial tunnel enlargement in ACL reconstruction with hamstring autograft: a prospective randomized controlled trial. Knee Surg Sports Traumatol Arthrosc 22:166–173
40. Lee YS, Nam SW, Sim JA, Lee BK (2014) Comparison of anatomic ACL reconstruction between selective bundle reconstruction and double-bundle reconstruction. Knee Surg Sports Traumatol Arthrosc 22:2803–2810
41. Ahn JH, Lee YS, Lee SH (2014) Creation of an anatomic femoral tunnel with minimal damage to the remnant bundle in remnant-preserving anterior cruciate ligament reconstruction using an outside-in technique. Arthrosc Tech 3:e175–e179
42. Noh JH, Yoon KH, Song SJ, Roh YH (2014) Re-tensioning technique to cover the graft with remnant in anterior cruciate ligament reconstruction. Arthrosc Tech 3:e679–e682
43. Sonnery-Cottet B, Freychet B, Murphy CG, Pupim BH, Thaunat M (2014) Anterior Cruciate Ligament reconstruction and preservation: the Single-Anteromedial Bundle Biological Augmentation (SAMBBA) technique. Arthrosc Tech 3:e689–e693
44. Muneta T, Koga H, Nakamura T, Horie M, Watanabe T, Yagishita K, Sekiya I (2015) A new behind-remnant approach for remnant-preserving double-bundle anterior cruciate ligament reconstruction compared with a standard approach. Knee Surg Sports Traumatol Arthrosc 23 (12):3743–3749
45. Kim MK, Lee SR, Ha JK, Ra HJ, Kim SB, Kim JG (2014) Comparison of second-look arthroscopic findings and clinical results according to the amount of preserved remnant in anterior cruciate ligament reconstruction. Knee 21:774–778
46. Taketomi S, Inui H, Sanada T, Nakamura K, Yamagami R, Masuda H, Tanaka S, Nakagawa T (2014) Remnant-preserving anterior cruciate ligament reconstruction using a three-dimensional fluoroscopic navigation system. Knee Surg Relat Res 26:168–176

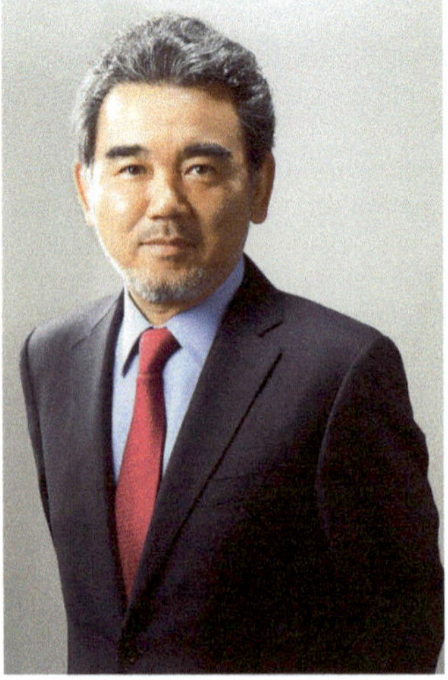

Mitsuo Ochi, M.D., Ph.D.,[1] President of Hiroshima University, Hiroshima, Japan.

Chapter 28
Surgical Technique of ACL Augmentation

Masataka Deie

Abstract Remnants of ACL have been reported to promote recovery of proprioceptive functions in a graft, resulting in the technique of ACL augmentation becoming accepted widely. We recommend that ACL augmentation is performed in the following cases: ACL remnant retained as a thick ACL remnant bridged between the intercondylar notch and tibia, partial rupture of the PL bundle, and partial rupture of the AM bundle. This procedure is usually performed using the three-portal technique, involving the anterolateral, central anteromedial, and far anteromedial (FAM) portals. The ACL femoral attachment is accessed anatomically through the FAM portal. To make the tibial bone tunnels, guide wires are inserted at the tibial attachment of the ACL remnant and then are over-drilled, making sure that the drill tip does not reach the ACL remnant fibers to minimize damage. Then, a passage is created through the slit made in the ACL remnants. After passing the graft tendon through the slit and checking the length change of the graft during knee flexion, the graft is fixed to the tibia using two staples. Currently, patients undergoing ACL augmentation go through the same postoperative rehabilitation as those undergoing ACL reconstruction.

Keywords Remnant • Augmentation • Mechanoreceptor • Far anteromedial portal

28.1 Objective

Restoration of normal biomechanical and biological function is the primary goal of anterior cruciate ligament (ACL) reconstruction, with the double-bundle ACL reconstruction considered to have greater potential to restore normal knee kinematics than the single-bundle technique [1, 2]. The double-bundle method aims to reconstruct both the anteromedial (AM) and posterolateral (PL) bundles of the native ACL at their sites of insertion. However, recent studies indicate that central anatomical single-bundle ACL reconstruction can also restore normal knee

M. Deie, M.D., PhD (✉)
Department of Orthopaedic Surgery, School of Medicine, Aichi Medical University, 1-1 Yasagokarimata, Nagakute, Aichi 480-1195, Japan
e-mail: masatakadeie@yahoo.co.jp; snm3@aichi-med-u.ac.jp

M. Ochi et al. (eds.), *ACL Injury and Its Treatment*,
DOI 10.1007/978-4-431-55858-3_28

function biomechanically [3–5]. Several clinical studies have directly compared these two reconstruction techniques, but have yielded conflicting results [1, 3, 5, 6].

It is established that early biological healing of the graft is an important and essential factor in obtaining a satisfactory clinical result after ACL reconstruction. An augmentation technique for treating the injured ACL has recently received attention because preserving the ACL remnant has several potential advantages [7–11]. The remnant of ACL can enhance the revascularization and cellular proliferation of the grafted tissues and promote the recovery of proprioceptive functions in the graft via reinnervation [12–19].

This chapter describes and illustrates our surgical technique of ACL augmentation.

28.2 Indications

Defining the indications for ACL augmentation is crucial for attaining satisfactory clinical results. Thus, the ACL remnant should be identified adequately before surgery using magnetic resonance imaging (MRI) and three-dimensional computed tomography (3D CT), with the final indication defined based on the arthroscopic findings.

We can divide the types of ACL remnants suitable for ACL augmentations [19] as follows (Fig. 28.1):

1. A thick ACL remnant remaining between the PCL and tibia, with complete loss of the original site of attachment of the ACL to the femur
2. A thick ACL remnant bridging the intercondylar notch and tibia, with no ligamentous continuous fibers in the normal attachment of the ACL to the femur
3. Partial rupture of the PL bundle
4. Partial rupture of the AM bundle
5. No substantial ACL remnants

Based on these categories, we believe that the indication for double-bundle ACL augmentation surgery is type (2), while single-bundle ACL augmentation surgery would be chosen for types (3) and (4). When the arthroscopic view shows type (1) or (5), the anatomical ACL reconstruction will be performed.

28.3 Surgical Procedures

28.3.1 Arthroscopic Portal Placement

We generally use a three-portal technique using the anterolateral portal, central anteromedial portal (CAM), and the far anteromedial portal (FAM) [20]. The anterolateral portal is positioned above the lateral meniscus, adjacent to the lateral border of the patellar tendon, and serves as a viewing portal for the tibial insertion,

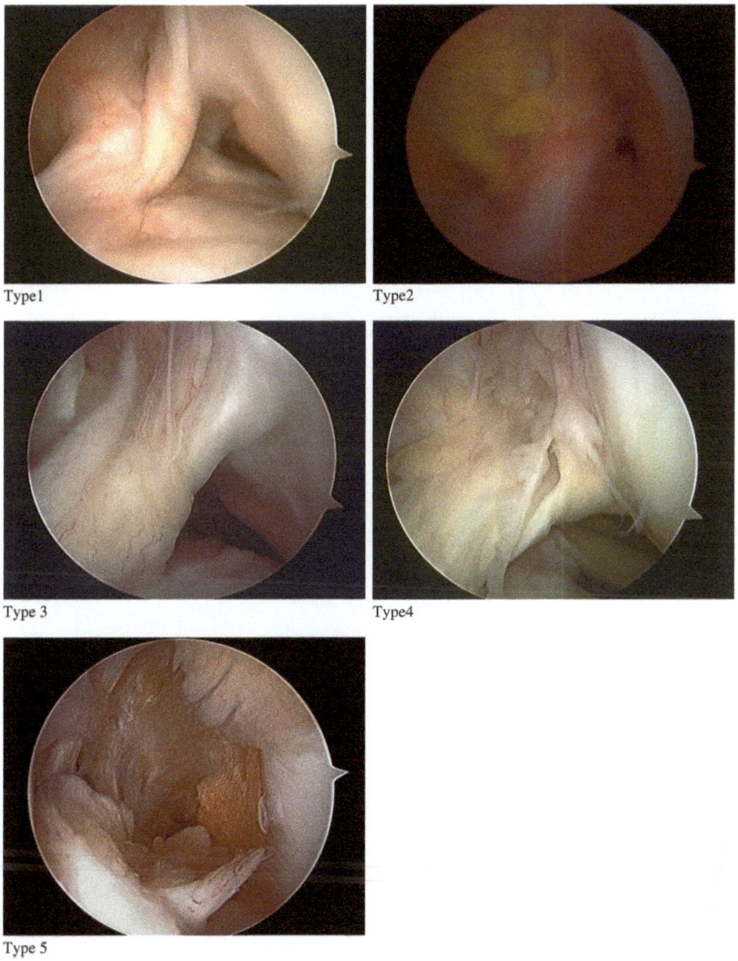

Fig. 28.1 Classification of ACL remnant
Type 1: a thick ACL remnant remaining between the PCL and tibia. The normal attachment of the ACL to the femur was entirely lost.
Type 2: a thick ACL remnant bridging the intercondylar notch and tibia. No ligamentous continuous fibers are apparent in the normal attachment of the ACL to the femur.
Type 3: partial rupture of the PL bundle.
Type 4: partial rupture of the AM bundle.
Type 5: no substantial ACL remnants

as well as a working portal. For creation of the FAM, 3D CT with specialized software [Virtual Place Raijin (Aze Ltd., Tokyo, Japan)] is used for preoperative assessment of the optimal position of the skin incision for this portal that allows the femoral tunnels to be created within the confines of the anatomical ACL femoral footprint (Fig. 28.2a), to avoid damaging the articular cartilage of the medial femoral condyle (Fig. 28.2c) [21]. Usually the skin incision for this portal is located just superior to the medial joint line about 2.5 cm medial to the medial border of the

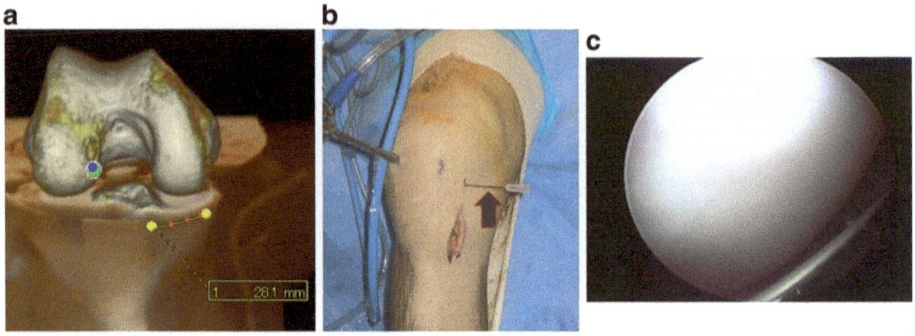

Fig. 28.2 (**a**) This figure shows a typical 3D CT view represented using specialized software [Virtual Place Raijin (Aze Ltd., Tokyo, Japan)]. Such imaging is used for preoperative assessment of the optimal position of the skin incision for this portal that would allow creation of the femoral tunnels within the confines of the anatomical ACL femoral footprint to avoid scuffing the articular cartilage of the medial femoral condyle. Usually the skin incision for this portal is located just superior to the medial joint line about 2.5 cm medial to the medial border of the patellar tendon. (**b**) FAM portal according to the 3D CT view. (**c**) Direction should be monitored when the guide needle is inserted, to avoid cartilage damage

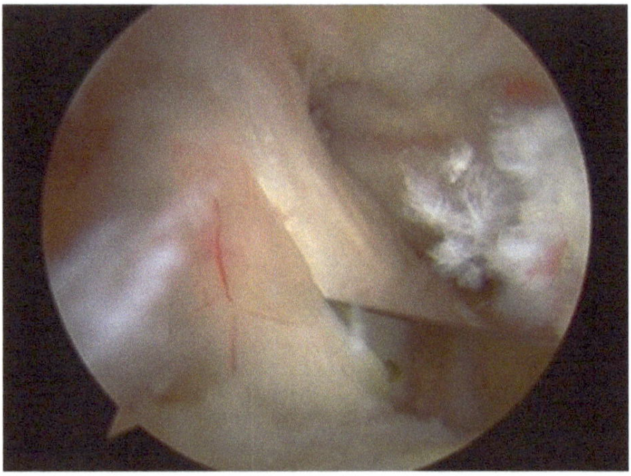

Fig. 28.3 Representation of the slit added to an ACL remnant using a No. 11 knife

patellar tendon (Fig. 28.2b), and using this FAM portal for instrumentation allows the CAM portal to be used for viewing the femoral insertion site of both the AM and PL bundle and the lateral wall of the intercondylar notch [11, 22–26]. The CAM portal is located above the joint line, adjacent to the edge of the inferomedial portion of the patellar tendon. This portal can be used also as a viewing or working portal [11, 22–26]. When the anterolateral portal is used as a viewing portal, the CAM portal can be used to make a longitudinal slit in the ACL remnant to accommodate the anatomically created tibial tunnels within the confines of the ACL tibial foot print (Fig. 28.3).

28.3.2 Arthroscopic Evaluation

We perform routine arthroscopic intra-articular inspections including the medial and lateral menisci and cartilage through the anterolateral and FAM portals with a 45° oblique arthroscopy with the knee flexed at 90° to identify any remaining ACL fibers and determine the nature of their attachment. For the arthroscopic diagnosis of a partial rupture and/or the state of ACL remnant, arthroscopic examination should be performed at various knee flexion angles to consider the different tension patterns of the two bundles. The state of the PL bundle femoral insertion can be evaluated with the knee in a figure-of-4 position for good visualization of the femoral attachment to the PL bundle [15, 16, 18, 27].

28.3.3 Bone Tunnel Placement

The tunnel placements should be made based on the normal anatomical attachments of ACL. Remnant preservation can be technically difficult, because it might actually hinder visualization of the tip of the guide pin used as the first step in creating the anatomical femoral and tibial tunnels

28.3.4 Femoral Bone Tunnel

Femoral bone tunnels are usually made through the FAM portal, which we consider easier to drill through within the ACL posterolateral bundle anatomical footprint. In fact, we extend the use of the FAM portal for anatomical creation of both femoral tunnels within the confines of the native ACL femoral footprint. FAM was verified intraoperatively by inserting a 23-gauge spinal needle under direct vision from the anterolateral portal into the point predetermined by 3D CT (Fig. 28.2) and examining its relation to the cartilage of the medial femoral condyle. Then, after cleaning the remaining portion of the anatomical femoral attachment site with a motorized shaver or a curette, a passing pin was directed through the FAM portal at the ACL anatomical femoral attachment sites for the AM and/or PL bundles. This passing pin is then drilled through the femur to emerge on the lateral aspect of the thigh, and after over-drilling with the 4.5-mm diameter EndoButton drill, the length of the femoral tunnel is calculated. Then the femoral bone socket is created using a cannulated reamer with the same diameter (usually 5–6 mm) as that of the proximal portion of the doubled semitendinosus tendon graft. During creation of the femoral tunnels through the FAM, the ACL remnant can be carefully retracted medially by a probe introduced through the medial portal.

28.3.5 Tibial Bone Tunnel

Harvesting the semitendinosus tendon to prepare the site for tibial tunnel creation is then performed. At the medial site of the tibia, the periosteum is exposed and the cortex of the tibia is explored, from the MCL attachment to the proximal of the tibial tuberosity [15, 16]. First, two 2.0-mm Kirschner wires are inserted through the anteromedial and the posterolateral portions of the slit made at the tibial attachment of the ACL remnant using the Pro-trac ACL guide system (Acufex, Smith & Nephew, Mansfield, MA) with an angle up to 63° to the tibial plateau to allow visualization of the wire tip (Figs. 28.3 and 28.4). The transverse intermeniscal ligament is used as a landmark for placement of the AM tibial tunnel close to its posterior edge. The positions of the guide wires are then checked with knee extension [28]. In a double-bundle augmentation, the PL tibial bundle tunnel would be made just behind the AM tunnel, and the appropriate Kirschner wire then over-drilled using a cannulated reamer to make a tibial tunnel with the same diameter as that of the distal portion of the doubled semitendinosus tendon, which was connected with EndoButton tape (Acufex, Smith & Nephew) (Fig. 28.5). Damage to the ACL remnant from the arthroscopic probe through the AL portal should be minimized while viewing through the AM and PL portal to drill the tibial tunnel by ensuring the tip of the drill pit does not reach the ACL remnant fibers.

28.3.6 Passing the Graft

Before the graft is passed into the bone tunnels, a passage is created through the longitudinal slit made in the ACL remnant using a curved hemostat to avoid impinging the reconstruction graft with the ACL remnant (Fig. 28.6).

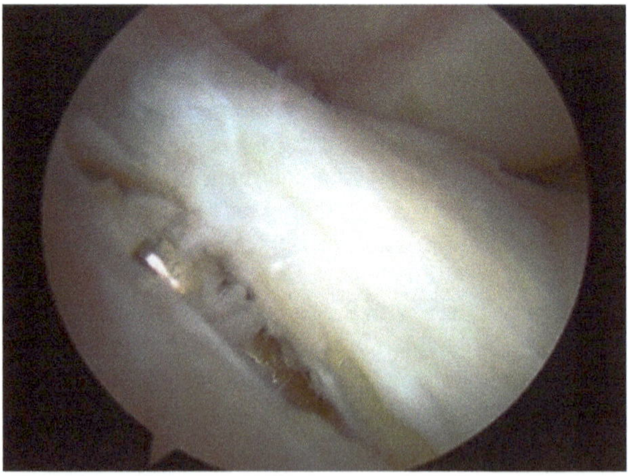

Fig. 28.4 A 2.0-mm Kirschner wire was inserted through the slit made at the tibial attachment of the ACL remnant using the Prot-trac ACL guide system with an angle up to 63° to the tibial plateau to allow visualization of the tip of the wire

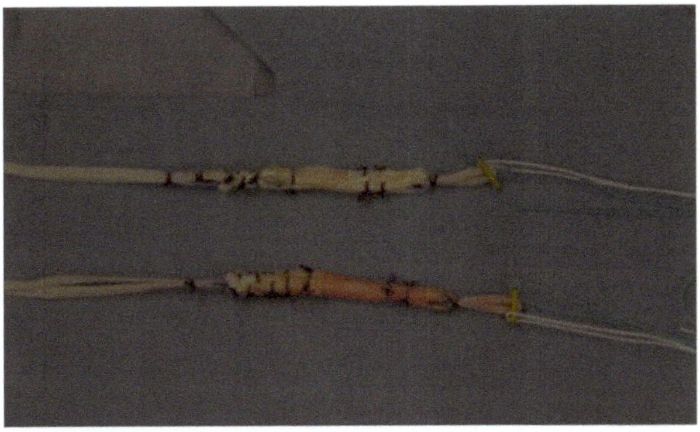

Fig. 28.5 Image showing the AM and PL substitutes. The upper panel shows the AM substitute of 6.0 mm diameter and 6 cm length; the lower panel shows the PL substitute of 5.5 mm diameter and 6 cm length

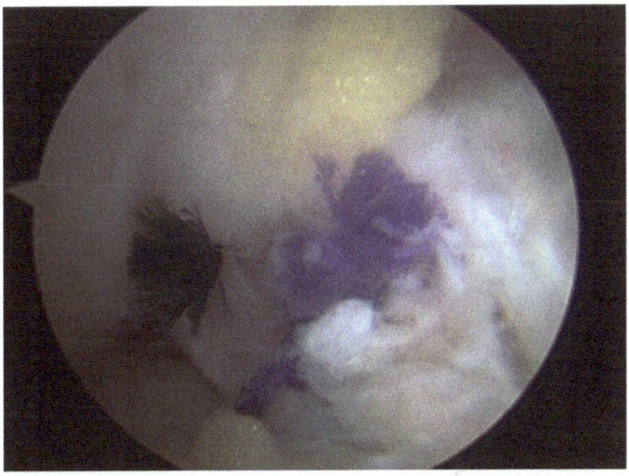

Fig. 28.6 This image represents the intra-articular view after the grafted tendon was fixed. The arrowhead shows the PL bundle augmentation, and the arrow indicates the preserved ACL remnant

In a double-bundle ACL augmentation, a curved hemostat is carefully passed through the slit in the midportion of the ACL remnant from the CAM portal to create a passage to the intra-articular aperture of the femoral tunnels. Then, two No. 5 Ethibond loops are passed through the FAM portal into the PL and AM femoral tunnels, respectively.

In a single-bundle ACL augmentation, a curved hemostat is carefully passed through the slit in the midportion of the ACL remnant to create a passage to the intra-articular aperture of the PL or AM femoral tunnels, and then a No. 5 Ethibond loop is passed into the femoral tunnel through the FAM portal.

Subsequently, each loop tie is retrieved by an arthroscopic grasper through the PL and/or AM tibial tunnel. The AM graft substitute is then passed above the ACL remnant, while the PL graft substitute only is passed through the slit in the ACL remnant.

After selecting an appropriate size of EndoButton-CL (Acufex, Smith & Nephew), the doubled semitendinosus tendon is connected with the EndoButton-CL for the femoral side and EndoButton tape for the tibial side.

28.3.7 *Fixing the Graft*

After passing the graft tendon through the tibial tunnel and the femoral tunnel, the graft is fixed to the lateral femoral cortex by flipping the EndoButton and pulling the graft distally. Then the knee is fully extended in order to examine impingement of the grafted tendons or preserved ACL remnant against the intercondylar notch. When impingement is found, the ACL remnant is shaved partially to avoid the possible development of cyclops lesion. After the length change of the graft during knee flexion is finalized, the EndoButton tape connected to the graft was fixed to the tibia using two staples (Meira, Nagoya, Japan) with a pulling force of 30 N.

In a single-bundle augmentation, the EndoButton tape connected to the graft is fixed to the tibia using two staples with a pulling force of 50 N

After graft fixation, the tensions of the grafted tendons should be checked arthroscopically, and then, the synovium is sutured over the graft-remnant composite to create a closed tube of the reconstructed ACL extending between the tibial and the femoral anatomical foot prints (Fig. 28.7). After skin closure, the knee is fixed with a soft knee brace. After surgery, the tunnel positions should be assessed using 3D CT. (Fig. 28.8).

28.3.8 *Postoperative Rehabilitation*

The rehabilitation after ACL augmentation is identical to that undertaken for ACL reconstruction. At 3 days after surgery, limited-range of motion exercise is initiated, and at 1 week after surgery, partial weight-bearing gait is allowed. At 4–5 months after surgery, jogging and light squatting exercise is introduced, and then after 10–12 months, patients are allowed to return to their original sport.

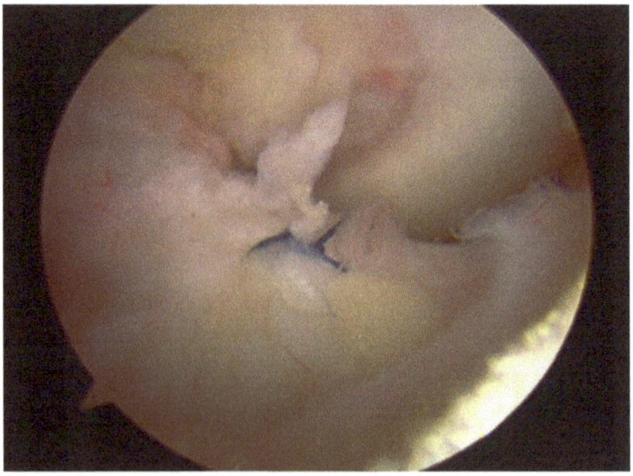

Fig. 28.7 After the graft was fixed, the slit lesion of preserving ACL remnant was sutured

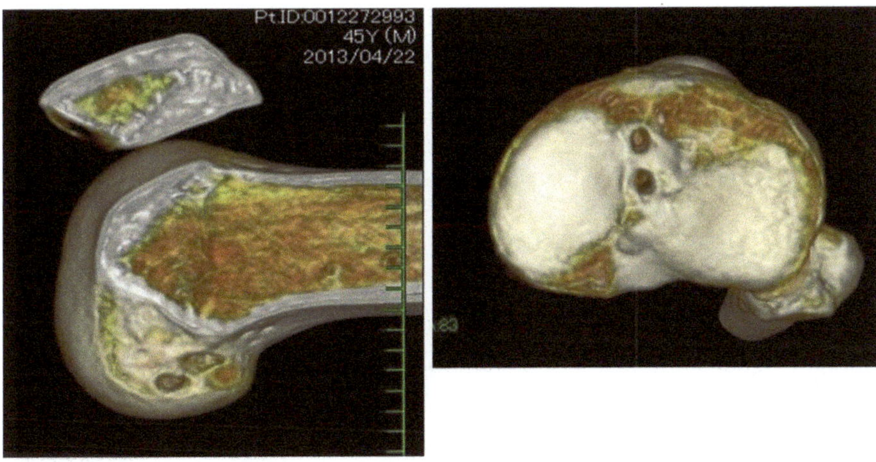

Fig. 28.8 After surgery, the grafted position was evaluated by 3D CT, as shown

28.4 Discussion

In this chapter we described the procedures of remnant-preserving ACL reconstruction. Such ACL remnants can conserve the mechanoreceptors and vessels that are beneficial to joint position sense and important in recovering neovascularity after surgery. Adachi et al. [13] observed a positive correlation between the number of mechanoreceptors and the accuracy of joint position sense. They even found mechanoreceptors in patients having a long interval between the ACL injury and the surgery and concluded that surgeons should consider preserving ACL remnants during any ACL reconstruction. Additionally, an ACL remnant with abundant vascularity could favorably influence revascularization of the grafted tendon [1, 2, 5, 16, 18, 19, 29], while Crain et al. [18] showed that resection of ACL remnants, especially those healed to the femur effectively crossing the joint, resulted in a measurable increase in passive anterior laxity in a group of ACL-deficient knees. Augmentation reconstruction was initially performed in cases of partial rupture of the ACL by creating a tunnel that complements the ACL remnant in the native femoral anatomical attachment site, and Ochi et al. [9] demonstrated the favorable clinical results of such augmentation reconstructive surgery using a one-incision technique.

Our technique of surgical ACL augmentation involves creating a longitudinal slit in the ACL remnant fibers, allowing the tip of the guide wire used for preliminary drilling of the tibial tunnel to be adequately visualized. We also use the transverse intermeniscal ligament as a landmark for creating the AM tibial tunnel, thus allowing for creation of the tibial tunnels within the native ACL tibial footprint under direct vision without the need to use an image intensifier to localize the tibial tunnel. Moreover, reconstruction of the femoral tunnels using the FAM portal, independent of the tibial tunnels, allows the angulation of the tibial tunnels to be increased from 45° to up to 65° to maximize visualization of the guide wire tip. In addition, making a passage using a curved hemostat through the slit in the ACL remnant to reach the intra-articular aperture of the femoral tunnel avoids impingement of the reconstruction graft against the ACL remnant and avoids notch overstuffing and the development of cyclops lesion. Finally, our technique of suturing the highly vascularized synovial folds over the reconstructed graft-remnant composite optimizes the biological potential for graft maturation [30, 31].

In this study, the FAM was used to create the femoral tunnels, while viewing through the central anteromedial portal. This resulted in the creation of a femoral tunnel within the anatomical femoral ACL attachment independent of the tibial tunnel [10, 11, 22–24]. Additionally we recommend using 3D CT for preoperative prediction of the optimal site of incision for the FAM portal to enable creation of femoral tunnels of optimal length and orientation without damaging the articular cartilage of the medial femoral condyle [21].

In our technique, the main part of the femoral attachment of the ACL is situated on the resident's ridge, and the remaining part is attached to the posterior portion of the ridge. However, in ACL reconstruction using hamstring tendons, the center of the femoral tunnel opening is not the central point of application of force, because the graft is pulled anteriorly. Therefore, the femoral bone tunnel should be created just behind the resident's ridge through the far anteromedial portal.

In an ongoing prospective clinical study, Ma et al. [32] compared three different ACL surgeries: single-bundle reconstruction, single-bundle augmentation, and double-bundle reconstruction. While this is only a 1-year study, the authors reported that the single augmentation and double-bundle reconstruction were superior to the single-bundle reconstruction with respect to anterior instability and balance ability. In the future, long-term prospective and retrospective clinical studies might be needed to prove the theoretical biological and biomechanical advantages of our procedure compared with the anatomical double-bundle ACL reconstruction with ACL remnant preservation. While currently, both procedures involve the same rehabilitation, we believe that postoperative rehabilitation after ACL augmentation could be shortened in the near future compared to those needed after ACL reconstruction.

28.5 Conclusions

We present a technique that combines the biological advantage of maximal preservation of the ACL remnant and the biomechanical advantage of performing anatomical ACL reconstruction.

References

1. Hussein M, van Eck CF, Cretnik A, Dinevski D, Fu FH (2012) Prospective randomized clinical evaluation of conventional single-bundle, anatomic single-bundle, and anatomic double-

bundle anterior cruciate ligament reconstruction: 281 cases with 3- to 5- year follow-up. Am J Sports Med 40:512–520
2. Komzák M, Hart R, Okál F, Safi A (2012) Does the posterolateral bundle influence rotational movement more than the anteromedial bundle in anterior cruciate ligament reconstruction?: a clinical study. J Bone Joint Surg (Br) 94-B:1372–1376
3. Ahldén M, Sernert N, Karlsson J, Kartus J (2013) A prospective randomized study comparing double- and single-bundle techniques for Anterior Cruciate Ligament reconstruction. Am J Sports Med 41:2484–2491
4. Ho JY, Gardiner A, Shah V, Steiner ME (2009) Equal kinematics between central anatomic single-bundle and double-bundle anterior cruciate ligament reconstructions. Arthroscopy 25:464–472
5. Kanaya A, Ochi M, Deie M, Adachi N, Nishimori M, Nakamae A (2009) Intraoperative evaluation of anteroposterior and rotational stabilities in anterior cruciate ligament reconstruction: lower femoral tunnel placed single-bundle versus double-bundle reconstruction. Knee Surg Sports Traumatol Arthrosc 17:907–913
6. Siebold R, Dehler C, Ellert T (2008) Prospective randomized comparison of double-bundle versus single-bundle anterior cruciate ligament reconstruction. Arthroscopy 24:137–145
7. Adachi N, Ochi M, Uchio Y, Sumen Y (2000) Anterior cruciate ligament augmentation under arthroscopy. A minimum 2-year follow-up in 40 patients. Arch Orthop Trauma Surg 120:128–133
8. Lee BI, Kwon SW, Kim JB, Choi HS, Min KD (2008) Comparison of clinical results according to amount of preserved remnant in arthroscopic anterior cruciate ligament reconstruction using quadrupled hamstring graft. Arthroscopy 24:560–568
9. Ochi M, Adachi N, Deie M, Kanaya A (2006) Anterior cruciate ligament augmentation procedure with a 1-incision technique: anteromedial bundle or posterolateral bundle reconstruction. Arthroscopy 22:463.e1–e5
10. Ochi M, Adachi N, Uchio Y et al (2009) A minimum 2-year follow-up after selective anteromedial or posterolateral bundle anterior cruciate ligament reconstruction. Arthroscopy 25:117–122
11. Siebold R, Fu FH (2008) Assessment and augmentation of symptomatic anteromedial or posterolateral bundle tears of the anterior cruciate ligament. Arthroscopy 24:1289–1298
12. Shidahara H, Deie M, Niimoto T et al (2011) Prospective study of kinesthesia after ACL reconstruction. Int J Sports Med 32:386–392
13. Adachi N, Ochi M, Uchio Y, Iwasa J, Ryoke K, Kuriwaka M (2002) Mechanoreceptors in the anterior cruciate ligament contribute to the joint position sense. Acta Orthop Scand 73:330–334
14. Denti M, Monteleone M, Berardi A, Panni AS (1994) Anterior cruciate ligament mechanoreceptors. Histologic studies on lesions and reconstruction. Clin Orthop Relat Res 308:29–32
15. Ochi M, Iwasa J, Uchio Y, Adachi N, Sumen Y (1999) The regeneration of sensory neurons in the reconstruction of the anterior cruciate ligament. J Bone Joint Surg (Br) 81-B:902–906
16. Ochi M, Iwasa J, Uchio Y, Adachi N, Kawasaki K (2002) Induction of somatosensory evoked potentials by mechanical stimulation in reconstructed anterior cruciate ligaments. J Bone Joint Surg (Br) 84-B:761–766
17. Mifune Y, Ota S, Takayama K et al (2013) Therapeutic advantage in selective ligament augmentation for partial tears of the anterior cruciate ligament: results in an animal model. Am J Sports Med 41:365–373
18. Crain EH, Fithian DC, Paxton EW, Luetzow WF (2005) Variation in anterior cruciate ligament scar pattern: does the scar pattern affect anterior laxity in anterior cruciate ligament-deficient knees? Arthroscopy 21:19–24
19. Nakamae A, Ochi M, Deie M et al (2010) Biomechanical function of anterior cruciate ligament remnants: how long do they contribute to knee stability after injury in patients with complete tears? Arthroscopy 26:1577–1585
20. Shino K, Horibe S, Hamada M et al (2002) Allograft anterior cruciate ligament reconstruction. Tech Knee Surg 1:78–85
21. Nishimori M et al (2014) Simulated ACL reconstruction with trans-medial portal technique using pre-operative 3D CT -Proposed optimum medial portal position. Knee Surg Sports Traumatol Arthrosc 22:1175–1181

22. Mae T, Shino K, Matsumoto N, Natsu-Ume T, Yoneda K, Yoshikawa H, Yoneda M (2010) Anatomic double-bundle anterior cruciate ligament reconstruction using hamstring tendons with minimally required initial tension. Arthroscopy 26:1289–1295
23. Araki D, Kuroda R, Kubo S, Fujita N, Tei K, Nishimoto K, Hoshino Y, Matsushita T, Matsumoto T, Nagamune K, Kurosaka M (2011) A prospective randomised study of anatomical single-bundle versus double-bundle anterior cruciate ligament reconstruction: quantitative evaluation using an electromagnetic measurement system. Int Orthop 35:439–446
24. Adachi N, Ochi M, Uchio Y, Iwasa J, Kuriwaka M, Ito Y (2004) Reconstruction of the anterior cruciate ligament, single- versus double-bundle multistranded hamstring tendons. J Bone Joint Surg (Br) 86:515–520
25. Lam MH, Fong DT, Yung PS, Ho EP, Fung KY, Chan KM (2011) Knee rotational stability during pivoting movement is restored after anatomic double bundle anterior cruciate ligament reconstruction. Am J Sports Med 39:1032–1038
26. Kopf S, Pombo MW, Shen W, Irrgang JJ, Fu FH (2011) The ability of 3 different approaches to restore the anatomic anteromedial bundle femoral insertion site during anatomic anterior cruciate ligament reconstruction. Arthroscopy 27:200–206
27. Sonnery-Cottet B, Lavoie F, Ogassawara R, Scussiato RG, Kidder JF, Chambat P (2010) Selective anteromedial bundle reconstruction in partial ACL tears: a series of 36 patients with mean 24 months follow-up. Knee Surg Sports Traumatol Arthrosc 18:47–51
28. Kongcharoensombat W, Ochi M, Abouheif M, Adachi N, Ohkawa S, Kamei G, Okuhara A, Shibuya H, Niimoto T, Nakasa T, Nakamae A, Deie M (2011) The transverse ligament as a landmark for tibial sagittal insertions of the anterior cruciate ligament: a cadaveric study. Arthroscopy 27:1395–1399
29. Nakamae A, Ochi M, Deie M, Adachi N, Shibuya H, Ohkawa S, Hirata K (2014) Clinical outcomes of second-look arthroscopic evaluation after anterior cruciate ligament augmentation: comparison with single- and double-bundle reconstruction. Bone Joint J 1325–1332
30. Chen CH (2009) Graft healing in anterior cruciate ligament reconstruction. Sports Med Arthrosc Rehabil Ther Technol 1:21
31. Kuo CK, Marturano JE, Tuan RS (2010) Novel strategies in tendon and ligament tissue engineering: advanced biomaterials and regeneration motifs. Sports Med Arthrosc Rehabil Ther Technol 2:20
32. Ma Y, Deie M, Iwaki D, Asaeda M, Fujita N, Adachi N, Ochi M (2014) Balance ability and proprioception after single-bundle, single-bundle augmentation, and double –bundle ACL reconstruction. Sci World J 2014:342012

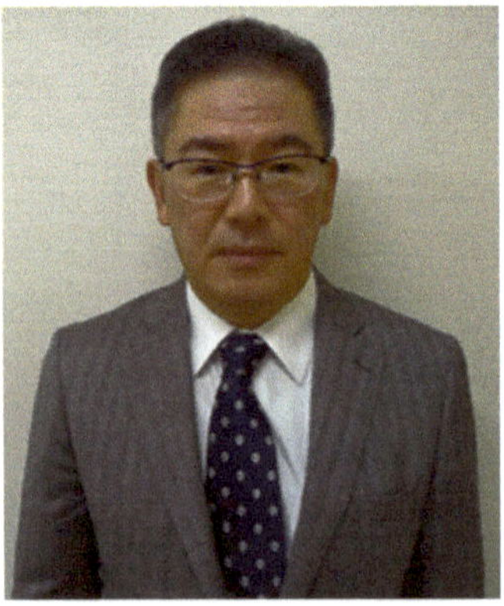

Masataka Deie, M.D., PhD, Department of Orthopaedic Surgery, School of Medicine, Aichi Medical University, Aichi, Japan.

Part VII
ACL Reconstruction Using Bone-Patella Tendon-Bone

Chapter 29
An Overview

Shuji Horibe and Ryohei Uchida

Abstract The BTB autograft, which is morphologically and biomechanically suitable in mimicking the native ACL, has long been considered the gold standard for ACL reconstruction. Although this technique provides good long-term clinical results, including a higher rate of returning to previous sporting levels, BTB ACL reconstruction is associated with many technical difficulties and high risks of donor-site morbidity and osteoarthritis. The abovementioned issues, however, could be reduced by modifying surgical techniques, such as anatomic graft placement, application of appropriate initial tension to the graft, use of fixation devices, and improved graft harvesting techniques.

Keywords Bone patellar tendon-bone graft • ACL reconstruction • Overview

29.1 Patellar Tendon Grafts

Since Hey Groves [1] first reported the use of an iliotibial band transplant for anterior cruciate ligament (ACL) reconstruction in 1917, many substitutes for ACL replacement have been reported, including autogenous tissues. In particular, patellar, hamstring, and quadriceps tendons have been used widely due to their ease of procurement and reliable clinical results. The bone-patellar tendon-bone (BTB) autograft technique has been considered the gold standard for ACL reconstruction, as it provides strength and early bone-to-bone healing with rigid interference screw fixation. Campbell [2] reported the first use of tendinous tissue from the medial border of the quadriceps and patellar tendon in 1936; however, this procedure was not widely adopted. In 1963, Jones reported a new technique for ACL reconstruction using the central one-third of the patellar tendon [3]. In this procedure, the patellar tendon was left attached distally, and the proximal part was removed from

S. Horibe, MD, PhD (✉)
Faculty of Comprehensive Rehabilitation, Osaka Prefecture University, 3-7-30 Habikino, Habikino, Osaka 583-8555, Japan
e-mail: s-horibe@rehab.osakafu-u.ac.jp

R. Uchida, MD, PhD
Department of Orthopaedic Sports Medicine, Seifu Hospital, Osaka, Japan

M. Ochi et al. (eds.), *ACL Injury and Its Treatment*,
DOI 10.1007/978-4-431-55858-3_29

the patella together with a small block of bone. Since then, ACL reconstruction with patellar tendon graft has become popular. In Europe, instead of using the central one-third of the patellar tendon, the medial one-third was used for ACL graft [4–6]. Tibia-based patellar tendon grafts were commonly used at that time, since vascularity was believed to be preserved from the tibia; however, there was no blood supply to the patellar tendon through the tibial attachment [7], and the pedicle graft was not sufficiently long for anatomical femoral placement. Franke was the first to advocate the use of a free graft from one-fourth of the patellar tendon with tibial and patellar bones [8]. Following this report, the use of free medial or the central third of the patellar tendon with both patellar and tibial bones was also reported [9–11].

Meanwhile, several animal studies have focused on the effect of preserved graft vascularity on the remodeling process [12–14]. Kondo reported that, in a comparative animal study, no biomechanical or histological differences were observed between pedicle and free grafts [12]. Clancy et al. compared pedicle grafts for ACL and free grafts for PCL using a rhesus model and found that revascularization was as complete in free grafts as in pedicle grafts [13]. Noyes et al. hypothesized that a biologic graft with a partly intact vascular supply might undergo less necrosis and remodeling, thereby achieving a higher mechanical strength with less risk of excessive deformation [15, 16]. However, an attempt to preserve vascularity to the patellar tendon graft did not help prevent the rapid adverse changes in mechanical properties observed in nonvascularized free grafts postoperatively [14]. Those experimental studies demonstrated that pedicle and vascularized grafts have no advantage over free grafts in facilitating the remodeling process [12–14].

Noyes et al. reported that the BTB graft was the strongest and was 1.6-fold stronger than the normal ACL [17]. Lambert originally described aperture fixation with interference screws on both sides [18]. Interference fit-screw fixation became popular after Kurosaka et al. reported that it was mechanically superior to other fixation methods [19]. In addition to the mechanical superiority of BTB grafts, rapid bone-to-bone healing at the insertion site allows aggressive rehabilitation and early return to sports activity. Then, with the development of arthroscopic instruments, arthroscopically assisted BTB ACL reconstruction gained popularity between the late 1980s and the early 1990s [20–23]. However, many surgeons gradually shifted toward using the hamstring tendon [24–28], likely due to the higher incidence of postoperative complications including donor-site morbidity, as well as the spread of anatomic double-bundle ACL reconstruction. Instead of the conventional technique using a single round tunnel, which renders the replacement of the BTB graft anatomically challenging, Shino et al. proposed anatomic rectangular-tunnel ACL reconstruction [29–31]. This technique mimics the natural ACL fiber arrangement by creating bone tunnels within areas of ACL insertion and provides restoration of normal laxity with small initial tension applied to the graft and early bony integration within the femoral tunnel by snug-fit fixation [31–33]. This technique may reduce postoperative complications such as knee motion loss and osteoarthritis.

29.2 BTB Graft Biomechanics

According to several cadaveric and clinical studies [34–39], the cross-sectional area (CSA) of 10-mm-wide BTB grafts ranged from 32.3 to 41.0 mm^2, which corresponds to 73–98 % of the normal ACL if the native ACL with a CSA between 42 and 44 mm^2 [17, 40] is used. In a pioneering study by Noyes et al., the central third of the patellar tendon averaged 168 % in strength relative to the normal ACL, more than twice the strength of other potential grafts [17]. However, BTB grafts used in that study were 14–15 mm in width, i.e., too large for clinical use. The ultimate tensile strength of 10-mm BTB grafts from young specimens was between 2300 N and 2977 N [34], that is, 106–140 % that of the normal ACL, based on the reported strength of the ACL of normal youth (2160 N, Woo et al.) [41]. The average stiffness of 10-mm-wide BTB grafts was 440 N/mm [34], which is 182 % that of the normal ACL (242 N/mm) [41]. Reportedly, the central one-third of the patellar tendon normally used for ACL reconstruction is biomechanically superior to the medial or lateral one-third [42, 43]. The reasons for this include its elliptical shape in the transverse plane [44] and relatively high collagen density, mean fibril diameter, and/or collagen cross-linking [42, 43]. Therefore, BTB grafts are considered morphologically and biomechanically suitable for mimicking the native ACL [31]. When a BTB graft is used for ACL reconstruction, however, surgeons should be aware of its biomechanical characteristics including the stiffness, as well as the regional and mechanical properties that may influence knee motion and laxity postoperatively.

29.3 BTB Graft Healing Within Bone Tunnels

Since BTB grafts have a unique composite structure, the healing process in each portion within the bone tunnel is different. With no gap between the bone plug of the graft and the wall of the bone tunnel, anchoring in the newly formed bone was observed after 3–6 weeks and complete incorporation by 12 weeks [45, 46]. However, if there was a space between the plug and the tunnel wall, granulation tissue remained even after 12 weeks. Following rectangular ACL reconstruction, which ensures that there will be no gap at the anterior interface between the bone plug and the femoral tunnel wall, bony integration was found to be almost complete by 8 weeks [32].

The basic structure of the original bone-tendon insertion of the graft is maintained, but degeneration of the bone-tendon junction progressed with time after 6 weeks [45, 46]. Ishibashi et al. examined biopsied specimens within the tibial tunnels from revision ACL cases and reported that a normal original bone-tendon junction was found in a 4-month revision case; there was no obvious structure in 6-month-old cases [47].

Disorganized fibrous tissue, including fibroblasts and inflammatory cells, has been observed, filling the interface between the tendinous portion and the wall of the bone tunnel at 1 week. The perpendicular collagen fibers resembling Sharpey's fibers appeared in granulation tissue around the intraosseous tendon portion [46] and became mature and organized with time [45].

29.4 Graft Harvest

Prior to BTB ACL reconstruction, abnormalities in the patella tendon including bone insertion sites and the size of the graft should be evaluated by preoperative X-P and MRI. Patellar tendon abnormalities such as Osgood-Schlatter disease and patellar tendinitis may preclude the use of BTB grafts. Since graft protrusion occasionally occurs in cases of excessively long patellar tendons [48–51] and the incidence of donor-site morbidity may increase if more than one-third of the graft is harvested [52, 53], BTB graft size should be predicted beforehand.

When making a longitudinal skin incision just medial to the patellar tendon, care should be taken to preserve the infrapatellar branches of the saphenous nerve over the patellar tendon to the extent possible. Subcutaneous tissue dissection is carried out to the level of the paratenon, which is incised sharply and then retracted to expose the inferior pole of the patella and the tibial tubercle. The central third of the patellar tendon measuring 10 mm in width is cut, along with the longitudinal fibers. A 15-mm long patellar plug is harvested in a triangular fashion, and a 20-mm tibial bone plug is cut in a trapezoidal fashion. After removal of the BTB graft, the paratenon is sutured without tendon closure.

29.5 Donor-Site Complication/Morbidity

Compared to open surgery, arthroscopically assisted ACL reconstruction is associated with less postoperative morbidity, including loss of knee motion and anterior knee pain. However, there still is a risk of disruption of the knee-extensor apparatus (e.g., patellar fracture, tendon rupture) resulting from patellar tendon graft harvest with bone plugs. Patellar fracture occurs either during or after surgery, at an incidence of 0.12–1.3 % [53–59]. The etiology of patellar fracture is multifactorial and can be attributed to the bone harvesting technique, patellar bone defect, aggressive rehabilitation, and trauma [55, 57]. As the bone weakens after removal of the anterior cortex of the patella, the portion most resistant to loading, caution should be exercised not to remove too much of the patellar bone and to avoid damage to the anterior cortex by using an electric bone saw [52, 53]. Moreover, while several reports [60–62] recommend bone grafting of the patellar bone defect to reduce the risk of patellar fracture and minimize donor-site pain, the risk of painful spur formation and heterotopic bone formation has been noted [63].

Although the incidence of patellar tendon rupture is reportedly low (0.06–0.24 %) [53, 59, 64], ruptured tendons are technically difficult to repair [65–69]. To prevent this, the patellar tendon should be cut along the longitudinal fibers so as to minimize the risk of tendon laceration under direct vision; the edges of the residual patellar tendon at the tibial insertion site should not be undermined [52, 53, 65, 70]. Also, use of a double parallel blade is recommended to avoid tendon laceration [52, 53]. It should be noted that, when the contralateral, normal knee is used as the donor site, early mobilization with limited weight bearing on the reconstructed side may overload the contralateral donor knee, leading to patellar fracture and tendon rupture [54]. Since disruption of the knee-extensor apparatus is a severe complication, both patellar fracture and patellar tendon rupture should be avoided to the extent possible.

Only few cases of heterotopic ossification of the patellar tendon, another complication following BTB graft harvest, have been reported [71–74]. Although the underlying mechanism is still unknown, bone debris and hematoma during aggressive rehabilitation may result, with time, in progressive bone formation in the bone bed and the tendon [71, 73]. Erdil et al. emphasized the need for the graft to be meticulously prepared, and any bone debris must not be left inside the operative field in order to avoid this complication [73].

The disadvantage of BTB grafts is a higher incidence of donor-site morbidity, which includes anterior knee pain, kneeling problems, tenderness of the donor site, and intraoperative injury to the infrapatellar branches of the saphenous nerve. The incidence of anterior knee pain is reportedly 4–60 % [75–79], of which the causes have yet to be determined [80]. Correlated with anterior knee pain are knee extension loss [81], bone removal [62], changes in the mechanical properties of the patellar tendon [82, 83], scar formation within the removed area [84], patellofemoral arthritis [85], fat pad fibrosis [84], hypesthesia due to injury to the infrapatellar branches of the saphenous nerve [86], and a cyclops lesion [87], to name a few.

BTB ACL reconstruction is associated with a higher risk of extension loss [88]. Postoperative extension loss leads to notch regrowth, cyclops lesions, and patellofemoral arthritis, which may occur during the rehabilitation period following ACL reconstruction. According to Shelbourne and Trumper [81], the incidence of anterior knee pain could be reduced by obtaining full postoperative knee extension. Thus, care should be taken to regain full extension immediately postoperatively. Moreover, appropriate initial tension should be applied to the graft to avoid overloading the transplanted graft, since BTB grafts are stiffer than the normal ACL.

To reduce anterior knee pain, several technical improvements have been introduced for harvesting BTB grafts, such as skin incisions, bone grafting, repair of the peritenon, and closure of the patellar tendon defect [62, 78, 89, 90]. Some have advocated patellar tendon suture with bone grafting [60], although this does not decrease the rate of postoperative anterior knee pain [91, 92]. In a cadaveric study, it was possible to harvest BTB grafts through two vertical 25-mm incisions, leaving the infrapatellar nerve undamaged [93]. This double-incision approach decreases the occurrence of sensory disorders and the extent of hypoesthesia and reduces the incidence of anterior knee pain [62, 78, 90]. Recently, Cervellin et al [94] reported the use of autologous platelet-rich plasma gel to effectively reduce subjective knee pain at the donor-site level. However, further studies are needed to determine the effectiveness of this approach and to elucidate the mechanism of pain reduction [94].

29.6 Remodeling After Graft Harvest

In animal models, complete filling and scarring of the defect after graft removal have been observed [82], and the mechanical properties of the remaining patellar tendon are significantly reduced for up to 6 months postoperatively [82, 83]. In humans, many postoperative MRI studies of the patellar tendon and histological studies of biopsied defect specimens have been performed. According to MRI studies, the defect in the patellar tendon heals with time after harvesting, but does not completely close in all cases [95–100]. Histologically, scarring around the defect progressively matures over time [97], but the patellar tendon does not normalize completely [101–103]. Encouraged by two studies on defect healing potential [82, 95], the use of a healed donor site was proposed for revision cases [104]. Since then, many have reported on cases of revision ACL reconstruction with reharvested BTB grafts [105–109]. Although reharvested grafts appeared to have ligamentization potential based on MRI and second-look arthroscopy with concomitant histological findings, clinical results have been unsatisfactory [108, 109].

29.7 Graft Fixation

Secure BTB graft fixation is essential to allow for early joint mobilization after surgery. Among the various BTB graft fixation methods, including metallic or bioresorbable interference screws, cortical suspensory graft fixation devices, post screws, and buttons, interference screws have been used the most widely. Since BTB grafts have bone plugs at both ends, interference screws provide rigid and osseous aperture fixation compared to other devices. However, potential disadvantages of this fixation method include divergent screw placement, difficulties with removal during revision surgery, and the risk of graft damage [58, 110, 111]. To circumvent these drawbacks, a hardware-free ACL reconstruction technique has been developed [112]. Since Hertel originally described the BTB press-fit technique, many modified techniques have been proposed [110, 113, 114]. These techniques, though technically challenging, provide fixation strength and long-term clinical outcomes comparable to conventional techniques [115].

29.8 Clinical Results

Long-term follow-up studies of endoscopic BTB ACL reconstruction have shown good subjective and objective clinical results over 10 years postoperatively [112, 116–120]. The percentage of normal or nearly normal overall IKDC grades ranged from 74 % to 91 % [112, 116, 117, 119] with a high patient satisfaction rate [117–120]. Good ligament stability was maintained in 82–100 % of patients over 10 postoperative years, and the average KT-1000 side-to-side difference ranged from 1.6 to 1.8 mm [112, 117, 118]. However, graft rerupture occurred in 5.1–13 % of cases during long-term follow-up periods [116–118, 120]. Maletis et al. reported that the revision rate per 100 years of observation was 0.66 % in a community-based sample of 2791 BTB reconstructed patients [121].

Many reports have compared clinical outcomes between BTB and hamstring tendon grafts widely used for ACL reconstruction. These include comparative studies [77, 122–127] as well as systematic reviews [88, 128–134]. BTB grafts provided good subjective outcomes that are comparable to those of hamstring tendon grafts [122–124, 126, 127, 131] while offering better static knee stability [88, 122, 129, 130] with a significantly lower rate of graft failure [121, 126, 128–130, 133]. However, patients with BTB ACL reconstruction had increased donor-site morbidity, including anterior knee pain, pain with kneeling and walking [77, 88, 125, 129–134], and a greater prevalence of osteoarthritis [123, 126, 134].

29.9 Summary

The BTB autograft, which is morphologically and biomechanically suitable in mimicking the native ACL, has long been considered the gold standard for ACL reconstruction. Although this technique provides good long-term clinical results, including a higher rate of returning to previous sporting levels, BTB ACL reconstruction is associated with many technical difficulties and high risks of donor-site morbidity and osteoarthritis. The abovementioned issues, however, could be reduced by modifying surgical techniques, such as anatomic graft placement, application of appropriate initial tension to the graft, use of fixation devices, and improved graft harvesting techniques.

References

1. Hey Groves EW (1917) Operation for the repair of cruciate ligament. Lancet 2:674–675
2. Campbell WC (1936) Repair of the ligaments of the knee. Surg Gynecol Obstet:62:964–968
3. Jones KG (1963) ACL reconstruction. A technique using the central one-third of the patellar ligament. J Bone Joint Surg Am 45:925–932
4. Brückner H (1966) Eine neue methode der Krueuzbandplasitk. Chirurg 37:413–414

5. Gillquist J, Lijedahl SO, Lindvall H (1971) Reconstruction for old rupture of the anterior cruciate ligament. A follow-up study. Injury 2:271–278
6. Eriksson E (1976) Reconstruction of the ACL. Orthop Clin N Am 7:167–179
7. Sccapinelli R (1968) Studies on the vasculature of the human knee joints. Acta Anat 70 (3):305–331
8. Franke K (1976) Clinical experience in 130 cruciate ligament reconstructions. Orthop Clin N Am 7:191–193
9. Clancy WGJ et al (1982) Anterior cruciate ligament reconstruction using one-third of the patellar ligament, augmented by extra-articular tendon transfers. J Bone Joint Surg Am 64:352–359
10. Clancy WGJ (1985) Intra-articular reconstruction of the ACL. Orhtop Clin N Am 16:181–189
11. Paterson FW, Trickey EL (1986) Anterior cruciate ligament reconstruction using part of the patellar tendon as a free graft. J Bone Joint Surg (Br) 68B:453–457
12. Kondo M (1979) An experimental study of reconstructive surgery of the anterior cruciate ligament. Nihon Seikeigeka Gakkai Zasshi 53:521–533
13. Clancy WGJ et al (1981) Anterior and posterior cruciate ligament reconstruction in rhesus monkeys. J Bone Joint Surg Am 63:1270–1284
14. Butler DL et al (1989) Mechanical properties of primate vascularized vs. nonvascularized patellar tendon grafts; changes over time. J Orthop Res 7:68–79
15. Noyes FR et al (1983) Intra-articular cruciate reconstruction I:perspectives on graft strength vascularization and immediate motion after replacement. Clin Orthop Relat Res 172:71–77
16. Paulos LE et al (1983) Intra-articular cruciate reconstruction II. Replacement with vascularized patellar tendon. Clin Orthop Relat Res 172:78–84
17. Noyes FR et al (1984) Biomechanical analysis of human ligament grafts used in knee-ligament repairs and reconstructions. J Bone Joint Surg Am 66A:344–352
18. Lambert KL (1983) Vascularized patellar tendon graft with rigid internal fixation for anterior cruciate ligament insufficiency. Clin Orthop Relat Res 172:85–89
19. Kurosaka M, Yoshiya S, Andrish JT (1987) A biomechanical comparison of different surgical techniques of graft fixation in anterior cruciate ligament reconstruction. Am J Sports Med 15:225–229
20. Wilcox PG, Jackson DW (1987) Arthroscopic ACLR. Clin Sports Med 6:513–524
21. Gillquist J, Odensten M (1988) Arthroscopic reconstruction of the anterior cruciate ligament. Arthroscopy 4:5–9
22. Jackson DW, JL/D (1988) Arthroscopically assisted reconstruction of the ACL using a patella tendon bone autograft. Clin Sports Med 7:785–800
23. Marder RA, Raskind JR, Carroll M (1991) Prospective evaluation of arthroscopically assisted anterior cruciate ligament reconstruction. Patellar tendon versus semitendinosus and gracilis tendons. Am J Sports Med 19:478–484
24. Chechik O et al (2013) An international survey on anterior cruciate ligament reconstruction practices. Int Orthop 37(2):201–206
25. Maletis GB, Inacio MC, Funahashi TT (2013) Analysis of 16,192 anterior cruciate ligament reconstructions from a community-based registry. Am J Sports Med 41(9):2090–2098
26. Middleton KK et al (2014) Anatomic anterior cruciate ligament (ACL) reconstruction: a global perspective. Part 1. Knee Surg Sports Traumatol Arthrosc 22(7):1467–1482
27. Kvist J et al (2014) Results from the Swedish national anterior cruciate ligament register. Arthroscopy 30(7):803–810
28. Rahr-Wagner L et al (2014) Comparison of hamstring tendon and patellar tendon grafts in anterior cruciate ligament reconstruction in a nationwide population-based cohort study: results from the danish registry of knee ligament reconstruction. Am J Sports Med 42 (2):278–284

29. Shino K et al (2005) Anatomically oriented anterior cruciate ligament reconstruction with a bone-patellar tendon-bone graft via rectangular socket and tunnel: a snug-fit and impingement-free grafting technique. Arthroscopy 21(11):1402
30. Shino K et al (2008) Rectangular tunnel double-bundle anterior cruciate ligament reconstruction with bone-patellar tendon-bone graft to mimic natural fiber arrangement. Arthroscopy 24 (10):1178–1183
31. Shino K, Mae T, Tachibana Y (2015) Anatomic ACL reconstruction: rectangular tunnel/ bone-patellar tendon-bone or triple-bundle/semitendinosus tendon grafting. J Orthop Sci 20 (3):457–468
32. Suzuki T et al (2011) Early integration of a bone plug in the femoral tunnel in rectangular tunnel ACL reconstruction with a bone-patellar tendon-bone graft: a prospective computed tomography analysis. Knee Surg Sports Traumatol Arthrosc 19(Suppl 1):S29–S35
33. Suzuki T et al (2014) Biomechanical comparison between the rectangular-tunnel and the round-tunnel anterior cruciate ligament reconstruction procedures with a bone-patellar tendon-bone graft. Arthroscopy 30(10):1294–1302
34. Cooper DE et al (1993) The strength of the central third patellar tendon graft. A biomechanical study. Am J Sports Med 21:818–824
35. Schatzmann L, Brunner P, Stäubli HU (1998) Effect of cyclic preconditioning on the tensile properties of human quadriceps tendons and patellar ligaments. Knee Surg Sports Traumatol Arthrosc 6(Suppl 1):S56–S61
36. Stäubli HU et al (1999) Mechanical tensile properties of the quadriceps tendon and patellar ligament in young adults. Am J Sports Med 27:27–34
37. Yoshiya S et al (2003) Cross-sectional area of a bone-patellar tendon-bone graft for anterior cruciate ligament reconstruction. J Knee Surg 16:75–78
38. Shimizu K et al (2007) Change in the cross-sectional area of a patellar tendon graft after anterior cruciate ligament reconstruction. Knee Surg Sports Traumatol Arthrosc 15 (5):515–521
39. Toritsuka Y et al (2003) Comparison between the cross-sectional area of bone-patellar tendon-bone grafts and multistranded hamstring tendon grafts obtained from the same patients. Knee Surg Sports Traumatol Arthrosc 11(2):81–84
40. Muneta T, Takakuda K, Yamamoto H (1999) Intercondylar notch width and its relation to the configuration and cross-sectional area of the anterior cruciate ligament. A cadaveric knee study. Am J Sports Med 25:69–72
41. Woo SL et al (1991) Tensile properties of the human femur-anterior cruciate ligament-tibia complex. The effects of specimen age and orientation. Am J Sports Med 19:217–225
42. Yanke AB et al (2013) Central-third bone-patellar tendon-bone allografts demonstrate superior biomechanical failure characteristics compared with hemi-patellar tendon grafts. Am J Sports Med 41(11):2521–2526
43. Yanke A et al (2015) Regional mechanical properties of human patellar tendon allografts. Knee Surg Sports Traumatol Arthrosc 23(4):961–967
44. Matava MJ, Hutton W (1995) A biomechanical comparison between the central one-third patellar tendon and the residual tendon. Br J Sports Med 29:178–184
45. Yoshiya S et al (2000) Graft healing in the bon tunnel in ACLR. Clin Orthop Relat Res 376:278–286
46. Tomita F et al (2001) Comparisons of intraosseous graft healing between the doubled flexor tendon graft and the bone-patellar tendon-bone graft in anterior cruciate ligament reconstruction. Arthroscopy 17(5):461–476
47. Ishibashi Y et al (2001) Graft incorporation within the tibial bone tunnel after anterior cruciate ligament reconstruction with bone-patellar tendon-bone autograft. Am J Sports Med 29:473–479
48. Denti M et al (1998) Graft-tunnel mismatch in endoscopic anterior cruciate ligament reconstruction. Intraoperative and cadaver measurement of the intra-articular graft length and the length of the patellar tendon. Knee Surg Sports Traumatol Arthrosc 6:165–168

49. Shaffer B, Gow W, Tibone JE (1993) Graft tunnel mismatch in endoscopic anterior cruciate ligament reconstruction: a new technique of intraarticular measurement and modified graft harvesting. Arthroscopy 9:633–646
50. Fowler BL, DiStefano VJ (1998) Tibial tunnel bone grafting a new technique for dealing with graft tunnel mismatch in endoscopic anterior cruciate ligament reconstruction. Arthroscopy 14:224–228
51. Grawe B, Smerina A, Allen A (2014) Avoiding graft-tunnel length mismatch in anterior cruciate ligament reconstruction: the single-bone plug technique. Arthrosc Tech 3(3):e417–e420
52. Malek MM, Kunkel KL, Knable KR (1996) Intraoperative complications of arthroscopically assisted ACLR using patellar tendon autograft. American Academy of Orthopaedic Surgeons. Instr Course Lect 45:297–302
53. Lee GH et al (2008) The incidence of acute patellar tendon harvest complications for anterior cruciate ligament reconstruction. Arthroscopy 24(2):162–166
54. Christen B, Jakob RP (1992) Fractures associated with patellar ligament grafts in cruciate ligament surgery. J Bone Joint Surg (Br) 74:617–619
55. Viola R, Vianello R (1999) Three cases of patella fracture in 1,320 anterior cruciate ligament reconstructions with bone-patellar tendon-bone autograft. Arthroscopy 15:93–97
56. Papageorgiou CD et al (2001) Patellar fractures associated with medial-third bone-patellar tendon-bone autograft ACL reconstruction. Knee Surg Sports Traumatol Arthrosc 9 (3):151–154
57. Stein DA et al (2002) The incidence and outcome of patella fractures after anterior cruciate ligament reconstruction. Arthroscopy 18(6):578–583
58. Almazan A et al (2006) Intraoperative incidents and complications in primary arthroscopic anterior cruciate ligament reconstruction. Arthroscopy 22(11):1211–1217
59. Milankov M et al (2013) Disruption of the knee extensor apparatus complicating anterior cruciate ligament reconstruction. Acta chirurgica iugoslavica 60(2):13–21
60. Ferrari JD, Bach BRJ (1998) Bone graft procurement for patellar defect grafting in anterior cruciate ligament reconstruction. Arthroscopy 14:543–545
61. Daluga D, Johnson C, Bach BRJ (1990) Primary bone grafting following graft procurement for anterior cruciate ligament insufficiency. Arthroscopy 6:205–208
62. Tsuda E et al (2001) Techniques for reducing anterior knee symptoms after ACLR using BTB autograft. Am J Sports Med 29:450–456
63. Kohn D, Sander-Beuermann A (1994) Donor-site morbidity after harvest of a bone-tendon-bone patellar tendon autograft. Knee Surg Sports Traumatol Arthrosc 2:219–223
64. Benner RW, Shelbourne KD, Freeman H (2011) Infections and patellar tendon ruptures after anterior cruciate ligament reconstruction: a comparison of ipsilateral and contralateral patellar tendon autografts. Am J Sports Med 39(3):519–525
65. Hardin GT, Bach BRJ (1992) Distal rupture of the infrapatellar tendon after use of central third for ACLR. Am J Knee Surg 5:140–143
66. Marumoto JM et al (1996) Late patellar tendon ruptures after removal of the central third for anterior cruciate ligament reconstruction. A report of two cases. Am J Sports Med 24:698–701
67. Miller MD, Nichols T, Butler CA (1999) Patella fracture and proximal patellar tendon rupture following arthroscopic anterior cruciate ligament reconstruction. Arthroscopy 15:640–643
68. Mickelsen PL et al (2001) Patellar tendon rupture 3 years after anterior cruciate ligament reconstruction with a central one third bone-patellar tendon-bone graft. Arthroscopy 17 (6):648–652
69. Milankov Ziva M et al (2008) Reconstruction of patellar tendon rupture after anterior cruciate ligament reconstruction: a case report. Knee 15(5):419–422
70. Hospodar SJ, Miller MD (2009) Controversies in ACL reconstruction bone-patellar tendon-bone anterior cruciate ligament reconstruction remains the gold standard. Sports Med Arthrosc Rev 17:242–246

71. Erdogan F et al (2004) Calcification of the patellar tendon after ACL reconstruction. A case report with long-term follow-up. Knee Surg Sports Traumatol Arthrosc 12(4):277–279
72. Valencia H, Gavin C (2007) Infrapatellar heterotopic ossification after anterior cruciate ligament reconstruction. Knee Surg Sports Traumatol Arthrosc 15(1):39–42
73. Erdil M et al (2012) Heterotopic bone formation following anterior cruciate ligament reconstruction with BPTB autograft. Acta Orthop Traumatol Turc 46(1):72–76
74. Camillieri G et al (2013) Patellar tendon ossification after anterior cruciate ligament reconstruction using bone-patellar tendon-bone autograft. BMC Musculoskelet Disord 14:164
75. Plancher K et al (1998) Reconstruction of the anterior cruciate ligament in patients who are at least forty years old. A long-term follow-up and outcome study. J Bone Joint Surg Am 80:184–197
76. Kartus J, Movin T, Karlsson J (2001) Donor-site morbidity and anterior knee problems after anterior cruciate ligament reconstruction using autografts. Arthroscopy 17(9):971–980
77. Shaieb MD et al (2002) A prospective randomized comparison of patellar tendon versus semitendinosus and gracilis tendon autografts for anterior cruciate ligament reconstruction. Am J Sports Med 30:214–220
78. Gaudot F et al (2009) Double-incision mini-invasive technique for BTB harvesting: its superiority in reducing anterior knee pain following ACL reconstruction. Orthop Traumatol Surg Res 95(1):28–35
79. Beaufils P et al (2011) Mini-invasive technique for bone patellar tendon bone harvesting: its superiority in reducing anterior knee pain following ACL reconstruction. Curr Rev Musculoskelet Med 4(2):45–51
80. Jones KJ et al (2015) Quantitative assessment of patellar vascularity following bone-patellar tendon-bone autograft harvest for ACL reconstruction. Knee Surg Sports Traumatol Arthrosc. 2015 Jan 22. [Epub ahead of print]
81. Shelbourne KD, Trumper RV (1997) Preventing anterior knee pain after anterior cruciate ligament reconstruction. Am J Sports Med 25:41–47
82. Burks RT, Haut RC, Lancaster RL (1990) Biomechanical and histological observations of the dog patellar tendon after removal of its central one-third. Am J Sports Med 18:146–153
83. Beynnon BD et al (1995) Biomechanical assessment of the healing response of the rabbit patellar tendon after removal of its central third. Am J Sports Med 23:452–457
84. Atkinson TS et al (1998) Patellar tendon and infrapatellar fat pad healing after harvest of an ACL graft. Surg Res 79:25–30
85. Shino K et al (1994) Deterioration of patellofemoral articular surfaces after anterior cruciate ligament reconstruction. Am J Sports Med 22:206–211
86. Kartus J et al (1997) Factors affecting donor-site morbidity after anterior cruciate ligament reconstruction using bone-patellar tendon-bone autografts. Knee Surg Sports Traumatol Arthrosc 5:222–228
87. Jackson DW, Schaefer RK (1990) Cyclops syndrome: loss of extension following intra-articular anterior cruciate ligament reconstruction. Arthroscopy 6:171–178
88. Goldblatt JP et al (2005) Reconstruction of the anterior cruciate ligament: meta-analysis of patellar tendon versus hamstring tendon autograft. Arthroscopy 21(7):791–803
89. Berg P, Mjöberg B (1991) A lateral skin incision reduces peripatellar dysaesthesia after knee surgery. J Bone Joint Surg (Br) 73:374–376
90. Kartus J et al (2000) Comparison of traditional and subcutaneous patellar tendon harvest. A prospective study of donor site-related problems after anterior cruciate ligament reconstruction using different graft harvesting techniques. Am J Sports Med 28:328–335
91. Brandsson S et al (1998) Closing patellar tendon defects after anterior cruciate ligament reconstruction. absence of any benefit. Knee Surg Sports Traumatol Arthrosc 62:82–87
92. Frank RM et al (2015) Closure of patellar tendon defect in anterior cruciate ligament reconstruction with bone-patellar tendon-bone autograft: systematic review of randomized controlled trials. Arthroscopy 31(2):329–338

93. Kartus J et al (1999) The localization of the infrapatellar nerves in the anterior knee region with special emphasis on central third patellar tendon harvest. A dissection study on cadaver and amputated specimens. Arthroscopy 15:577–586
94. Cervellin M et al (2012) Autologous platelet-rich plasma gel to reduce donor-site morbidity after patellar tendon graft harvesting for anterior cruciate ligament reconstruction: a randomized, controlled clinical study. Knee Surg Sports Traumatol Arthrosc 20(1):114–120
95. Coupens SD et al (1992) Magnetic resonance imaging evaluation of the patellar tendon after use of its central one-third for anterior cruciate ligament reconstruction. Am J Sports Med 20:332–335
96. Meisterling RC et al (1993) Morphologic changes in the human patellar tendon after bone-tendon-bone anterior cruciate ligament reconstruction. Clin Orthop Relat Res 289:208–212
97. Nixon RG et al (1995) Reconstitution of the patellar tendon donor site after graft harvest. Clin Orthop Relat Res 317:162–171
98. Liu SH et al (1996) MRI and morphology of the insertion of the patellar tendon after graft harvesting. J Bone Joint Surg (Br) 78:823–826
99. Bernicker JP et al (1998) Patellar tendon defect during the first year after anterior cruciate ligament reconstruction appearance on serial magnetic resonance imaging. Arthroscopy 14:804–809
100. Koseoglu K et al (2004) MRI evaluation of patellar tendon defect after harvesting its central third. Eur J Radiol 50(3):292–295
101. Kartus J et al (2000) A radiographic and histologic evaluation of the patellar tendon after harvesting its central third. Am J Sports Med 28:218–226
102. Svensson M et al (2007) Ultrastructural collagen fibril alterations in the patellar tendon 6 years after harvesting its central third. Am J Sports Med 35(2):301–306
103. Svensson M et al (2005) A long-term serial histological evaluation of the patellar tendon in humans after harvesting its central third. Knee Surg Sports Traumatol Arthrosc 13 (5):398–404
104. Karns DJ et al (1994) Case report: revision anterior cruciate ligament reconstruction. Arthroscopy 10:148–151
105. Colosimo AJ et al (2001) Revision anterior cruciate ligament reconstruction with a reharvested ipsilateral patellar tendon. Am J Sports Med 29:746–750
106. Noyes FR, Barber-Westin SD (2001) Revision anterior cruciate surgery with use of bone-patellar tendon-bone autogenous grafts. J Bone Joint Surg Am 83-A:1131–1143
107. O'Shea JJ, Shelbourne KD (2002) Anterior cruciate ligament reconstruction with a reharvested bone-patellar tendon-bone graft. Am J Sports Med 30:208–213
108. Liden M et al (2006) The course of the patellar tendon after reharvesting its central third for ACL revision surgery: a long-term clinical and radiographic study. Knee Surg Sports Traumatol Arthrosc 14(11):1130–1138
109. Stener S et al (2012) The reharvested patellar tendon has the potential for ligamentization when used for anterior cruciate ligament revision surgery. Knee Surg Sports Traumatol Arthrosc 20(6):1168–1174
110. Gobbi A et al (2002) Patellar tendon anterior cruciate ligament reconstruction with conical press-fit femoral fixation: 5-year results in athletes population. Knee Surg Sports Traumatol Arthrosc 10(2):73–79
111. Zeng C et al (2013) Methods and devices for graft fixation in ACLR. Cochrane Syst Rev 9:1–14
112. Hertel P et al (2005) ACL reconstruction using bone-patellar tendon-bone press-fit fixation: 10-year clinical results. Knee Surg Sports Traumatol Arthrosc 13(4):248–255
113. Boszotta H (1997) Arthroscopic anterior cruciate ligament reconstruction using a patella tendon graft in press-fit technique surgical technique and follow-up. Arthroscopy 13:332–339
114. Felmet G (2010) Implant-free press-fit fixation for bone-patellar tendon-bone ACL reconstruction: 10-year results. Arch Orthop Trauma Surg 130(8):985–992

115. Lee YH, Siebold R, Paessler HH (2014) Implant-free ACL reconstruction: a review. Arch Orthop Trauma Surg 134(3):395–404
116. Salmon LJ et al (2006) Long-term outcome of endoscopic anterior cruciate ligament reconstruction with patellar tendon autograft: minimum 13-year review. Am J Sports Med 34 (5):721–732
117. Lebel B et al (2008) Arthroscopic reconstruction of the anterior cruciate ligament using bone-patellar tendon-bone autograft: a minimum 10-year follow-up. Am J Sports Med 36 (7):1275–1282
118. Ahn JH et al (2012) Long-term results of anterior cruciate ligament reconstruction using bone-patellar tendon-bone: an analysis of the factors affecting the development of osteoarthritis. Arthroscopy 28(8):1114–1123
119. Gerhard P et al (2013) Long-term results of arthroscopically assisted anatomical single-bundle anterior cruciate ligament reconstruction using patellar tendon autograft: are there any predictors for the development of osteoarthritis? Knee Surg Sports Traumatol Arthrosc 21 (4):957–964
120. Rodriguez-Merchan EC et al (2014) Arthroscopic BPTB graft reconstruction in ACL ruptures: 15-year results and survival. Knee 21(5):902–905
121. Maletis GB et al (2013) Reconstruction of the anterior cruciate ligament association of graft choice with increased risk of early revision. Bone Joint J 95-B:623–628
122. Anderson AF, Snyder RB, Lipscomb JAB (2001) ACLR: a prospective randomized study of three surgical methods. Am J Sports Med 29:272–279
123. Sajovic M et al (2006) A prospective, randomized comparison of semitendinosus and gracilis tendon versus patellar tendon autografts for anterior cruciate ligament reconstruction: five-year follow-up. Am J Sports Med 34(12):1933–1940
124. Liden M et al (2007) Patellar tendon or semitendinosus tendon autografts for anterior cruciate ligament reconstruction: a prospective, randomized study with a 7-year follow-up. Am J Sports Med 35(5):740–748
125. Barenius B et al (2010) Quality of life and clinical outcome after anterior cruciate ligament reconstruction using patellar tendon graft or quadrupled semitendinosus graft: an 8-year follow-up of a randomized controlled trial. Am J Sports Med 38(8):1533–1541
126. Leys T et al (2012) Clinical results and risk factors for reinjury 15 years after anterior cruciate ligament reconstruction: a prospective study of hamstring and patellar tendon grafts. Am J Sports Med 40(3):595–605
127. Gifstad T et al (2013) Long-term follow-up of patellar tendon grafts or hamstring tendon grafts in endoscopic ACL reconstructions. Knee Surg Sports Traumatol Arthrosc 21 (3):576–583
128. Yunes M et al (2001) Patellar versus hamstring tendons in anterior cruciate ligament reconstruction. Arthroscopy 17(3):248–257
129. Freedman KB et al (2003) Arthroscopic anterior cruciate ligament reconstruction: a metaanalysis comparing patellar tendon and hamstring tendon autografts. Am J Sports Med 31:2–11
130. Reinhardt KR, Hetsroni I, Marxm RG (2010) Graft selection for ACLR A level II systematic review comparing failure rates and functional outcomes. Orthop Clin N Am 41:249–262
131. Mohtadi NG et al (2011) Patellar tendon versus hamstring tendon autograft for anterior cruciate ligament rupture in adults. Cochrane Database Syst Rev 9:CD005960
132. Li S et al (2012) A systematic review of randomized controlled clinical trials comparing hamstring autografts versus bone-patellar tendon-bone autografts for the reconstruction of the anterior cruciate ligament. Arch Orthop Trauma Surg 132(9):1287–1297
133. Xie X et al (2015) A meta-analysis of bone-patellar tendon-bone autograft versus four-strand hamstring tendon autograft for anterior cruciate ligament reconstruction. Knee 22 (2):100–110

134. Xie X et al (2015) Increased incidence of osteoarthritis of knee joint after ACL reconstruction with bone-patellar tendon-bone autografts than hamstring autografts: a meta-analysis of 1,443 patients at a minimum of 5 years. Eur J Orthop Surg Traumatol 25(1):149–159

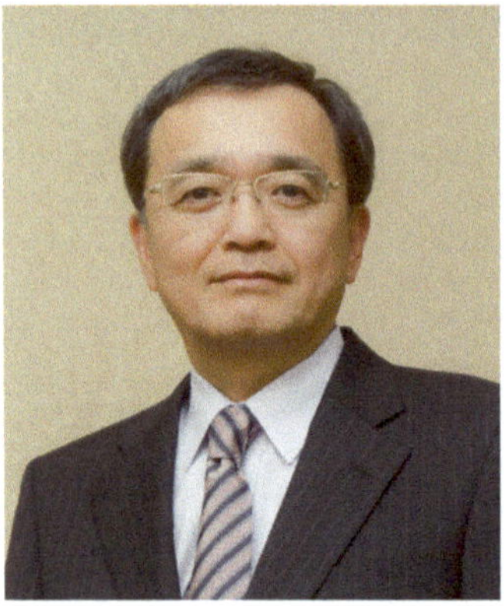

Shuji Horibe, MD., PhD, Faculty of Comprehensive Rehabilitation, Osaka Prefecture University, Osaka, Japan.

Chapter 30
Anatomical Rectangular Tunnel ACL Reconstruction with a Bone-Patellar Tendon-Bone Graft

Konsei Shino and Tatsuo Mae

Abstract The anatomical rectangular tunnel ACL reconstruction with a bone-patellar tendon-bone (BTB) graft (ART BTB ACLR) to mimic natural ACL fiber arrangement was developed. This technique has the following advantages: (1) to mimic fiber orientation inside the native ACL with a single BTB graft, (2) to maximize the graft-tunnel contact area, (3) to keep the tunnel apertures inside the ACL attachment areas, (4) to prevent improper rotation of the graft inside the tunnels during or after its fixation, and (5) to preserve the notch anatomy. This procedure has been making it possible to overcome instability due to loss of ACL without loss of motion.

Keywords Bone-patellar tendon-bone (BTB) graft • Far anteromedial portal • Rectangular tunnel • Notchplasty • Resident's ridge

30.1 Introduction

It is needless to say that our goal for ACL reconstruction (ACLR) is to restore stability without loss of motion. For achieving this goal, we believe it is very important to mimic the native ACL with a graft as closely as possible. This makes it possible for the graft to avoid impingement to the intercondylar notch or the posterior cruciate ligament (PCL). Thus, it is mandatory to select a suitable graft and to place it in strictly anatomical tunnels.

An autogenous bone-patellar tendon-bone (BTB) graft is one of the most suitable tissues for ACLR [1]. The procedure with the graft of 10 mm width is one of most frequently performed procedures, while it has been aiming at achieving

K. Shino, M.D., PhD (✉)
Sports Orthopaedic Center, Yukioka Hospital, 2-2-3 Ukita, Kita-ku, Osaka 530-0021, Japan
e-mail: shinok0220@gmail.com

T. Mae
Department of Orthopaedic Surgery, Osaka University Medical School, Osaka, Japan

M. Ochi et al. (eds.), *ACL Injury and Its Treatment*,
DOI 10.1007/978-4-431-55858-3_30

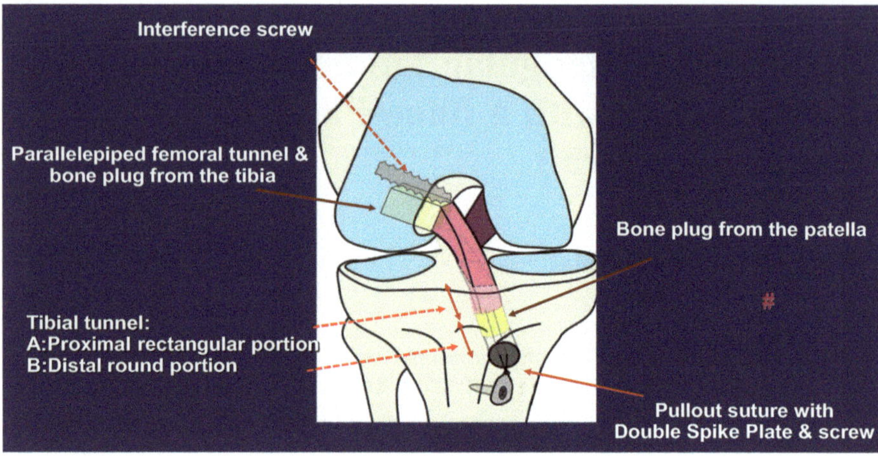

Fig. 30.1 Schema of the anatomical rectangular tunnel (ART) BTB ACL reconstruction via rectangular femoral and half rectangular tibial tunnels. For femoral side fixation, 6-mm interference screw is applied. For tibial side, pullout suture fixation technique using the double spike plate (*DSP*) and a screw is used

a single bundle reconstruction through round tunnels [2]. In this procedure, the following issues yet remained unsolved: (1) The graft could not mimic the natural fiber arrangement inside the ACL; (2) there is unfavorable space between a trapezoid or triangular pillar bone plug and the round femoral tunnel; (3) there is disadvantageous space between the proximal portion of the round tibial tunnel and tendinous portion of the graft. In order to overcome these issues, the anatomical rectangular tunnel (ART) ACLR was developed. In this procedure [3, 4], the BTB graft is placed to mimic fiber arrangement inside the normal ACL [4], as well as to maximize the graft-tunnel contact area. Concretely, parallelepiped tunnels are created in accordance with the rectangular cross section of the graft. Furthermore, half rectangular/round tibial tunnel makes it possible for the distal tendinous portion of the graft to fit the tibial tunnel wall (Fig. 30.1). The instruments for the procedure were developed in cooperation with Smith & Nephew, Andover, MA (Fig. 30.2).

30.2 Rationale for Anatomic Grafting

1. The attachment areas should not thoroughly be filled out with the grafts, because grafts used for ACLR become hypertrophic after implantation [5] and because they are greater in mechanical properties than the native ACL [6].

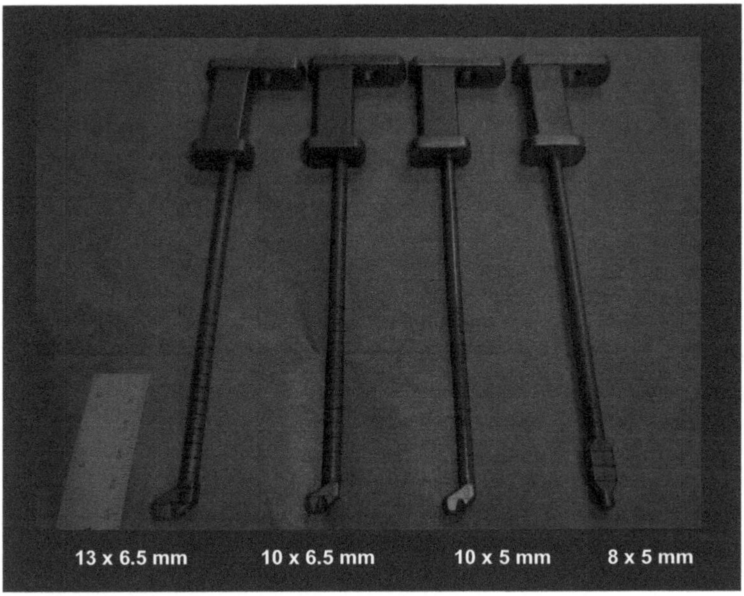

Fig. 30.2 Set of rectangular dilators: 13 × 6.5, 10 × 6.5, 10 × 5, and 8 × 5 mm

2. Grafts must be off-centered inside the areas for them to properly function stabilize the knee, as the grafts deforms according to tensile force.
3. Tunnel apertures should be created inside the attachment areas not only for mimicking the native ACL but also for keeping them inside the areas of thicker cortex to make the apertures robust [7].

30.3 Indications for BTB Grafting

The BTB graft is suitable not only in shape but in mechanical properties, as described previously. However, people should be aware that BTB graft harvest site morbidity is relatively high, as a few of our female patients were suffering from arthrofibrosis postoperatively. However, the integration of bone plug to bone tunnel wall is very early in the anatomical rectangular tunnel (ART) ACLR procedure [8]. Therefore, this graft may be selected for the following population: male athletes with high motivation for returning strenuous/contact sports including football or judo.

30.4 Surgical Technique

30.4.1 Bone-Patellar Tendon-Bone (BTB) Graft Harvest and Preparation

While the width of the patellar tendon is relatively consistent among people, a 10-mm-wide graft is suitable for more than 90 % of our patients. Thus, the 10-mm-wide graft harvesting is described in this section. However, an 8-mm graft is applied for small female patients, while a 13-mm graft is used for large male patients.

The graft is harvested through 5–6-cm longitudinal skin incision just medial to the patellar tendon from the central portion of the medial half of the patellar tendon. As the central portion of the tendon is shorter than the lateral or medial side, the graft has longer and shorter side in its tendinous portion. The former is assigned to anteromedial portion of the graft, and the shorter one is to the posterolateral portion (Fig. 30.3).

The harvested graft is prepared as follows: the bone plug from the tibia is shaped into a parallelepiped of 5 mm thick × 10 mm wide × 15 mm long and used for the femoral tunnel. The patellar bone block is left as a triangular pillar for the tibial tunnel (Fig. 30.3)

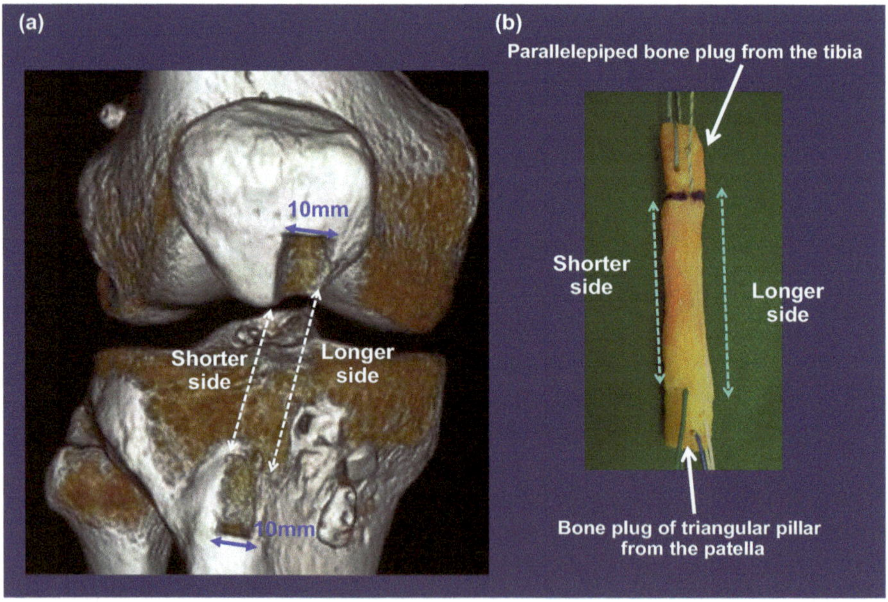

Fig. 30.3 Graft harvest and preparation. (**a**) BTB graft harvest site of the *central* portion of the medial half of the patellar tendon of the *right* knee. The tendinous portion of the graft has longer and shorter sides. (**b**) Prepared graft of 10-mm in width of the *right* knee. The parallelepiped bone plug from the tibia of 5 mm thick × 10 mm wide × 15 mm long is for the rectangular femoral tunnel, while patellar bone block of a triangular pillar is for the distal round portion of the tibial tunnel

To minimize the graft harvest site morbidity, the defect in the tibial tubercle due to bone plug harvesting should be filled with cancellous bone obtained at the time of creating the tibial tunnel.

30.4.2 Setup and Arthroscopic Portals (Fig. 30.3)

The thigh is routinely kept horizontal with a leg holder to obtain a consistent view of the intercondylar notch, while the calf is hung down with gravity. In addition to the regular anterolateral and anteromedial portals, the far anteromedial (FAM) portal which is 2–2.5 cm posterior to the anteromedial portal and just above the medial meniscus is routinely created. This portal makes it possible for instruments to get more perpendicular access to the ACL femoral attachment area on the lateral wall of the notch [9].

30.4.3 Femoral Tunnel Preparation

30.4.3.1 Exposure of the ACL Femoral Attachment Area

Viewing the posterior third of the lateral wall of the notch via the anteromedial portal, the fibrous tissues including ACL stump on superior-posterior half of the lateral wall of the intercondylar notch is thoroughly removed using a radiofrequency device through the FAM portal. Mechanical shavers are not utilized in order to preserve subtle undulation of the bony surface around the attachment area. After cleaning up, the crescent-shaped attachment area is clearly delineated by the resident's ridge, anteriorly; upper cartilage margin, superiorly; and posterior cartilage margin, posteriorly (Fig. 30.4) [10–12].

30.4.3.2 Creation of the Femoral Tunnel

Inside-Out Technique Through the FAM Portal

After marking two points with 5-mm distance in the center of the attachment area along its long axis using a micro-fracture awl or RF device (Fig. 30.4), two guide pins are parallelly drilled from these points to the lateral femoral cortex via the FAM portal with the knee flexed over 140 °. The proximal pin is over-drilled with a 5.0-mm cannulated drill bit to the lateral femoral cortex, while the distal one is over-drilled to 20 mm in depth. The continuous two round holes are dilated into a $5 \times 10 \times 22$-mm parallelepiped socket with the 5 x 10-mm cannulated dilator. Then the socket is rasped to make the wall smooth and flat.

Notchplasty is not required unless marginal osteophytes are formed.

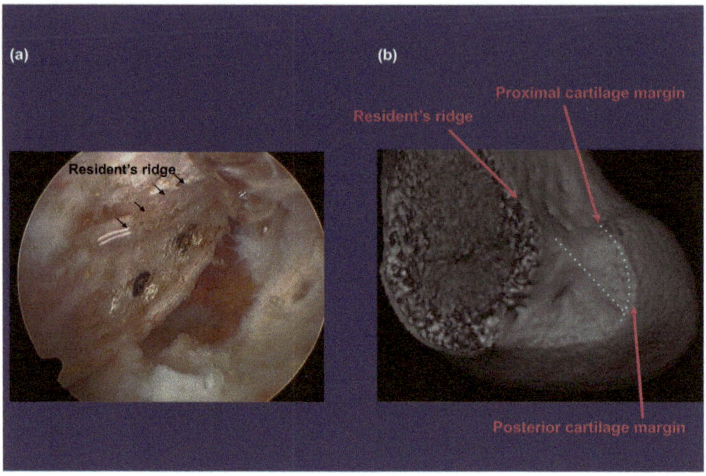

Fig. 30.4 ACL femoral attachment area of the *right* knee. (**a**) Arthroscopic view via the anteromedial portal with a 45 °arthroscope; (**b**) 3D CT view. There are three landmarks to identify the attachment area: resident's ridge, *proximal* cartilage margin, posterior cartilage margin

Outside-In Technique Through the Lateral Incision

For the knee of passive flexion less than 140 °, this approach is recommended to avoid blowout of the tunnel. Viewing the ACL femoral attachment area via the anteromedial portal, a central guide pin is drilled into the center of the area from the lateral femoral cortex with the anterolateral entry femoral guide (Smith & Nephew # 6901189 or 7210984) via the anterolateral portal. A 10-mm skin protection cannula is installed over the guide pin via 2-cm lateral femoral incision. With the aid of a 10-mm Offset Drill Guide, two guide pins are drilled parallel to the central pin along the long axis of the attachment area or the resident's ridge. After the central pin is removed, two guide pins are over-drilled with 5-mm drill bit. With the dilator of 5 × 10 mm from the lateral femoral cortex, the two drill holes are dilated into one rectangular tunnel in outside-in fashion (Fig. 30.6a).

30.4.4 Tibial Tunnel Preparation

30.4.4.1 Marking of the Tunnel Aperture Area Inside the ACL Tibial Attachment

Viewing down the ACL tibial remnant and/or attachment area via the anteromedial portal, the stump is cut to 3–5 mm in length with a shaver. Viewing the anterior and medial margin of the residual fibers of ACL, and the anterior horn of the lateral

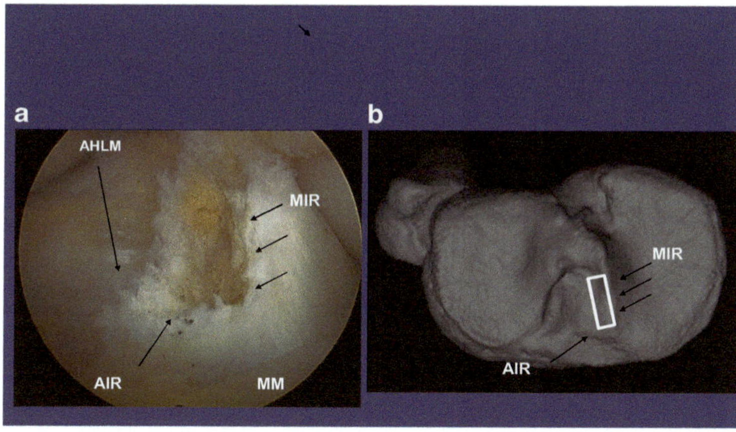

Fig. 30.5 ACL tibial attachment area of the *right* knee. (**a**) Arthroscopic view via the anteromedial portal with a 45 °arthroscope; (**b**) 3D CT view. There are three landmarks to identify the attachment area: medial intercondylar ridge (*MIR*), anterior intercondylar ridge (*AIR*), and anterior horn of the lateral meniscus (*AHLM*). *MM* medial meniscus

meniscus, the targeted tunnel aperture area along the medial intercondylar ridge inside the tibial attachment is marked with RF device [1, 10] (Fig. 30.5).

30.4.4.2 Outside-In Creation of the Half Rectangular/Round Tibial Tunnel

Viewing down the attachment area via the anteromedial portal, the tip of the tibial drill guide through the FAM portal is placed at the center of the area. The pin is over-drilled halfway or 2–2.5 cm with a 10-mm cannulated drill bit or a bone dowel harvester for a bone plug to be grafted to defects in the graft harvest site. The anterior and posterior pins are drilled in line with the medial intercondylar ridge with 5-mm distance using an Offset Pin Guide. After removing the central pin, they are over-drilled with a 5.0-mm cannulated drill bit, respectively, followed by dilation into a 5 x 10-mm rectangle (Fig. 30.6b).

30.4.5 Graft Tensioning and Fixation

With two leading sutures, the graft is passed from the tibial tunnel to the femoral socket with its parallelepiped bone plug kept on the top, and with its cancellous bone surface maintained anteriorly.

For femoral fixation, a 6-mm × 20–30-mm interference screw is used in outside-in fashion through the 5-mm hole from the lateral femoral cortex to the bottom of

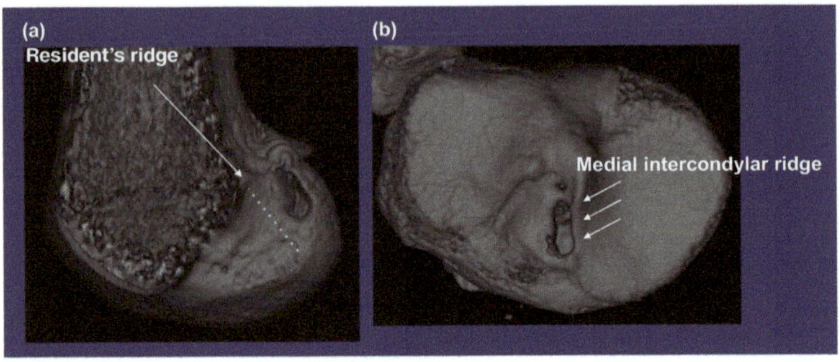

Fig. 30.6 3D CT views on tunnel apertures after ART ACLR (*right* knee) (medial half of the femur is removed). (**a**) Femoral tunnel aperture; (**b**) tibial tunnel aperture

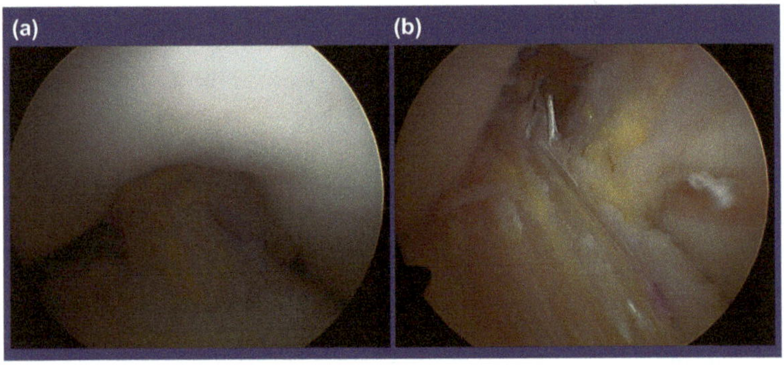

Fig. 30.7 An anatomically placed BTB graft of the right knee viewed through the anterolateral portal; (**a**) in extension; (**b**) in flexion. Note no graft impingement to the notch or PCL

the socket using a 6.5-mm skin protector (Smith & Nephew #6901106) via an additional small lateral femoral incision. For inside-out interference fixation, the screw is introduced through the FAM portal. Otherwise, the other pullout techniques including DSP (Double Spike Plate, MEIRA, Aichi, Japan) and screw through an additional lateral skin incision of 3–4 cm are utilized [13].

After the femoral fixation, the relationship between the notch in extension or the posterior cruciate ligament (PCL) in flexion should be observed. If the graft is placed anatomically correct, there is no impingent of the graft against the notch or PCL (Fig. 30.7).

Tibial fixation is achieved with a modified pullout suture technique using the DSP system at an optional/predetermined amount of the initial tension. According to our cadaveric experiment, the mean laxity match tension for the ART ACLR knees was 8.6 ± 4.8 N, the recommended initial tension to the graft at the time of its final fixation could be reasonably assumed to 10 to 20 N [13].

The tensioning sutures distally connected to DSP are tied to a tensioner mounted on the metal shell boot fixed to the tibia with a bandage. Then the creep of the construct is meticulously removed by repetitive manual pulls of the graft suture with knee flexed 15–20 °. After the reading of the tensioner is stabilized at the intended level of 10–20 N for 2 min, the graft is temporarily fixed by hammering DSP bottom spikes into the tibial cortex, and the DSP is secured with a screw. Care is taken to remove the periosteum where the DSP is placed.

30.5 Postoperative Rehabilitation

The knee is splint immobilized at 10 ° flexion for 1 week, followed by passive and active ROM exercises. Partial weight bearing is allowed at 2 weeks followed by full weight bearing at 4–5 weeks. Full extension or flexion exceeding 130 ° is not permitted until 5 weeks. Jogging is recommended at 3 months. Return to strenuous activity is not allowed until 6 months.

30.6 Discussion

Data on patient's outcomes after the current procedure have been accumulated for submission to be published.

Unless the patients sustained the graft rupture due to trauma, our goal of restoration of stability without loss of motion has been achieved in more than 95 % of the patients. Furthermore, tunnel expansion following the current procedure is much less than that after the reconstruction using hamstring tendons [14].

There is a concern on higher graft rupture rate following the anatomic ACLR compared to that after less anatomic ACLRs in the last century [15], while subsequent meniscal damage after ACLR decreased drastically. The more strenuous sports patients returned with totally stable knee, the higher the graft rupture rate could be. Improved rehabilitation or proprioceptive training may be required to prevent secondary ACL injury, while it is important to let the patients know the risk management on it.

30.7 Conclusion

ACL reconstruction should be performed to mimic the native ACL by grafting (Fig. 30.8). Thus, the surgery should be anatomy based. The emphasis is on tunnel apertures inside the attachment areas, proper graft choice and preparation, correct orientation of the graft, and appropriate graft tensioning and fixation. Our goal is to restore healthy knee by the real anatomic ACL grafting.

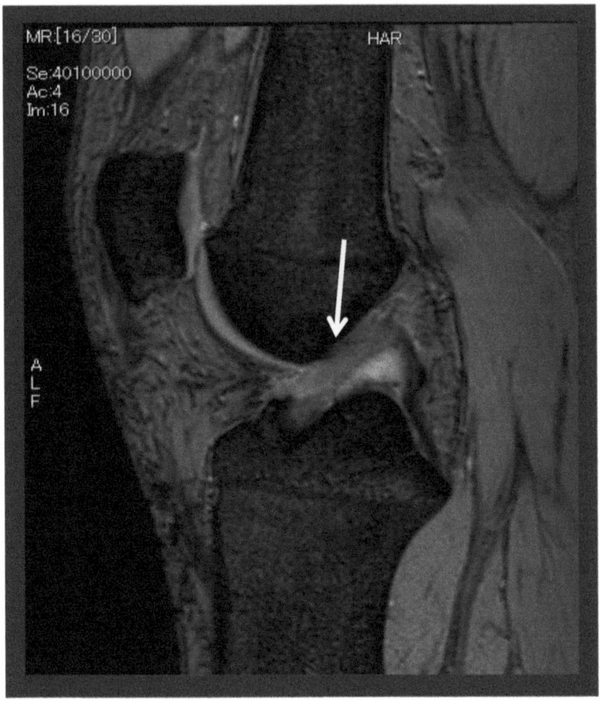

Fig. 30.8 An example of 1-year-old ART BTB ACL graft shown in T2-weighted sagittal MR image. The graft is running along the Blumensaat's line like the native ACL in extention, while the femur-tibia relationship is normally maintained

References

1. Siebold R, Schumacher P, Fernandez F, Smigielski R, Fink C, Brehmer A, Kirsch J (2015) Flat midsubstance of the anterior cruciate ligament with tibial "C"-shaped insertion site. Knee Surg Sports Traumatol Arthosc 23:3136–3142
2. Suzuki T, Shino K, Otsubo H, Suzuki D, Mae T, Fujimiya M, Yamashita T, Fujie H (2014) Biomechanical comparison between the rectangular-tunnel and the round-tunnel anterior cruciate ligament reconstruction procedures with a bone patellar tendon bone graft. Arthroscopy 30:1294–1302
3. Shino K, Nakata K, Nakamura N, Toritsuka Y, Nakagawa S, Horibe S (2005) Anatomically-oriented ACL reconstruction with a bone-patellar tendon graft via rectangular socket/tunnels: a snug-fit and impingement-free grafting technique. Arthroscopy 21:1402.e1–1402.e5
4. Shino K, Nakata K, Horibe S, Nakamura N, Toritsuka Y, Nakagawa S, Suzuki T (2008) Rectangular tunnel double-bundle anterior cruciate ligament reconstruction with bone–patellar tendon–bone graft to mimic natural fiber arrangement. Arthroscopy 24:1178–1183
5. Hamada M, Shino K, Horibe S, Mitsuoka T, Toritsuka Y, Nakamura N (2005) Changes in cross-sectional area of hamstring anterior cruciate ligament grafts as a function of time following transplantation. Arthroscopy 21:917–922
6. Noyes FR, Butler DL, Grood ES, Zernicke RF, Hefzy MS (1984) Biomechanical analysis of human ligament grafts used in knee-ligament repairs and reconstructions. J Bone Joint Surg 66-A:344–352

7. Hutchinson MR, Ash SA (2003) Resident's ridge: assessing the cortical thickness of the lateral wall and roof of the intercondylar notch. Arthroscopy 19:931–935
8. Suzuki T, Shino K, Nakamura N, Iwahashi T, Nakata K, Tanaka Y, Nakagawa S, Kinugasa K, Yamashita T (2011) Early integration of a bone plug in the femoral tunnel in rectangular tunnel ACL reconstruction with a bone-patellar tendon-bone graft: a prospective computed tomography analysis. Knee Surg Sports Traumatol Arthrosc 19(Suppl 1):S29–S35
9. Shino K, Horibe S, Hamada M, Nakamura N, Nakata K, Mae T, Toritsuka Y (2002) Allograft anterior cruciate ligament reconstruction. Tech Knee Surg 1:78–85
10. Purnell ML, Larson AI, Clancy WG (2008) Anterior cruciate ligament insertions on the tibia and femur and their relationships to critical bony landmarks using high-resolution volume-rendering computed tomography. Am J Sports Med 36:2083–2090
11. Iwahashi T, Shino K, Nakata K, Otsubo H, Suzuki T, Amano H, Nakamura N (2010) Direct ACL insertion to the femur assessed by histology and three-dimensional volume-rendered computed tomography. Arthroscopy 26:S13–S20
12. Shino K, Suzuki T, Iwahashi T, Mae T, Nakata K, Nakamura N, Nakagawa S (2010) The resident's ridge as an arthroscopic landmark for anatomical femoral tunnel drilling in ACL reconstruction. Knee Surg Sports Traumatol Arthosc 18:1164–1168
13. Shino K, Mae T, Maeda A, Miyama T, Shinjo H, Kawakami H (2002) Graft fixation with pre-determined tension using a new device, the double spike plate. Arthroscopy 18:908–911
14. Tachibana Y, Mae T, Shino K, Kanamoto T, Sugamoto K, Yoshikawa H, Nakata K (2015) Morphological changes in femoral tunnels after anatomic anterior cruciate ligament reconstruction. Knee Surg Sports Traumatol Arthrosc 23(12):3591–3600
15. Mae T, Shino K, Matsumoto N, Yoneda K, Yoshikawa H, Nakata K (2014) Risk factors for ipsi-lateral graft rupture or contralateral anterior cruciate ligament tear after anatomic double-bundle reconstruction. A-P SMART 1:90–95

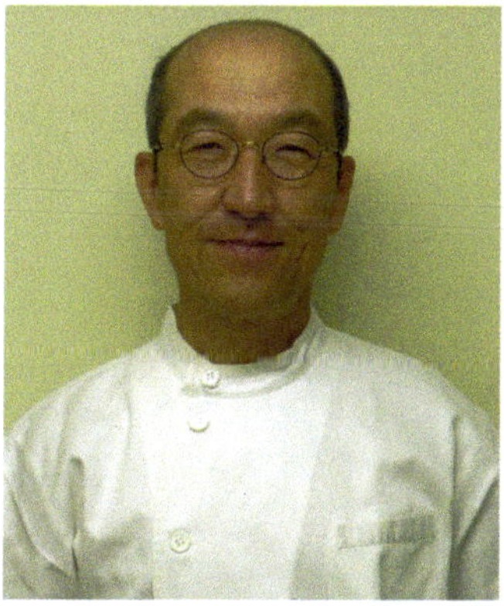

Konsei Shino, M.D., PhD, Sports Orthopaedic Center, Yukioka Hospital, Osaka, Japan.

Chapter 31
Rectangular vs. Round Tunnel

Tomoyuki Suzuki and Konsei Shino

Abstract There are several advantages of the rectangular tunnel over the round tunnel anterior cruciate ligament reconstruction (ACLR). First, the rectangular tunnel procedure enables the placing of a 10-mm wide bone–patellar tendon–bone (BPTB) graft in the tunnel within the anatomic attachment area. Second, the bone plug can be matched to the parallelepiped bone tunnel with subsequent interference screw fixation. This enables earlier integration of the bone plug to the femoral tunnel wall by maximizing the interface of the graft and tunnel wall. Finally, there are better biomechanical performances: (1) the mean laxity match pretension for the rectangular tunnel ACL-reconstructed knees is 8.6 ± 4.8 N, whereas that for the round tunnel ACL-reconstructed knees is 34.8 ± 9.3 N. (2) The rectangular tunnel ACLR knees demonstrate significantly higher stability against combined rotatory loads following laxity match tensioning. (3) The kinematics of rectangular tunnel ACLR knees far closely resembles the kinematics of normal knees compared with that of the round tunnel ACLR knees following laxity match pretensioning of the graft.

Keywords Anterior cruciate ligament reconstruction (ACLR) • Rectangular tunnel ACLR • Round tunnel ACLR • Bone–patellar tendon–bone (BPTB) graft

31.1 Introduction

Shino developed the anatomic rectangular tunnel ACLR using a bone–patellar tendon–bone (BPTB) graft to mimic the natural fiber arrangement inside the native ACL and to minimize the tunnel size [1, 2]. With this technique, ACLR based on the double-bundle concept with a single BPTB graft can be achieved. Because the crescent-shaped ACL femoral attachment area located at the posterior superior

T. Suzuki, M.D. (✉)
The Department of Orthopaedic Surgery, Sapporo Medical University Graduate School of Medicine, South 1 West 16, Chuo-ku, Sapporo, Hokkaido 060-8456, Japan
e-mail: suzutomo@sapmed.ac.jp

K. Shino
Sports Orthopaedic Center, Yukioka Hospital, 2-2-3 Ukita, Kita-ku, Osaka 530-0021, Japan

M. Ochi et al. (eds.), *ACL Injury and Its Treatment*,
DOI 10.1007/978-4-431-55858-3_31

margin of the lateral wall of the notch is <10 mm wide [3, 4], this technique enables us to create a robust tunnel aperture inside the attachment area with greater cortical thickness [5, 6].

31.2 ACL Attachment Area and Optimized Tunnels for ACLR

It has been proved that the bony ridge termed "resident's ridge" (lateral intercondylar ridge) is an important landmark as the anterior border of the femoral attachment of the ACL [3, 4, 7]. Iwahashi et al. reported the ACL femoral attachment area is 17.4 ± 0.9 mm (mean ± SD) in length, 8.0 ± 0.5 mm in width, and 128.3 ± 10.5 mm^2 in area [7]; therefore, as depicted in Fig. 31.1, a 10-mm diameter round tunnel for a 10-mm wide bone plug cannot be created posterior to the resident's ridge. Therefore, for the round tunnel ACLR in our biomechanical study, a round femoral tunnel proximal to the isometric point is created using the transtibial approach. Furthermore, on the tibial side, a 10-mm round tunnel within the ACL attachment area may damage the insertion of the lateral meniscus [7, 8], as observed in Fig. 31.1. In contrast, with the rectangular tunnel ACLR, in which the femoral and tibial tunnels are individually created inside the attachment areas, the graft placement closely replicating the native ACL can be achieved [1, 2, 9].

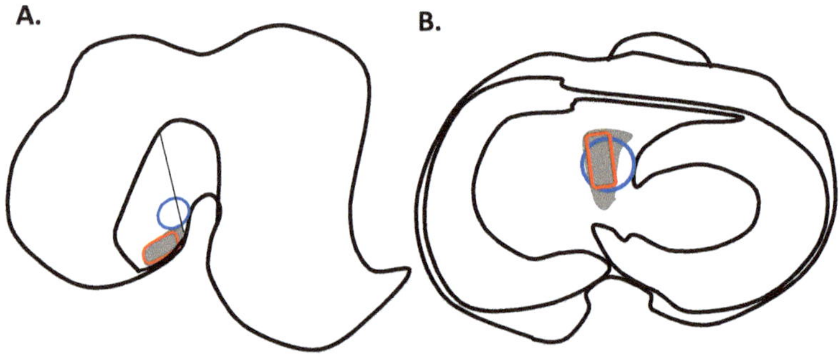

Fig. 31.1 Tunnel position on the femur. (**a**) The *shaded area* represents the original ACL attachment area on the femur. The *red area* indicates the 5 × 10 mm rectangular aperture. The *blue circle* indicates the point at which a 10-mm diameter round tunnel is drilled. (**b**) The shaded area represents the area where the original ACL is attached to the tibia. Because of its proximity to the insertion of the lateral meniscus, the attachment area is narrow. The *red area* represents the 5 × 10 mm rectangular aperture. The *blue circle* indicates the point at which a 10-mm diameter round tunnel is drilled

31.3 Early Integration of a Bone Plug

The BPTB graft during the rectangular tunnel ACLR is placed not only to mimic the natural fiber arrangement of normal ACL following the double-bundle reconstruction concept but also to maximize graft-tunnel contact area [1, 2, 9]. Thus, a parallelepiped femoral tunnel with a rectangular aperture is created according to the rectangular cross section of the graft, enabling accelerated graft–bone integration in the femoral tunnel (Fig. 31.2). Thus, we evaluated minute changes in bone plug integration to the femoral tunnel wall using macroscopic analysis of slices using computed tomography (CT) with multiplanar reconstruction (MPR) images and examined macroscopically undetectable changes using CT values [10] (Fig. 31.3). In our study, 20 patients underwent multidetector CT-MPR first at 3–5 weeks and then again at 7–8 weeks, postoperatively. During the first postoperative week (days 2 and 4), all slices were macroscopically "incomplete" with a clear gap, resulting in a classification of "poor" integration. Excellent integration of the bone plug was observed in 55% of the cases at 4 weeks and 80% at 8 weeks postoperatively. The normalized change in the CT value [shown in Hounsfield units (HU)] at the border of the bone plug tunnel at 8 weeks was significantly lower than that at 4 weeks. Thus, it could be assumed that the bone plugs were mostly integrated into the femoral tunnel by 8 weeks after the rectangular tunnel ACLR using a BPTB graft (Fig. 31.3). Clancy et al. [11] reported that the bone plug in a round bone tunnel

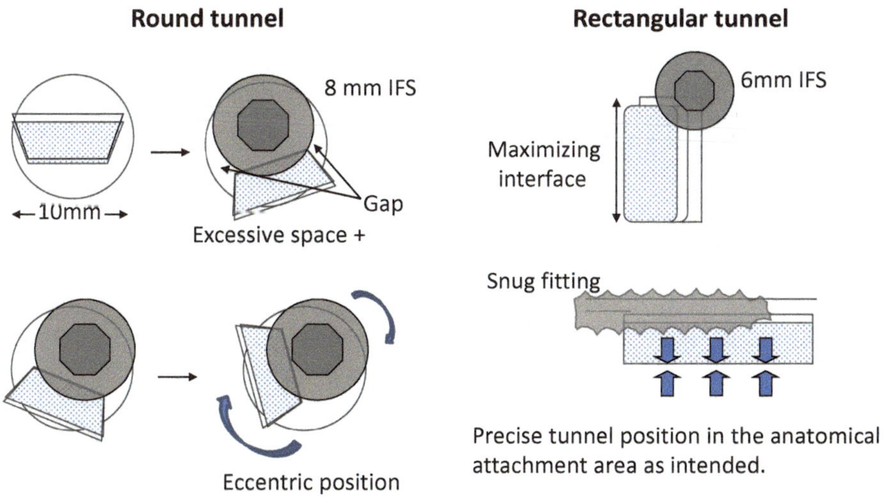

Fig. 31.2 Conventional interference screw fixation to a round bone tunnel may create excessive bone gap at the graft–bone tunnel interface. Moreover, it may be difficult to fix the graft in the anatomical position as intended. In contrast, the rectangular tunnel procedure provides advantages, such as permitting precise tunnel drilling in the anatomical position as intended and providing a snug fit of the bone plug in the tunnel, enabling contact bone healing, and accelerating graft-tunnel integration as demonstrated in this study

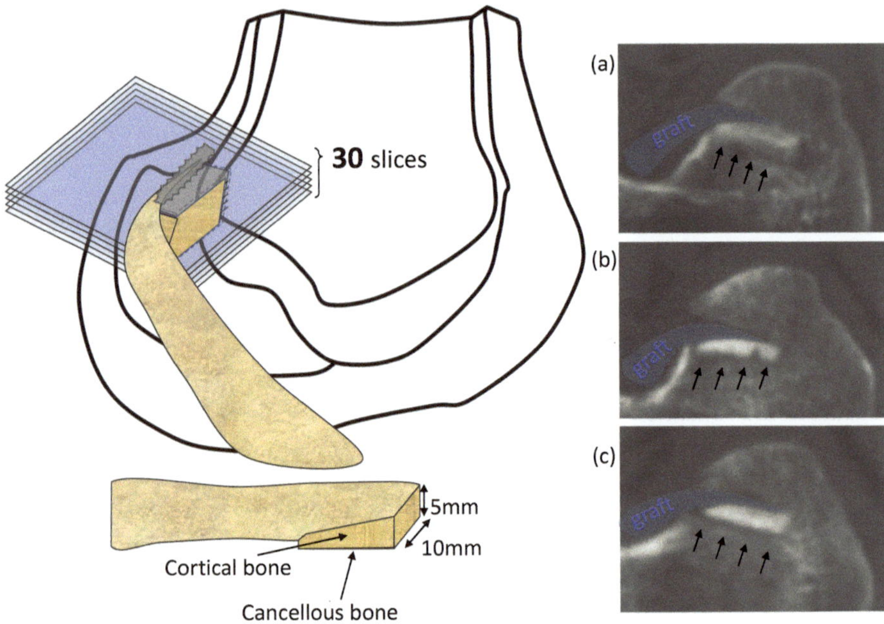

Fig. 31.3 The femoral bone plug is prepared from the tibial tubercle. The tendinous portion is placed posteriorly. The graft is fixed with an interference screw exactly posterior superior to the bone plug, enabling the reconstruction of the final bone–tendon junction at the femoral joint that can successfully mimic the native ACL fiber arrangement. There are 30 slices that are reconstructed using multiplanar reconstruction, parallel to the long axis of the bone plug as indicated above. This permits the evaluation of the anterior interface at all slices. On morphological CT evaluation, 30 reconstructed slices are divided into the following three phases: (1) "complete" shows no border between the plug and tunnel wall, and it does not exhibit trabecular continuity. (2) "Incomplete" has a visible hairline of <1 mm. (3) "Gap" has a visible gap of >1 mm. Further, results are classified into three groups by number of "complete" slices

established histological fixation at 8 weeks postoperatively in rhesus monkeys. In clinical studies, Lomasney used CT images to demonstrate successful fixation in 28.6% of cases at 8 weeks postoperatively after conventional surgery with a BPTB graft and a round bone tunnel [12]. Thus, the 8-week period for bone plug integration into the femoral tunnel after the rectangular tunnel ACLR with a BPTB graft could be assumed to be shorter than that after the conventional round tunnel ACLR.

There are two types of healing processes following a bone plug within the tunnel [13–15]. In indirect healing, granulation tissue is generated between bone segments, resulting in callus development. This is followed by an increase in the gap between bone segments, which is finally filled by neonatal bone [13, 14]. In contrast, direct healing proceeds without the generation of callus at the boundary or the bone absorption at the bone edge at the interface; thus, the gap is not formed in a mechanically stable environment. Our morphological CT evaluation indicated that direct healing occurred following the surgical technique used in our study, indicating that early biological fixation is likely with this technique. If a gap was formed at the interface, a postoperative period of 8 weeks will be insufficient to fill the gap.

31.4 Biomechanical Study: Rectangular Versus Round Tunnel ACLR

31.4.1 Laxity Match Pretension

A key factor for successful ACLR is the initial graft tension. There is a close correlation between the initial tension required to control abnormal anterior laxity and the tunnel position [17–20]. Thus, the biomechanical study on human cadaveric knees was conducted to determine the desirable graft tension in the rectangular tunnel ACLR in which the femoral tunnel creation is independent of the tibial tunnel or the round tunnel ACLR in which the femoral tunnel is created via the transtibial tunnel [16] (Fig. 31.4). We found that at 15° of flexion, the mean laxity match pretension for the rectangular tunnel ACL-reconstructed knees was 8.6 ± 4.8 N, whereas that for the round tunnel ACL-reconstructed knees was 34.8 ± 9.3 N. Thus, initial graft tension required to restore normal anteroposterior

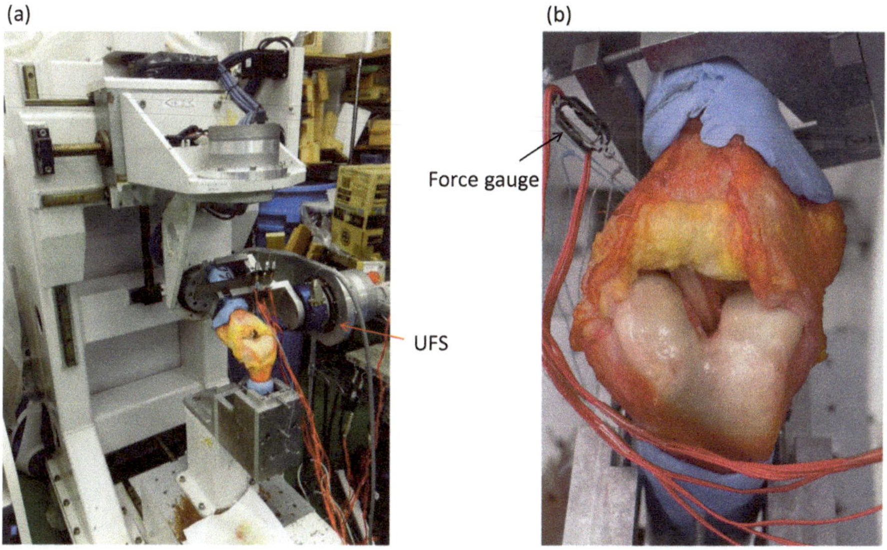

Fig. 31.4 (**a**) Robotic/universal force–moment sensor (UFS) testing system showing a *left knee* mounted for testing. (**b**) *Right knee*, after the removal of the extensor mechanism. Because the robotic arm fitted with the UFS comprises the upper part of the system, the femur is fixed to the *bottom* and the tibia is held on *top*. The custom-made force gauge is fixed on the tibia

(AP) laxity for the rectangular tunnel ACLR is smaller than that for the round tunnel ACLR, suggesting that the rectangular tunnel ACLR can control AP instability more efficiently than the round tunnel ACLR.

31.4.2 Kinematics and External Load Test

Three-dimensional paths were recorded to clarify the knee joint kinematics. If the graft is placed in the isometric position during the round tunnel ACLR, initial graft tension should be increased to restore normal AP stability, resulting in abnormal knee kinematics. Thus, in the round tunnel ACL-reconstructed knees with a higher initial graft tension, the tibia moved posterolaterally with external and valgus rotation, suggesting abnormal joint kinematics. Furthermore, we found that the amount of displacement in the rectangular tunnel ACL-reconstructed knees was <1 mm compared with that in the normal knees in all flexion angles, with a slight over-tightness while approaching extension and slight looseness during flexion. In contrast, the round tunnel ACL-reconstructed knees demonstrated looseness while approaching extension and over-tightness during flexion.

An external load test was conducted to compare the biomechanical behavior of the rectangular tunnel ACL-reconstructed knee with that of the round tunnel ACL-reconstructed knee (Fig. 31.4). The mean anterior laxity of rectangular tunnel ACL-reconstructed knees at 30° flexion with 5 Nm of internal rotation and 10 Nm of valgus moment load was 0.4 mm greater than that of the normal knee, whereas the mean anterior laxity of the round tunnel ACL-reconstructed knees under the same conditions was 0.8 mm greater than that of the normal knee.

31.5 Conclusion

The rectangular tunnel ACLR is superior to the round tunnel ACLR in biological and biomechanical aspects, mimicking the native ACL or to pursue the primary goal of ACLR.

References

1. Shino K, Nakata K, Nakamura N, Toritsuka Y, Nakagawa S, Horibe S (2005) Anatomically-oriented ACL Reconstruction with a bone–patellar tendon graft via rectangular socket/tunnels: a snug-fit and impingement-free grafting technique. Arthroscopy 21(11):1402
2. Shino K, Nakata K, Horibe S, Nakamura N, Toritsuka Y, Nakagawa S, Suzuki T (2008) Rectangular tunnel double-bundle anterior cruciate ligament reconstruction with bone–patellar tendon–bone graft to mimic natural fiber arrangement. Arthroscopy 24(10):1178–1183

3. Ferretti M, Ekdahl M, Shen W, Fu FH (2007) Osseous landmarks of the femoral attachment of the anterior cruciate ligament: an anatomic study. Arthroscopy 11:1218–1225
4. Shino K, Suzuki T, Iwahashi T et al (2010) The resident's ridge as an arthroscopic landmark for anatomical femoral tunnel drilling in ACL reconstruction. Knee Surg Sports Traumatol Arthrosc 18:1164–1168
5. Hutchinson MR, Ash SA (2003) Resident's ridge: assessing the cortical thickness of the lateral wall and roof of the intercondylar notch. Arthroscopy 19:931–935
6. Shino K, Mae T, Nakamura N (2012) Revision ACL reconstruction with rectangular tunnel technique. Clin Orthop Relat Res 470(3):843–852
7. Iwahashi T, Shino K, Nakata K, Otsubo H, Suzuki T, Amano H, Nakamura N (2010) Direct ACL insertion to the femur assessed by histology and three-dimensional volume-rendered computed tomography. Arthroscopy 26(9 Suppl):S13–S20
8. Otsubo H, Shino K, Suzuki D et al (2012) The arrangement and the attachment areas of three ACL bundles. Knee Surg Sports Traumatol Arthrosc 20:127–134
9. Shino K, Mae T, Tachibana Y (2015) Anatomic ACL reconstruction: rectangular tunnel/bone–patellar tendon–bone or triple-bundle/semitendinosus tendon grafting. J Orthop Sci 20:457–468
10. Suzuki T, Shino K, Nakamura N, Iwahashi T, Nakata K, Tanaka Y, Nakagawa S, Kinugasa K, Yamashita T (2011) Early integration of a bone plug in the femoral tunnel in rectangular tunnel ACL reconstruction with a bone–patellar tendon–bone graft: a prospective computed tomography analysis. Knee Surg Sports Traumatol Arthosc 19(Suppl 1):S29–S35
11. Clancy WG, Narechania RG, Lange TA (1981) Anterior and posterior cruciate ligament reconstruction in rhesus. J Bone Joint Surg Am 63:1270–1284
12. Lomasney LM, Tonino PM, Coan MR (2006) Evaluation of bone incorporation of patellar tendon autografts and allografts for ACL reconstruction using CT. Orthopedics 30:152–157
13. Claes L, Augat P, Wilke HJ (1997) Influence of size and stability of the osteotomy gap on the success of fracture healing. J Orthop Res 15:577–584
14. Claes LE, Heigele CA (1999) Magnitudes of local stress and strain along bony surfaces predict the course and type of fracture healing. J Biomech 32:255–266
15. Rahn BA, Gallinaro P, Perren SM (1971) Primary bone healing: an experimental study in the rabbit. J Bone Joint Surg Am 53:783–786
16. Suzuki T, Shino K, Otsubo H, Suzuki D, Mae T, Fujimiya M, Yamashita T, Fujie H (2014) Biomechanical comparison between the rectangular-tunnel and the round-tunnel anterior cruciate ligament reconstruction procedures with a bone patellar tendon bone graft. Arthroscopy 30(10):1294–1302
17. Mae T, Shino K, Matsumoto N et al (2006) Force sharing between two grafts in the anatomical two-bundle anterior cruciate ligament reconstruction. Knee Surg Sports Traumatol Arthrosc 14:505–509
18. Markolf KL, Burchfield DM, Sharpio MM, Davis BR, Finerman GAM, Slauterbeck JL (1996) Biomechanical consequences of replacement of the anterior cruciate ligament with a patellar ligament allograft. Part I: insertion of the graft and anterior-posterior testing. J Bone Joint Surg Am 78:1720–1727
19. Markolf KL, Burchfield DM, Sharpio MM et al (1996) Biomechanical consequences of replacement of the anterior cruciate ligament with a patellar ligament allograft. Part II: forces in the graft compared with forces in the intact ligament. J Bone Joint Surg Am 78:1728–1734
20. Markolf KL, Hame S, Hunter DM et al (2002) Effects of femoral tunnel placement on knee laxity and forces in an anterior cruciate ligament graft. J Orthop Res 20:1016–1024

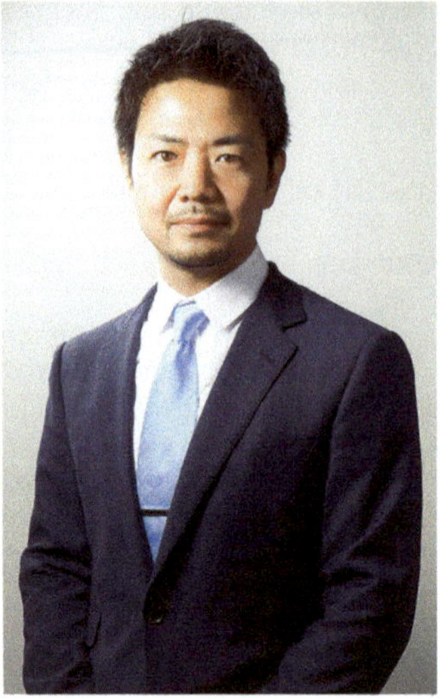

Tomoyuki Suzuki, M.D., Department of Orthopaedic Surgery, Sapporo Medical University Graduate School of Medicine, Hokkaido, Japan.

Part VIII
Computer-Assisted Navigation in ACL Reconstruction

Chapter 32
Intraoperative Biomechanical Evaluation Using a Navigation System

Yuji Yamamoto and Yasuyuki Ishibashi

Abstract Originally, the navigation system for anterior cruciate ligament (ACL) reconstruction has been a tool for increasing the precision of surgical procedures, especially for bone tunnel placement. In addition to assisting the surgeon to decide the proper tunnel position, the navigation system has the supplementary ability to assess knee kinematics during surgery; therefore, the navigation system could be a tool to evaluate knee kinematics or laxity in ACL-deficient knees. In this article, we introduce the navigation process and also describe our intraoperative biomechanical studies using an image-free navigation system, including intraoperative kinematics changes before and after double-bundle ACL reconstruction with hamstrings graft, effect of the different ACL bundles on knee kinematics in double-bundle reconstruction, and the effect of ACL remnant on knee kinematics. Finally, we also describe the quantification of the pivot shift phenomenon using a navigation system with noninvasive surface markers.

Keywords Anterior cruciate ligament (ACL) • ACL reconstruction • Navigation • Biomechanical evaluation • Knee kinematics

32.1 Introduction

Anterior cruciate ligament (ACL) reconstruction using hamstrings or bone-patellar tendon-bone graft is widely used and is as the most common surgical procedure for ACL injuries. Biomechanical study has demonstrated that tunnel placement affected kinematics of ACL-reconstructed knee [1]. Clinical studies have also demonstrated that proper tunnel placement is a key factor for successful clinical outcome after ACL reconstruction [2, 3]. Considerable variation in tunnel placement during conventional ACL reconstruction has been reported [4, 5]. Furthermore, in ACL revision study cohort, femoral tunnel malposition was rated as the most common technical failure, followed by tibial tunnel malposition [6, 7]. Therefore,

Y. Yamamoto, MD, PhD (✉) • Y. Ishibashi, MD, PhD
Dept. of Orthopaedic Surgery, Hirosaki University Graduate School of Medicine, 5 Zaifu-cho, Hirosaki, Aomori 036-8562, Japan
e-mail: yuji1112@hirosaki-u.ac.jp

M. Ochi et al. (eds.), *ACL Injury and Its Treatment*,
DOI 10.1007/978-4-431-55858-3_32

computer-assisted surgery such as using a navigation system has the potential to improve clinical outcomes by reducing variability of tunnel placement and allowing for more accurate tunnel placement [8]. Although image-based navigation system using preoperative computed tomography or intraoperative fluoroscopy has been available [9, 10], image-free navigation system has become popular and has been introduced in ACL reconstruction in our institutes since 2003 [11]. The navigation system has been used as a tool for intraoperative evaluation of knee kinematics as well as proper tunnel placement during ACL reconstruction. In this article, we introduce the navigation process of OrthoPilot (B. Braun Aesculap, Tuttlingen, Germany) as an example and also describe our intraoperative biomechanical study using the navigation system.

32.2 Navigation Process

OrthoPilot, image-free, wireless navigation system is currently used in our institutes. The latest version, OrthoPilot ACL version 3.0, has been adapted to include double-bundle ACL reconstruction.

32.2.1 Registration

The image-free navigation system uses intraoperative data acquisition to build a computer model of the patient anatomy, without preoperative computed tomography or intraoperative fluoroscopy. For the navigation process, transmitters with reflective markers were firmly fixed to the femur and tibia via metal pin fixators. Both anatomical landmarks and knee kinematics were registered. Anatomical landmarks consisted of the tibial tuberosity, the anterior edge of the tibia, and the medial and lateral point of the tibia plateau. ACL footprints in both femoral (more than five points on the circumference) and tibial sides (anterior, medial, lateral, and posterior borders) were also registered. The knee kinematics between 0° and 90° of knee flexion were registered. After registration of both anatomical landmarks and knee kinematics, real-time information on knee kinematic data are available to the surgeon.

32.2.2 Tibial Tunnel Placement

During tunnel placement, information about tunnel positions and angles is displayed on the navigation screen, helping to insert the guidewire. In case of double-bundle reconstruction, navigation helps to avoid tunnel overlap because the distance between two tunnels is also displayed with the second tunnel placement.

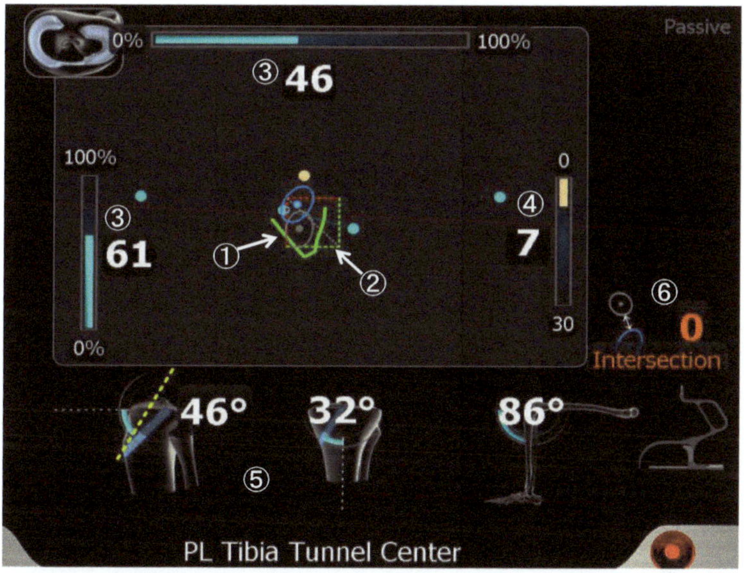

Fig. 32.1 Navigation for tibial tunnels (double-bundle technique).
1. ACL tibial footprint (*dotted box*).
2. Anterior notch boundary in extension projected onto the tibial plateau.
3. Width and depth of the tibial plateau (width in A-P view in % from medial to lateral, depth in lateral view in % from anterior to posterior).
4. Distance to the PCL anterior edge in mm.
5. Angle of the tibial tunnel in sagittal and frontal planes in degrees.
6. Distance between two tunnels in mm

Information about tibial tunnels on the navigation screen include (1) ACL tibial footprint; (2) anterior notch boundary in extension projected onto the tibial plateau (roof impingement); (3) width and depth of the tibial plateau (width in anterior-posterior (A-P) view in % from medial to lateral, depth in lateral view in % from anterior to posterior); (4) distance to the PCL anterior edge in mm; (5) angle of the tibial tunnel in sagittal and frontal planes in degrees; and (6) the distance between the two tunnels in mm (Fig. 32.1). In deciding the tibial tunnel position, because the tibia may be displaced anteriorly in ACL-deficient knee, there is a risk that the tunnel may be placed in the posterior setting when only the roof impingement is paid attention to. Therefore, the ACL footprint and other landmarks on the navigation screen must also be used as references for making the tunnels in the anatomical position [12].

32.2.3 Femoral Tunnel Placement

Information about femoral tunnels on navigation screen includes (1) ACL femoral footprint; (2) Blumensaat's line, (3) tunnel position in % from over the top to

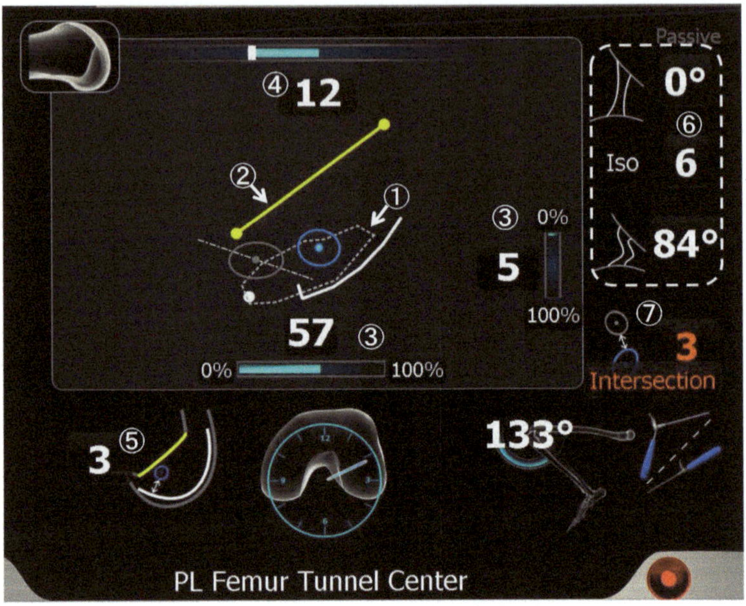

Fig. 32.2 Navigation in femoral tunnels (double-bundle technique).
1. ACL femoral footprint (*dotted line*).
2. Blumensaat's line.
3. Tunnel position in % from over the top to anterior notch outlet (*deep-shallow*) and from over the top to the bottom of lateral condyle (*high-low*).
4. Femoral offset from over-the-top in mm.
5. Distance to the posterior cartilage border in mm.
6. Isometry value (flexion angle at the graft experiences the greatest tension, in degrees, isometry value in mm; flexion angle at the graft experiences the least tension, in degrees).
7. Distance between two tunnels in mm.
PL tunnel (*blue*) is shown high position on the screen; surgeon can move it to *lower* position

anterior notch outlet (deep-shallow) and % from over-the-top to bottom of the lateral condyle (high-low); (4) femoral offset from over-the-top in mm; (5) distance to the posterior cartilage border in mm; (6) isometry value (flexion angle at the graft experiences the greatest tension, in degrees, isometry value in mm; flexion angle at the graft experiences the least tension, in degrees), and (7) the distance between two tunnels in mm (Fig. 32.2).

Femoral tunnel position is displayed as deep-shallow (% from over-the-top to anterior notch outlet) and high-low (% from over the top to bottom of lateral condyle) position for convenience in arthroscopic view [13]. For reference to navigation data mentioned above, the femoral tunnel position can be decided. In the case of double-bundle reconstruction, the second tunnel (usually for posterolateral (PL) bundle) position can be adjusted in reference to the first tunnel position (usually for anteromedial (AM) bundle).

32.3 Biomechanical Evaluation of Knee Kinematics During Surgery

Originally, the navigation system for ACL reconstruction has been a tool for increasing the precision of surgical procedure, especially for bone tunnel placement. In addition to assisting the surgeon to decide the proper tunnel position, the navigation system has the supplementary ability to assess knee kinematics during surgery; therefore, the navigation system could be a tool to evaluate knee kinematics or laxity in ACL-deficient knees. There are several publications which reported knee kinematics measured using the navigation system in ACL-deficient or ACL-reconstructed knees during surgery [14–18, 21].

32.3.1 Evaluation of Double-Bundle ACL Reconstruction

In our clinical study using a navigation system, we reported intraoperative kinematics changes before and after double-bundle ACL reconstruction with hamstring graft and anatomically oriented reconstruction with patellar tendon graft [18]. The effect of the different ACL bundles on knee kinematics in double-bundle reconstruction was also reported. Before ACL reconstruction, manual maximum anterior-posterior (A-P) forces were applied to the tibia in neutral rotation, and A-P displacement of the tibia at each angle of knee flexion was measured using the navigation system (OrthoPilot ACL version 2.0). After the PL bundle or AM bundle was temporarily fixed during double-bundle reconstruction, A-P displacement of the tibia was also measured to assess the function of each bundle. After double-bundle reconstruction or anatomically oriented reconstruction with patellar tendon, knee laxity was measured in the same manner.

Both double-bundle reconstruction and anatomically oriented reconstruction similarly improved knee laxity compared with before reconstruction in all knee flexion angles (Figs. 32.3 and 32.4). Regarding the function of the AM and PL bundles in double-bundle reconstruction, the two grafts showed contrasting behavior. A-P displacement after PL bundle fixation was significantly smaller than that after AM bundle fixation at only 15° of knee flexion and significantly larger than after more than 30° of knee flexion (Fig. 32.3). Although the PL bundle has an important role in the extension position, the AM bundle is more important in the flexion position. These results were consistent with the previous biomechanical studies [19, 20]. On the basis of this study, both bundles should be reconstructed to improve knee laxity throughout knee range of motion. Furthermore, we believe that, even with single-bundle reconstruction using a patellar tendon, anatomic reconstruction might improve knee laxity similar to double-bundle reconstruction.

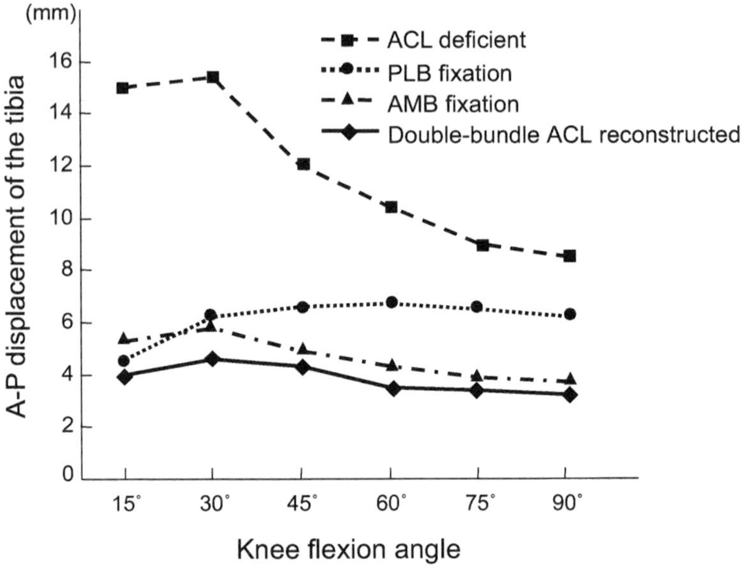

Fig. 32.3 Anterior-posterior (A-P) displacement of the tibia before and after double-bundle ACL reconstruction. ACL-deficient knee was most unstable at 30° of knee flexion. Double-bundle ACL reconstruction achieved stable knees compared to both PL and AM bundle fixation at all flexion angles

32.3.2 Evaluation of Pivot Shift Test

In another study, both tibial internal rotation and anterior translation under the pivot shift test were measured using a navigation system (OrthoPilot ACL version 2.0) before ACL reconstruction, after PL bundle fixation, after AM bundle fixation, and after double-bundle reconstruction [21] (Fig. 32.5). Before ACL reconstruction, average (± standard deviation) tibial internal rotation and anterior translation under the pivot shift test were 23.7° ± 6.1° and 5.2 ± 2.4 mm. They were significantly decreased to 20.9° ± 6.4° and 2.3 ± 1.1 mm after PL bundle fixation and also decreased to 22.2° ± 5.7° and 2.4 ± 1.1 mm after AM bundle fixation. There was no significant difference between the groups. After double-bundle reconstruction, tibial internal rotation and anterior translation improved to 20.3° ± 6.3° and 2.0 ± 1.0 mm. Results indicated that both the PL and the AM bundle similarly control both anterior translation and internal rotation during pivot shift testing.

Navigation data that were compared with clinical grades of manual test include Lachman, anterior drawer, and pivot shift test in ACL-deficient knees, and correlation between clinical grading and navigation data were also analyzed using OrthoPilot version 2.0 [22]. It was shown that there were positive correlations between clinical grading and A-P displacement in the Lachman and anterior drawer tests. Although positive correlations between clinical grading and A-P displacement in pivot shift test were found, there were no correlations between clinical

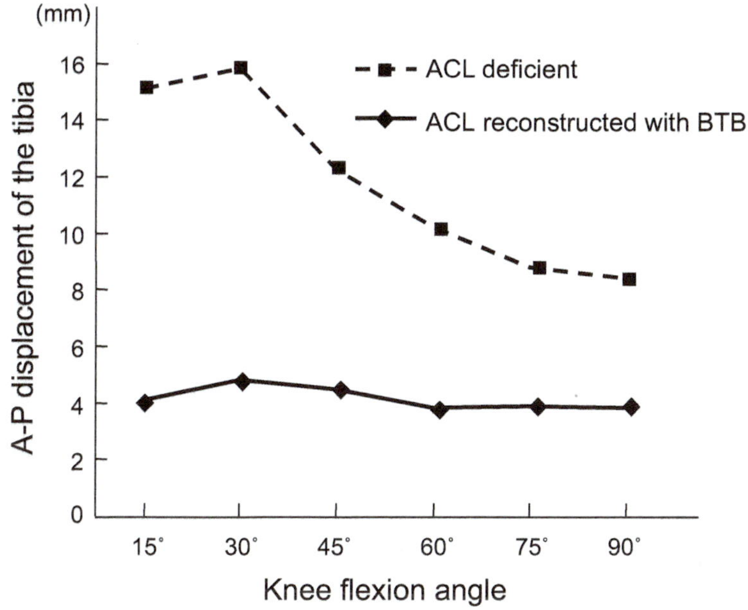

Fig. 32.4 Anterior-posterior (A-P) displacement of the tibia before and after anatomical ACL reconstruction with bone-patellar tendon-bone graft. A-P displacements after reconstruction were significantly decreased at all knee flexion angles compared to before reconstruction and were not statistically different from those after double-bundle ACL reconstruction

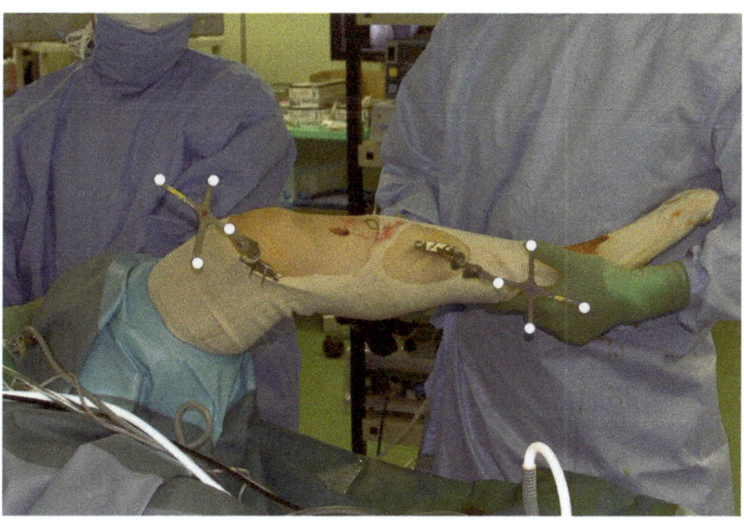

Fig. 32.5 The pivot shift test during surgery with the navigation system.
The transmitters were affixed to the femur and tibia via metal pin fixators. The pivot shift test was performed before and after ACL reconstruction

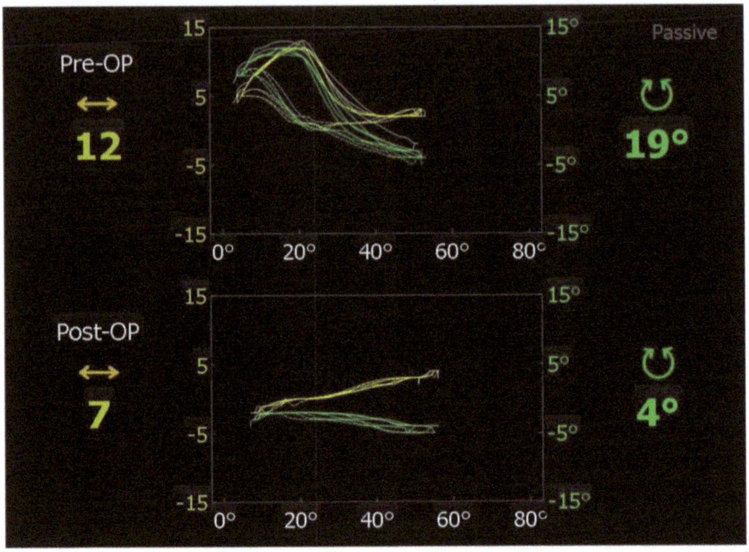

Fig. 32.6 A typical navigation screen of a positive pivot shift test.
The pivot shift test is repeated 2 to 3 times preoperatively. Subluxation and reduction of the tibia occur during pivot shift test (x-axis, knee flexion angles in degree; y-axis, A-P translation and rotation of the tibia in relation to the femur). Pivot shift phenomenon does not occur after ACL reconstruction (*lower figure*)

grading and tibial rotation. We concluded that in response to A-P force, the navigation system can provide the surgeon with correct objective data for knee laxity in ACL-deficient knees, and, during the pivot shift test, physicians may grade according to the displacement of the tibia, rather than rotation.

However, OrthoPilot version 2.0 could only assess statistically at the selected knee angles during pivot shift test [22]. The latest version, OrthoPilot version 3.0, can evaluate dynamic or sudden movement of the knee such as pivot shift phenomenon. It automatically shows a chart of tibial anterior-posterior displacement and internal-external rotation on the navigation screen and records the knee kinematics (tibial translation and rotation) during the pivot shift test. A typical example of a positive pivot shift test patient is shown in Fig. 32.6. Since graphs during pivot shift test before and after ACL reconstruction are displayed at the same screen, it is easy to recognize that the pivot shift phenomenon disappears after reconstruction.

32.3.3 Evaluation of ACL Remnant

The effect of ACL remnants on knee laxity was assessed in 83 knees undergoing primary ACL reconstruction using a computer navigation system [23]. ACL remnants were classified into four morphologic types based on the arthroscopic findings: type 1, bridging between the posterior cruciate ligament and tibia; type 2, bridging between the roof of the intercondylar notch and tibia; type 3, bridging between the lateral wall of the intercondylar notch and tibia; and type 4, no substantial ACL remnants (Fig. 32.7). Anterior tibial translation (ATT) and range of internal-external rotation of the tibia (total rotation) at 15°, 30°, 45°, 60°, 75°, and 90° of knee flexion were measured before and after resection of the ACL remnants. The different morphologic types of the ACL remnants were as follows: 12 knees for type 1; 16 knees for type 2; 51 knees for type 3; and 4 knees for type 4. There were no significant differences in the mean ATT before and after resection at any knee flexion angle in type 1, 2, or 4 knees. In type 3 knees, the mean ATT at 15° of knee flexion before resection significantly increased after resection. There were no significant differences in the mean total rotation before and after resection at any knee flexion angle for each type. After resection of the ACL remnants, 12 knees (14.5%) in the type 3 showed an increased ATT by 3 mm or more. This study suggests that the ACL remnant does not play a major role in stabilization of the knee. Although type 3 ACL remnants significantly decreased anterior knee laxity in the knee extension position, the knee stability provided by the ACL remnants was not adequate.

Nakamae et al. also evaluated the biomechanical function of ACL remnants using a navigation system for anteroposterior and rotational knee stability in patients with a complete ACL injury [24]. Patients in groups 1 (bridging between the posterior cruciate ligament and tibia) and 2 (bridging between the intercondylar

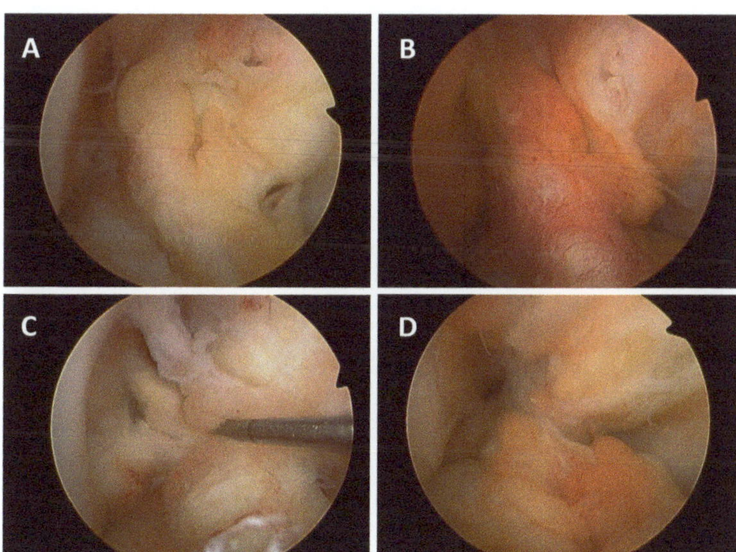

Fig. 32.7 Arthroscopic findings of ACL remnants:
(**a**) type 1, bridging between the posterior cruciate ligament and tibia; (**b**) type 2, bridging between the roof of the intercondylar notch and tibia; (**c**) type 3, bridging between the lateral wall of the intercondylar notch and tibia; and (**d**) type 4, no substantial ACL remnants

notch and tibia) underwent intraoperative arthrometry with a navigation system before and immediately after resection of the ACL remnant. They found that chronicity had a significant effect on changes in anteroposterior knee laxity evaluated at 30° of knee flexion after resection of the ACL remnant (change in laxity of 2.22 mm for chronicity <1 year and 0.17 mm for chronicity >1 year). However, biomechanical function of remnant in groups 3 (partial rupture of PL bundle) and 4 (partial rupture of AM bundle) was not evaluated because ACL augmentation procedures with preservation of remnant were performed on these patients. They concluded that in groups 1 and 2, ACL remnants contributed to anteroposterior knee stability evaluated at 30° of knee flexion for up to 1 year after injury, beyond which this biomechanical function was lost.

32.3.4 Evaluation with Noninvasive Surface Markers

Navigation system has been developed and proposed for the evaluation and quantification of the pivot shift test [21, 22]. However, the navigation system is difficult to use in clinical practice because of the invasive nature of the transmitter attachment. The use of noninvasive surface markers for navigation system could be a solution. Therefore, we validated laxity measurements during the pivot shift test by using a navigation system with noninvasive surface markers (Fig. 32.8) and compared these measurements with those obtained using commercial pin-fixed markers. The pivot shift test results using navigation system were also compared with the

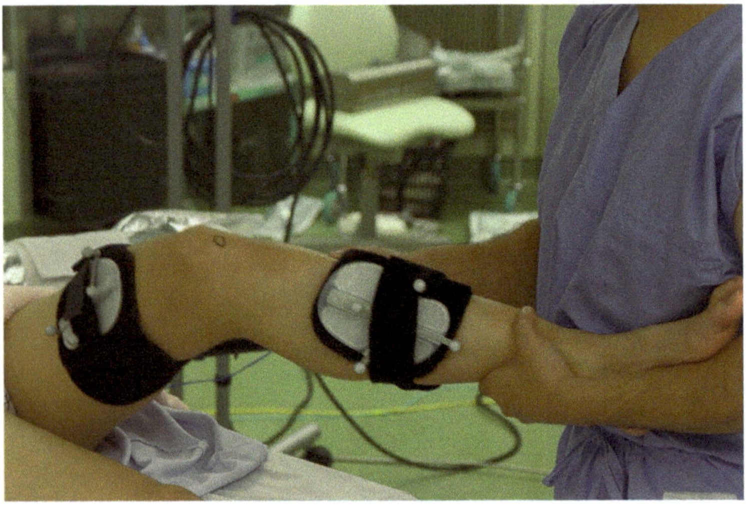

Fig. 32.8 Surface markers for the navigation system.
(**a**) Commercial transmitters are placed on soft polyethylene plates and affixed to the skin with elastic bandages and Velcro tape. (**b**) Surface markers were affixed to the thigh and shin, and the pivot shift test was performed by applying valgus and internal torque to the knee

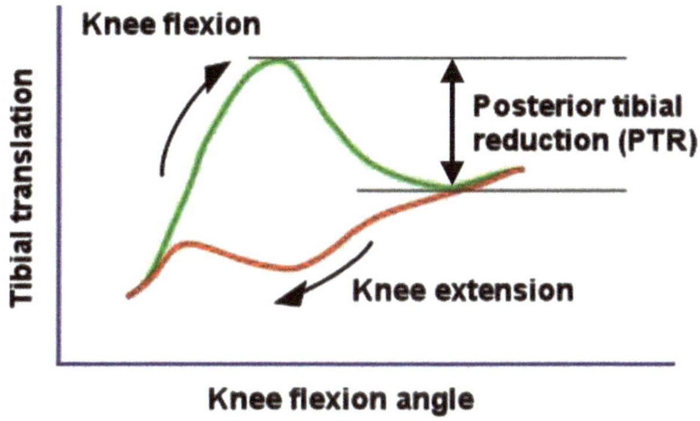

Fig. 32.9 Simplified navigation screen. Posterior tibial reduction (PTR) is suddenly observed as the knee is passively flexed during the pivot shift test. This sudden reduction of the tibial plateau is the pivot shift phenomenon, and the PTR can be calculated using the navigation system

clinical grades of the pivot shift test. Laxity measurements during the pivot shift test were performed in 70 patients who had undergone ACL reconstruction using the OrthoPilot ACL version 3.0. Because a sudden reduction of the tibial plateau is the pivot shift phenomenon, the posterior tibial reduction (PTR) was measured from the chart of the navigation system. PTR was defined as the distance of posterior tibial reduction after maximum anterior translation of the tibia during passive knee flexion (Fig. 32.9).

The average PTR measured with surface markers and pin-fixed markers was 4.6 ± 2.3 mm and 5.2 ± 2.8 mm, respectively. A statistically moderate correlation was found between the PTRs, as measured using the two methods ($\rho = 0.524$, $p < 0.001$). There were statistically moderate correlations between the clinical grades recorded and the PTRs measured using surface markers ($\rho = 0.522$, $p < 0.001$), as well as between the clinical grades and PTRs measured using pin-fixed markers ($\rho = 0.645$, $p < 0.001$). The average PTRs measured, respectively, with the surface and pin-fixed markers, for each clinical grade, were grade 1+ (2.8 ± 1.3 mm, 2.7 ± 1.6 mm), grade 2+ (3.9 ± 1.6 mm, 4.4 ± 1.8 mm), and grade 3+ (6.1 ± 2.4 mm, 7.3 ± 2.6 mm). There were statistically significant differences in the PTRs measured with surface markers between all grades, except between grades 1+ and 2+. Similarly, there were significant PTR differences between all clinical grades when the pin-fixed markers were used.

As a limitation of this system (OrthoPilot ACL version 3.0), the sampling rate of the navigation system (sampling rate, 12 Hz) used was lower than that of other quantitative instruments for the pivot shift test (accelerometer, 198 Hz; electromagnetic system, 60 Hz). Therefore, PTR measured with surface markers moderately correlated with both the PTR obtained using pin-fixed markers and with the clinical grade of the pivot shift test in this study. If the sampling rate of this navigation system is increased by improving the software and camera system, the accuracy of quantification of the pivot shift test may be improved. However, results suggest that the use of a navigation system and surface markers, using modified commercial transmitters, might be able to quantify the pivot shift phenomenon in clinical situations. To increase the accuracy of this measurement method, improved surface markers and the development of dedicated software are also desirable.

32.4 Future Direction

In the "Clinical Practice Guideline on the Management of ACL Injury" supervised by Japanese Orthopaedic Association [25], for the clinical question about the efficacy of using computer-assisted navigation system in ACL reconstruction, it was summarized that there was no consensus of efficacy on tunnel placement and there was no benefit of postoperative knee stability. Currently, randomized controlled trials on the use of navigation in ACL reconstruction have failed to demonstrate a clinical benefit, including radiographic evaluation, knee stability, and clinical outcome. [26–31]. However, a navigation system for the ACL reconstruction is still developing; if more useful information is provided for a surgeon by progress of the future technology and development of new software, it may lead to better anatomical tunnel placement or improved clinical results. The navigation system that could be used as a tool for basic and clinical researches such as the effect of different surgical techniques on knee kinematics, and new ideas for ACL reconstruction may be generated. Furthermore, the use of navigation system as an educational tool for young doctors may lead to better understanding of ACL anatomy and surgical procedure in ACL reconstruction and improve their skill.

References

1. Musahl V, Plakseychuk A, VanScyoc A et al (2005) Varying femoral tunnels between the anatomical footprint and isometric positions: effect on kinematics of the anterior cruciate ligament-reconstructed knee. Am J Sports Med 33(5):712–718
2. Khalfayan EE, Sharkey PF, Alexander AH, Bruckner JD, Bynum EB (1996) The relationship between tunnel placement and clinical results after anterior cruciate ligament reconstruction. Am J Sports Med 24(3):335–341
3. Sommer C, Friederich NF, Müller W (2000) Improperly placed anterior cruciate ligament grafts: correlation between radiological parameters and clinical results. Knee Surg Sports Traumatol Arthrosc 8(4):207–213
4. Kohn D, Busche T, Carls J (1998) Drill hole position in endoscopic anterior cruciate ligament reconstruction. Results of an advanced arthroscopy course. Knee Surg Sports Traumatol Arthrosc 6(Suppl 1):S13–S15
5. Picard F, DiGioia AM, Moody J, Martinek V, Fu FH, Rytel M et al (2001) Accuracy in tunnel placement for ACL reconstruction. Comparison of traditional arthroscopic and computer-assisted navigation techniques. Comput Aided Surg 6:279–289
6. Descriptive epidemiology of the Multicenter ACL Revision Study (MARS) cohort. MARS Group, Wright RW, Huston LJ, Spindler KP, Dunn WR, Haas AK, Allen CR, Cooper DE, DeBerardino TM, Lantz BB, Mann BJ, Stuart MJ (2010) Descriptive epidemiology of the Multicenter ACL Revision Study (MARS) cohort. Am J Sports Med 38(10):1979–1986.

7. Getelman MH, Friedman MJ (1999) Revision anterior cruciate ligament reconstruction surgery. J Am Acad Orthop Surg 7(3):189–198
8. Jalliard R, Lavallée S, Dessenne V (1998) Computer assisted reconstruction of the anterior cruciate ligament. Clin Orthop Relat Res 354:57–64
9. Hiraoka H, Kuribayashi S, Fukuda A, Fukui N, Nakamura K (2006) Endoscopic anterior cruciate ligament reconstruction using a computer-assisted fluoroscopic navigation system. J Orthop Sci 11(2):159–166
10. Nakagawa T, Takeda H, Nakajima K, Nakayama S, Fukai A, Kachi Y, Kawano H, Miura T, Nakamura K (2008) Intraoperative 3-dimensional imaging-based navigation-assisted anatomic double-bundle anterior cruciate ligament reconstruction. Arthroscopy 24(10):1161–1167
11. Ishibashi Y, Tsuda E, Fukuda A, Tsukada H, Toh S (2006) Future of double-bundle anterior cruciate ligament (ACL) reconstruction: incorporation of ACL anatomic data into the navigation system. Orthopedics 29(10 Suppl):S108–S112
12. Tsukada H, Ishibashi Y, Tsuda E et al (2008) Anatomical analysis of the anterior cruciate ligament femoral and tibial footprints. J Orthop Sci 13(2):122–129
13. Watanabe S, Satoh T, Sobue T et al (2005) Three-dimensional evaluation of femoral tunnel position in anterior cruciate ligament reconstruction (in Japanese). J Jpn Knee Soc 30:253–256
14. Martelli S, Bignozzi S, Zaffagnini S, Visani A (2007) Validation of a new protocol for navigated intraoperative assessment of knee kinematics. Comput Biol Med 37(6):872–878
15. Ferretti A, Monaco E, Labianca L, Conteduca F, De Carli A (2008) Double-bundle anterior cruciate ligament reconstruction: a computer-assisted orthopaedic surgery study. Am J Sports Med 36(4):760–766
16. Song EK, Seon JK, Park SJ, Hur CI, Lee DS (2009) In vivo laxity of stable versus anterior cruciate ligament-injured knees using a navigation system: a comparative study. Knee Surg Sports Traumatol Arthrosc 17(8):941–945
17. Lopomo N, Bignozzi S, Martelli S, Zaffagnini S, Iacono F, Visani A, Marcacci M (2009) Reliability of a navigation system for intra-operative evaluation of antero-posterior knee joint laxity. Comput Biol Med 39(3):280–285
18. Ishibashi Y, Tsuda E, Fukuda A, Tsukada H, Toh S (2008) Intraoperative biomechanical evaluation of anatomic anterior cruciate ligament reconstruction using a navigation system: comparison of hamstring tendon and bone-patellar tendon-bone graft. Am J Sports Med 36 (10):1903–1912
19. Yagi M, Wong EK, Kanamori A, Debski RE, Fu FH, Woo SL (2002) Biomechanical analysis of an anatomic anterior cruciate ligament reconstruction. Am J Sports Med 30(5):660–666
20. Yamamoto Y, Hsu WH, Woo SL-Y, Van Scyoc AH, Takakura Y, Debski RE (2004) Knee stability and graft function after anterior cruciate ligament reconstruction: a comparison of a lateral and an anatomic femoral tunnel placement. Am J Sports Med 32(8):1825–1832
21. Ishibashi Y, Tsuda E, Yamamoto Y, Tsukada H, Toh S (2009) Navigation evaluation of the pivot-shift phenomenon during double-bundle anterior cruciate ligament reconstruction: is the posterolateral bundle more important? Arthroscopy 25(5):488–495
22. Yamamoto Y, Ishibashi Y, Tsuda E, Tsukada H, Maeda S, Toh S (2010) Comparison between clinical grading and navigation data of knee laxity in ACL-deficient knees. Sports Med Arthrosc Rehabil Ther Technol 2:27
23. Maeda S, Ishibashi Y, Tsuda E, Yamamoto Y, Toh S (2011) Intraoperative navigation evaluation of tibial translation after resection of anterior cruciate ligament remnants. Arthroscopy 27(9):1203–1210
24. Nakamae A, Ochi M, Deie M, Adachi N, Kanaya A, Nishimori M, Nakasa T (2010) Biomechanical function of anterior cruciate ligament remnants: how long do they contribute to knee stability after injury in patients with complete tears? Arthroscopy 26(12):1577–1585
25. The Clinical Practice Guideline Committee of Japanese Orthopaedic Association (2012) In: Japanese Orthopaedic Association (ed) Clinical practice guideline on the management of ACL injury, 2nd edn. Nankodo Co., Ltd., Tokyo, 139–140

26. Plaweski S, Cazal J, Rosell P, Merloz P (2006) Anterior cruciate ligament reconstruction using navigation: a comparative study on 60 patients. Am J Sports Med 34(4):542–552
27. Mauch F, Apic G, Becker U, Bauer G (2007) Differences in the placement of the tibial tunnel during reconstruction of the anterior cruciate ligament with and without computer-assisted navigation. Am J Sports Med 35(11):1824–1832
28. Hart R, Krejzla J, Sváb P, Kocis J, Stipcák V (2008) Outcomes after conventional versus computer-navigated anterior cruciate ligament reconstruction. Arthroscopy 24(5):569–578
29. Chouteau J, Benareau I, Testa R, Fessy MH, Lerat JL, Moyen B (2008) Comparative study of knee anterior cruciate ligament reconstruction with or without fluoroscopic assistance: a prospective study of 73 cases. Arch Orthop Trauma Surg 128(9):945–950
30. Endele D, Jung C, Becker U, Bauer G, Mauch F (2009) Anterior cruciate ligament reconstruction with and without computer navigation: a clinical and magnetic resonance imaging evaluation 2 years after surgery. Arthroscopy 25(10):1067–1074
31. Meuffels DE, Reijman M, Verhaar JAN (2012) Computer-assisted surgery is not more accurate or precise than conventional arthroscopic ACL reconstruction: a prospective randomized clinical trial. J Bone Joint Surg Am 94(17):1538–1545

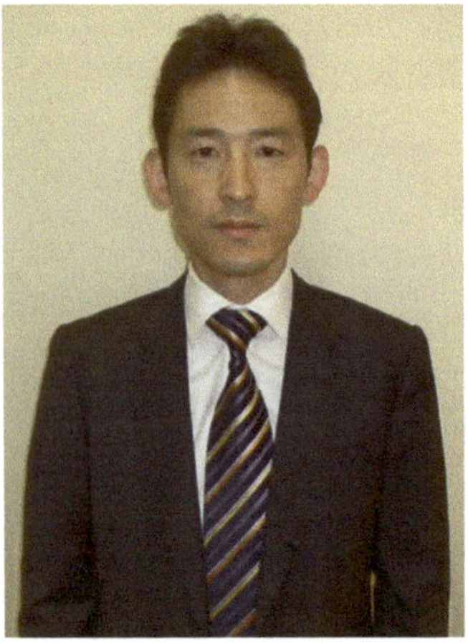

Yuji Yamamoto, MD, PhD, Dept. of Orthopaedic Surgery, Hirosaki University Graduate School of Medicine, Aomori, Japan.

Chapter 33
Application of Computer-Assisted Navigation

Takumi Nakagawa and Shuji Taketomi

Abstract Tunnel malposition is known to be major cause of failure after ACL reconstruction. Three -dimensional fluoroscopic computer navigation has been used to further improve the accuracy of femoral tunnel placement. After a reference frame is securely fixated to the femur, intraoperative image of the distal femur is obtained, which is reconstructed into a 3-D image. During placement of guide pins through far anteromedial portal, navigation guidance allows surgeon to place them inside original attachment area which is located behind resident's (lateral intercondylar) ridge. The virtual femoral tunnel on the navigation monitor assists surgeon to notice the risk of posterior cortical blowout and the estimated tunnel exit on the lateral femoral cortex. The navigation is also applied to remnant-preserving ACL reconstruction in which anatomical tunnel placement is more challenging because of poor arthroscopic visualization of femoral insertion site. This technology is more powerful in revision ACL reconstruction which is accompanied by several technical challenges such as previous bone tunnels, preexisting implants, or bone defect due to tunnel expansion.

Keywords Computer-assisted navigation • Anatomical ACL reconstruction • Remnant preservation • Revision ACL reconstruction

33.1 Three-Dimensional (3-D) Fluoroscopic Navigation-Assisted ACL Reconstruction

Anterior cruciate ligament reconstruction (ACLR) is one of the most common sports injuries in active young people, requiring surgical reconstruction to allow patients to return to an active lifestyle and prevent secondary meniscus or cartilage injuries. However, inaccurate placement of either the femoral or the tibial tunnel

T. Nakagawa, M.D., Ph.D (✉)
Department of Orthopaedic Surgery, Teikyo University, 2-11–1 Kaga, Itabashi–ku, Tokyo 173-8605, Japan
e-mail: takumin-tky@umin.ac.jp

S. Taketomi, M.D., PhD
Department of Orthopaedic Surgery, The University of Tokyo, Tokyo, Japan

M. Ochi et al. (eds.), *ACL Injury and Its Treatment*,
DOI 10.1007/978-4-431-55858-3_33

may occur in up to 15 % of procedures using standard surgical techniques; this may result in laxity, instability, suboptimal clinical results, and increased revision rates [1]. Computer-assisted navigation offers surgeons real-time feedback of the surgical field, enabling them to adjust the surgical technique to improve postoperative outcomes and decrease intraoperative errors [2]. Based on the method of referencing information, computer-assisted navigation systems are further classified into computed tomography (CT) based, fluoroscopy based, and imageless. Imageless navigation systems consist of a computer platform, a tracking system, and a set of infrared markers. Imageless navigation is used to restore normal knee kinematics by measuring graft isometry in ACLR. Computed tomography-based navigation use CT scans of the area of interest. The CT scans are performed either pre- or intraoperatively and used to reconstruct three-dimensional (3-D) images. To improve the accuracy and reproducibility of femoral tunnel placement, 3-D fluoroscopy-based navigation has been used since 2007 in our institution [3].

33.1.1 Surgical Procedure

33.1.1.1 Fixation of a Reference Frame to Femur and Acquisition of 3-D Images

The patient was placed in the supine position in such a way that the break in the operating table is just distal to the leg holder, keeping the distal thigh horizontal. A tourniquet is applied to the proximal thigh. At the beginning of the surgery, the reference frame must be fixated rigidly to the femur using two half pins monocortically. To minimize muscle load especially in muscular male patients, pins are placed with the knee in 90° of flexion (Fig. 33.1a). Intraoperative 3-D images were acquired with C-arm of Arcadis Orbic 3-D (Siemens AG, Erlangen, Germany) of which isocentric design and 190° orbital movement provide the prerequisites for 3-D imaging (Fig. 33.1b). The C-arm of the image intensifier was equipped with a wireless tracker (Stealth Active wireless tracker S/N 130, Medtronic, Louisville, CO) for navigation registration. After the distal femur was positioned in the isocenter of the C-arm using the image intensifier, a radiation-free manual test run was performed to ensure that the unit will not collide with other objects during the automated scan. The system is equipped with a stepper motor to realize a high-precision orbital rotation around the distal femur, and the automatic scan was initiated via the foot switch [3, 4].

The acquired image data are transferred to the navigation computer (StealthStation TRIA^{TM} *plus*, Medtronic, Louisville, CO) (Fig. 33.1c), and the 3-D image of the distal femur was reconstructed on the computer monitor. The medial half of the 3-D reconstructed distal femur was deleted using the computer software for a better view of the lateral wall of the intercondylar notch. Resident's (lateral intercondylar) ridge, anterior border of ACL femoral attachment area, can be confirmed easily on the navigation display (Fig. 33.1d).

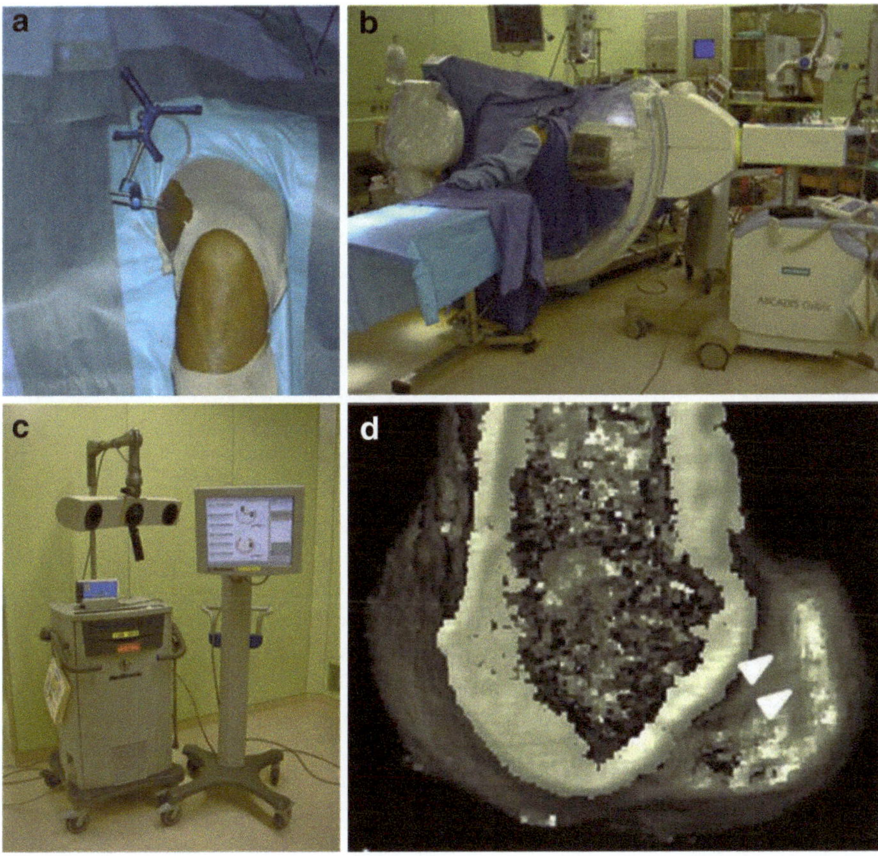

Fig. 33.1 (**a**) Reference frame is securely fixed to the femur with two half pins before acquiring images
(**b**) Intraoperative 3-D images are acquired with C-arm of an Arcadis Orbic 3-D (Siemens AG) and transferred to a navigation computer. The C-arm of the image intensifier is equipped with a wireless tracker
(**c**) Medtronic StealthStation TRIA plus navigation system
(**d**) A 3-D reconstructed image of the distal femur on the navigation monitor. The medial half of the distal femur was removed using the navigation software. The *white triangles* show resident's (lateral intercondylar) ridge

33.1.1.2 3-D Fluoroscopic Navigation-Assisted Femoral Guide Pin Placement

In case the remnant tissue's quality is poor, the fibrous tissue including the ACL stump on the superior-posterior half of the lateral wall of the intercondylar notch is thoroughly cleaned up with a radio-frequency device. Special care is taken to expose the lateral intercondylar ridge, the upper cartilage margin, and the posterior cartilage margin. A femoral guide equipped with a tracking device is used to identify anatomical entry points both on the navigation screen and the arthroscopic monitor. Once the correct entry points are identified under the guidance of the navigation, a microfracture awl is used to mark two points in the center of attachment area along its long axis. The distance between the two marked points is 5 mm in creating rectangular femoral tunnel for bone-patellar tendon-bone graft and is more than 5 mm in making two round tunnels for double-bundle hamstring grafts depending on the graft diameter. While viewing the lateral wall of the notch through anteromedial portal, the two guide pins are inserted through far anteromedial portal. The placement of guide pins for two femoral tunnels was performed with a femoral guide equipped with a tracker. The tip of the femoral guide is placed at the marked point, and the image-interactive navigation assisted the surgeons to confirm the anatomically correct placement of the femoral guide's tip on the 3-D reconstructed image (Fig. 33.2a). Once the femoral guide is placed at the center of femoral insertion site, the tail of the aimer is tapped into the bone with a mallet for provisional fixation. Keeping the femoral guide's tip at the planned entry point, the knee is flexed to 130–140° (Fig. 33.2b). On the navigation display, the 3-D image of the distal femur is rotated to face the posterior aspect of the femur. The diameter of the virtual femoral tunnel is set to the real diameter of graft (BTB graft 5 mm; hamstring grafts 6–7 mm on average), and the risk of the blowout through the posterior condyle is checked (Fig. 33.2c). The flexion angle of the knee and the trajectory of the femoral aimer are adjusted while monitoring posterior cortical blowout. The 3-D image is further rotated 90° to face the lateral aspect of the distal femur on the navigation monitor. The virtual femoral tunnel exit on the lateral femoral cortex enables to estimate the length of the femoral tunnel (Fig. 33.2d). Once the guide pins are placed, its correct positioning can be confirmed on the navigation computer. The guide pins are drilled with a cannulated drill of the diameter of the graft for an adequate length, and the lateral femoral cortex is drilled through using an Endobutton drill (Smith & Nephew, Andover, MA) for a suspensory fixation. For rectangular tunnel BTB ACL reconstruction, the continuous two round holes are dilated into a rectangular socket using the 5 × 10 mm dilator (Smith & Nephew) [5].

33.1.2 Remnant-Preserving Anterior Cruciate Ligament Reconstruction Using a 3-D Fluoroscopic Navigation

Theoretically, remnant preservation of ACL is supposed to enhance graft maturation via revascularization, cell proliferation, and recovery of proprioception. Remnant-preserving ACL reconstruction has been increasingly performed to achieve better knee stability and function. However, the remnant-preserving surgery is more technically demanding because arthroscopic visualization of ACL bony attachment is difficult due to existence of relatively thick and abundant ACL remnant tissue. Therefore, the femoral tunnels after remnant-preserving ACL

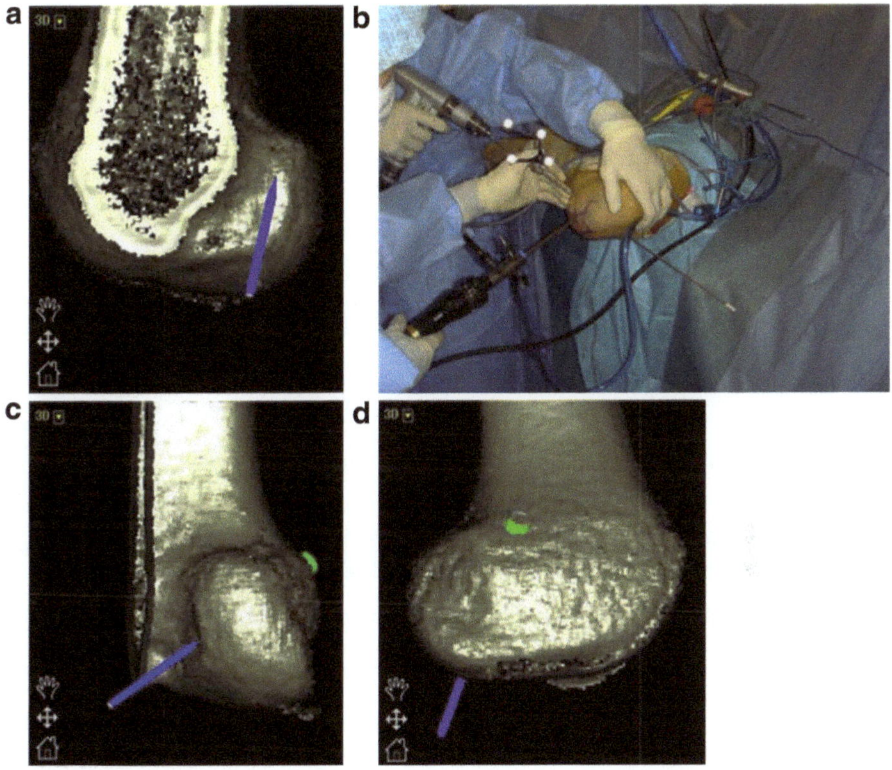

Fig. 33.2 (**a**) The tip of femoral guide with the tracking device is shown on the 3-D image navigation screen in real-time fashion
(**b**) Keeping the tip of the femoral guide placed at the target entry point, the knee is deeply flexed (130–140°) by an assistant
(**c**) A virtual femoral tunnel in the 3-D femoral image without posterior cortical blowout
(**d**) The exit of the virtual femoral tunnel on the lateral femoral cortex can be seen on the navigation screen, and the length of the femoral tunnel is measured on the navigation before drilling the guide pin

reconstruction tend to be positioned suboptimal. Three-dimensional fluoroscopic navigation enables surgeons to identify ACL attachment area even with minimum debridement of the fibrous tissue [6]. With the assistance of navigation, anatomic ACL reconstruction can be performed reproducibly with minimal damage to the remnant bundle of the femoral attachment (Fig. 33.3a–f).

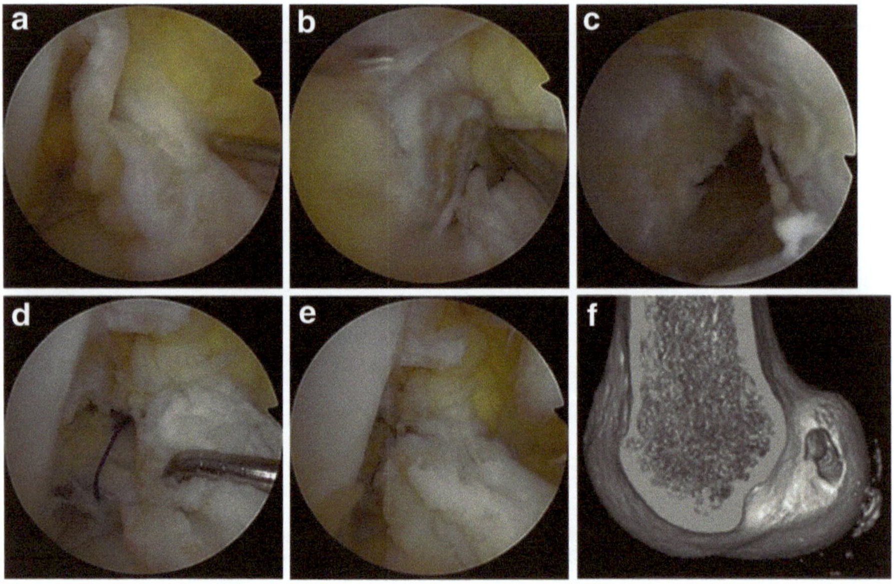

Fig. 33.3 (**a**) An ACL is ruptured near its femoral insertion. Its midsubstance and its tibial insertion are preserved
(**b**) After minimally debridement of its femoral attachment area with radio-frequency device, two guide pins were placed anatomically with the assistance of 3-D navigation
(**c**) The rectangular-shaped femoral tunnel aperture created with minimum damage to the remnant tissue
(**d**) The probe is seated on the remnant tissue for better visualization of the anatomically placed BTB graft
(**e**) The remnant-preserved BTB ACL graft viewed through the anterolateral portal
(**f**) 3-D CT image of femoral tunnel aperture after remnant-preserved anatomical rectangular tunnel BTB ACLR at 1 week postoperatively

33.1.3 Femoral Tunnel Creation in Revision ACL Reconstruction Using 3-D Fluoroscopic Navigation

Revision ACL reconstruction is accompanied by several technical challenges which need to be addressed, such as preexisting hardware, bone tunnel defects, or primary tunnel malposition. Technical errors have been found to be a common cause of failure of primary reconstruction, and above all femoral tunnel malposition seems to be the most common cause. Thus, it is frequently difficult to create a new femoral tunnel at an ideal position in revision ACL reconstructions because it may be impacted by the location of the previous femoral tunnel.

Our Preferred Technique The BTB graft is our current preference for revision ACL reconstruction because direct bone-to-bone healing is expected, resulting in secure and consistent fixation. The femoral bone plug is usually shaped 5-mm thick, 10-mm wide, and 15-mm long for a rectangular tunnel placement, except in cases with prior femoral aperture widening. Because the cross-sectional area of the tunnels required for rectangular ACL reconstruction is less than that for the round tunnel technique, this method is advantageous as it allows surgeons to consistently avoid overlap with tunnels from prior surgery [7].

33.1.3.1 3-D Fluoroscopic Navigation Guidance in Creation of Anatomic Femoral Tunnel in Revision ACL Reconstruction

It is essential to perform preoperative planning using 3-D computed tomography (CT) images before every revision procedure. The previous femoral tunnel position can be classified into three types based on the 3-D CT image depending on the location of the femoral tunnel relative to the lateral intercondylar ridge, as described by Magnussen et al. [8]. The principle is to create a new femoral socket for a BTB graft or two independent sockets for hamstring tendon grafts inside the original femoral attachment area. If the primary rectangular BTB femoral or double hamstring tendon apertures were created anatomically, the revision can be performed in the same way as in a primary rectangular tunnel BTB ACL reconstruction without the assistance of the navigation system. In this case, the prior anatomically placed aperture(s) can be easily expanded with a 5 × 10-mm dilator (Smith & Nephew Endoscopy, Andover, MA) into a single rectangular tunnel. If the previous tunnels on the femoral side were significantly improperly placed, a new femoral socket can be independently created anatomically in the same manner as in a primary ACL reconstruction with the assistance of the computer navigation (Fig. 33.4a–f). A case with slightly malpositioned femoral tunnel or previously expanded femoral tunnel aperture is the most technically challenging because overlap between the original tunnel aperture and the newly created one is sometimes inevitable. In such case, a divergent tunnel can be created with the assistance of the navigation system [9]. If a large femoral tunnel bone defect existed, a BTB graft with trapezoidal bone block is used as a substitute for rectangular-shaped graft.

33.2 Accuracy and Clinical Outcome After 3-D Fluoroscopic Navigation-Assisted Double-Bundle ACL Reconstruction

The positions of the femoral tunnel apertures were evaluated using 3-D CT model taken 1 week after the surgery in 34 anatomic double-bundle ACL reconstruction patients performed with assistance of 3-D fluoroscopic navigation [10]. Measurement of the anteromedial (AM) and posterolateral (PL) femoral socket on the 3-D CT images using the quadrant method showed that the center of the AM tunnel aperture was located at a depth of 21.0 ± 4.1 % and a height of 30.5 ± 9.3 % and that

a b c d e

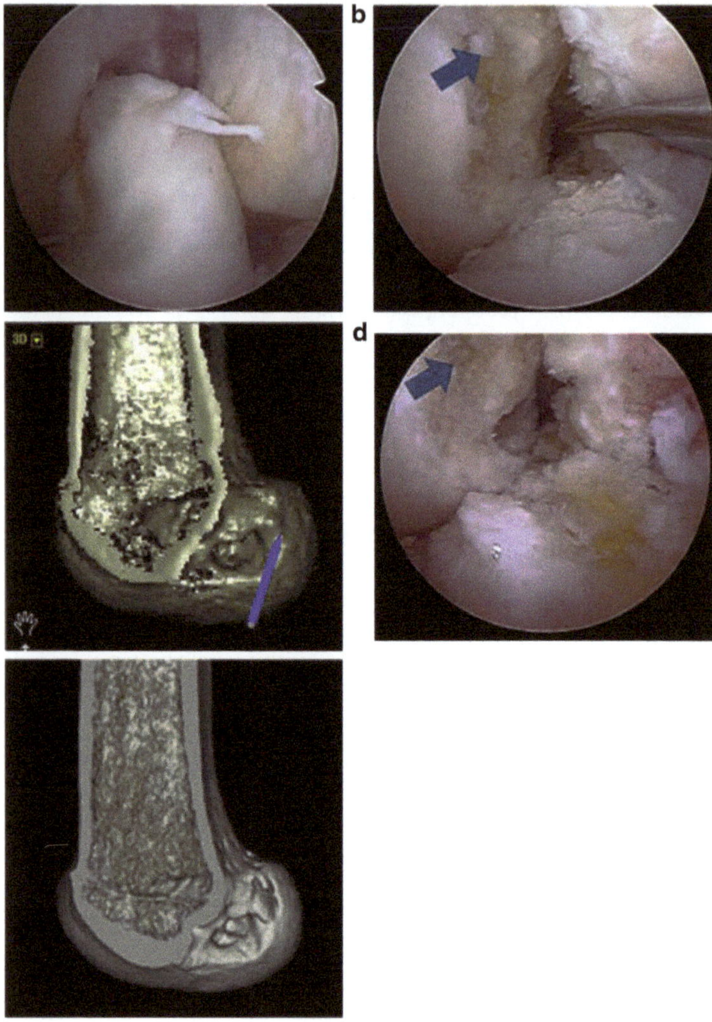

Fig. 33.4 (**a**) A hamstring ACL primary graft sustaining PCL impingement. The maximum flexion angle of the knee was 100° before revision surgery
(**b**) After the impinged ACL graft was debrided, the lateral intercondylar ridge is identified
(**c**) A navigation view of right knee shows anteriorly and distally placed (near high noon position) primary femoral tunnel aperture. The tip of the femoral guide is placed at an anatomical position without overlapping the original tunnel aperture. The *blue arrow* shows the previous tunnel aperture
(**d**) Rectangular-shaped femoral tunnel aperture created anatomically. The *blue arrow* shows the previous tunnel aperture
(**e**) 3-D CT image of femoral tunnel aperture after revision ACL reconstruction taken 1 week after the surgery

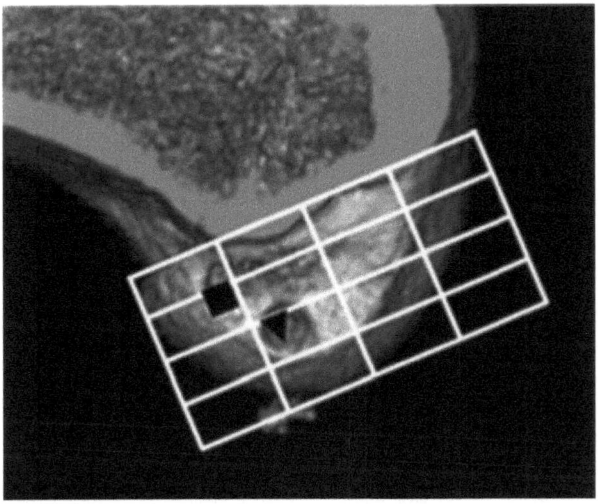

Fig. 33.5 Center of the anteromedial (*AM*) and the posterolateral (*PL*) tunnel aperture location calculated using the quadrant method after three-dimensional fluoroscopic navigation-assisted ACLR. The *black square* shows the location of the center of the AM tunnel aperture, and the *black triangle* shows the location of PL tunnel aperture

of the PL socket aperture was located at a depth of 31.3 ± 5.8 % and a height of 57.2 ± 7.7 % (Fig. 33.5). The femoral socket locations were considered as anatomic in accordance with previous cadaveric studies examining the positions of ACL femoral insertion site. With regard to the clinical results, 26 knees (76 %) were objectively graded as normal, 8 (24 %) as nearly normal, and 0 (0 %) as abnormal or severely abnormal in IKDC objective scores. Postoperative side-to-side anterior translation measured with a KT-2000 arthrometer averaged 0.7 ± 1.2 mm. The short-term clinical results were satisfactory.

33.3 Complications

In comparison to conventional ACL reconstruction, additional fixation of the reference tracker to the femur using two half pins is necessary in the navigated procedure. No serious complication related to the fixation of the tracker to the femur was encountered. The reference tracker must be rigidly fixated to the femur for accurate navigation. The loosening or bending of the half pins brings about complications such as malpositioning of the femoral tunnel or posterior cortical blowout due to inaccurate navigation.

References

1. Endele D et al (2009) Anterior cruciate ligament reconstruction with and without computer navigation: a clinical and magnetic resonance imaging evaluation 2 years after surgery. Arthroscopy 25(10):1067–1074

2. Mavrogenis AF et al (2013) Computer-assisted navigation in orthopedic surgery. Orthopedics 36(8):631–642
3. Nakagawa T et al (2008) Intraoperative 3-dimensional imaging-based navigation-assisted anatomic double-bundle anterior cruciate ligament reconstruction. Arthroscopy 24 (10):1161–1167
4. Taketomi S et al (2011) Anatomical placement of double femoral tunnels in anterior cruciate ligament reconstruction: anteromedial tunnel first or posterolateral tunnel first? Knee Surg Sports Traumatol Arthrosc 19(3):424–431
5. Shino K et al (2008) Rectangular tunnel double-bundle anterior cruciate ligament reconstruction with bone-patellar tendon-bone graft to mimic natural fiber arrangement. Arthroscopy 24 (10):1178–1183
6. Taketomi S et al (2014) Remnant-preserving anterior cruciate ligament reconstruction using a three-dimensional fluoroscopic navigation system. Knee Surg Relat Res 26(3):168–176
7. Shino K, Mae T, Nakamura N (2012) Surgical technique: revision ACL reconstruction with a rectangular tunnel technique. Clin Orthop Relat Res 470(3):843–852
8. Magnussen RA et al (2012) A CT-based classification of prior ACL femoral tunnel location for planning revision ACL surgery. Knee Surg Sports Traumatol Arthrosc 20(7):1298–1306
9. Taketomi S et al (2012) Three-dimensional fluoroscopic navigation guidance for femoral tunnel creation in revision anterior cruciate ligament reconstruction. Arthrosc Tech 1(1): e95–e99
10. Taketomi S et al (2014) Clinical outcome of anatomic double-bundle ACL reconstruction and 3D CT model-based validation of femoral socket aperture position. Knee Surg Sports Traumatol Arthrosc 22(9):2194–2201

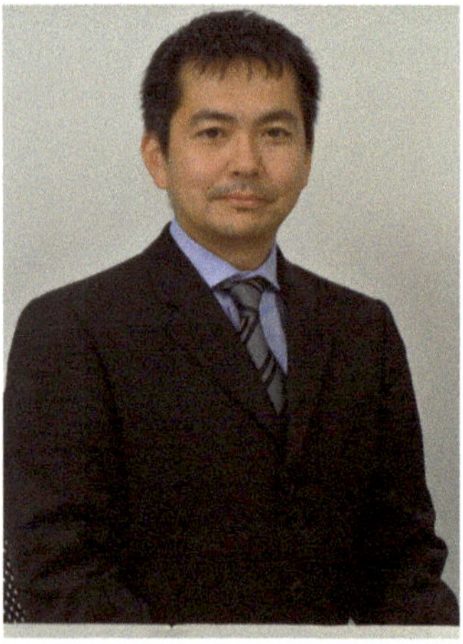

Takumi Nakagawa, M.D., Ph.D, Department of Orthopaedic Surgery, Teikyo University, Tokyo, Japan.

Part IX
ACL Injury in Patients with Open Physes

Chapter 34
ACL Reconstruction with Open Physes

Hiroyuki Koizumi, Masashi Kimura, and Keiji Suzuki

Abstract The surgical management of anterior cruciate ligament (ACL) injuries in patients with open physes is a controversial issue. Different techniques for ACL reconstruction (ACLR) have been described in patients with open physes, including the transphyseal and physeal-sparing techniques. ACLRs that are performed in adolescents with open physes in a manner that is similar to that in adults risk causing injuries to the physes and may result in an angular deformity of the knee or a leg length discrepancy after surgery. We devised two ACLRs for patients with open physes based on several previous clinical studies and animal experiments. The first operation is a partial transphyseal single-bundle ACLR with a bone socket of 8 mm in diameter created in the epiphysis of the tibia through the physes using a 3.5 mm drill and with a transepiphyseal tunnel in the femur that avoids the physes. This ACLR ensures that damage to the physes is prevented to the maximum possible extent. The second operation is a physeal-sparing double-bundle ACLR with transepiphyseal tunnels in the tibia and an over-the-top route for the anteromedial bundle and a transepiphyseal tunnel for the posterolateral bundle on the femur. This technique is used, when the proximal epiphysis on the tibia is of sufficient thickness to allow the creation of two transepiphyseal tunnels. Both ACLRs can lead to good clinical outcomes in patients with open physes that are similar to the outcomes that are expected in adult patients without growth abnormalities.

Keywords Anterior cruciate ligament • Reconstruction • Open physes

H. Koizumi, MD (✉) • M. Kimura • K. Suzuki
Gunma Sports Medicine Research Center, Zenshukai Hospital, 1381 Ninomiya-cho, Maebashi, Gunma 379-2117, Japan
e-mail: kimura@zenshukai.com

M. Ochi et al. (eds.), *ACL Injury and Its Treatment*,
DOI 10.1007/978-4-431-55858-3_34

34.1 Introduction

Recent studies show that double-bundle anterior cruciate ligament reconstruction (ACLR) is associated with better results in adults than other types of ACLR [1, 2]. However, the management of anterior cruciate ligament (ACL) injuries in adolescents with open physes remains a controversial issue.

Nonoperative treatments have been unsuccessful in preventing instability or further meniscal damage and cartilage degeneration in patients with open physes [3–6]. Different ACLR techniques, such as transphyseal or physeal-sparing techniques, have been described in patients with open physes. Extra-articular ACLR can avoid damaging the physes, but it is a non-anatomical technique, which is associated with poor clinical outcomes [4, 5]. The reports appear to indicate that intra-articular ACLR, which seeks to preserve the physes, may lead to clinical outcomes that are superior to those associated with nonoperative treatment or extra-articular ACLR.

Lipscomb and Anderson [7] reported a series of 24 skeletally immature patients who were treated by transphyseal ACLR using a hamstring tendon. They reported that one patient showed a significant limb length discrepancy. There are also some reports on ACLRs in adolescents [8, 9]. ACLRs that are performed in adolescents with open physes in a manner that is similar to that in adults risk causing injuries to the physes and may result in an angular deformity of the knee or a leg length discrepancy after surgery. On animal experiments, Houle et al. performed transphyseal ACLR in skeletally immature rabbits. Physis growth was observed to be arrested in 8 of 11 rabbits. The author did not recommend the placement of tunnels involving $\geq 1\,\%$ of the area across the tibial and femoral physes in ACLRs in children with a high level of skeletal immaturity [10]. Seil et al. evaluated the risk of growth disturbances of transphyseal ACLR with a 5 mm drill using a soft tissue graft in a sheep model. They concluded that transphyseal ACLR did not lead to clinically relevant growth disturbances [11]. Stadelmaier et al. examined the ability of a soft tissue graft to inhibit the formation of a bony bridge within tunnels that were drilled across open physes in a canine model. They found that a soft tissue graft of the fascia lata placed in the drill holes across the open physes prevented the formation of a bony bridge [12].

Janarv et al. [13] reported 15 skeletally immature patients who underwent over-the-top ACLR procedures using a hamstring autograft in which the physes were avoided by way of a tibial tunnel that was created by the transepiphyseal technique. Anderson [14] performed ACLR with a hamstring tendon graft using the transepiphyseal technique on both the femur and tibia in skeletally immature patients. These ACLRs are considered to be physeal-sparing techniques in that they avoid both the distal femoral and the proximal tibial physes. ACLRs using an over-the-top position or the transepiphyseal technique on the femur and the transphyseal technique on the tibia have also been performed in patients with open physes [15–17]. These ACLRs are considered to be partial transphyseal techniques, which avoid the distal femoral physis and pass through the proximal tibial physis. Guzzanti et al. [18] performed physeal-sparing ACLR with the use of a hamstring tendon in five Tanner stage 1 pediatric patients. They reported that ACLR using physis-preserving surgical techniques led to good clinical outcomes and that no clinically significant growth abnormalities were observed. As noted previously, the surgical techniques and timing described in the literature are heterogeneous. Moreover, some of these reports involve small study populations or pediatric patients whose Tanner stages are not clearly described. In addition, there is a tendency for the number of patients at the Tanner stages of 1 and 2 to be relatively small and for many of the patients to be near physeal closure. The surgical management of ACL injuries in patients with open physes has remained a controversial issue because of the risks associated with surgery, which may include angular deformities of the knee and leg length discrepancies. In particular, when the distal femoral physis is damaged, it may lead to a valgus deformity of the lower extremity.

Based on these considerations, we herein attempt to fully explain the need for exercise restriction in patients with wide-open physes and to recommend nonoperative treatment as the initial treatment for ACL injuries in adolescents. For patients who are found to be nearing physeal closure and who want an early return to athletic activity, we suggest two ACLRs using a hamstring autograft to prevent damage to the physes to the maximum possible extent. Specifically, when a preoperative T2-gradient-recalled echo MRI shows very high-signal bands of the physes (no drop-out sign) (Fig. 34.1), we perform a partial transphyseal single-bundle ACLR or a physeal-sparing double-bundle ACLR. In a partial transphyseal single-bundle ACLR, a bone socket of 8 mm in diameter is created in the epiphysis of the tibia through the physis using a 3.5 mm drill, with a transepiphyseal tunnel in the femur that avoids the physis (Fig. 34.2). This technique prevents damage to the physes to the maximum possible extent.

In cases where the proximal epiphysis on the tibia is of sufficient thickness to allow the creation of two transepiphyseal tunnels, we perform a physeal-sparing double-bundle ACLR with transepiphyseal tunnels in the tibia and an over-the-top route or a transepiphyseal tunnel in the femur (Fig. 34.3) [19]. We herein describe the two abovementioned surgical methods and present their respective postoperative results for comparison.

34.2 The Partial Transphyseal ACLR Surgical Technique

We perform single-bundle ACLR using a semitendinosus tendon. In this technique, a femoral tunnel is created avoiding the distal femoral physis. The tibial tunnel is created through the proximal tibial physis with a 3.5 mm drill, after which the bone socket is completed with an 8 mm retrograde drill in the epiphysis of the tibia

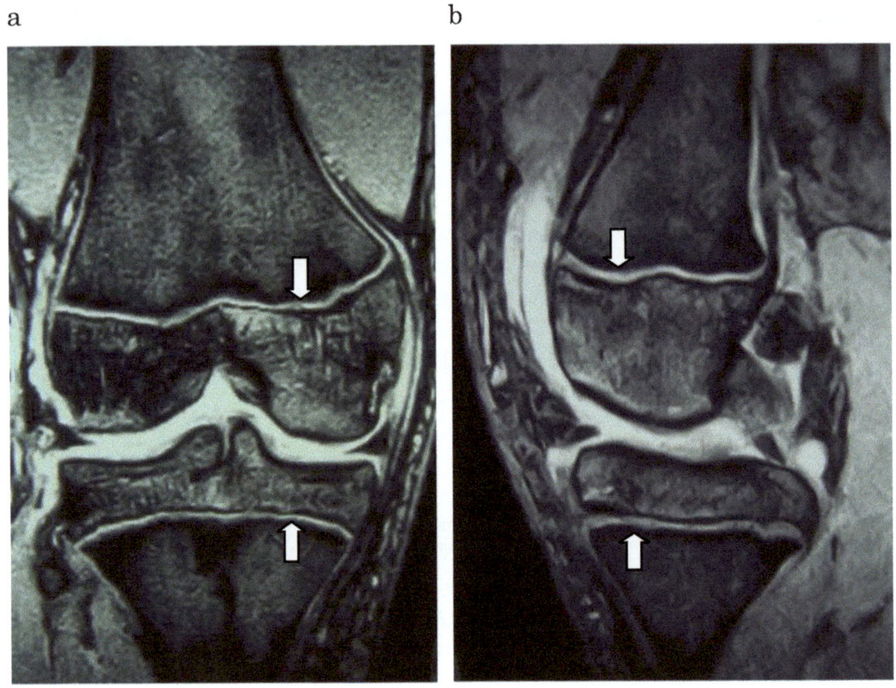

Fig. 34.1 Preoperative T2-gradient-recalled echo MRI of the knee in the coronal plane (**a**) and the sagittal plane (**b**). The images show the very high-signal bands of the physes (no drop-out signs) [19]

(Fig. 34.2). The tendon graft is placed in the anatomic position using the native ACL footprint as a positioning guide.

On the femoral side, using the mini-open approach, a longitudinal incision of approximately 2 cm in length is made from the lateral condyle of the femur to a more distal region. An outside-in guide is placed at the footprint of the anteromedial bundle (AMB), and a guide wire of 2.4 mm in diameter is inserted into the region that is more distal to the femoral physis. An intraoperative X-ray is performed to check the positional relationship between the physis and the guide wire in order to confirm that the physis will not be damaged by drilling with a drill of up to 8 mm in diameter (Fig. 34.4). After confirmation, a bone tunnel with a diameter of 8 mm is created.

On the tibial side, we make a small incision 1 cm medial of the tibial tuberosity. In the joint, the tip of a drill guide is placed just behind the Parsons' knob, slightly medial from the center of the ACL footprint. This position corresponds to the anatomical AMB in adults. A guide wire of approximately 2.4 mm in diameter is introduced through the physis. The appropriate positioning of the guide wire should

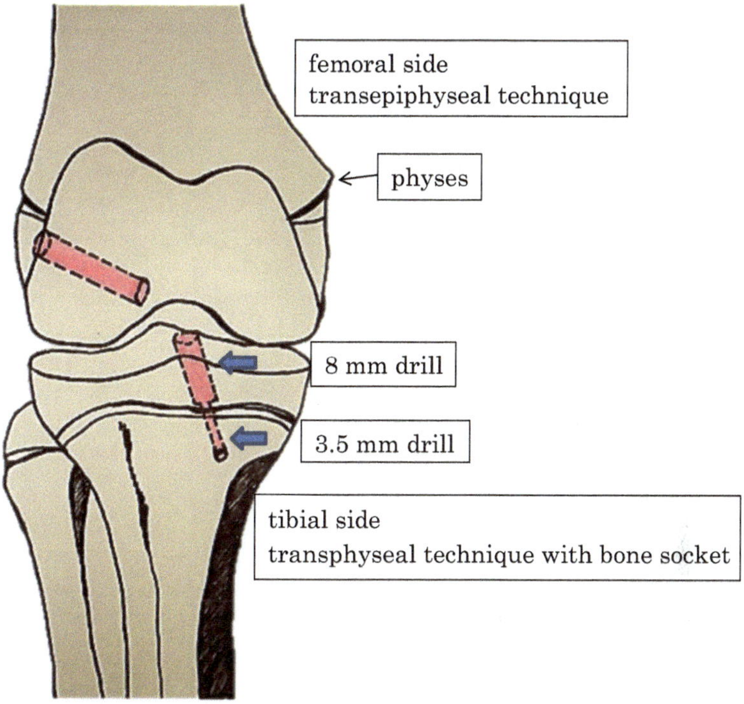

Fig. 34.2 A schematic illustration of a single-bundle ACL reconstruction using the partial transphyseal technique [20]

be confirmed on an intraoperative X-ray (Fig. 34.4). Next, a bone tunnel is created through the physis from the outside of the joint with a 3.5 mm drill. Under radioscopy, drilling is performed from the inside of the joint using an 8 mm FlipCutter®. At that time, drilling is performed just up to the edge of the physis to complete a bone socket (Fig. 34.5).

A quadrupled semitendinosus tendon graft of 6 cm in length is prepared (Fig. 34.6), and the passage is performed with a tight graft-tunnel interface, allowing no room between the graft and bone. A fiber wire or a Telos artificial ligament® should be tied to both ends of the tendon graft. After the induction thread is pushed through the bone tunnel, the tendon graft is introduced from the femoral side into the joint. The tendon graft is then pulled strongly until the distal part of the graft is placed in the bone socket of the tibia.

Firstly, on the tibial side, the fixation is performed in the metaphysis using an EndoButton®, away from the proximal physis. Then, on the femoral side, after load relaxation is achieved by repeating the manual traction (manual max) of the tendon graft approximately ten times, fixation is performed in the epiphysis using a SutureButton® set at 30 N of tension with 20° of knee flexion (Fig. 34.7).

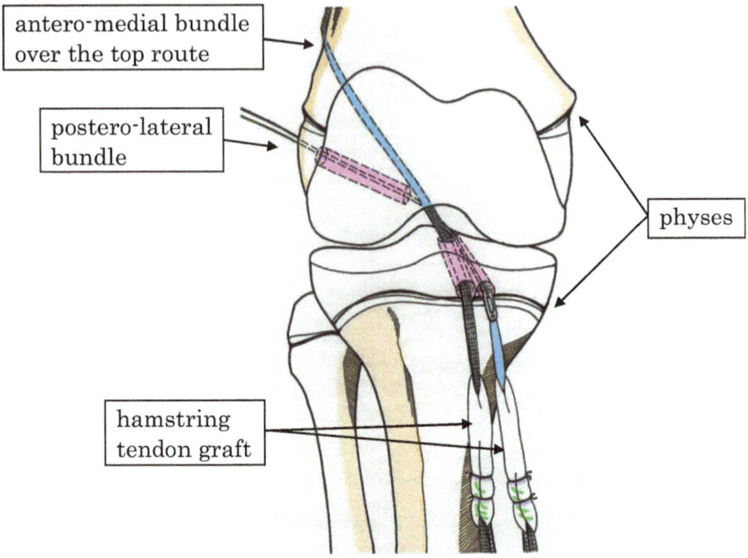

Fig. 34.3 A schematic illustration of a double-bundle ACL reconstruction using the physeal-sparing technique [19]

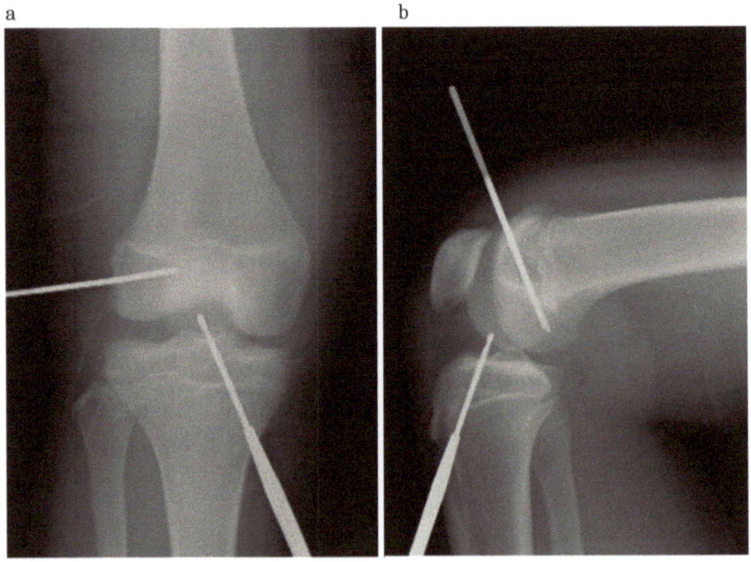

Fig. 34.4 Intraoperative radiographs of the knee in the (**a**) anteroposterior and (**b**) lateral views after guide wires were inserted using the partial transphyseal technique

a

b

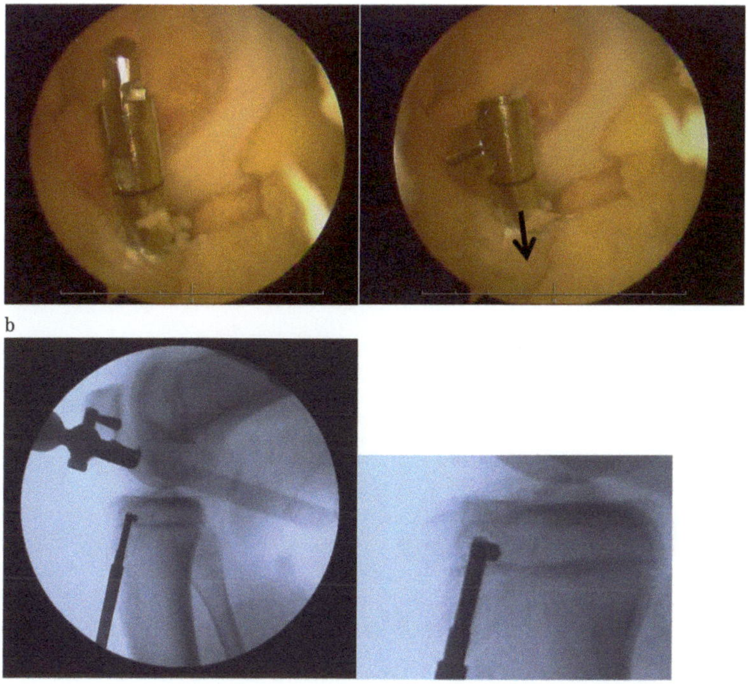

Fig. 34.5 An intraoperative arthroscopic image of the knee (a) and intraoperative fluoroscopy of the proximal tibial physis (b). The bone socket can be created in the epiphysis with an 8 mm retrograde drill

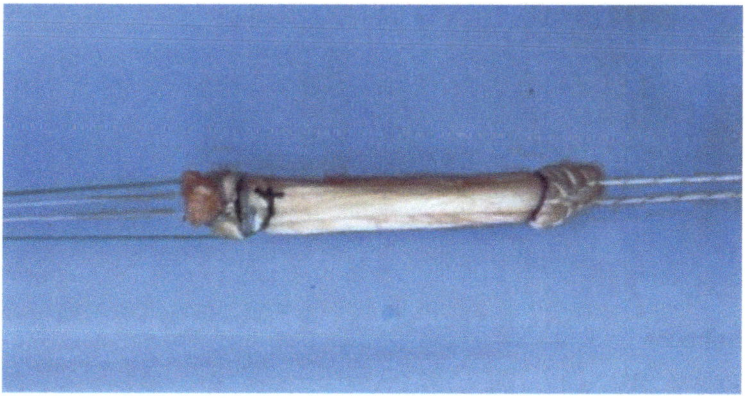

Fig. 34.6 A quadrupled semitendinosus tendon graft measuring 6 cm in length is prepared for a partial transphyseal single-bundle ACLR

a b

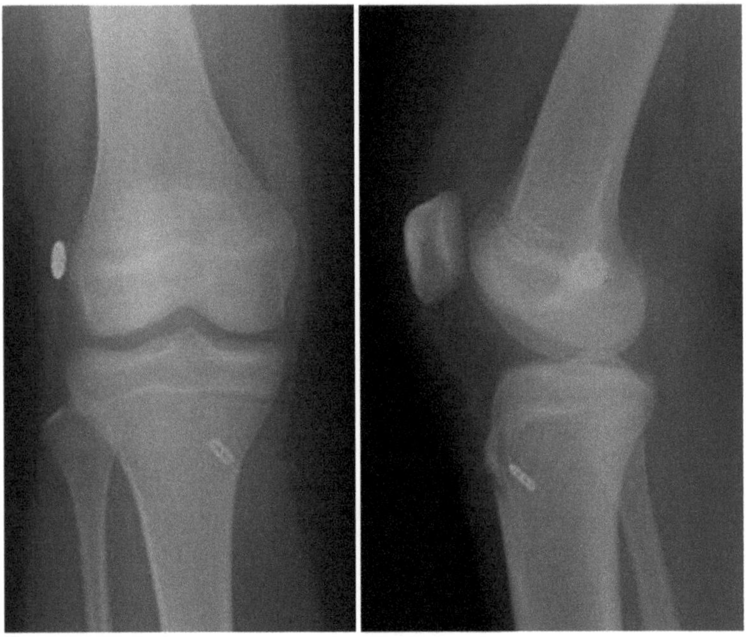

Fig. 34.7 (**a**) Anteroposterior and (**b**) lateral postoperative radiographs of a partial transphyseal single-bundle ACLR

34.3 The Physeal-Sparing ACLR Surgical Technique

A double-bundle ACLR is performed using a hamstring tendon. The AMB on the femur is located in an over-the-top femoral position without a tunnel and the femoral tunnel for the posterolateral bundle (PLB). Tibial tunnels are created to avoid both the distal femoral and proximal tibial physes (Fig. 34.3). The AMB and PLB on the tibia are placed in the anatomic position of each bundle using the native ACL footprint as a positioning guide.

On the femoral side, we make a longitudinal incision of 3 cm in length to a more proximal region from the lateral condyle of the femur, along the posterior border of the iliotibial band. We push the lateral gastrocnemius muscle inward, and the posterior capsule of the joint is detached using the fingers. A crooked forceps is inserted into the posterior part from the medial infrapatellar portal. We touch the forceps with fingers from the posterior articular capsule. The articular capsules should be punctured with the forceps in the outer region and the more proximal region; this is defined as the over-the-top region for the AMB. The PLB is anatomically positioned by the outside-in technique (Fig. 34.8). With an outside-in guide placed in the PMB footprint, a guide wire of 2.4 mm in diameter is inserted distal to the femoral physis. An intraoperative X-ray is performed to check the positional relationship between the physes and the guide wire in order to confirm

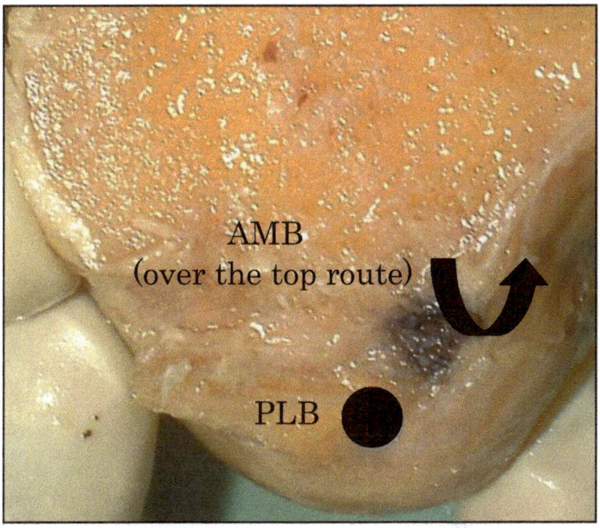

Fig. 34.8 The placements, in the femoral over-the-top route, of the AMB and the femoral tunnel for the PLB in a physeal-sparing double-bundle ACLR [19]

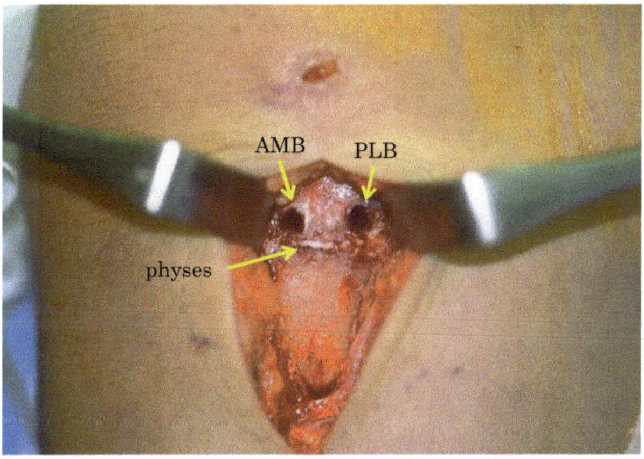

Fig. 34.9 The periosteum is exfoliated and the proximal tibial physis is exposed. Two guide wires are inserted for a physeal-sparing double-bundle ACLR, while the location of the proximal tibial physis is confirmed

that the physis is not damaged by the drilling. After confirmation, the femoral tunnel for the PLB is created using the transepiphyseal technique with a 5–6 mm drill.

On the tibial side, we make a longitudinal incision of 3 cm in length, 1 cm medial of the tibial tuberosity. We exfoliate the periosteum and expose the proximal tibial physis (Fig. 34.9). From outside the joint, the drill guide is placed in the epiphysis, 1 cm medial of the tibial tuberosity in order to avoid damaging the proximal tibial physis. In the joint, the tip of the drill guide is placed just behind the Parsons' knob, slightly medial from the center of the ACL footprint. This position corresponds to the anatomical position of the AMB in adults. A guide wire with a diameter of 2.4 mm is introduced into the proximal tibial physis. Then, the guide wire for the

PLB is inserted. Outside the joint, the drill guide is placed a fingerbreadth from the medial side of the AMB in order to avoid damaging the proximal tibial physis. In the joint, the tip of the drill guide is inserted 7–8 mm posterior from the AMB, facing outward at an angle of 10–20°. Following this technique, bone tunnels are created in the epiphysis. Therefore, careful attention should be paid in order to avoid inserting the guide wire at a shallow angle and damaging the articular surface of the tibia. Moreover, special care should be paid in the placement of the guide to avoid damaging the physes in drilling. We recommend that two guide wires be inserted for the AMB and PLB while directly confirming the location of the proximal tibial physis (Fig. 34.9). After the proper positioning of the inserted guide wires is confirmed by intraoperative X-ray, the tibial tunnel is created with the use of the transepiphyseal technique with a 6 mm drill for the AMB and a 5–6 mm drill for the PLB.

Two doubled hamstring tendon grafts of 6 cm in length are prepared, and the graft passage is performed with a tight graft-tunnel interface that allows no room between the graft and bone. A Telos artificial ligament® or a fiber wire is preliminarily tied to each end of the tendon grafts. After an induction thread is introduced through the bone tunnel, each of the tendon grafts (first the PLB and then AMB) is inserted from the tibial side to the inside of the joint.

On the femoral side, the AMB is fixed in the metaphysis, away from the distal physis, with double staples, and the PLB is fixed by an EndoButton® in the epiphysis. Successively, on the tibial side, after load relaxation is achieved by repeating the manual traction (manual max) of the tendon graft approximately ten times, both the AMB and PLB are fixed simultaneously by double staples with a tension of 30 N at 20° of knee flexion in the metaphysis away from the proximal physis.

34.4 Postoperative Rehabilitation

Both of the surgical techniques follow the same postoperative rehabilitation protocol. The use of a continuous passive motion (CPM) machine is initiated from postoperative day 2. Weight bearing (one-third of body weight) is permitted from week 2. Full weight bearing is permitted from week 4. Jogging is permitted from 4 months after surgery, and full-speed running is allowed after 6 months. A complete return to competitive sports is allowed at 8–10 months.

34.5 Results

During the postoperative follow-up period, no clinically significant growth abnormalities were observed with either the partial transphyseal techniques or the physeal-sparing techniques. One out of the 10 patients and 2 out of the 15 patients who underwent surgery with the partial transphyseal and physeal-sparing techniques, respectively, showed positive results on a Lachman test (n.s.). One out of the 10 patients and 3 out of the 15 patients who underwent surgery with the partial transphyseal and physeal-sparing techniques showed positive results on a pivot shift test (n.s.). The mean side-to-side differences in KT-2000 (MED metric Corp. San Diego, CA) measurements using the partial transphyseal and physeal-sparing techniques were 1.2 ± 1.5 mm and 1.5 ± 1.5 mm, respectively (n.s.). The mean IKDC scores using the partial transphyseal and physeal-sparing techniques were 95.7 and 96.7, respectively. Finally, the mean Lysholm knee scoring scales using the partial transphyseal and physeal-sparing techniques were 97.5 and 99, respectively (n.s.). Both techniques led to good clinical outcomes in patients with open physes with results that were similar to those in adult patients without growth abnormalities.

References

1. Branch TP, Siebold R, Freedberg HI, Jacobs CA (2011) Double-bundle ACL reconstruction demonstrated superior clinical stability to single-bundle ACL reconstruction: a matched-pairs analysis of instrumented tests of tibial anterior translation and internal rotation laxity. Knee Surg Sports Traumatol Arthrosc 19:432–440
2. Järvelä T, Suomalainen P (2011) ACL reconstruction with double-bundle technique: a review of clinical results. Phys Sportsmed 39:85–92
3. Kannus P, Jarvinen M (1988) Knee ligament injuries in adolescents: eight year follow-up of conservative management. J Bone Joint Surg (Br) 70:772–776
4. McCarroll JR, Rettig AC, Shelbourne KD (1988) Anterior cruciate ligament injuries in the young athlete with open physes. Am J Sports Med 16:44–47
5. Graf BK, Lange RH, Fujisaki CK, Landry GL, Saluja RK (1992) Anterior cruciate ligament tears in skeletally immature patients: meniscal pathology at presentation and after attempted conservative treatment. Arthroscopy 8:229–233
6. Mizuta H, Kubota K, Shiraishi M, Otsuka Y, Nagamoto N, Takagi K (1995) The conservative treatment of complete tears of the anterior cruciate ligament in skeletally immature patients. J Bone Joint Surg (Br) 77:890–894
7. Lipscomb AB, Anderson AF (1986) Tears of the anterior cruciate ligament in adolescents. J Bone Joint Surg Am 68:19–28
8. Koman JD, Sanders JO (1999) Valgus deformity after reconstruction of the anterior cruciate ligament in a skeletally immature patient. J Bone Joint Surg Am 81:711–715
9. Robert HE, Casin C (2010) Valgus and flexion deformity after reconstruction of the anterior cruciate ligament in a skeletally immature patient. Knee Surg Sports Traumatol Arthrosc 18:1369–1373
10. Houle JB, Letts M, Yang J (2001) Effects of a tensioned tendon graft in a bone tunnel across the rabbit physis. Clin Orthop 391:275–281
11. Seil R, Pape D, Kohn D (2008) The risk of growth changes during transphyseal drilling in sheep with open physes. Arthroscopy 24:824–833
12. Stadelmaier DM, Arnoczky SP, Dodds J, Ross H (1995) The effect of drilling and soft tissue grafting across open growth plates: a histologic study. Am J Sports Med 23:431–435
13. Janarv PM, Nystrom A, Werner S, Hirsch G (1996) Anterior cruciate ligament injuries in skeletally immature patients. J Pediatr Orthop 16:673–677
14. Anderson AF (2003) Transepiphyseal replacement of the anterior cruciate ligament in skeletally immature patients. J Bone Joint Surg Am 85:1255–1263

15. Bisson LJ, Wickiewicz T, Levinson M, Warren R (1998) ACL reconstruction in children with open physes. Orthopedics 21:659–663
16. Henry J, Chotel F, Chouteau J, Fessy MH, Berard J, Moyen B (2009) Rupture of the anterior cruciate ligament in children: early reconstruction with open physes or delayed reconstruction to skeletal maturity? Knee Surg Sports Traumatol Arthrosc 17:748–755
17. Lo IK, Kirkley A, Fowler PJ, Miniaci A (1997) The outcome of operatively treated anterior cruciate ligament disruptions in the skeletally immature child. Arthroscopy 13:627–634
18. Guzzanti V, Falciglia F, Stanitski CL (2003) Physeal-sparing intraarticular anterior cruciate ligament reconstruction in preadolescents. Am J Sports Med 31:949–953
19. Koizumi H, Kimura M, Kamimura T, Hagiwara K, Takagishi K (2013) The outcomes after anterior cruciate ligament reconstruction in adolescents with open physes. Knee Surg Sports Traumatol Arthrosc 21:950–956
20. Suzuki K, Kimura M, Koizumi H et al (2013) J Kanto District Soc Study Knee Joint 29(1): 17–21

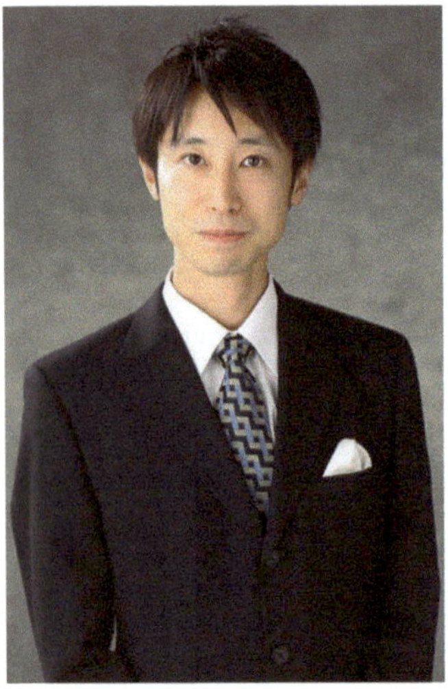

Hiroyuki Koizumi, MD, Gunma Sports Medicine Research Center, Zenshukai Hospital, Gunma, Japan.

Chapter 35
Avulsion Fracture of the ACL

Takehiko Matsushita and Ryosuke Kuroda

Abstract Avulsion fracture of the anterior cruciate ligament (ACL) is seen in pediatric patients and infrequently in adult patients. It primarily occurs during sports activities and trauma. Inadequate treatment can cause pain, range of motion limitation, and instability with subsequent deterioration of the knee joint. Therefore, it is important to provide appropriate treatment to prevent such significant complications. Treatments are generally chosen according to the extent of fragment displacement and criteria of the fracture classification systems used for determining treatment strategy. Surgical methods have varied among surgeons. Currently, no gold standard surgical method exists; however, most of the reported results are satisfactory. Surgeons need to consider the advantages and disadvantages of each surgical method. The prognosis for patients with avulsion fracture of the ACL appears to be good if appropriate treatments are applied. In this chapter, injury etiology, mechanism, diagnosis, classification, treatments, and surgical methods, including the author's technique, will be described and discussed.

Keywords Avulsion fracture • Anterior cruciate ligament • Open epiphyses

35.1 Introduction

Avulsion fracture of the anterior cruciate ligament (ACL) is a fracture of the tibial attachment site of the ACL, which is pulled out, rather than a tear in the substance of the ACL. It is also called an "intercondylar eminence fracture of the tibia," "tibial eminence fracture," "tibial eminentia fracture," or "tibial spine fracture." Although a previous report suggested that ACL fibers could become elongated and damaged when avulsion fractures occur [1], the ACL substance is well preserved in most cases. Avulsion fractures of the ACL are seen in pediatric patients and infrequently in adult patients. Patients manifest symptoms similar to those of patients with ACL tears. Inadequate treatment can result in pain, range of motion limitation, and joint

T. Matsushita, M.D., PhD (✉) • R. Kuroda
Department of Orthopaedic Surgery, Kobe University Graduate School of Medicine, 7-5-1 Kusunoki-cho, Chuo-ku, Kobe, Hyogo 650-0017, Japan
e-mail: matsushi@med.kobe-u.ac.jp

M. Ochi et al. (eds.), *ACL Injury and Its Treatment*,
DOI 10.1007/978-4-431-55858-3_35

instability. Therefore, it is important to provide appropriate treatment to prevent such significant complications, especially in young patients. Avulsion fracture of the ACL often requires surgical treatment if the fragment is displaced although surgical methods have varied among surgeons. Currently, no gold standard surgical method exists; however, most reported results are satisfactory. In this chapter, injury etiology, mechanism, diagnosis, classification, treatments, and surgical methods, including the author's technique, will be described and discussed.

35.2 Etiology, Mechanisms

Avulsion fracture of the ACL occurs during sports activities and traffic accidents. Generally, it is seen more often in children than in adults, most likely because the ACL attachment site on the bone is immature and biomechanically weak in children [2]. Avulsion fracture of the ACL often occurs in children between ages 6 and 17 years [3–5]. Previous reports have suggested that the mechanism of injury is direct force, with hyperextension of the knee and injury patterns similar to ACL tears [6–9].

35.3 Classification

The fracture classification system of Meyers and McKeever [10, 11] is commonly used. Their system classifies fracture patterns into three different types on the basis of the displacement of the fragment (Fig. 35.1). Type I fractures are those with a non-displaced or minimally displaced fragment. Type II fractures are those in which the anterior part of the fragment is partially displaced superiorly without complete displacement of the whole fragment. Type III fractures are completely displaced fractures. Zaricznyj further divided type III fractures into subtypes IIIA, IIIB, and IV (Fig. 35.1) [12]. Type IIIA fractures include completely displaced

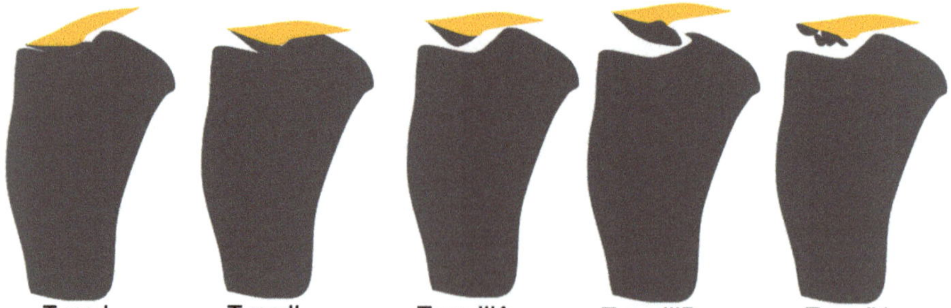

Fig. 35.1 Classification of anterior cruciate ligament avulsion fractures

fragments of the ACL insertion area. Type IIIB fractures include fragments from non-ACL insertion areas, such as the whole intercondylar eminence, and fragment rotation. Type IV fractures are comminuted fractures. These classifications are useful for determining treatment choice, such as conservative treatment vs. surgery, and for choosing surgical methods.

35.4 Diagnosis

Patients with avulsion fracture of the ACL usually exhibit swelling and hemarthrosis. Manual tests for detecting ACL injuries, such as the Lachman test and pivot shift test, can be positive. The Lachman test shows an unclear end point, as is usual with ACL injury, and the examiner will feel an increased anteroposterior translation of the tibia during the test. The pivot shift test may be difficult to perform because of pain in the acute phase.

Displaced fragments can be detected by the standard anteroposterior view, tunnel view, and lateral view on plain radiographs. Generally, the lateral view is best for diagnosing avulsion fractures (Fig. 35.2). Computed tomography (CT) is useful for evaluating fragment size and degree of displacement, and three-dimensional CT (3D-CT) images assist with surgical planning, providing a whole view of the fragment and fracture site (Fig. 35.3). Magnetic resonance imaging (MRI) facilitates evaluation of the ACL mid-substance and other combined injuries, such as meniscal and chondral injuries (Fig. 35.4). Johnson et al. reviewed

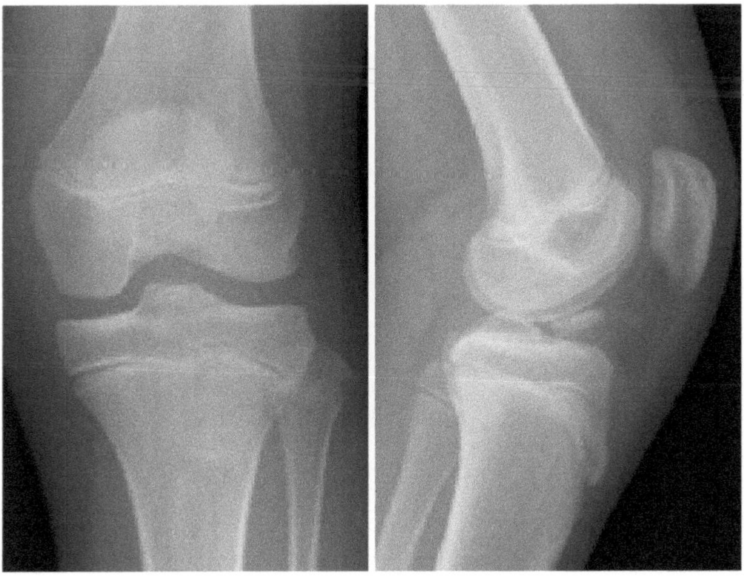

Fig. 35.2 X-rays of a 12-year-old girl. Anteroposterior view (*left*). Lateral view (*right*)

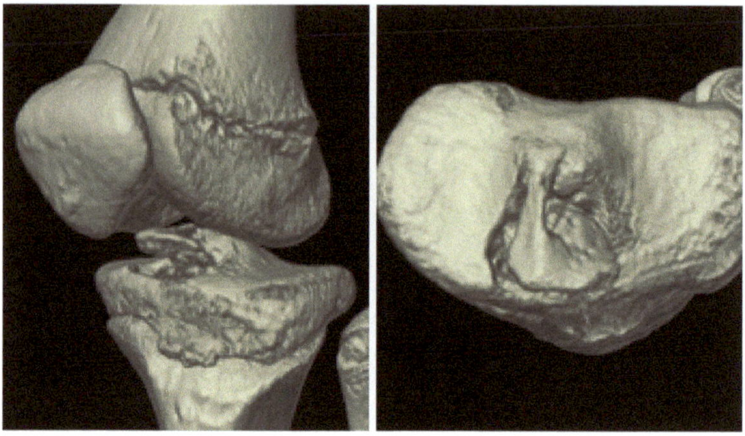

Fig. 35.3 Computed tomography. Three-dimensional computed tomography image shows the displaced fragment and fracture site

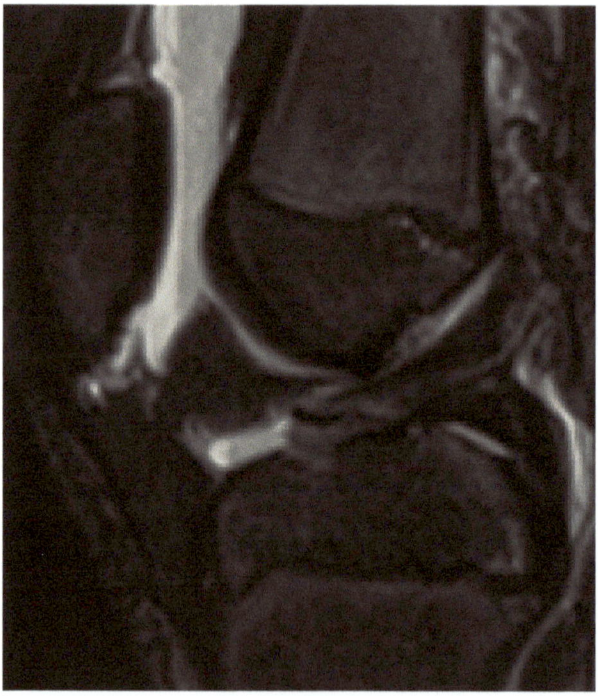

Fig. 35.4 Magnetic resonance imaging. Magnetic resonance imaging shows continuity of the anterior cruciate ligament fiber attached to the displaced fragment

20 pediatric tibial eminence fractures and found that six patients had associated meniscal tears, which were seen more frequently in type III than in type II fractures [13]. MRI also helps to detect non-displaced fracture. In most cases, the tibial

intercondylar eminence is avulsed. However, the femoral attachment site can also be avulsed [14] and should be assessed carefully.

35.5 Treatments

Type I fractures can be treated conservatively. However, the treatment of type II fractures is controversial. Some authors report acceptable results after conservative treatment [15], while surgical treatment may promote faster progression of rehabilitation. Type III and IV fractures generally require surgical treatment, and various surgical methods have been reported [16]. It has been suggested that the transverse meniscal ligament can interpose within the fracture site and block reduction of the fragment [17]. Therefore, the fracture site should be carefully observed and checked to determine whether proper reduction can be obtained. Previous reports have described techniques using screw fixation, suture anchor fixation, and pullout suture fixation under open arthrotomy or arthroscopy [18–27]. Recently, hybrid technique has been also reported [28, 29]. Each surgical method has advantages and disadvantages, and surgeons need to consider the potential complications associated with each method. For example, screw fixation is a relatively simple technique but may not be suitable for comminuted fractures and requires a second surgery for screw removal if metal screws are used. In addition, impingement at near full extension may occur. Pullout suture techniques are technically more demanding but are preferred for treatment of comminuted fractures and fractures with small fragments, such as type IV fractures.

35.5.1 Conservative Treatment

Conservative treatment is usually immobilization of the knee by applying a cast. Previous reports have recommended keeping the knee in maximum extension to reduce the fragment for 4–8 weeks. Weight bearing is permitted 4–6 weeks after the immobilization [30]. Keeping the knee in hyperextension for more than 4 weeks may not be practical; therefore, a slightly flexed knee position of 10–20° can be used if reduction of the fragment is maintained. Caution is needed when determining the knee position because the ACL becomes tight in extension, and maximum extension may worsen the extent of the displacement.

35.5.2 Screw Fixation

Once proper reduction is achieved, the fragment can be temporarily fixed in place with a guide wire transligamentally or from a superomedial position. The position of the guide wire is carefully checked by an image intensifier. After measuring the length of the screw, drilling is performed over the guide wire, and a 4.0–4.5-mm cannulated cancellous screw with or without washer is inserted anterior to posterior, taking care not to damage the epiphyseal plate. Screw removal is necessary if a metal screw is used. Screw fixation techniques using Herbert screw has been also reported [31].

35.5.3 Pullout Fixation

Pullout fixation can be performed via arthrotomy or arthroscopy, with sutures placed in ACL fibers just above the fragment through a mini-open incision. Arthroscopically, sutures are placed with a suture hook. However, one of the problems with using a suture hook is that the size of the hook is relatively large, and the ACL fibers may be damaged when they are pierced. Therefore, a smaller hook is recommended as described below in the author's preferred method. Strong sutures, such as FiberWire® and No. 2 Ethibond, are safest for holding the fragment securely; however, absorbable or nonabsorbable sutures can also be used [32]. If the fragment is temporarily fixed with a K-wire percutaneously, suture placement will be easier. The sutures are once retrieved through a portal. Using a drill guide for ACL reconstruction, a 2.4-mm K-wire is drilled. A suture retriever is inserted into the K-wire hole, and the sutures placed in the ACL fiber are retrieved. Sutures are tied over the tibial cortex.

35.6 Biomechanical Studies

To compare the initial strength of different methods of fixation, biomechanical studies were conducted in ACL avulsion fracture models. Bong et al. compared arthroscopic suture fixation with cannulated screw fixation using human cadaveric knees. For the suture fixation, three No. 2 FiberWire® sutures were passed through the tibial base of the ACL and tied over bone tunnels on the anterior tibial cortex. For the screw fixation, a cannulated screw was used. The fixation with FiberWire® showed a significantly higher mean ultimate strength than that of fixation with a cannulated screw [33]. Anderson et al. compared the biomechanical strength of the following four physeal-sparing techniques: (1) ultrahigh molecular weight polyethylene suture–suture button, (2) suture anchor, (3) polydioxanone suture–suture button (PDS/SB), and (4) screw fixation technique using skeletally immature porcine knees. They reported that the ultrahigh molecular weight polyethylene suture–suture button technique was biomechanically superior to the other techniques [34]. Senekovic et al. compared metal cannulated screw and washer fixation with absorbable suture fixation in human cadaveric knees. The suture fixation was found to be stronger than fixation with the cannulated screw and washer [35]. These reports suggest that fixation with sutures may have a biomechanical advantage compared with screw fixations. However, conflicting results were reported by other studies. In et al. examined the initial stability of a suture anchor fixation, comparing with a screw fixation and pullout suture fixation in human cadaveric knees. They reported that the failure strength of the suture anchor fixation was significantly higher than that of the pullout suture fixation but it was not significantly different from that of the screw fixation. In addition, they reported that the initial displacement of the suture anchor fixation was lower than that of the screw fixation and the pullout suture fixation, suggesting an advantage of the suture anchor fixation over the other techniques [36]. Tsukada et al. examined the initial strength of three different techniques, pullout suture fixation, and antegrade and retrograde screw fixations in response to a tensile cyclic load in human cadaveric knees. The anterior tibial translation was significantly increased in the pullout suture fixation compared with the antegrade screw fixation, suggesting that antegrade fixation is biomechanically more reliable than pullout suture fixation [37].

These biomechanical studies provided useful information in the surgical treatment choice for ACL avulsion fractures. However, the cadavers used in the reported studies were of advanced age, and the fracture models were not the same as the fractures seen in patients. Therefore, results may differ in patients.

35.7 Clinical Outcomes in the Literature

A number of clinical outcomes after treatment for ACL avulsion fractures in children and adults have been reported.

35.7.1 Conservative Treatment

Wilfinger et al. reported clinical outcomes after nonoperative treatment of fractures of the tibial intercondylar eminence in 43 pediatric patients < 17 years (range 6–16 years) of age. The injuries comprised 14 type I, 13 type II, and 16 type III fractures. Patients were treated with a long leg cast with the knee hyperextended for 3 weeks followed by casting at 10–15° flexion for another 2–3 weeks. Only one patient showed a delayed union and needed surgical treatment; none of the patients reported pain or "giving way" in their daily life. Therefore, the authors recommended conservative treatment as a primary treatment choice for intercondylar eminence fractures in children [15].

35.7.2 Arthroscopic Reduction with Cast

Prince and Moyer described a technique using arthroscopic reduction and casting and reported a good postoperative outcome. The authors concluded that arthroscopic reduction of the tibial eminence followed by cast immobilization is a good treatment choice because it eliminates the risk of damaging the physis and does not require subsequent surgery for hardware removal [38]. McLennan reported outcomes of 35 patients, whose injuries included 20 type IIIA fractures and 15 type IIIB fractures, treated with arthroscopic reduction combined with either casting with the knee in extension or percutaneous pin fixation. He concluded that arthroscopic reduction combined with percutaneous pin fixation was an effective treatment although lack of extension persisted in some patients [30]. Hallam et al. performed an anatomical study creating an intercondylar eminence fracture model using human cadaveric knees and found that the transverse meniscal ligament tended to block reduction of the fragment. On the basis of this observation, they performed arthroscopic reduction followed by immobilization in a cast with the knee in hyperextension for 6 weeks on eight adolescents (mean age, 12.6 years) with type II or type III fractures and reported good clinical outcomes [17].

35.7.3 Screw Fixation/Suture Fixation/Suture Anchor Fixation

Senekovic and Veselko assessed the 5-year results of arthroscopic reductions followed by anterograde fixations with a cannulated screw in 32 patients with type II, III, and IV fractures. The authors reported that the average value for KT-1000 after surgery was 1.1 mm, and overall results were successful. In addition, they reported that the fixation was stable enough, even in type IV fractures, to allow early range of motion exercise [22]. Wiegand et al. treated eight children with type II or III fractures using 3.9-mm Herbert screws in a physeal-sparing manner and reported successful results without major complications [31].

Hunter et al. examined clinical outcomes of 17 patients, age 7–60 years. Of these, eight patients received suture fixations, and nine patients received screw fixations. All patients had satisfactory results; however, skeletally immature patients with suture fixation had better clinical outcomes [19]. Huang et al. reported outcomes of 36 patients (age 17–73 years) who received an arthroscopic suture fixation with four No. 5 Ethibond polyester sutures and reported that all patients obtained union within 3 months without major complications [20].

Louis et al. treated 17 pediatric patients (age 6–16 years) with type II fractures by open reduction and internal fixation with sutures or a suture anchor. They reported that none of the patients showed obvious instability, and all patients were able to return to their original sports activities. The authors, therefore, recommended surgical treatment for type II tibial intercondylar eminence fractures in children [39]. Casalonga et al. retrospectively examined 32 children with avulsion fractures of the ACL, including 8 type I, 17 type II, 5 type III, and 2 type IV fractures, who were treated both conservatively and surgically, with a mean follow-up of 9 years. Type I and II fractures were treated conservatively, and types III and IV were treated by open reduction and fixation with either sutures or a screw. The mean side-to-side anteroposterior difference on KT-1000 testing was 0.88 mm for type I fractures, 0.82 mm for type II, and 0.30 mm for types III and IV together; patients treated surgically showed better objective scores, such as IKDC score and muscle power, than patients treated conservatively [4]. Tudisco et al. examined long-term clinical outcomes in a group of 14 patients with avulsion fracture of the ACL, including four type I, three type II, and seven type III fractures according to the Meyers and McKeever classification. Seven patients were treated conservatively, and seven patients were treated surgically, either by open reduction and internal fixation or arthroscopic reduction and internal fixation. Thirteen patients showed no obvious instability and returned to their original sports activity level, whereas one patient with a type III fracture who was treated conservatively developed gross instability. Other authors have concluded that good results can be obtained by conservative treatment in type I fractures, whereas surgical treatments are recommended for type II and III fractures [40].

35.8 Author's Preferred Surgical Method

My colleagues and I prefer to treat ACL avulsion fractures using a pullout suture technique under arthroscopy. We believe that the pullout suture technique can be applied in most cases, including those with comminuted fractures. Our surgical method is described below.

35.8.1 Procedure

Standard anterolateral and medial portals are created. Arthroscopic lavage is performed to wash out the hematoma and obtain a clear view. The displaced fragment and the location of the origin are carefully evaluated. We usually debride the backside of the fragment and fragment bed. This helps reduce the fragment to its original location. If surgery is delayed for some reason, the fragment may not fit the original fragment bed, and an excessive debridement may be necessary. Sometimes the medial meniscus will interfere with reduction of the fragment; therefore, the position and orientation of the fragment must be carefully observed. Once reduction of the fragment is estimated, a 2.4-mm K-wire or Hewson pins are inserted, using a drill guide for ACL reconstruction, in the tibia at the margin of the fracture site. Usually, penetrating the epiphysis with 2.4-mm K-wire does not cause growth disturbance. However, if avoiding violation of the epiphysis is considered safer, the position of the epiphysis needs to be determined under fluoroscopy. We usually insert four wires, aiming at the corner of the fragment bed. Anterior pins can be inserted without penetrating the epiphysis, but this may be difficult to achieve with posterior pins. Next, the K-wires are replaced with suture retrievers. Two sutures (No. 2 FiberWire®) are inserted into the ACL using a suture hook (SutureLasso™, Arthrex, Inc., Naples, FL, USA). Sutures can be inserted in the position, anterior

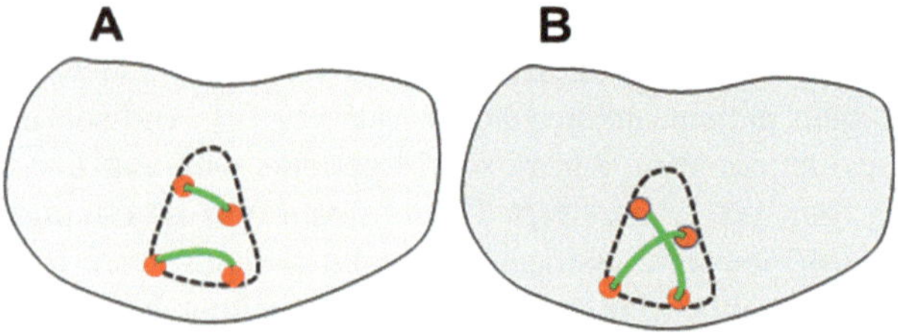

Fig. 35.5 Position of drill holes and sutures. *Red dots* show the position of the drill holes. *Green line* shows sutures. (**a**) Sutures place in vertical positions. (**b**) Sutures placed in a crisscross position

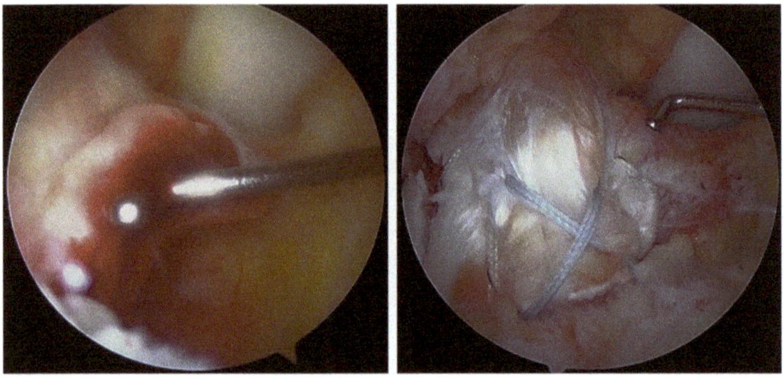

Fig. 35.6 Arthroscopic views. The probe shows the fragment peeled off the attachment site (*left*). The pullout suture fixation is placed in figure-8 configuration (*right*)

and posterior in vertical positions or a crisscross position (Fig. 35.5). Sutures also can be placed in a figure-8 configuration if the fragment is comminuted, as reported by Zao et al. [41] (Fig. 35.6). Each suture is then placed in the suture retriever and pulled out. Sutures are tied on the periosteum of the tibia. A button can be used, if necessary, to avoid cutting out the bone bridge. After the fixation is complete, the knee is moved to check whether the fixation is rigid. Because the ACL becomes tight in extension, careful observation of the status of the fragment during maximum extension is necessary. If rigid fixation is not obtained, a suture may be added anteriorly, or the progression of postoperative rehabilitation should be delayed. A similar operative procedure has been reported by Su et al. [21].

35.8.2 Postoperative Protocols

Immobilization with a cast or knee brace may be safest after surgery. The period of immobilization depends on the stability of the fragment during the surgery. A knee brace is applied for 2–4 weeks. The range of motion exercise is allowed 2–3 weeks after surgery. Partial weight bearing is started 2–3 weeks after surgery with a knee brace in children. Full weight bearing is allowed 6 weeks after surgery. Activity may be increased, depending on the status of the union. Jogging is usually permitted 3 months after surgery, and sports activity is permitted 4–6 months after surgery.

35.9 Conclusion

Avulsion fracture of the ACL is one of the common injuries seen in children. Minimally displaced fractures can be treated conservatively, whereas displaced fragments should be reduced properly and fixed with careful attention to the epiphyseal plate. Various surgical methods have been reported, and surgeons should know the advantages and disadvantages of each procedure. The prognosis for patients with avulsion fracture of the ACL is acceptable if proper treatments are applied.

References

1. Noyes FR, DeLucas JL, Torvik PJ (1974) Biomechanics of anterior cruciate ligament failure: an analysis of strain-rate sensitivity and mechanisms of failure in primates. J Bone Joint Surg Am 56:236–253
2. Woo SL, Hollis JM, Adams DJ, Lyon RM, Takai S (1991) Tensile properties of the human femur-anterior cruciate ligament-tibia complex. The effects of specimen age and orientation. Am J Sports Med 19:217–225
3. Gronkvist H, Hirsch G, Johansson L (1984) Fracture of the anterior tibial spine in children. J Pediatr Orthop 4:465–468
4. Casalonga A, Bourelle S, Chalencon F, De Oliviera L, Gautheron V, Cottalorda J (2010) Tibial intercondylar eminence fractures in children: the long-term perspective. Orthop Traumatol Surg Res 96:525–530. doi:10.1016/j.otsr.2010.01.012
5. Song EK, Seon JK, Park SJ, Yoon TR (2009) Clinical outcome of avulsion fracture of the anterior cruciate ligament between children and adults. J Pediatr Orthop B 18:335–338. doi:10.1097/BPB.0b013e32832f06bd
6. Ahmad CS, Stein BE, Jeshuran W, Nercessian OA, Henry JH (2001) Anterior cruciate ligament function after tibial eminence fracture in skeletally mature patients. Am J Sports Med 29:339–345
7. Kendall NS, Hsu SY, Chan KM (1992) Fracture of the tibial spine in adults and children. A review of 31 cases. J Bone Joint Surg (Br) 74:848–852
8. Accousti WK, Willis RB (2003) Tibial eminence fractures. Orthop Clin North Am 34:365–375
9. White EA, Patel DB, Matcuk GR, Forrester DM, Lundquist RB, Hatch GF 3rd, Vangsness CT, Gottsegen CJ (2013) Cruciate ligament avulsion fractures: anatomy, biomechanics, injury patterns, and approach to management. Emerg Radiol 20:429–440. doi:10.1007/s10140-013-1121-0
10. Meyers MH, Mc KF (1959) Fracture of the intercondylar eminence of the tibia. J Bone Joint Surg Am 41-A:209–220; discussion 220–202
11. Meyers MH, McKeever FM (1970) Fracture of the intercondylar eminence of the tibia. J Bone Joint Surg Am 52:1677–1684

12. Zaricznyj B (1977) Avulsion fracture of the tibial eminence: treatment by open reduction and pinning. J Bone Joint Surg Am 59:1111–1114
13. Johnson AC, Wyatt JD, Treme G, Veitch AJ (2014) Incidence of associated knee injury in pediatric tibial eminence fractures. J Knee Surg 27:215–219. doi:10.1055/s-0033-1360656
14. Tohyama H, Kutsumi K, Yasuda K (2002) Avulsion fracture at the femoral attachment of the anterior cruciate ligament after intercondylar eminence fracture of the tibia. Am J Sports Med 30:279–282
15. Wilfinger C, Castellani C, Raith J, Pilhatsch A, Hollwarth ME, Weinberg AM (2009) Nonoperative treatment of tibial spine fractures in children-38 patients with a minimum follow-up of 1 year. J Orthop Trauma 23:519–524. doi:10.1097/BOT.0b013e3181a13fe4
16. Lubowitz JH, Elson WS, Guttmann D (2005) Part II: Arthroscopic treatment of tibial plateau fractures: intercondylar eminence avulsion fractures. Arthroscopy 21:86–92. doi:10.1016/j.arthro.2004.09.031
17. Hallam PJ, Fazal MA, Ashwood N, Ware HE, Glasgow MM, Powell JM (2002) An alternative to fixation of displaced fractures of the anterior intercondylar eminence in children. J Bone Joint Surg (Br) 84:579–582
18. Lu XW, Hu XP, Jin C, Zhu T, Ding Y, Dai LY (2010) Reduction and fixation of the avulsion fracture of the tibial eminence using mini-open technique. Knee Surg Sports Traumatol Arthrosc 18:1476–1480. doi:10.1007/s00167-010-1045-0
19. Hunter RE, Willis JA (2004) Arthroscopic fixation of avulsion fractures of the tibial eminence: technique and outcome. Arthroscopy 20:113–121. doi:10.1016/j.arthro.2003.11.028
20. Huang TW, Hsu KY, Cheng CY, Chen LH, Wang CJ, Chan YS, Chen WJ (2008) Arthroscopic suture fixation of tibial eminence avulsion fractures. Arthroscopy 24:1232–1238. doi:10.1016/j.arthro.2008.07.008
21. Su WR, Wang PH, Wang HN, Lin CJ (2011) A simple, modified arthroscopic suture fixation of avulsion fracture of the tibial intercondylar eminence in children. J Pediatr Orthop B 20:17–21. doi:10.1097/BPB.0b013e32832d8452
22. Senekovic V, Veselko M (2003) Anterograde arthroscopic fixation of avulsion fractures of the tibial eminence with a cannulated screw: five-year results. Arthroscopy 19:54–61. doi:10.1053/jars.2003.50012
23. Reynders P, Reynders K, Broos P (2002) Pediatric and adolescent tibial eminence fractures: arthroscopic cannulated screw fixation. J Trauma 53:49–54
24. Doral MN, Atay OA, Leblebicioglu G, Tetik O (2001) Arthroscopic fixation of the fractures of the intercondylar eminence via transquadricipital tendinous portal. Knee Surg Sports Traumatol Arthrosc 9:346–349. doi:10.1007/s001670100235
25. In Y, Kim JM, Woo YK, Choi NY, Moon CW, Kim MW (2008) Arthroscopic fixation of anterior cruciate ligament tibial avulsion fractures using bioabsorbable suture anchors. Knee Surg Sports Traumatol Arthrosc 16:286–289. doi:10.1007/s00167-007-0466-x
26. Kwon OS, Kamath AF, Kelly JD (2012) Arthroscopic treatment of an anterior cruciate ligament avulsion fracture in a skeletally immature patient. Orthopedics 35:589–592. doi:10.3928/01477447-20120621-04
27. Mann MA, Desy NM, Martineau PA (2012) A new procedure for tibial spine avulsion fracture fixation. Knee Surg Sports Traumatol Arthrosc 20:2395–2398. doi:10.1007/s00167-012-1906-9
28. Kim JI, Kwon JH, Seo DH, Soni SM, Munoz M, Nha KW (2013) Arthroscopic hybrid fixation of a tibial eminence fracture in children. Arthrosc Tech 2:e117–e120. doi:10.1016/j.eats.2012.12.005
29. Gans I, Babatunde OM, Ganley TJ (2013) Hybrid fixation of tibial eminence fractures in skeletally immature patients. Arthrosc Tech 2:e237–e242. doi:10.1016/j.eats.2013.02.013
30. McLennan JG (1982) The role of arthroscopic surgery in the treatment of fractures of the intercondylar eminence of the tibia. J Bone Joint Surg (Br) 64:477–480

31. Wiegand N, Naumov I, Vamhidy L, Not LG (2014) Arthroscopic treatment of tibial spine fracture in children with a cannulated Herbert screw. Knee 21:481–485. doi:10.1016/j.knee.2013.12.004
32. Verdano MA, Pellegrini A, Lunini E, Tonino P, Ceccarelli F (2014) Arthroscopic absorbable suture fixation for tibial spine fractures. Arthrosc Tech 3:e45–e48. doi:10.1016/j.eats.2013.08.016
33. Bong MR, Romero A, Kubiak E, Iesaka K, Heywood CS, Kummer F, Rosen J, Jazrawi L (2005) Suture versus screw fixation of displaced tibial eminence fractures: a biomechanical comparison. Arthroscopy 21:1172–1176. doi:10.1016/j.arthro.2005.06.019
34. Anderson CN, Nyman JS, McCullough KA, Song Y, Uppuganti S, O'Neill KR, Anderson AF, Dunn WR (2013) Biomechanical evaluation of physeal-sparing fixation methods in tibial eminence fractures. Am J Sports Med 41:1586–1594. doi:10.1177/0363546513488505
35. Senekovic V, Balazic M (2014) Bioabsorbable sutures versus screw fixation of displaced tibial eminence fractures: a biomechanical study. Eur J Orthop Surg Traumatol 24:209–216. doi:10.1007/s00590-013-1176-3
36. In Y, Kwak DS, Moon CW, Han SH, Choi NY (2012) Biomechanical comparison of three techniques for fixation of tibial avulsion fractures of the anterior cruciate ligament. Knee Surg Sports Traumatol Arthrosc 20:1470–1478. doi:10.1007/s00167-011-1694-7
37. Tsukada H, Ishibashi Y, Tsuda E, Hiraga Y, Toh S (2005) A biomechanical comparison of repair techniques for anterior cruciate ligament tibial avulsion fracture under cyclic loading. Arthroscopy 21:1197–1201. doi:10.1016/j.arthro.2005.06.020
38. Prince AR, Moyer RA (1995) Arthroscopic treatment of an avulsion fracture of the intercondylar eminence of the tibia. Case report. Am J Knee Surg 8:114–116
39. Louis ML, Guillaume JM, Launay F, Toth C, Jouvre JL, Bollini G (2008) Surgical management of type II tibial intercondylar eminence fractures in children. J Pediatr Orthop B 17:231–235. doi:10.1097/BPB.0b013e32830b61f4
40. Tudisco C, Giovarruscio R, Febo A, Savarese E, Bisicchia S (2010) Intercondylar eminence avulsion fracture in children: long-term follow-up of 14 cases at the end of skeletal growth. J Pediatr Orthop B 19:403–408. doi:10.1097/BPB.0b013e32833a5f4d
41. Zhao J, Huangfu X (2007) Arthroscopic treatment of nonunited anterior cruciate ligament tibial avulsion fracture with figure-of-8 suture fixation technique. Arthroscopy 23:405–410. doi:10.1016/j.arthro.2006.12.008

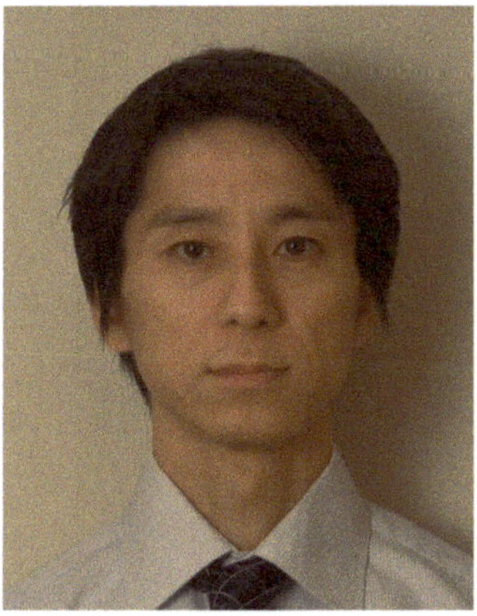

Takehiko Matsushita, M.D., PhD, Department of Orthopaedic Surgery, Kobe University Graduate School of Medicine, Hyogo, Japan.

Part X
Revision ACL Reconstruction

Chapter 36
Double-Bundle Technique

Takeshi Muneta and Hideyuki Koga

Abstract A recent operative technique of our revision double-bundle (DB) anterior cruciate ligament (ACL) surgery with a four-strand semitendinosus (ST) tendon is described in detail in this chapter. The use of the ST tendon is more patient friendly than that of the bone-patellar tendon-bone, and the DB technique is more reliable for achieving knee stability. Femoral tunnel creation is also important for the revision surgery. The outside-in technique is generally recommended in the revision DB surgery because of the adequate room for arthroscopic observation and procedures. The recent behind-remnant technique is anatomically more reproducible for creating femoral tunnels. Tibial tunnel creation inevitably overlaps to the previous tunnel at the aperture to the joint. Anterior aperture to the tibia should be different from the previous tunnel in order to be placed in the fresh bony structure. The outcome of the revision DB surgery is inferior to that of the primary reconstruction. It is partly because the patients who require revision surgery have a higher number of combined meniscus injuries and articular cartilage damages as well as laxity of the secondary restraint.

Keywords Revision anterior cruciate ligament reconstruction • Double-bundle reconstruction • Semitendinosus tendon • Operative details

36.1 Introduction

Anterior cruciate ligament (ACL) injury is well known as an injury that requires surgical treatment and occurs frequently in athletes. It has been reported that the incidence of anterior cruciate ligament reconstruction (ACLR) increased between 1994 and 2006, particularly in females younger than 20 years as well as those 40 years or older in the United States [1]. The prevalence of the ACL revision has

T. Muneta, M.D., PhD (✉) • H. Koga, M.D., PhD
Department of Orthopaedic Surgery, Tokyo Medical and Dental University Medical Hospital, 1-5-45 Yushima, Bunkyo-ku, Tokyo 113-8510, Japan

Department of Joint Surgery and Sports Medicine, Graduate School, Tokyo Medical and Dental University, 1-5-45 Yushima, Bunkyo-ku, Tokyo 113-8510, Japan
e-mail: muneta.orj@tmd.ac.jp

M. Ochi et al. (eds.), *ACL Injury and Its Treatment*,
DOI 10.1007/978-4-431-55858-3_36

not decreased in Sweden. The number of ACLR and revision surgeries has also not changed between 2009 and 2012 in Sweden [2]. According to the Danish registry for knee ligament reconstructions, the 5-year revision ACL reconstruction rate was 4.1 %. Revision occurred most frequently after 1–2 years [3].

Knee stability after our ACL reconstruction has been improved over these years due to our efforts [4]. However, additional surgeries after ACL reconstruction including revision surgery after primary surgery, primary ACL reconstruction for contralateral injury, and secondary surgeries for meniscus injury and hardware removal are still common problems for the knee ligament surgeons. The number of ACL reinjuries and revision surgeries after ACL reconstruction has not decreased worldwide. The outcome of the revision ACL surgery should be improved; in addition, researchers should take an increased interest in ACL injury prevention. In reality, the outcome of revision surgery is worse than that of the primary surgery [5].

We continue to perform a double-bundle (DB) reconstruction using a four-strand semitendinosus tendon (ST) as our standard option for more than 20 years for a patient who sustained an ACL injury [6]. As a revision surgery, a DB reconstruction using the ST tendon is also our selection [7]. In this chapter, recent operative details are described and discussed. The outcome of the revision surgery using ST, since we started to perform anatomic DB reconstruction, is summarized.

36.2 Double-Bundle Technique Using Four-Strand Semitendinosus Tendon

36.2.1 Indication for Double-Bundle Revision Surgery Using Semitendinosus Tendon

A prospective comparison study of ACL reconstruction using autologous ST and bone-patellar tendon-bone (BTB) grafts was performed in Tokyo Medical and Dental University Medical Hospital more than 20 years ago. ACL reconstruction with ST tendon resulted in more cases with better subjective evaluation, while a higher number of cases with worse postoperative stability were observed in ACL reconstruction with ST [8, 9]. Arthrofibrosis causing patients difficulty of kneeling and increased pain in activities has been indicated after BTB reconstruction [10]. Therefore, subjectively favorable tendon selection is thought to be more appropriate in the revision ACL surgery. Less joint fibrosis occurs after hamstring tendon ACL reconstruction, which will be patient-oriented graft selection. Moreover, use of the ST tendon alone for the reconstruction will give less morbidity to the patient than both ST and gracilis tendon harvest [11]. Autologous tendon is always used in Japan.

It is well known that the outcome of the revision ACL reconstruction is inferior to that of the primary one [5]. It may be partly because a higher number of cases with complicated lesions of meniscus and articular cartilage cause a poor outcome subjectively and objectively [12]. In some cases, prolonged unstable conditions will change the normal knee kinematics accompanied by laxity of the secondary restraints before the revision surgery. Some patients will heal poorly even though the primary surgery was appropriately performed [13], while others were too aggressive and too early to return to sports after the primary surgery. The operative technique with the better stabilized function will be more preferable for the revision cases, so that a DB reconstruction using the four-strand ST tendon is the standard technique for us in the revision cases [7, 14].

However, another tendon is necessary for the revision surgery; therefore, the contralateral ST tendon has to be harvested. While lacking scientific data, we suspect that surgeons will hesitate to perform the revision surgery with the same operative method using the same tendon. The cases with poor graft healing would end up with the same poor outcome, especially in patients with a low level of activity. The other aspect is that a patient will not want to have an incision in the healthy limb. Therefore, our standard graft choice for the revision ACL reconstruction after primary reconstruction using hamstring tendons without apparent technical errors is a bone-patellar-bone (BTB) graft.

The current indications of the revision DB ACLR using an ST tendon in our group are patients after primary BTB reconstruction, failure of the primary hamstring tendon reconstruction due to apparent technical errors, and patients willing to participate in repetitive jumping.

36.2.2 One- or Two-Stage Surgery

We have no experience in two-stage revision surgery so far, because the majority of revision cases with nonanatomic high noon femoral tunnels did not show any prominent tunnel expansion. Additionally, we lack research in regard to the importance and efficacy of bone grafting for the expanded tunnel. However, bony defects with a diameter greater than 15 mm will need two-stage surgery [15].

36.2.3 Operative Details of Double-Bundle Revision Surgery Using Four-Strand ST Tendon

36.2.3.1 Basic Consensus for the Technique

The basic operative method is the same as the primary one. We began using a more reproducible and remnant-preserving DB technique of the behind-remnant approach for femoral tunnel creation in 2012 [16]. During the remnant-preserving DB technique of the behind-remnant approach for femoral tunnel creation, ACL remnant is observed from the anteromedial portal and is not removed at all. Two femoral tunnels are created in the anatomic insertion area with the knee positioned at 90° flexion. In a revision case, normal ACL anatomy is not easily observed or reproduced; however, the remnant tissue including the previous ACL graft is preserved as much as possible.

The most proximal portion of the femoral insertion of the normal ACL is converged to the anterior proximal portion to the lateral wall of the intercondylar notch as fibrous convergence (Fig. 36.2a, white line). The fibrous convergence is a marker of the anterior limit of the AM graft. The distance from the articular surface and the position of the posterior end of the articular surface are also the landmarks for the AM tunnel creation. The PL tunnel is created as the perpendicular line of the deepest point of the articular cartilage at 90° flexion is the proximal limit marker of the PL tunnel, and the insertion remnant and distance from the articular surface are also used as landmarks.

36.2.3.2 Femoral Tunnel Creation

Situations regarding previous femoral tunnels are classified into the following six categories: (1) nonanatomic anteriorly created femoral tunnels regardless of the procedures, (2) obviously expanded femoral tunnel by artificial ligament reconstruction, (3) less expanded femoral tunnel by artificial ligament reconstruction, (4) anatomic single-bundle reconstruction, (5) anatomic double-bundle reconstruction, and (6) BTB reconstruction. How to create femoral tunnel is indicated based on each femoral tunnel situation. It is better to create the femoral tunnel in the fresh bone that does not communicate a previous tunnel with the tendon.

Actual Procedures of Femoral Tunnel Creation

The creation of an anatomically correct femoral tunnel is possible through any femoral tunnel creation method, such as transtibial, transportal, and outside-in techniques.

However, to practice the behind-remnant approach more easily, the outside-in technique will be the best because adequate room for arthroscopic procedures and observation can be achieved [16].

Two femoral tunnels are created on the basis of anatomic structures as original femoral attachment suggested by synovial change, most proximal end of the articular surface, and articular surface (Fig. 36.1). The procedures are undergone in a figure-four position. The anteromedial (AM) tunnel should be created not too posteriorly but in the middle portion on the basis of the most proximal portion of the articular surface because the original remnant of the AM portion could be observed. On the other hand, because posterolateral (PL) tunnel is inclined to move anteriorly and distally after reconstruction [17], it is recommended to create the PL tunnel in the posterior portion of the original anatomic attachment. The distal and posterior positioning is also supported with less graft length change.

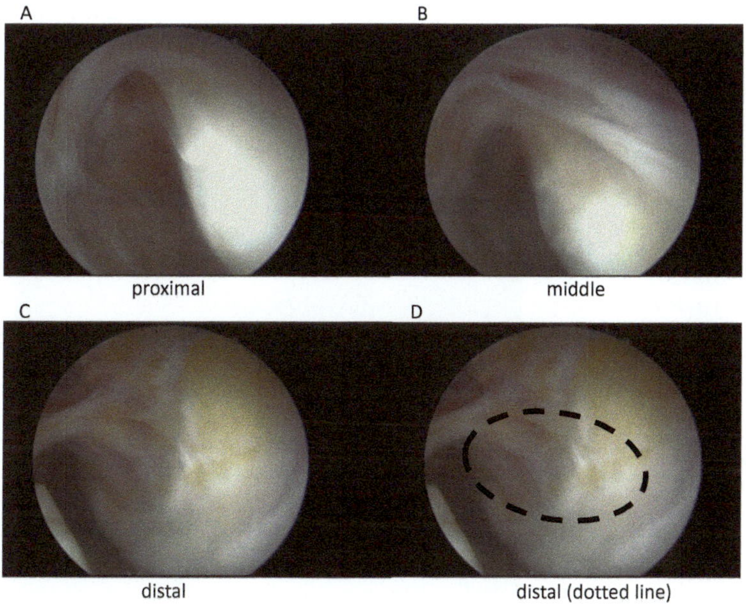

Fig. 36.1 Behind-remnant observation of the reinjured ACL femoral remnant. (**a**) Proximal portion of the remnant, (**b**) middle portion, and (**c**) distal-middle portion. (**d**) Even after reinjury of the reconstruction, the original femoral attachment can be identified arthroscopically

Normal ACL femoral attachment has a wide variety of anatomy in individuals. It has been reported that bony landmarks are not always constant and reliable [18, 19]. Now, we determine the tunnel positioning to reflect the anatomical structures, such as residual tissue of the normal femoral attachment and articular surface, from the behind remnant. The remnant tissue is usually preserved as much as possible even when the previous graft was inserted in a nonanatomic position [17].

Nonanatomic Anteriorly Created Femoral Tunnels Regardless of the Procedures

In such cases, two isolated anatomic tunnels can be usually created apart from the previous tunnel even if the tunnel expanded to some extent. We recently experienced a case where primary thick slack graft disturbed the outside-in femoral guide in reaching the anatomic femoral position, and the approach was converted to the transportal technique (Fig. 36.3). The most proximal fibrous convergence of the normal ACL (Fig. 36.2a, white line) is a marker of the anterior limit of the AM graft with the behind-remnant observation. The distance from the articular surface and the position of the posterior end of the articular surface are also the landmarks for the AM tunnel creation. The proximal to distal axis of the normal ACL insertion is

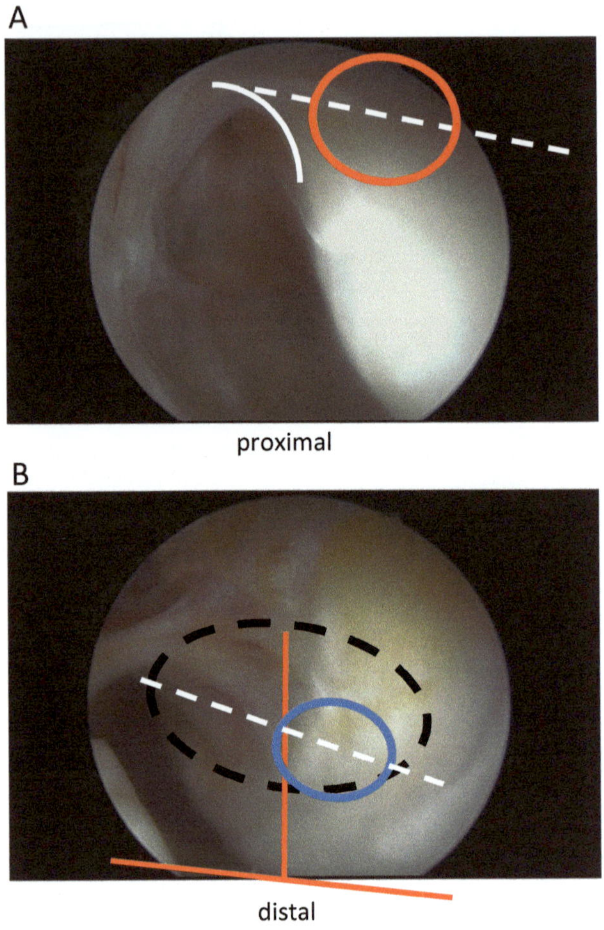

Fig. 36.2 Landmarks of femoral tunnel placement by the behind-remnant approach
(**a**) *White line* indicates the fibrous convergence of the ACL as the center of the most proximal portion of the ACL. *Dotted white line* indicates the assumed proximal to distal axis of the ACL. *Red circle* indicates presumable placement of the AM tunnel.
(**b**) *Black dotted circle* indicates the normal femoral insertion of the ACL. *Dotted white line* indicates the assumed proximal to distal axis of the ACL. *Red line* is perpendicular from the deepest portion of the femoral joint surface. *Blue circle* indicates presumable placement of the PL tunnel

assumed at the posterior limit of the direct insertion (Fig. 36.2a, b). The center of the AM tunnel is put on the line with good margin to the articular surface and the fibrous convergence as a landmark of the anterior limit. The PL tunnel is created with the perpendicular line of the deepest point of the articular cartilage at 90° flexion as the proximal limit. The insertion remnant and distance from the articular surface are appreciated as landmarks. Also, an assumed proximal to distal axis of the normal ACL insertion at the posterior limit and the distance from the articular surface are also used as a landmark for the PL tunnel (Fig. 36.2b).

Obviously Expanded Femoral Tunnel by Artificial Ligament Reconstruction

When the previous reconstruction with an artificial ligament results in significant expansion of the tunnel, two-stage surgery could be considered to prevent the new

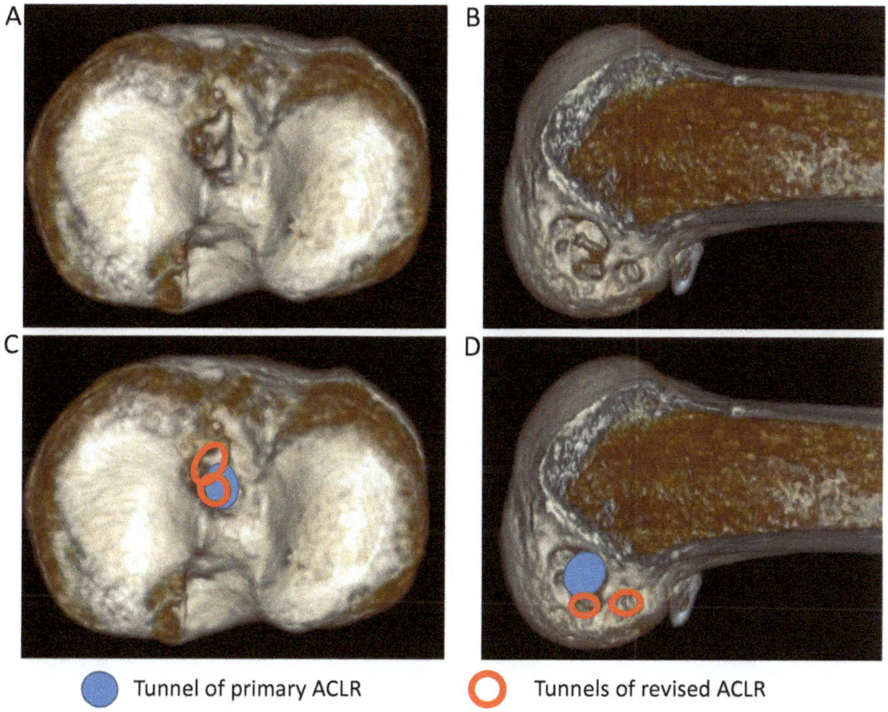

Fig. 36.3 Revision after a nonanatomic anteriorly created femoral tunnel. (**a, b**) 3-D CT presentation of tibial and femoral tunnel post-revision surgery. (**c, d**) Tunnel of the primary surgery and tunnels of the revision surgery are indicated by the *blue area* and *red circles*, respectively

tunnel from merging to the expanded tunnel. Polyethylene mesh artificial ligament rarely presents such a problem because of good cooperation of the ligament to adjacent bony tissue, such that a one-stage approach is usually selected regardless of the previous tunnel position.

Less Expanded Femoral Tunnel by Artificial Ligament Reconstruction

Two anatomic femoral tunnels can be created without being disturbed by the previous tunnel [7]. That is, two tunnels can be created at the margin of the previous tunnel. By changing the direction of the new tunnels to the original tunnel, the bone tunnel is refreshed for better healing of the graft tendon-bone junction.

Anatomic Single-Bundle Reconstruction

Even after an anatomic single-bundle reconstruction with some tunnel enlargement, two anatomic tunnels can usually be created without compromising graft function with the new tunnel merging to the previous one (Fig. 36.4–1, 36.4–2, 36.4–3, 36.4–4). In a case of previous anatomic single-bundle reconstruction, preoperative

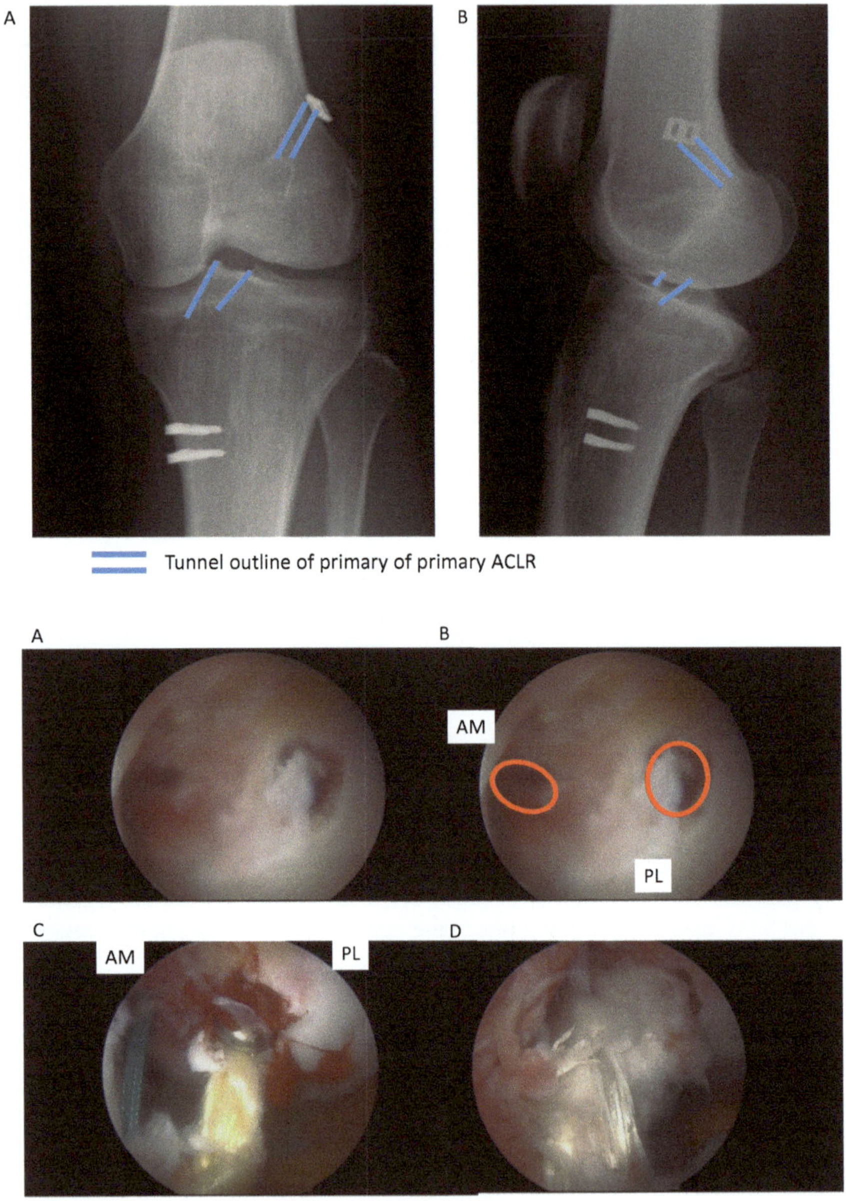

Fig. 36.4 Revision after an anatomic single-bundle reconstruction.
(1) Preoperative two-directional radiographs. (**a**) Anterior-posterior view. (**b**) Lateral view. Primary tunnel placement is indicated by *blue lines*.
(2) Arthroscopic findings during the revision ACL reconstruction performed by portal technique. (a) Created two tunnels in the anatomic femoral attachment. (**b**) *Red circles* point out the two femoral tunnels more clearly. (**c**) AM graft insertion. EndoButton of PL graft is seen. (**d**) Final findings after two grafts inserted.
(3) 3D CT indicates the position of the three tunnels of both primary and revision ACLRs. (**a**) and (**b**) show the position of femoral and tibial tunnels, respectively. In (**c**) and (**d**), the *blue area* indicates the position of the primary ACLR and *red circles* those of the revision ACLR.
(4) Post-revision two-directional radiographs. (**a**) Anterior-posterior view. (**b**) Lateral view. Tunnel placement of femoral and tibial tunnels is indicated by *red lines*

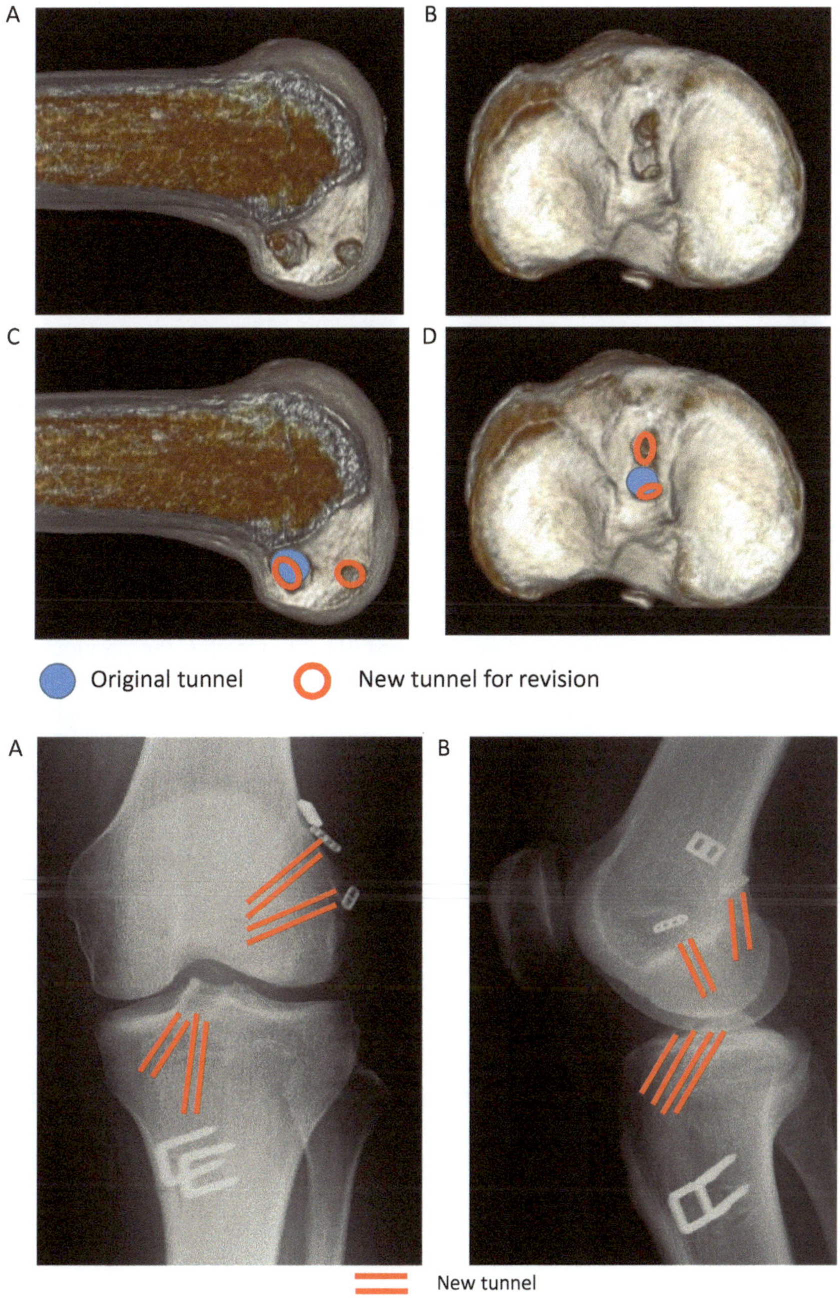

Fig. 36.4 (continued)

radiographs suggested the original single tunnel positioned in the anatomic AMB area. The AM tunnel during revision surgery was planned in the posterior part of the original position with different tunnel orientations using a portal technique. Arthroscopic observation did not indicate an original tunnel orifice. With the behind-remnant approach, AM guide wire was inserted successfully at the bony structure of the posterior part of the original single tunnel. The postoperative 3-D CT indicated that the newly created two tunnels were in the anatomic femoral attachment position.

However, for the AM tunnel creation, creating an over-the-top route is another option. An over-the-top route becomes more isometric by making a groove in the lateral corner of the intercondylar notch, which will facilitate the tendon healing to the bone.

Anatomic Double-Bundle Reconstruction

Careful preoperative planning is important in regard to using the same tunnel with some overdrilling, or making a new route to the over-the-top route instead of the previous AM tunnel, or performing two-stage surgery. We have not yet experienced such a case where two-stage surgery is required.

Based on the preoperative radiographs and 3D CT, whether the previous bone tunnel should be overdrilled or not had been determined for each AM and PL tunnel. When the previous tunnel will be overdrilled, the new femoral tunnel should be created by the other femoral tunnel creation technique. That is, if the previous femoral tunnels were created by transtibial technique, the new tunnels had better be created by portal or outside-in technique. Changed femoral tunnel creation technique will make the femoral tunnel direction change with refreshed bone tunnel walls. When the position of the previous femoral tunnels was determined to change, the new guide pin can be put on the edge of the previous tunnels or outer.

BTB Reconstruction

After BTB reconstruction, femoral tunnel expansion and bony defect of the lateral wall of the intercondylar notch are not too much problematic because BTB graft has two bony ends of its characteristics. Therefore, usual anatomic DB surgery is performed regardless of where the previous tunnel was created.

36.2.3.3 Tibial Tunnel Creation

Situations regarding previous tibial tunnels are classified into the following three categories: (1) massive tunnel enlargement, (2) anatomic tibial tunnel creation, and (3) nonanatomic tibial tunnel creation posteriorly or laterally. Even when the previous surgery was performed by a BTB graft, the aperture of the tunnel is

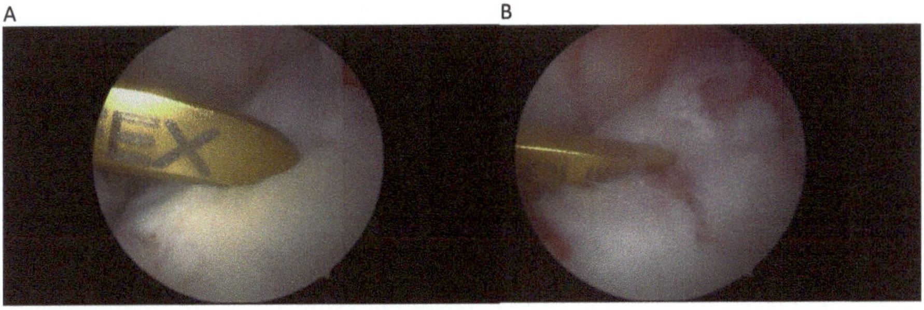

Fig. 36.5 Tibial drill guide for AM and PL tunnels.
(**a**) Tibial drill guide for AM tunnel. (**b**) Tibial drill guide for PL tunnel; note the tip of the guide sinks into the tibial tunnel

usually not filled with a bony tissue. Two tibial tunnels should be placed in the anatomic position.

However, the aperture of the previous tibial tunnel is usually in the anatomic position anyhow. Making new isolated anatomic tunnels is impossible in the majority of cases. We try to change the tunnel route to make a new entrance to the tibial surface for each bundle (Fig. 36.4). When the tibial tunnel expansion is obvious and the tibial tunnel fixation seems unstable, two-stage surgery could be considered. We have not experienced such a case so far. To take care not to move the graft laterally, new tibial tunnel aperture to the joint should be in the center of the medial intercondylar eminence. Technically, it should be noted that the tip of the tibial drill guide often sinks into the previous tibial tunnel; therefore, care should be taken for the guide wire not to be placed posterior to the intended position (Fig. 36.5).

36.2.3.4 Graft Fixation

As refraining from overlapping the new tibial tunnels to the previous one is impossible, the graft length should be as long as possible in the tibial tunnels. The new tibial drill holes should be created from more distal portion of the anteromedial side of the tibia. For such a purpose, transtibial technique should not be employed. At least 20 mm long graft is managed to be put in the bone tunnel. Only semitendinosus tendon is harvested from the contralateral limb. The tendon is cut into the halves and folded into two double-strand grafts. The least intraarticular length of the AM and PL grafts is assumed to be 30 mm and 25 mm, respectively. Pretension of the grafts is applied sufficiently manually and kept tensioned on a graft preparing device.

Fixation Device

A suspensory fixation device such as EndoButton (Smith & Nephew Endoscopy, Andover, MA, USA) is usually used for the femoral fixation. Pullout fixation method using two fixation staples (anchor staple; Meira, Nagoya, Japan) is employed for the tibial fixation. Sometimes, due to poor bone quality, stability of tibial device fixation is not secure. In such cases, it is better to fix the tibial fixation device in a more distal portion than usual, or an anchor screw can be used. With such bone quality and tibial tunnel placement, it is not recommended to use soft tissue interference fixation for this procedure. In many cases, the previous tibial fixation device is removed.

Initial Graft Tensioning

Each graft is fixed to the tibial anchor staple with the cross-sectional area-matched tension (the AM graft first, then the PL graft) at 20° of knee flexion. When the diameter of the graft is 6 mm, 25 N tension is applied with a calibrated spring scale. The initial tension is matched to the diameter of the graft as 30, 25, 21, and 17 N to the graft diameter of 6.5, 6.0, 5,5, and 5.0 mm, respectively [20]. After initial fixation, the balance and tension change of the two grafts are checked by probing. Equal tensioning is proven at 20° of flexion without exception. It has been suggested that balanced tension between two grafts is important [21].

36.2.3.5 Postoperative Management After Revision Surgery

Patients for revision ACL reconstruction have more frequent combined meniscus injuries and articular cartilage damages, which cause knee kinematic changes during physical activity [12]. Anterior tibial displacement is observed in some cases preoperatively. Therefore, after re-stabilization by a revision surgery, prolonged joint inflammation is more often experienced postoperatively. Such joint inflammation is also experienced when a patient returns to sports. On the other hand, general joint laxity and/or hyperextended knee are observed in patients with revision surgery. They are apt to show a high pain threshold and poor muscle strength recovery. Each patient's knee condition as well as his/her personal characteristics, such as poor healer or knee abuser, should be carefully evaluated. Usually, the knee of a patient who required the revision surgery tends to become loose. A longer period of knee brace wearing and prolonged crutch usage should be considered for preventing recurrence of knee instability in the early period after surgery. Another issue for patients of revision surgery is in respect to damaged structures of the meniscus and articular cartilage. Prolonged crutch usage, Cox-2 inhibitor prescription, and hyaluronan knee injection are considered to prevent progression of osteoarthritis.

To prevent reinjury after the revision, more careful and repetitive exercises are necessary. Exercises involving single-leg activities such as squatting and jumping are very important. Biofeedback exercises are important to make patients aware of their strength recovery. Core training and strengthening limb exercises are also important after revision surgeries compared to usual primary reconstructions. Stereotype progression of the postoperative schedule is less important for patients after revision surgery. Preventing patient knees from becoming loose again should be prioritized during the first several months after the revision surgery. Patient goals for having a surgery vary more in patients of revision surgery than in those with the usual primary surgery.

36.2.4 Clinical Results of the Revision Anatomic Double-Bundle Reconstruction Using Four-Strand Semitendinosus Tendon

Summarized outcomes of the revision ACL reconstruction are as follows. The cases included were between July 2002 and December 2013. The anatomic DB reconstruction began in June 2002 in our group. The total number of revision surgeries was 25. Out of 25, eight patients were excluded from the summary: five bilaterally injured cases and three patients who were followed up for less than 12 months. The remaining 17 patients were ten males and seven females with an average age of 26 ± 12 years at the time of revision. One was a tri-revision case. Average follow-up period was 33 months. The median follow-up was 24 months (range, 12–84).

The difference between the revised and the uninjured limbs was as follows: Lachman test, negative 14, 1+ 3, and 2+ 0; anterior drawer test, negative 12, 1+ 4, and 2+ 1; pivot shift (N-test maneuver), negative 10, 1+ 7, and 2+ 0; anterior laxity measured by the KT-1000 (KT measurements), 2.4 ± 2.0 mm (average ± SD); Lysholm knee score, 92 ± 6 points (average ± SD); sports performance recovery, 81 ± 14 % (average ± SD of 10 patients who participated in some sports); and subjective recovery, 86 ± 11 % (average ± SD).

The outcomes of rotational stability, KT measurements, Lysholm scale, and sports performance recovery seemed inferior to those of the primary cases. In the patient cases after July 2002, sports activities seem lower than in those of our previous publication in 2010 [7].

References

1. Mall NA, Chalmers PN, Moric M, Tanaka MJ, Cole BJ, Bach BR Jr, Paletta GA Jr (2014) Incidence and trends of anterior cruciate ligament reconstruction in the United States. Am J Sports Med 42(10):2363–2370
2. Swedish ACL Register (2012) http://www.artroclinic.se/scripts/cgiip.exe/WService=skreg/xb_index?land=US
3. Lind M, Menhert F, Pedersen AB (2012) Incidence and outcome after revision anterior cruciate ligament reconstruction: results from the Danish registry for knee ligament reconstructions. Am J Sports Med 40(7):1551–1557
4. Muneta T (2015) Twenty-year experience of a double-bundle anterior cruciate ligament reconstruction. Clin Orthop Surg 7(2):143–151
5. Wright RW, Gill CS, Chen L, Brophy RH, Matava MJ, Smith MV, Mall NA (2012) Outcome of revision anterior cruciate ligament reconstruction: a systematic review. J Bone Joint Surg Am 94(6):531–536
6. Muneta T, Sekiya I, Yagishita K, Ogiuchi T, Yamamoto H, Shinomiya K (1999) Two-bundle reconstruction of the anterior cruciate ligament using semitendinosus tendon with endobuttons: operative technique and preliminary results. Arthroscopy 15(6):618–624
7. Muneta T, Hara K, Ju YJ, Mochizuki T, Morito T, Yagishita K, Sekiya I (2010) Revision anterior cruciate ligament reconstruction by double-bundle technique using multi-strand semitendinosus tendon. Arthroscopy 26(6):769–781
8. Muneta T, Sekiya I, Ogiuchi T, Yagishita K, Yamamoto H, Shinomiya K (1998) Effects of aggressive early rehabilitation on the outcome of anterior cruciate ligament reconstruction with multi-strand semitendinosus tendon. Int Orthop 22(6):352–356
9. Muneta T, Sekiya I, Ogiuchi T, Yagishita K, Yamamoto H, Shinomiya K (1998) Objective factors affecting overall subjective evaluation of recovery after anterior cruciate ligament reconstruction. Scand J Med Sci Sports 8(5 Pt 1):283–289
10. Lidén M, Ejerhed L, Sernert N, Laxdal G, Kartus J (2007) Patellar tendon or semitendinosus tendon autografts for anterior cruciate ligament reconstruction: a prospective, randomized study with a 7-Year follow-up. Am J Sports Med 35(5):740–748
11. Tashiro T, Kurosawa H, Kawakami A, Hikita A, Fukui N (2003) Influence of medial hamstring tendon harvest on knee flexor strength after anterior cruciate ligament reconstruction. A detailed evaluation with comparison of single- and double-tendon harvest. Am J Sports Med 31(4):522–529
12. Wyatt RW, Inacio MC, Liddle KD, Maletis GB (2014) Prevalence and incidence of cartilage injuries and meniscus tears in patients who underwent both primary and revision anterior cruciate ligament reconstructions. Am J Sports Med 42(8):1841–1846
13. Chen JL, Allen CR, Stephens TE, Haas AK, Huston LJ, Wright RW, Feeley BT, Multicenter ACL Revision Study (MARS) Group (2013) Differences in mechanisms of failure, intraoperative findings, and surgical characteristics between single- and multiple-revision ACL reconstructions: a MARS cohort study. Am J Sports Med 41(7):1571–1578
14. Muneta T, Koga H, Mochizuki T, Ju YJ, Hara K, Nimura A, Yagishita K, Sekiya I (2007) A prospective randomized study of 4-strand semitendinosus tendon anterior cruciate ligament reconstruction comparing single-bundle and double-bundle techniques. Arthroscopy 23 (6):618–628
15. Giron F, Losco M, Giannini L, Buzzi R (2014) Femoral tunnel in revision anterior cruciate ligament reconstruction. Joints 1(3):126–129
16. Muneta T, Koga H, Nakamura T, Horie M, Watanabe T, Yagishita K, Sekiya I (2015) A new behind-remnant approach for remnant-preserving double-bundle anterior cruciate ligament reconstruction compared with a standard approach. Knee Surg Sports Traumatol Arthrosc 23(12):3743–3749
17. Araki D, Kuroda R, Matsumoto T, Nagamune K, Matsushita T, Hoshino Y, Oka S, Nishizawa Y, Kurosaka M (2014) Three-dimensional analysis of bone tunnel changes bone

tunnel after anatomic double-bundleanterior cruciate ligament reconstruction using multidetector-row computed tomography. Am J Sports Med 42(9):2234–2241
18. Mochizuki T, Fujishiro H, Nimura A, Mahakkanukrauh P, Yasuda K, Muneta T, Akita K (2014) Anatomic and histologic analysis of the mid-substance and fan-like extension fibres of the anterior cruciate ligament during knee motion, with special reference to the femoral attachment. Knee Surg Sports Traumatol Arthrosc 22(2):336–344
19. Tsukada S, Fujishiro H, Watanabe K, Nimura A, Mochizuki T, Mahakkanukrauh P, Yasuda K, Akita K (2014) Anatomic variations of the lateral intercondylar ridge: relationship to the anterior margin of the anterior cruciate ligament. Am J Sports Med 42(5):1110–1117
20. Koga H, Muneta T, Yagishita K, Ju YJ, Sekiya I (2012) The effect of graft fixation angles on anteroposterior and rotational knee laxity in double-bundle anterior cruciate ligament reconstruction: evaluation using computerized navigation. Am J Sports Med 40(3):615–623
21. Muneta T, Koga H, Ju YJ, Yagishita K, Sekiya I (2011) Effects of different initial bundle tensioning strategies on the outcome of double-bundle ACL reconstruction: a cohort study. Sports Med Arthrosc Rehabil Ther Technol 3:15

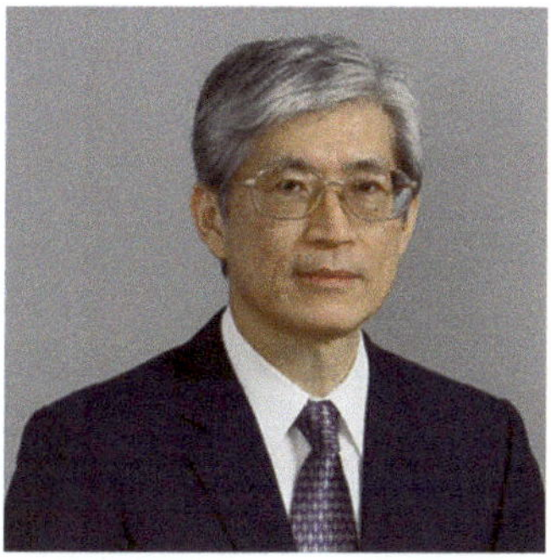

Takeshi Muneta, M.D., PhD, Department of Orthopaedic Surgery, Tokyo Medical and Dental University Medical Hospital, Tokyo, Japan.

Department of Joint Surgery and Sports Medicine, Graduate School Tokyo Medical and Dental University, Tokyo, Japan.

Chapter 37
Bone-Patellar Tendon-Bone Graft via Round Tunnel

Yasuo Niki

Abstract Revision anterior cruciate ligament (ACL) reconstruction with bone-patellar tendon-bone graft through a round tunnel has been perceived as a reliable technique. Some patients present with marked expansion of the bone tunnel, but the most important point is to reconstruct the ACL within the anatomical footprint, followed addressing large bone defects. Preoperative three-dimensional planning can help in understanding the degree of bone defect and precise tunnel direction. Cartilage and meniscus damage at the time of surgery negatively affect subjective outcomes due to persistent pain and a low rate of return to original sporting activities. Surgical skill and flexibility are needed to tailor measures to the context of the individual patient.

Keywords Anterior cruciate ligament • Bone-patellar tendon-bone • Revision • Bone tunnel enlargement • Bone grafting

37.1 Why Is the Bone-Patellar Tendon-Bone (BPTB) Graft Preferred in Revision Anterior Cruciate Ligament (ACL) Reconstruction?

The outcomes of revision ACL reconstruction have been considered inferior to those of primary ACL reconstruction [1–4]. As surgical techniques continue to improve and hardware options increase, recent reports on revision ACL reconstruction have described satisfactory results comparable to primary ACL reconstruction [5, 6]. In revision ACL reconstruction, graft choice is an important issue, especially for young, active patients. Because the use of ipsilateral autografts without disturbing the contralateral knee benefits the patient by avoiding injury to the normal healthy knee, ipsilateral BPTB might offer the best substitute for the ACL when hamstring autograft was used in primary ACL reconstruction, particularly in countries where clinical use of allograft is unavailable. In the setting of pre-existing

Y. Niki, M.D., PhD (✉)
Department of Orthopaedic Surgery, Keio University, 35 Shinanomachi, Shinjuku-ku, Tokyo 160-8582, Japan
e-mail: y-niki@keio.jp

M. Ochi et al. (eds.), *ACL Injury and Its Treatment*,
DOI 10.1007/978-4-431-55858-3_37

bone tunnel enlargement, soft tissue grafts are inappropriate because of concerns about poor tunnel fixation of the graft. In this context, graft sources available for bone-to-bone healing, such as BPTB and quadriceps tendon, will be selected to allow rigid fixation within the bone tunnels.

The past clinical evidences show that primary ACL reconstruction sometimes offers effective measures in the revision setting. Some studies have demonstrated a higher incidence of instrumental instability associated with hamstrings, when compared with BPTB autograft [7–9]. A meta-analysis concluded that BPTB autograft was associated with few failures and achieved better stability as compared to hamstring tendon autograft [10]. Indeed, numerous authors have preferred BPTB autograft or allograft for revision ACL reconstruction, because of the possibility of filling enlarged bone tunnels with attached bone plugs [1, 4, 11–13], but anterior knee pain has been perceived as an unavoidable postoperative morbidity of this graft [14].

This chapter reviews revision ACL reconstruction using conventional BPTB graft via a round tunnel and focuses on where this technique generally stands in the current situation of revision ACL reconstruction. In addition, our preferred procedure of one-stage revision is described with a representative case of post-synthetic ligament failure associated with a large bone defect in the femur.

37.2 Technical Tips for Revision ACL Reconstruction Using Conventional BPTB Graft via a Round Tunnel

37.2.1 Preoperative Planning

Prior to revision ACL reconstruction, surgeons should decide on the graft type, tunnel creation method, and necessity of bone grafting. If bone grafting is needed, a decision is needed whether to perform a one- or two-stage procedure. In practical preoperative planning, the most important information needed for the decision-making process prior to revision ACL reconstruction is the three-dimensional (3D) position of the original bone tunnel. Using both MRI and computed tomography (CT) may allow a better understanding of the 3D position of the original tunnel in relation to the ideal anatomical footprint. The original bone tunnel can be categorized into three different patterns based on the placement in relation to the ideal ACL footprint: correct position, indicating that the new bone tunnel should be made using the same position and direction; complete malposition, indicating that the original bone tunnel does not overlap with the ideal ACL footprint; and partial malposition, indicating that the original bone tunnel partially overlaps with ideal ACL footprint, and tunnel enlargement will definitely occur after new bone tunnel creation. This last pattern sometimes requires bone graft from the tibia or iliac crest in a one- or two-stage procedure.

37.2.2 *Bone Grafting*

The degree of tunnel expansion and whether bone graft is needed to fix the graft successfully should be considered prior to surgery. When tunnel expansion is sufficiently large to preclude satisfactory fixation of the graft in a one-stage revision procedure, one author has reported the superiority of two-stage procedures of revision ACL reconstruction with prior bone grafting to the tunnel, providing fixation conditions comparable to primary reconstruction [15]. Delivery and impaction of bone graft into the femoral tunnel are technically difficult using arthroscopic techniques, and the osteochondral autologous transfer system (OATS) grafting instruments (Arthrex, Naples, FL) is useful for femoral and tibial tunnel impaction grafting in two-stage procedures [16]. However, we fundamentally prefer a one-stage procedure in any situation where sufficient fixation of the graft can be achieved. Two-stage surgery on two separate anesthetic sessions might represent a heavy burden for young, active patients.

In cases of post-synthetic ligament failure, newly created bone tunnels might be enlarged after removal of synthetic material from former bone tunnels. In such cases, secure graft fixation can be achieved by harvesting the lateral side of the patellar tendon with bone plugs sized and trimmed as necessary to fill the enlarged tunnel without bone grafting. Using this strategy, 20 cases of one-stage ACL revision yielded favorable anteroposterior stability comparable to that of primary ACL, even for post-synthetic ligament failure [17]. Although ACL revision in post-synthetic ligament failure is a complicated and challenging operation, two-stage procedure might not be needed by using BPTB graft.

Mounting evidence has been accumulated that an increased time to revision correlates with increased meniscal and chondral lesions and development of radiographic osteoarthritis [18, 19]. Moreover, surgeons can easily imagine that the longer a patient continues to experience instability, the more frequently cartilage damage and subsequent osteoarthritis will occur. ACL revision for patients with a large bone defect might thus be caught in a dilemma between one- and two-stage revision procedures.

37.2.3 *Bone Tunnel Creation Technique*

Along with assessments of the original position and degree of enlargement of the bone tunnel, the direction of the bone tunnel should also be considered prior to surgery. Three major methods have been used for bone tunnel creation in the femur, including transtibial, transportal, and outside-in techniques (Fig. 37.1). When the previous surgery was performed using a transtibial or outside-in technique, a transportal technique is inevitably selected for the revision. Conversely, when the transportal technique was used in the original procedure, the outside-in technique should be used. When the bone tunnel has been enlarged or the anatomical ideal

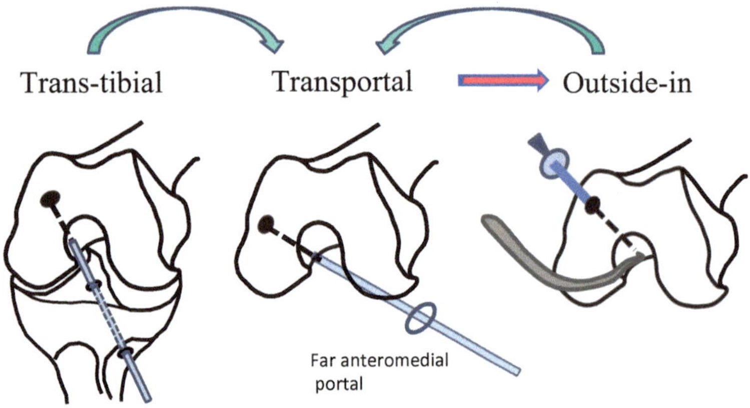

Fig. 37.1 Three types of femoral tunnel creation technique. Bone tunnel direction should be switched to an appropriate direction to ensure mutual divergence of the old and new tunnels, if the old bone tunnel aperture partially overlaps with the anatomical footprint

tunnel position overlaps the original tunnel position, a different tunnel direction allows for rigid fixation of the bone plug in BPTB, regardless of graft fixation devices, including various types of suspension devices and interference screws. In this context, using the outside-in technique is an appropriate strategy to maintain divergence between the original and new bone tunnels, since bone tunnel direction can be arbitrarily controlled without disturbing the intraarticular entry point of drilling. When an inside-out drilling technique through the far medial portal is used, changing the knee flexion angle at the time of drilling can control the bone tunnel direction and achieve mutual divergence between the original and new bone tunnels (Fig. 37.2).

37.2.4 Osteophytectomy and Synovectomy

In the case of synthetic ligament failure, transient joint effusion due to wear debris-induced synovitis is one factor associated with deterioration of subjective scores such as Lysholm score, both before and after surgery [17, 20]. Concomitant synovectomy and debridement of synthetic materials is necessary in this context. If the original bone tunnels are positioned in ideal anatomical position, the tunnels are reamed with a larger diameter to fresh cancellous bone, ensuring removal of synthetic ligament debris and sclerotic margins in the tunnels. As most revision cases possess varying degrees of osteophyte formation as a result of the progression of osteoarthritis, osteophytes formed around the intercondylar notch should be removed to prevent impingement of the ACL graft with the knee in extension. Both medial and lateral marginal osteophytes should be removed (Fig. 37.3), because anatomical positioning of the femoral bone tunnel aperture is prone to causing impingement of the graft against the lateral wall of the intercondylar notch [21].

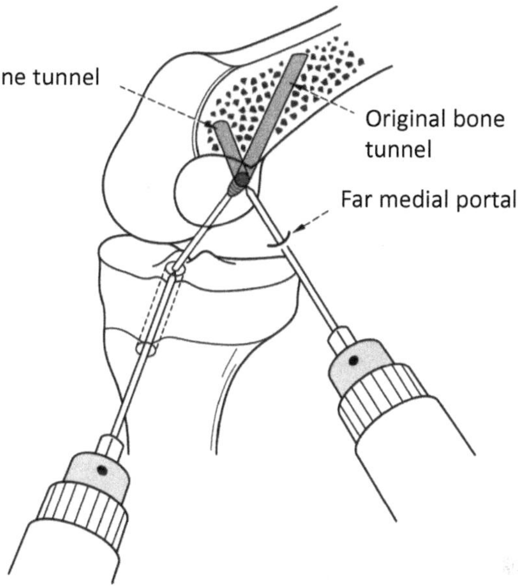

Fig. 37.2 Strategy to change bone tunnel direction.
When the original bone tunnel is made using a transtibial technique, the transportal technique should be used in revision ACL reconstruction. Knee flexion angle at the time of drilling affects mutual divergence of the old and new tunnels, as well as position of the tunnel outlet in the femoral cortex [22]

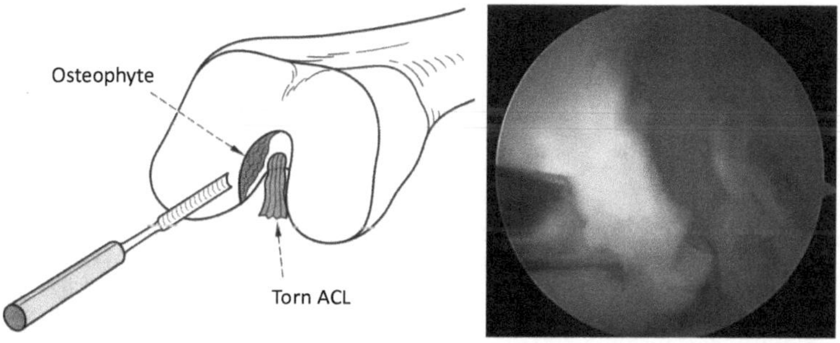

Fig. 37.3 Osteophytectomy of the intercondylar notch. Medial and lateral marginal osteophytes of the intercondylar notch should be removed using an osteotome to prevent graft-wall impingement

37.2.5 Graft Fixation

Current ACL revision aims to create new bone tunnels within the anatomical footprint, so the length of the femoral bone tunnel might be short, especially when the inside-out technique is adopted. As the femoral bone tunnel is around 25 mm long in patients of small stature, the socket for the bone plug should be made as short as possible, ideally 15–20 mm. In this context, the same length of interference screw or adjustable suspension device can be used to secure the BPTB graft. An adjustable suspension device may only allow the BPTB graft to be inserted into the bone tunnel as deep as needed for the bone plug length of the graft. When the original bone tunnel partially overlaps with the anatomical footprint of the ACL, the surgeons have to address substantial degrees of graft-tunnel mismatch. For mismatch <5 mm, metal or biodegradable interference screws can repair the defect. If mismatch ≥ 5 mm or a cylindrical bone defect exists after removal of the previous interference screw, iliac crest autograft or synthetic dowel graft can fill cylindrical bone defects without the need for allograft on one-stage revision ACL reconstruction [23].

37.3 Clinical Results of Revision ACL Reconstruction with BPTB Graft

Variations in concomitant pathological changes including collateral ligament, cartilage or meniscus injury, and surgical techniques including graft choices make it difficult to investigate clinical results of revision ACL reconstruction. Variations of graft choice may also complicate clinical assessment and make clear conclusions difficult to draw. Historically, clinical results for revision ACL reconstruction have been assessed using three perspectives: clinical laxity as measured with a KT-1000/2000 arthrometer, pivot shift test, or Lachman test; clinical scoring such as IKDC, Lysholm score, and the Knee Injury Osteoarthritis Outcome Score (KOOS); and radiographic changes progressing toward OA. To date, successful achievement of stability after revision ACL reconstruction with BPTB graft has been reported when assessed by KT-1000/2000, but subjective scores for revision procedures were relatively poor compared to scores for the primary procedure, since a higher incidence of associated injuries such as cartilage damage and meniscus tear may cause pain and subsequent muscle weakness and atrophy [24]. As in the graft maturation after primary ACL reconstruction, MRI signals of the BPTB graft reflect maturation of the ligament after the revision procedure. Graft intensity of the mid-substance increases from 3 months postoperatively, peaking at 6 months and decreasing thereafter (our unpublished data), quite comparable to primary ACL reconstruction. Increased intensity of the BPTB graft reportedly reflects the amount of synovial tissue embracing the graft and also correlates with hypervascularity and cellularity of the graft itself [25, 26]. Further improvement of imaging modalities such as MRI and CT might allow for monitoring of the graft maturation process and occasional detection of biological failure during the postoperative course of the reconstruction.

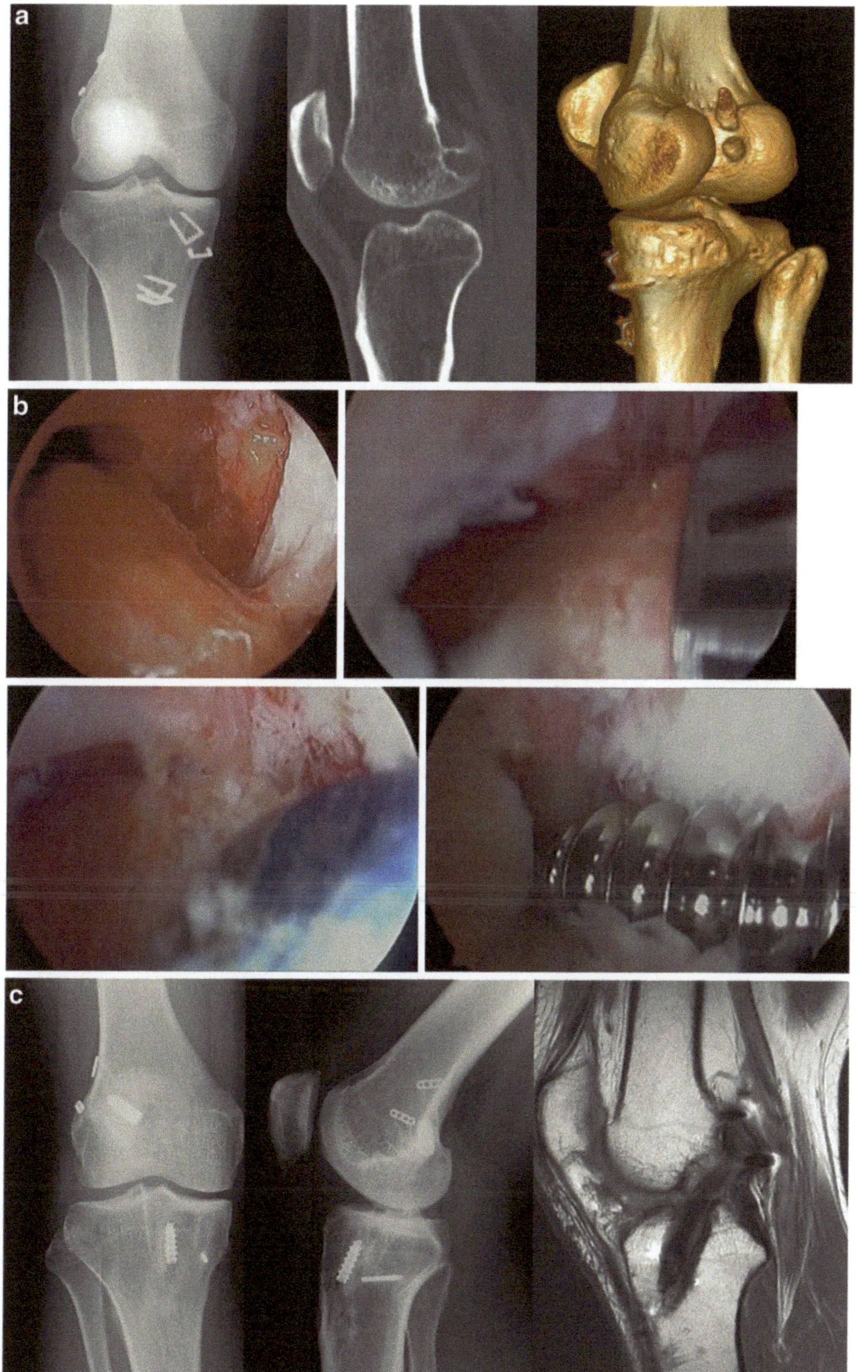

Fig. 37.4 Revision ACL reconstruction combined with one-stage bone grafting. (**a**) Based on the preoperative radiograph and 3D CT, the bone tunnel for the anteromedial bundle shows blowout of

37.4 Representative Case: BPTB Revision with One-Stage Bone Grafting

The patient was a 34-year-old, male recreational soccer player. He presented with an unstable feeling in the right knee, after reinjuring his knee during a soccer game 5 years after an ACL reconstruction. The primary procedure had been a double-bundle ACL reconstruction using synthetic ligament (Leeds-Keio ligament) and lateral meniscus repair. After the primary surgery, he had rapidly recovered and returned to the original sports activity of recreational soccer by 4 months postoperatively, due to the virtues of synthetic ligament. After reinjury, the patient suffered gross knee instability. On examination, anteroposterior laxity as measured by the KT-2000 arthrometer was 9 mm in side-to-side difference, and Lysholm score was 65. According to preoperative CT, the intraarticular apertures of the two bone tunnels were placed in acceptable positions, but the tunnel aperture of the anteromedial bundle was positioned slightly deep, resulting in blowout of the posterior cortex (Fig. 37.4a). Large bone tunnel expansion necessitating massive bone grafting was anticipated, but the patient was in denial about two-stage surgery. Revision ACL reconstruction was therefore performed using a BPTB graft, and one-stage bone graft from iliac crest was simultaneously performed with OATS grafting instruments (Arthrex, Naples, FL). After drilling a bone tunnel 11 mm long and introducing the BPTB graft to the tunnel, two cylindrical grafts (8 mm in diameter) harvested from the iliac crest were impacted to the enlarged bone tunnel through a far anteromedial portal (Fig. 37.4b). This bone grafting technique is fundamentally the same as the aforementioned two-stage technique. A metal interference screw was finally inserted to completely secure the BPTB graft. On the tibial side, the graft was also secured with the metal interference screw. After 4 years, the patient continued to play soccer, and MRI indicated very low intensity signal of the entire graft (Fig. 37.4c). On examination, anteroposterior laxity showed 2.0 mm of side-to-side difference, and Lysholm score was 90.

37.5 Conclusions

Revision ACL reconstruction with conventional BPTB graft through the round tunnel has been perceived as a reliable technique, especially after primary ACL reconstruction with hamstring tendons. Results of graft stability and the rate of negative pivot shift test are satisfactory, but subjective scoring is inferior to primary

---

Fig. 37.4 (continued) the posterior cortex of the femur. (**b**) Large bone defect is apparent even after introducing the BPTB graft (*left upper panel*). The first cylindrical bone plug (*right upper panel*) and second bone plug (*left lower panel*) are introduced to the defect using OATS grafting instruments. A metal interference screw is inserted to secure the graft rigidly. (**c**) At 4 years postoperatively, radiographs and MRI indicate good placement and low signal intensity of the graft

ACL reconstruction due to persistent pain and a low rate of return to original sports activities, likely associated with a high incidence of cartilage and meniscus damage at the time of revision surgery. Surgeon skill and flexibility in taking measures suited to each context are required. The point is how to reconstruct the ACL within the anatomical footprint while addressing the large bone defect. Preoperative 3D planning will help in understanding the degree of bone defect and appropriate tunnel direction. With improving hardware to facilitate rigid graft fixation, appropriate hardware is a key factor in successful graft incorporation and maturation after revision ACL reconstruction.

References

1. Harilainen A, Sandelin J (2001) Revision anterior cruciate ligament surgery: a review of the literature and results of our own revisions. Scand J Med Sci Sports 11:163–169
2. Allen CR, Giffin JR, Harner CD (2003) Revision anterior cruciate ligament reconstruction. Orthop Clin North Am 34:79–98
3. Fox JA, Pierce M, Bojchuk J, Hayden J, Bush-Joseph CA, Bach BR Jr (2004) Revision anterior cruciate ligament with nonirradiated fresh-frozen patellar tendon allograft. Arthroscopy 20:787–794
4. Safran MR, Harner CD (1996) Technical considerations of revision anterior cruciate ligament surgery. Clin Orthop Relat Res 323:50–64
5. Fules PJ, Madhav RT, Goddard RK, Mowbray MA (2003) Revision anterior cruciate ligament reconstruction using autografts with a polyester fixation device. Knee 10:335–340
6. Weiler A, Schmeling A, Stohr I, Kaab MJ, Wagner M (2007) Primary versus single-stage revision anterior cruciate ligament reconstruction using autologous hamstring tendon grafts. A prospective matched-group analysis. Am J Sports Med 35:1643–1652
7. Beynnon BD, Johnson RJ, Fleming BC, Kannus P, Kaplan M, Samani J, Renström P (2002) Anterior cruciate ligament replacement: comparison of bone-patellar tendon-bone grafts with two-strand hamstring grafts. A prospective, randomized study. J Bone Joint Surg 84-A:1503–1513
8. Feller JA, Webster KE (2003) A randomized comparison of patellar tendon and hamstring tendon anterior cruciate ligament reconstruction. Am J Sports Med 31:564–573
9. Spindler KP, Kuhn JE, Freedman KB, Matthews CE, Dittus RS, Harrell FE Jr (2004) Anterior cruciate ligament reconstruction autograft choice: bone-tendon-bone versus hamstring: does it really matter? A systematic review. Am J Sports Med 32:1986–1995
10. Freedman KB, D'Amato MJ, Nedeff DD, Kaz A, Bach BR Jr (2003) Arthroscopic anterior cruciate ligament reconstruction: a meta-analysis comparing patellar tendon and hamstring tendon autografts. Am J Sports Med 31:2–11
11. Bach B (2003) Revision anterior cruciate ligament surgery. Arthroscopy 19:14–29
12. Greis P, Johnson D, Fu F (1993) Revision anterior cruciate ligament surgery: causes of graft failure and technical considerations of surgery. Clin Sports Med 12:839–852
13. Harner CD, Giffin JR, Dunteman RC, Annunziata CC, Friedman MJ (2000) Evaluation and treatment of recurrent instability after anterior cruciate ligament reconstruction. J Bone Joint Surg Am 82:1652–1664
14. Niki Y, Hakozaki A, Iwamoto W, Kanagawa H, Matsumoto H, Toyama Y, Suda Y (2012) Factors affecting anterior knee pain following anatomic double bundle anterior cruciate ligament reconstruction. Knee Surg Sports Traumatol Arthrosc 20:1543–1549

15. Thomas NP, Kankate R, Wandless F, Pandit H (2005) Revision anterior cruciate ligament reconstruction using a 2-stage technique with bone grafting of the tibial tunnel. Am J Sports Med 33:1701–1709
16. Said HG, Baloch K, Green M (2006) A new technique for femoral and tibial tunnel bone grafting using the OATS harvesters in revision anterior cruciate ligament reconstruction. Arthroscopy 22:796.e1–796.e3
17. Niki Y, Matsumoto H, Enomoto H, Toyama Y, Suda Y (2010) Single-stage anterior cruciate ligament revision with bone-patellar tendon-bone: a case-control series of revision of failed synthetic anterior cruciate ligament reconstructions. Arthroscopy 26:1058–1065
18. Diamantopoulos AP, Lorbach O, Paessler HH (2008) Anterior cruciate ligament revision reconstruction: results in 107 patients. Am J Sports Med 36:851–860
19. Ohly NE, Murray IR, Keating JF (2007) Revision anterior cruciate ligament reconstruction: timing of surgery and the incidence of meniscal tears and degenerative change. J Bone Joint Surg 89B:1051–1054
20. Klein W, Jensen KU (1992) Synovitis and artificial ligaments. Arthroscopy 8:116–124
21. Udagawa K, Niki Y, Enomoto H, Toyama Y, Suda Y (2014) Factors influencing graft impingement on the wall of the intercondylar notch after anatomic double-bundle anterior cruciate ligament reconstruction. Am J Sports Med 42:2219–2225
22. Niki Y (2009) MB Orthopaedics 22(11): 63–67
23. Barrett GR, Brown TD (2007) Femoral tunnel defect filled with a synthetic dowel graft for a single-staged revision anterior cruciate ligament reconstruction. Arthroscopy 23:796.e1–796.e4
24. Wright RW, Gill CS, Chen L, Brophy RH, Matava MJ, Smith MV, Mall NA (2012) Outcome of revision anterior cruciate ligament reconstruction: a systematic review. J Bone Joint Surg 94A:531–536
25. Ntoulia A, Papadopoulou F, Ristanis S, Argyropoulou M, Georgoulis AD (2011) Revascularization process of the bone-patellar tendon-bone autograft evaluated by contrast-enhanced magnetic resonance imaging 6 and 12 months after anterior cruciate ligament reconstruction. Am J Sports Med 39:1478–1486
26. Ntoulia A, Papadopoulou F, Zampeli F, Ristanis S, Argyropoulou M, Georgoulis A (2013) Evaluation with contrast-enhanced magnetic resonance imaging of the anterior cruciate ligament graft during its healing process: a two-year prospective study. Skelet Radiol 42:541–552

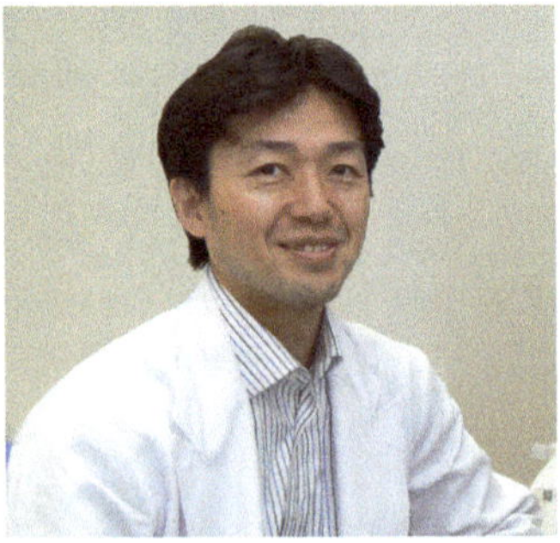

Yasuo Niki, M.D., PhD, Orthopaedic Surgery, Keio University School of Medicine, Tokyo, Japan.

Chapter 38
Anatomical Revision ACL Reconstruction with Rectangular Tunnel Technique

Konsei Shino and Yasuhiro Take

Abstract Revision ACL reconstruction (ACLR) is technically difficult because of pre-existing tunnels in the primary ACLR. We developed the anatomical rectangular tunnel ACL reconstruction (ART ACLR) with a bone-patellar tendon-bone (BTB) graft to mimic fiber arrangement inside the native ACL via smaller tunnels. With a 10-mm wide graft, the cross-sectional area of the tunnels of 50 mm^2 in ART ACLR is less than that of 79 mm^2 in a traditional 10-mm round tunnel procedure, suggesting that tunnel encroachment would be less of a problem at the time of revision ACLR with this novel technique. Thus, the ART ACLR technique could be most frequently applied to the patients suffering from failed nonanatomical primary ACLR. In this chapter, the indication and technical considerations for ART ACLR as one-stage revision ACLR were described.

Keywords Anatomic rectangular tunnel ACL reconstruction (ART ACLR) • Bone-patellar tendon-bone (BTB) graft • Nonanatomical primary ACLR • One-stage revision ACLR

38.1 Introduction

As the native ACL is oblong in cross section of its midsubstance, a bone-patellar tendon-bone (BTB) graft with rectangular cross section is one of the morphologically suitable ones to mimic the native ACL for revision or primary ACLR [1]. Biomechanically, a 10-mm wide BTB graft has sufficient maximum tensile load (1.2 × that for the normal ACL) with bone-tendon junctions and bone plugs [2]. We developed the anatomic rectangular tunnel ACL reconstruction (ART ACLR) with a BTB graft to mimic natural fiber arrangement inside the native

---

One of the authors (Konsei Shino) has received funding from Smith & Nephew Inc., MA, USA

K. Shino (✉)
Sports Orthopaedic Center, Yukioka Hospital, 2-2-3 Ukita, Kita-ku, Osaka 530-0021, Japan
e-mail: shinok0220@gmail.com

Y. Take
Department of Orthopaedic Surgery, Osaka University Medical School, Osaka, Japan

M. Ochi et al. (eds.), *ACL Injury and Its Treatment*,
DOI 10.1007/978-4-431-55858-3_38

ACL and to minimize tunnel size [3–5]. Thus the technique makes it possible to create the tunnel aperture inside the attachment area. Biomechanically this reconstruction technique is superior to the conventional transtibial tunnel single-bundle procedure [6].

Revision ACL reconstruction (ACLR) is technically difficult because of pre-existing tunnels in the primary ACLR [7]. The cross-sectional area of the tunnels of 50 mm^2 (5 × 10 mm) in ART ACLR is less than that of 79 mm^2 in a conventional 10-mm round tunnel technique, if a 10-mm wide BTB graft is utilized. For revision ACLR, therefore, the ART procedure is advantageous to leave more space between the previous tunnels and the new ones. Since tunnel encroachment would hypothetically be less of a problem, the ART ACLR technique could be more frequently applied as one-stage revision procedure to the patients after failed primary ACLR [8].

38.2 Surgical Principles

1. Create rectangular tunnels (parallelepiped tunnels with rectangular apertures) inside the anatomic attachment areas regardless of pre-existing nonanatomic tunnels (Fig. 38.1). If the distance between the revision tunnel aperture and the primary one is less than 3 mm, the latter is filled with an interference screw and/or bone graft.

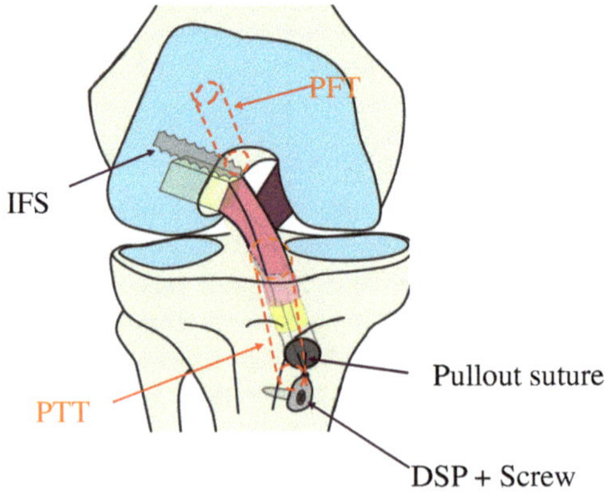

Fig. 38.1 Schema of revision rectangular tunnel ACL reconstruction with a BTB graft. The bone plug is fixed to the femur with a modified pullout suture technique using the DSP (double-spike plate) and a screw or an interference screw (*IFS*), while tibial fixation is achieved with the pullout suture technique using the DSP and a screw. New anatomic femoral tunnel can be properly placed in most cases without overlapping tunnels regardless of the previous anterior femoral tunnel (*PFT*). A new tibial tunnel is created to the aperture of the previous vertical tibial tunnel (*PTT*) in most cases

2. Reuse the pre-existing tunnel apertures if they were in the anatomic attachment areas.

38.3 For Graft Choice

With this procedure, autogenous or allogeneic tendon grafts with or without bone plugs can be used. As we are located in Japan where allogeneic tissues are not readily available, our primary graft choice for revision is a BTB graft from the contralateral knee or the one from the ipsilateral knee if it had not been used at the time of the primary ACLR. However, the BTB graft may not be indicated for every patient. For example, some judo wrestlers would not accept the BTB graft harvest from the contralateral knee. They tend to prefer an unbalanced dominant leg to well-balanced bilateral legs because of their sport event. For these patients, the ART technique could be applied with semitendinosus tendon or quadriceps tendon-bone graft if the double-/triple-bundle procedure might be compromised because of pre-existing tunnel(s) [9]. On the contrary, rugby or American football players may be good candidates for use of the contralateral BTB graft, because muscle imbalance between legs could be dissolved. However, extremely careful postoperative rehabilitation has to be taken to minimize anterior knee pain or thigh muscle weakness after harvesting BTB graft from the healthy knee.

38.4 Surgical Technique and Technical Considerations

First, the primary graft should be thoroughly removed. Then, the revision technique is exactly the same as the primary ART ACLR (Chaps. 7, 8, 9, 10, 11, 12, 13,14, 15, 16, 17, 18, 19, 20, 21, 22, 23, 24, 25, 26, 27, 28, 29, and 30).

38.4.1 With Properly Placed Previous Tunnels

After ART ACLR with BTB graft, the revision can be performed as the primary ART ACLR using any type of graft: two double-looped semitendinosus tendon grafts, quadriceps tendon-bone (QTB), or the contralateral BTB graft.

For failure cases following anatomic double-bundle ACLR using soft tissue grafts including semitendinosus tendon, a new rectangular tunnel can be easily created by dilating previous two tunnels. For those with mildly enlarged femoral tunnel, the extra space may be filled with an interference screw of greater than 7 mm.

However, for those with severely widened tunnels after repeated ACLRs, grafting via over the top of the lateral femoral condyle as well as bone graft behind the revision graft in the tibial tunnel may be considered.

38.4.2 With Improperly Placed Previous Tunnels

On the femoral side, the distance between the aperture rim of the previous tunnel and that of the new tunnel is 5 mm or greater; the new femoral tunnel is created as the primary ACLR leaving the primary tunnel. If the distance is less than 5 mm, however, the primary tunnel may be filled with a titanium interference screw of appropriate size.

On the tibial side, a tunnel placed too anteriorly is easily revisable by creating a new tunnel behind the previous one. With the tunnel placed properly in the attachment or malpositioned by 1 cm or less posteriorly, a divergent tunnel technique should be applied to obtain a new tunnel wall of fresh cancellous bone. When the tunnels were posteriorly malpositioned exceeding 1 cm, however, the previous tunnel should be filled with a bone graft or its substitute, as shown in Case 1.

38.4.3 Considerations at the Time of Graft Fixation

A 6-mm or larger interference screw may be used for femoral fixation (Fig. 38.1). However, cortical suspensory fixation may also be considered with a small lateral incision added, if the fixation is neither satisfactory nor applicable due to the previous tunnel, thin tunnel wall or bone atrophy. Tibial fixation is achieved with a modified pullout suture technique using DSP (Double Spike Plate; Smith-Nephew Endoscopy, Andover, MA) and a screw in the same manner as the primary ART ACLR [10].

38.5 Postoperative Rehabilitation

The postoperative rehabilitation is performed in the same manner as the primary ART ACLR (Chaps. 7, 8, 9, 10, 11, 12, 13, 14, 15, 16, 17, 18, 19, 20, 21, 22, 23, 24, 25, 26, 27, 28, 29, and 30).

An Illustrative Case

Case 1 with a previous surgery of single-bundle ACLR with hamstring tendon graft via high/improper femoral tunnels and a posterior tibial tunnel (Fig. 38.2).

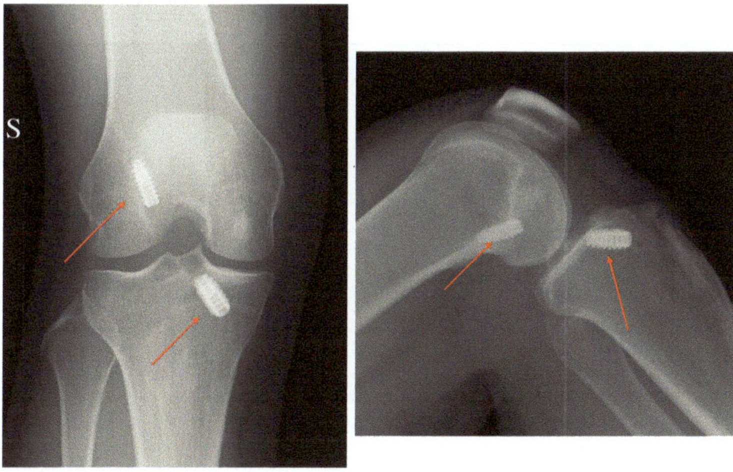

Fig. 38.2 Plain lateral radiographs of Case 1 who has been suffering from instability for years after the primary ACLR. Note the interference screw for fixation (*solid arrows*)

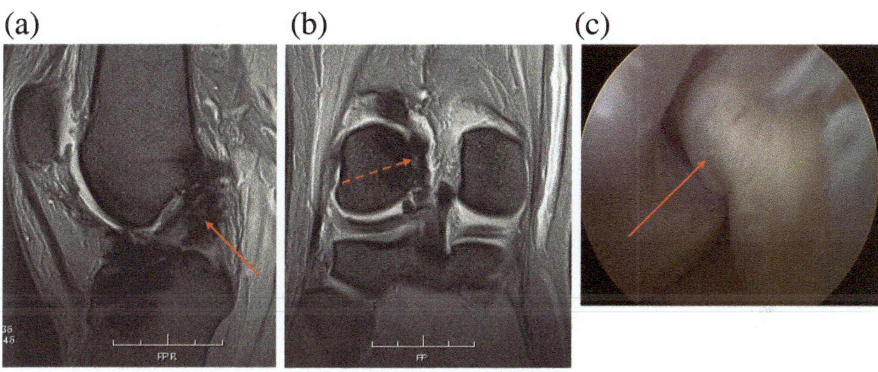

Fig. 38.3 Appearances of the failed graft of Case 1. (**a**) Sagittal T2-weighted image showing the continuity of the graft (*solid arrow*). (**b**) Coronal T2-weighted image showing wavy and irregular appearance of the graft (*dotted arrow*). (**c**) Arthroscopic appearance of wavy and irregular appearance in its proximal 1/3

A 33-year-old female former basketball player who had undergone a single-bundle ACLR by the other surgeon was suffering from persistent instability of her right knee for years (Fig. 38.3). She underwent the revision ART ACLR using the ipsilateral BTB graft, as well as medial meniscus repair, and restored stability without loss of motion (Figs. 38.4, 38.5, 38.6, 38.7).

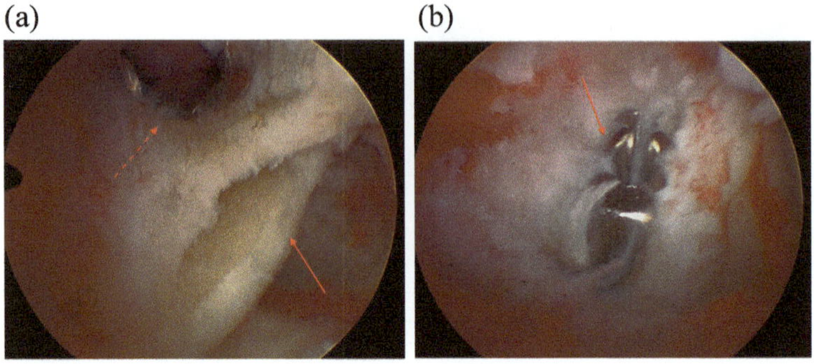

Fig. 38.4 Revision ACLR for Case 1. (**a**) Arthroscopic appearance of the new rectangular femoral tunnel aperture located in the anatomic attachment area (*solid arrow*) viewed via the anteromedial portal. Note the interference screw for the primary failed ACLR to be removed (*dotted arrow*). (**b**) The tip of the dilator showing the new rectangular tibial tunnel aperture just anterior to the previous one (*solid arrow*) viewed down from the anteromedial portal

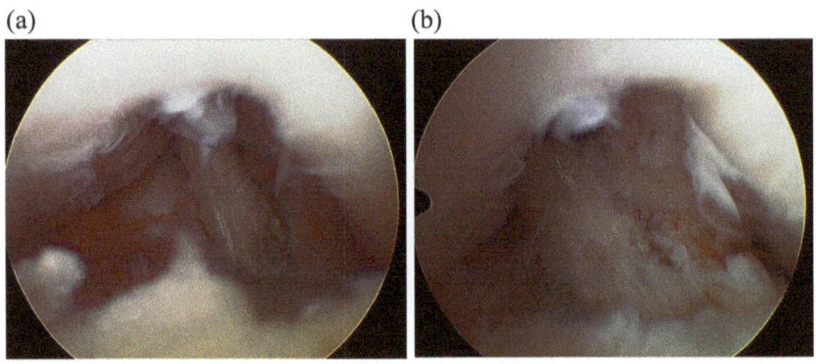

Fig. 38.5 Arthroscopic appearances of the revision anatomic ACL graft for Case 1. (**a**) No graft-notch impingement in extension. (**b**) No graft-PCL impingement in flexion

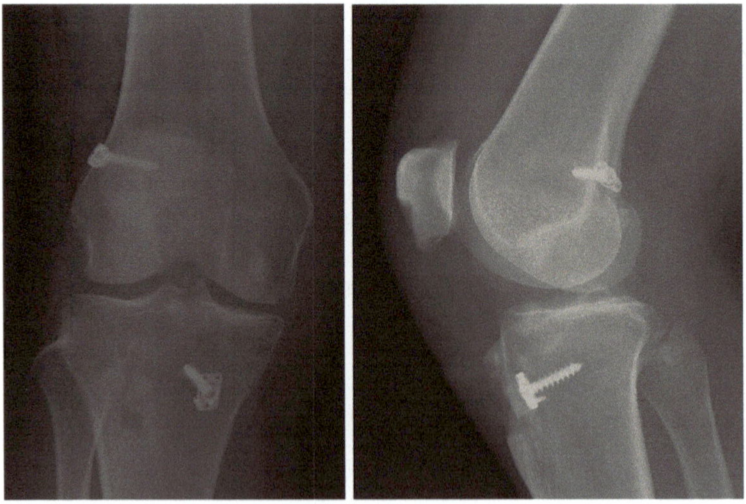

Fig. 38.6 Plain radiographs after the revision ACLR for Case 1. Note the DSPs and screws for fixation on the femur as well as on the tibia

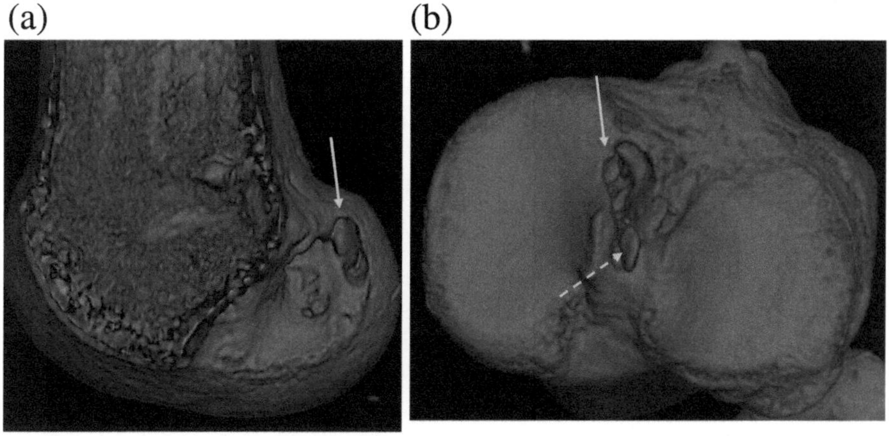

Fig. 38.7 3-D CT pictures showing femoral and tibial tunnel apertures after the revision ACLR for Case 1. (**a**) Note the new anatomic rectangular femoral tunnel aperture (*solid arrow*) with the bone plug inside (*solid arrow*). (**b**) Note the new rectangular tibial tunnel aperture just anterior to the previous one (*solid arrow*). Note the bone graft behind the tunnel to fill out the primary tunnel (*dotted arrow*)

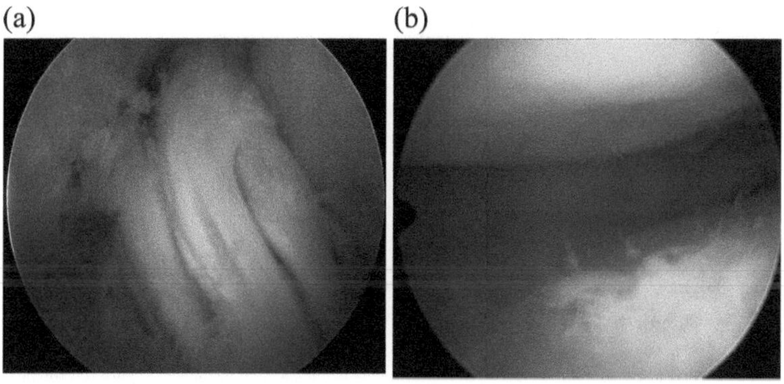

Fig. 38.8 Arthroscopic findings of Case 2. Note lax nonfunctioning ACL graft (**a**), loss of medial meniscus, and damaged articular surface of the medial compartment (**b**). He had to give up sports activity in fear of progression to severe joint degeneration after the revision

Case 2 with a previous surgery of double-bundle ACLR with hamstring tendon graft via improper nonanatomical femoral and tibial tunnels (Fig. 38.8).

A 17-year-old male soccer football player, who had undergone a single-bundle ACLR on his right knee by the other surgeon 18 months ago, was suffering from multiple subsequent surgeries including meniscectomy followed by persistent pain and instability. Arthroscopy revealed lax nonfunctioning ACL graft, loss of medial meniscus, and damaged articular surface of the medial compartment. He underwent the revision ART ACLR using the ipsilateral BTB graft and restored stability, while he had to give up sports activity in fear of progression to severe joint degeneration (Fig. 38.8).

38.6 Summary of Clinical Results

The ART ACLR technique made it possible to create a femoral tunnel in the anatomic attachment area in 30 of the 31 patients who had undergone the revision in the author's own practice between 2004 and 2008. The remaining one with severe tunnel widening had undergone the grafting via over the top of the lateral condyle. The tibial tunnel was successfully created without tunnel overlapping within the tibial attachment area in 29 of the 30 patients, whereas the remaining one required bone grafting to fill out the previous tunnel because of its posterior location. None of the patients underwent staged surgeries. Of the 18 patients directly followed for a minimum of 24 months, none reported giving way, subjective instability, or loss of motion, while one had retorn the graft at 28 months. Quantitative anterior laxity measurement with KT-1000 showed the mean side-to-side difference at maximum manual force improved from 6.8 ± 3.2 mm to 1.1 ± 1.4 mm with a range from -1 to 4 mm. One had sustained a tear of the revision graft and underwent a second revision ACLR with the quadriceps tendon-bone graft via the same tunnels [15].

However, it should be noted that the unstable knee due to failed ACL surgery destroys the cartilage as well as meniscus over time, as nonfunctioning ACL graft does not protect the cartilage or prevent early osteoarthritis (Case 2). Failed ACL surgery should be anatomically revised as soon as possible.

38.7 Conclusion

The revision anatomic rectangular tunnel ACLR is one of the useful options to manage unstable knee after failed ACL reconstruction.

References

1. Siebold R, Schumacher P, Fernandez F, Smigielski R, Fink C, Brehmer A, Kirsch J (2015) Flat midsubstance of the anterior cruciate ligament with tibial "C"-shaped insertion site. Knee Surg Sports Traumatol Arthrosc 23:3136–3142
2. Noyes FR, Butler DL, Grood ES, Zernicke RF, Hefzy MS (1984) Biomechanical analysis of human ligament grafts used in knee-ligament repairs and reconstructions. J Bone Joint Surg 66-A:344–352
3. Friedrich NF, O'Brien WR (1992) Functional anatomy of the cruciate ligaments. In: Jakob RP, Staeubli H-U (eds) The knee and the cruciate ligaments. Springer, Berlin, pp 78–91
4. Shino K, Nakata K, Nakamura N, Toritsuka Y, Nakagawa S, Horibe S (2005) Anatomically-oriented ACL reconstruction with a bone-patellar tendon graft via rectangular socket/tunnels: a snug-fit and impingement-free grafting technique. Arthroscopy 21:1402.e1–1402.e5

5. Shino K, Nakata K, Horibe S, Nakamura N, Toritsuka Y, Nakagawa S, Suzuki T (2008) Rectangular tunnel double-bundle anterior cruciate ligament reconstruction with bone–patellar tendon–bone graft to mimic natural fiber arrangement. Arthroscopy 24:1178–1183
6. Suzuki T, Shino K, Otsubo H, Suzuki D, Mae T, Fujimiya M, Yamashita T, Fujie H (2014) Biomechanical comparison between the rectangular-tunnel and the round-tunnel anterior cruciate ligament reconstruction procedures with a bone patellar tendon bone graft. Arthroscopy 30:1294–1302
7. Bach BR Jr (2003) Revision anterior cruciate ligament surgery. Arthroscopy 19(Suppl 1): 14–29
8. Shino K, Mae T, Nakamura N (2012) Revision ACL reconstruction with rectangular tunnel technique. Clin Orthop Relat Res 470:843–852
9. Shino K, Nakata K, Nakamura N, Mae T, Ohtsubo H, Iwahashi T, Nakagawa S (2005) Anatomic ACL reconstruction using two double-looped hamstring tendon grafts via twin femoral and triple tibial tunnels. Oper Tech Orthop 15:130–134
10. Shino K, Mae T, Maeda A, Miyama T, Shinjo H, Kawakami H (2002) Graft fixation with pre-determined tension using a new device, the double spike plate. Arthroscopy 18:908–911

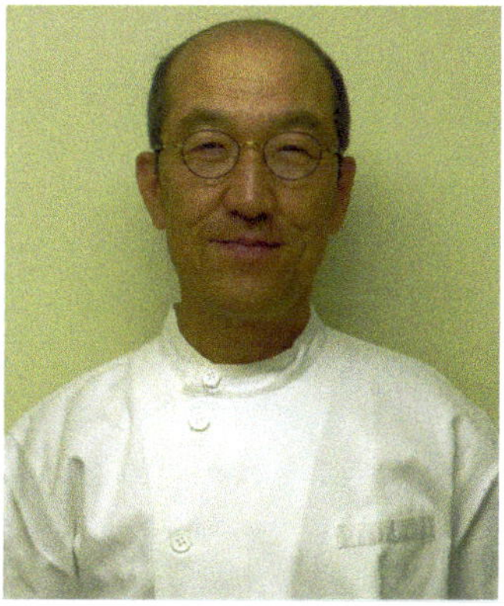

Konsei Shino, M.D., PhD, Sports Orthopaedic Center, Yukioka Hospital, Osaka, Japan.

Chapter 39
One- vs. Two-Stage Revision Anterior Cruciate Ligament Reconstruction

Shuji Taketomi, Hiroshi Inui, and Takumi Nakagawa

Abstract Revision surgery for failed anterior cruciate ligament (ACL) reconstruction is usually performed in a one- or two-stage procedure. Although a one-stage revision procedure should be performed whenever proper or anatomical tunnel creation and secure graft fixation can be achieved, in cases with incompletely placed previous tunnel(s) or large bone defect, a staged procedure is sometimes required. Revision ACL surgery after failed primary ACL reconstruction requires careful preoperative planning using three-dimensional (3D) computed tomography. An individualized approach should be used for each patient who needs a revision ACL procedure according to not only previous tunnel location and bone defect but also social background. A 3D fluoroscopy-based navigation system is a useful option in one-stage revision ACL reconstruction for technically demanding cases.

Keywords Revision anterior cruciate ligament reconstruction • One-stage • Two-stage • Bone grafting • Navigation

39.1 Introduction

Anterior cruciate ligament (ACL) reconstruction has become an increasingly common orthopedic surgery. With the increasing number of primary ACL reconstructions, revision procedures are likely to become more frequent. Although the approach to revision ACL reconstruction should ideally follow the same fundamental principles as those applied to primary ACL reconstruction, several issues need to be addressed, such as pre-existing implants, bone defects, and/or primary tunnel malposition in cases with failed ACL reconstruction. In particular, a revision procedure after failed primary ACL reconstruction with a synthetic ligament is a technically challenging surgery because of not only the complicated removal

S. Taketomi, MD, PhD (✉) • H. Inui, MD
Department of Orthopaedic Surgery, The University of Tokyo, 7-3-1 Hongo, Bunkyo-ku, Tokyo 113-0033, Japan
e-mail: takeos-tky@umin.ac.jp

T. Nakagawa, MD, PhD
Department of Orthopaedic Surgery, Teikyo University, Tokyo, Japan

M. Ochi et al. (eds.), *ACL Injury and Its Treatment*,
DOI 10.1007/978-4-431-55858-3_39

process for synthetic ligaments within the primary tunnels but also enlargement of bone tunnels [1].

Revision surgery for failed ACL reconstruction is usually performed in a one- or two-stage procedure. In cases with tunnel widening and/or removal of the previous implant, which leaves large bone defects, the staged procedure is sometimes required. The first stage includes graft and/or implant removal and bone grafting to the bone defect. After incorporation of the bone graft, revision ACL surgery can be performed [2, 3]. The strongest advantage of the two-stage procedure is that after the bone graft incorporation, any revision procedure can be performed as the primary ACL reconstruction using any type of grafts in the second-stage surgery. Meanwhile, the two-stage procedure has the following disadvantages: prolonged treatment period, additional costs, and the risk for potential inherent complications related to separate surgeries. Therefore, we think that one-stage revision ACL reconstruction should be performed as far as possible whenever proper or anatomical tunnel placement and stable graft fixation can be achieved. However, the one-stage revision procedure often requires various options to resolve problems which are pointed out above associated with failed primary ACL reconstruction.

Denti et al. reported 5 of 66 patients who underwent isolated revisions of ACL reconstruction failures that needed two-stage operations [4]. Five two-stage operations were for arthrolysis (four cases) and prior tibial and femoral bone grafting (one case). More than 90 % of revision cases could be performed as a one-stage operation.

Preoperative planning for a revision procedure is essential for a successful outcome. A preoperative three-dimensional (3D) computed tomography (CT) scan is a valuable and mandatory tool for evaluating previous tunnel location and bone defect due to tunnel widening and/or removal of the previous implant. The careful assessment of the cause of failed primary ACL reconstruction must also be made. It should not be preliminarily determined whether a one- or two-stage procedure is chosen, but it should be determined depending on the individual case based on careful preoperative planning. An individualized approach should be used for each patient who needs a revision ACL procedure according to not only previous tunnel location and bone defect but also social background. Becoming familiar with various sorts of techniques for revision procedures and graft fixation is key to success in revision ACL reconstruction.

The surgical approach is largely dependent on the previous tunnel location [5] and bone defect. Therefore, in this chapter, we describe appropriate revision procedures according to previous tunnel locations and bone defects due to tunnel widening and/or previous implant removal. Moreover, we will introduce a surgical technique using a navigation system for femoral tunnel creation in technically demanding one-stage revision ACL reconstruction.

39.2 Femoral Tunnel Creation

39.2.1 Previous Anatomical Femoral Tunnel Without Tunnel Widening

39.2.1.1 One-Stage Revision

In patients after anatomical double-bundle ACL reconstruction using hamstring tendon grafts without large tunnel widening (Fig. 39.1a), one-stage revision surgery can be performed using previous tunnels with contralateral hamstring grafts (Fig. 39.1b). For such cases, one-stage anatomical rectangular tunnel revision ACL reconstruction can also be performed with a bone-patellar tendon-bone (BPTB) graft by dilating the previous two tunnels (Fig. 39.1c).

In patients after anatomical rectangular tunnel ACL reconstruction using BPTB graft without tunnel widening (Fig. 39.1d), one-stage revision can be easily performed as the primary anatomical rectangular tunnel procedure using a contralateral BPTB graft (Fig. 39.1e).

39.2.1.2 Two-Stage Revision

In such cases, a two-stage procedure is not required.

39.2.2 Previous Completely Malpositioned Femoral Tunnel

39.2.2.1 One-Stage Revision

In patients in whom previous femoral tunnels were significantly non-anatomically placed and there was no bone defect within the femoral ACL footprint (Fig. 39.2a), a new femoral tunnel(s) can be independently created anatomically in the same manner as that in a primary ACL reconstruction with any type of graft (Fig. 39.2b, c).

39.2.2.2 Two-Stage Revision

In such cases, a two-stage procedure is not required. Even if bone grafting is needed for bone defects due to the previous tunnel or implant removal, bone grafting and a revision procedure can be simultaneously performed.

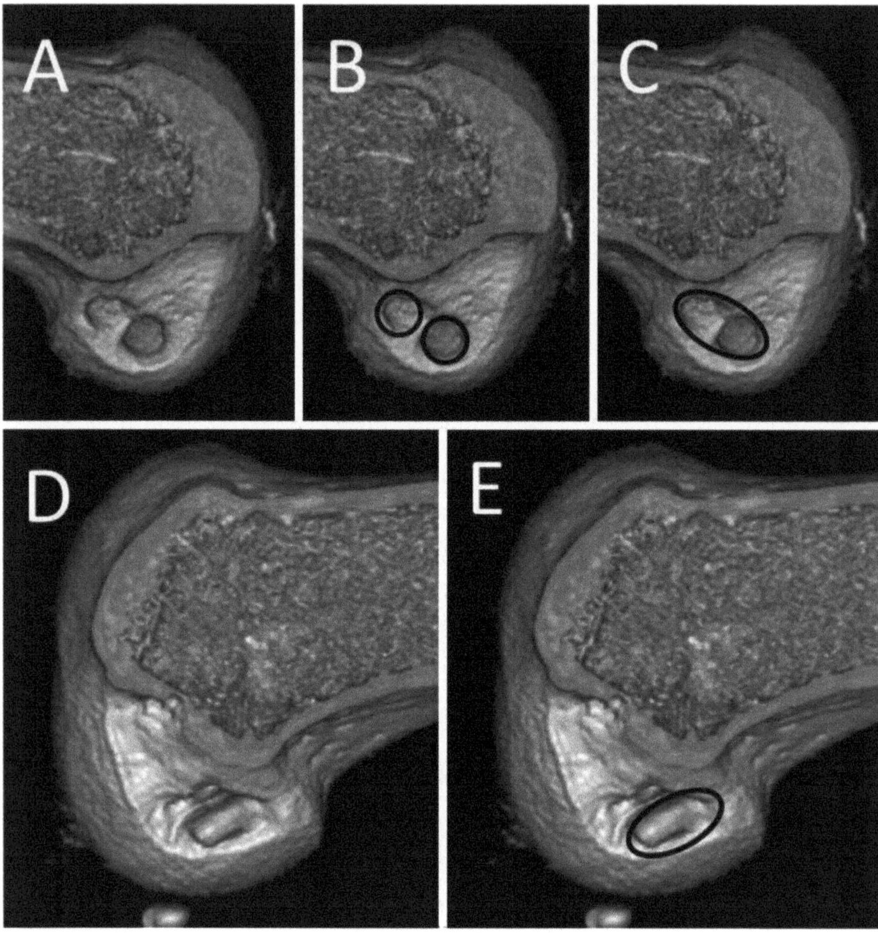

Fig. 39.1 (**a–c**) Preoperative three-dimensional (3D) computed tomography (CT) images of the *left knee* demonstrating anatomical positioned femoral tunnels without tunnel widening. (**b**) Two anatomical tunnels in a revision procedure using hamstring tendon grafts are marked. The previous tunnels can be used. (**c**) The *black ellipse* shows anatomical rectangular tunnel position in a revision procedure with bone-patellar tendon-bone (BPTB) graft by dilating the previous two previous tunnels. (**d, e**) Preoperative 3D CT images of the *right knee* demonstrating an anatomical positioned femoral rectangular tunnel without tunnel widening. (**e**) The *black ellipse* shows a new anatomical rectangular tunnel in a revision procedure with a BPTB graft

39.2.3 Previous Incompletely Malpositioned Femoral Tunnel

A previous incompletely malpositioned femoral tunnel is a common and technically difficult situation encountered in revision procedures after failed primary ACL reconstruction. Because the femoral tunnel is incompletely malpositioned and a part of the previous tunnel exists within the anatomical footprint, it is difficult to

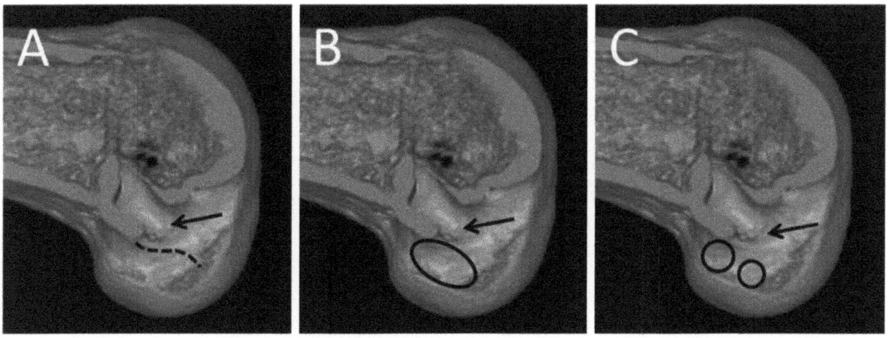

Fig. 39.2 Preoperative three-dimensional (3D) computed tomography (*CT*) images of the *left knee* showing a completely malpositioned femoral tunnel (*black arrow*). (**a**) The *broken line* shows a lateral intercondylar ridge which was not destroyed by the previous tunnel. (**b**) The *black ellipse* shows a new anatomical rectangular tunnel location in a revision procedure with bone-patellar tendon-bone graft without communication with the previous tunnel. (**c**) Two anatomical tunnels in a revision procedure using hamstring tendon grafts without communication with the previous tunnel are marked

create a new femoral tunnel in the location without communication with the previous femoral tunnel(s). (Fig. 39.3a)

39.2.3.1 One-Stage Revision

Shino et al. developed the anatomic rectangular tunnel ACL reconstruction with a BPTB graft to mimic natural fiber arrangement inside the native ACL and to minimize tunnel size [6, 7]. They applied this technique to patients after a failed primary ACL reconstruction [8, 9]. Because the cross-sectional area of the tunnels in their technique was less than that in a conventional round tunnel technique, the rectangular tunnel ACL reconstruction could be more often performed as a one-stage revision procedure. This technique is suitable for cases in which there is a previous incompletely malpositioned femoral tunnel and there is not enough space remaining for creating a new conventional tunnel. In cases in which there is a previous incompletely malpositioned femoral tunnel and the distance between the aperture rim of the previous femoral tunnel and posterior cartilage margin is more than 5 mm, a rectangular tunnel can be created. (Fig. 39.3b) Shino et al. reported that the femoral tunnel was created in the anatomic attachment area in 30 of the 31 patients who underwent revision procedures. We also used this technique for one-stage revision procedures. The details on this are described later. If the distance between the aperture rim of the previous tunnel and posterior cartilage margin is less than 5 mm, overlap between the previous tunnel aperture and the newly created one is inevitable. In such cases, a BPTB graft with the largest possible trapezoidal bone block can be used as a substitute for rectangular BPTB reconstruction. A

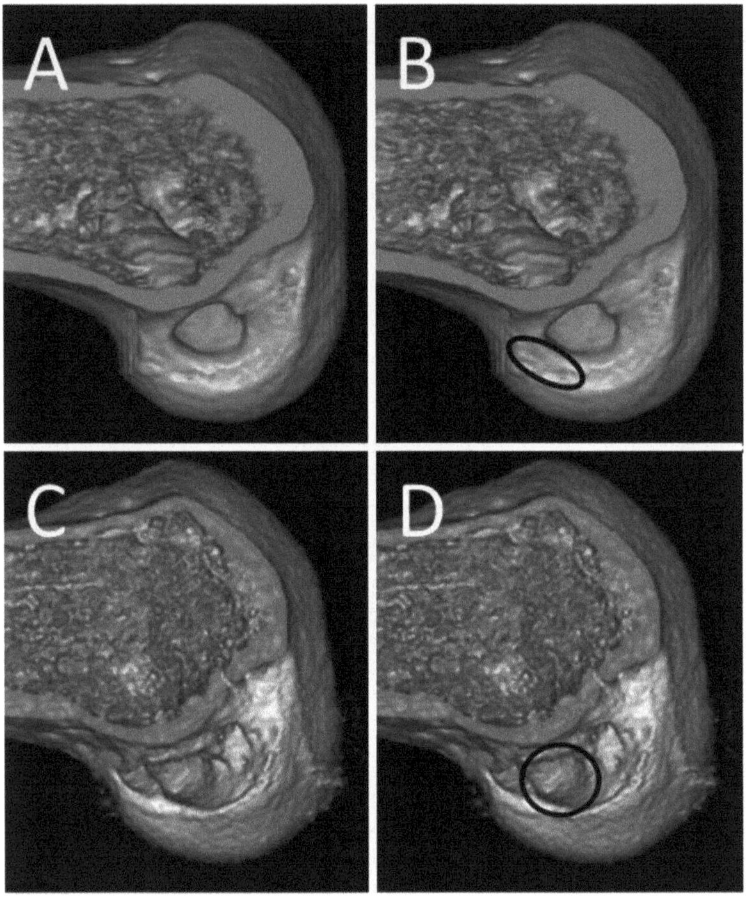

Fig. 39.3 (**a**, **b**) Preoperative three-dimensional (3D) computed tomography (CT) images of the *left knee* showing a previous incompletely malpositioned femoral tunnel. (**b**) The *black ellipse* shows a new anatomical rectangular tunnel location in a revision procedure with a bone-patellar tendon-bone (BPTB) graft without communication with the previous tunnel. (**c**, **d**) Preoperative 3D CT images of the *left knee* showing an anatomical positioned femoral tunnel with large tunnel widening. (**d**) The *black circle* shows a tunnel position in a revision procedure using a BPTB graft with the largest possible trapezoidal bone block as a substitute for rectangular BPTB reconstruction

rectangular BPTB graft can also be used, and the remaining bone defect just needs to be filled with an interference screw.

In cases in which the over-the-top procedure is primarily performed, although there is a small bone defect within the femoral footprint, a large bone defect is not usually observed (Fig. 39.6a, b). A rectangular tunnel procedure can be performed with BPTB graft in one-stage revision for such cases (Fig. 39.6c, d).

39.2.3.2 Two-Stage Revision

For cases in which revision procedures using BPTB or quadriceps tendon graft with bone plug are not feasible and there is not enough space remaining for creating a new tunnel for a double-bundle procedure, two-stage revision surgery is needed. During the first surgery, bone grafting of the bone defects with autografting is performed. Then, second-stage surgery can only be performed after bone-to-bone healing has occurred. According to the literature, incorporation of the bone grafts can take 10 weeks to 6 months [2, 10, 11]. Once the bone grafts incorporate with the femoral condyle, any revision procedure can be performed as the primary ACL reconstruction using any type of graft.

39.2.4 Previous Anatomical Femoral Tunnel with Large Bone Defect

In patients in whom previous femoral tunnels were anatomically placed and there was a large bone defect in the lateral femoral condyle due to tunnel widening and/or previous implant removal (Fig. 39.3c), it is difficult to choose between one- or two-stage revisions.

39.2.4.1 One-Stage Revision

A BPTB graft with the largest possible trapezoidal bone block can be used as a substitute for rectangular BPTB reconstruction (Fig. 39.3d). A divergent tunnel may lead to early bone-to-graft healing and secure graft fixation. A remaining bone defect can sometimes be filled with a bioabsorbable or metal interference screw. An impacted bone graft can also be used [12]. In such cases, creating bone tunnel (s) within the anatomical position and using a soft tissue graft may result in failure of a graft fixation.

In cases in which anatomical tunnel creation is not feasible because of a bone defect in the lateral femoral condyle, an over-the-top procedure may be considered. Usman et al. stated that the over-the-top route procedure was a valuable option for revision ACL reconstruction for cases in which the bone tunnel could not be created in an anatomical position because of tunnel enlargement and overlap with the malpositioned tunnel of primary reconstruction [13]. Over-the-top ACL reconstruction involves placing a graft by routing it through the notch and around, posterior to the lateral femoral condyle. As a result, bone grafting and creating new femoral tunnels can be avoided in the revision procedure. They concluded that the clinical results of the over-the-top route procedure were almost equivalent to those of anatomical single-bundle revision reconstruction in their study. Hofbauer et al. also used one-stage revision ACL reconstruction using the over-the-top technique for patients who have extensive expansion of anatomically placed femoral tunnels [10]. Prior to passing the graft, they created a groove with a rasp to guide the graft around the posterior aspect of the medial wall of the lateral condyle as well as to induce bleeding for theoretically improved healing of the soft tissue graft to the bone.

39.2.4.2 Two-Stage Revision

In the same way as the case with a previous incompletely malpositioned femoral tunnel, two-stage revision surgery may be chosen. If the surgeon or patient prefers soft tissue grafts and would like to avoid the over-the-top procedure, bone grafting is needed as the first-stage surgery.

39.3 Tibial Tunnel Creation

Severe tibial tunnel malposition is less common than femoral tunnel malposition. However, a staged revision procedure is required only in a case with a large bone defect or incompletely malpositioned tibial tunnel.

39.3.1 Tibial Tunnel Creation in One-Stage Revision

If the previous tibial tunnel is created too much to the anterior or posterior side, a new tibial tunnel(s) can be independently created in the same manner as that in a primary ACL reconstruction with any type of graft.

In patients after anatomical double-bundle ACL reconstruction using hamstring tendon grafts without large tunnel widening, one-stage revision surgery can be performed using previous tunnels with contralateral hamstring grafts. One-stage anatomical rectangular tunnel revision ACL reconstruction can also be performed with a BPTB graft by dilating the previous two tunnels or in cases following anatomical rectangular tunnel ACL reconstruction using a BPTB graft without large tunnel widening.

If the previous tibial tunnel is incompletely non-anatomically located, in particular posteriorly, one-stage anatomical rectangular tunnel revision ACL reconstruction can be performed with a BPTB graft. For such cases, a new tibial tunnel should be divergently created to the previous tunnel. If a bone defect more than 10 mm remains behind the new tunnel, the previous tunnel should be filled with a bone graft [9]. These techniques are hard to be applied to a revision procedure using a soft tissue graft.

When there are two previous tibial tunnels after double-bundle primary ACL reconstruction and one of two tunnels is anatomically located, a one-stage procedure can be performed by dilating the previously placed tunnel.

39.3.2 Tibial Tunnel Creation in a Two-Stage Revision

In cases in which anatomical tunnel creation is not feasible because of a large bone defect or in which overlapping of a new tibial tunnel and the previous tunnel is inevitable and a BPTB graft or other graft with a bone plug cannot be used, two-stage revision surgery is needed. In the same way as that for femoral tunnel creation, bone grafting of the bone defects is performed as a first stage. After bone-to-bone healing, second-stage surgery can be performed.

39.4 Bone Grafting Device

Refilling of a bone defect usually requires bone harvesting from the iliac crest. Said et al. described a technique for femoral and tibial tunnel impaction grafting in a two-stage revision procedure using the osteochondral autologous transfer system (OATS; Arthrex, Naples, FL) [14]. According to the authors, the appropriately sized OATS harvester was chosen 1 mm larger than the tunnel size and was used to harvest a bone graft from the iliac crest through a percutaneous approach. They concluded that the second stage can be performed 6–10 weeks after the first stage. Grote et al. developed a procedure combining minimally invasive intramedullary bone harvesting from the proximal femur using a reamer-irrigator-aspirator system with arthroscopic tunnel refilling [15]. Franceschi et al. used autologous bone from the medial tibial metaphyseal safe zone to manage femoral bone defects [16]. Wong et al. described a simple technique using the elasticity and transparent properties of a chest drain, which effectively delivers the bone graft to the femoral tunnel defect [3].

39.5 A One-Stage Femoral Tunnel Creation Procedure Using a Navigation System for Technically Demanding Cases (Author's Technique)

Computer-assisted surgery has recently been introduced to improve the accuracy and reproducibility of tunnel creation during ACL reconstruction [17–19]. We have been using a 3D fluoroscopy-based navigation system for accurate and reproducible placement of the femoral tunnel(s) in primary ACL reconstruction [20, 21]. This computer navigation is particularly useful for revision ACL reconstruction because it enables visualization of the whole previous femoral tunnel or the pre-existing hardware inside the femoral bone, which is not arthroscopically visible [22]. Osseous landmarks, such as the lateral intercondylar ridge or lateral bifurcate ridge, which are crucial to the identification of the femoral insertion of the ACL, cannot often be identified because of previous femoral tunnel(s) in a revision procedure. Using this imaging system, orientation of the lateral wall and the roof of the femoral intercondylar notch can be easily identified even if the natural morphology of the intercondylar notch was destroyed in the previous procedure. Here we describe a surgical technique using a 3D fluoroscopic-based navigation system for femoral tunnel creation in technically demanding one-stage revision ACL reconstruction.

39.5.1 Graft Selection and Preoperative Planning

The BPTB graft is our current preference for revision ACL reconstruction because direct bone-to-bone healing is expected, resulting in secure and consistent fixation. In addition, even if a bone defect exists, a BPTB graft with a large bone plug can fill the bone defect. Hamstring tendon grafts or quadriceps tendon grafts can also be used. The femoral bone plug is usually 5–6 mm thick, 10 mm wide, and 15 mm long for a rectangular tunnel placement as described by Shino et al. [6, 7], except in cases with a large femoral bone defect. As previously mentioned, because the cross-sectional area of the tunnels required for rectangular ACL reconstruction is less than that for the round tunnel technique, this method is advantageous as it allows surgeons to consistently avoid overlap with tunnels from prior surgeries.

Again, it is essential to perform preoperative planning using 3D CT images before every revision procedure. The principle is to create a new femoral tunnel for a BPTB graft inside the anatomic footprint. This navigation system works best for cases with previous incompletely malpositioned femoral tunnels and previous anatomical femoral tunnels with a bone defect. In case in which there is a previous incompletely malpositioned femoral tunnel and the distance between the aperture rim of the previous femoral tunnel and posterior cartilage margin is more than 5 mm, a rectangular tunnel can be created. On the other hand, when there is a previous incompletely malpositioned femoral tunnel and the distance is less than 5 mm, overlap between the previous tunnel aperture and the newly created one is inevitable. In such a case, a divergent tunnel can be created with the assistance of the navigation system. If a large femoral tunnel bone defect exists, a BPTB graft with a trapezoidal bone block is used as a substitute for rectangular BPTB reconstruction to fill the bone defect.

39.5.2 Intraoperative Image Data Acquisition

At the beginning of the surgery, the reference frame (Orthopaedic Frame HC; Medtronic, Louisville, CO) is attached rigidly to the femur with two half pins (Fig. 39.4a). Intraoperative 3D images are acquired with the C-arm of Arcadis Orbic 3D (Siemens AG, Erlangen, Germany) (Fig. 39.4b). The C-arm of the image intensifier is equipped with a wireless tracker (Stealth Active wireless tracker S/N 130; Medtronic) for navigation registration. The acquired image data are transferred to the navigation computer (StealthStation TRIA plus; Medtronic) (Fig. 39.4c), and a 3D image of the distal femur is reconstructed on the computer display screen. The medial half of the 3D reconstructed distal femur is deleted using computer software for a better view of the lateral wall and the roof of the femoral intercondylar notch (Fig. 39.5b). The obtained 3D model can be rotated and viewed from an arbitrary angle on the navigation monitor [22].

39.5.3 Computer Navigation-Assisted Femoral Tunnel Creation

Any metal hardware inside or outside the femoral bone is removed in case it may interfere with the creation of the new anatomical femoral tunnels(s). However, because navigation view allows the surgeon to create a new femoral tunnel without any interference with the retained hardware, it does not need to be removed in most cases. The insertion of guide wires for the femoral tunnel is performed using a femoral guide equipped with a tracker (SureTrak2 Universal Tracker, Large Passive Fighter; Medtronic). With an arthroscope introduced through a medial portal, the tip of the femoral guide can be arthroscopically placed through a far anteromedial portal [23] at the designated location. The navigation enables the surgeon to confirm the position of the femoral guide tip on the 3D reconstructed image in real time (Fig. 39.5b).

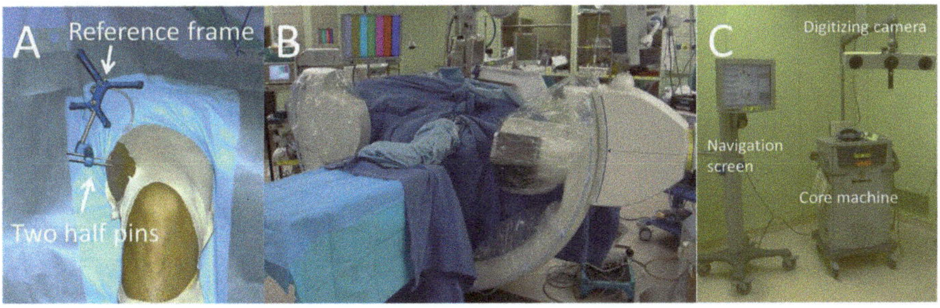

Fig. 39.4 Three-dimensional fluoroscopy-based navigation system. (**a**) Reference frame fixed with two half pins inserted into the *right femur*. (**b**) Intraoperative three-dimensional images are acquired with the C-arm. (**c**) The acquired image data are downloaded to the navigation computer

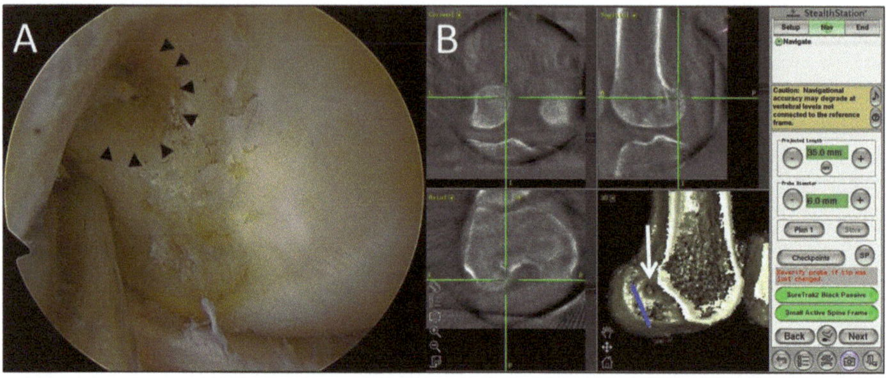

Fig. 39.5 Arthroscopic and navigation views of the lateral femoral condyle and the femoral guide in the *left knee*. (**a**) Arthroscopic view of the lateral wall of the femoral intercondylar notch can be obtained through the anteromedial portal with the knee at 90° flexion. The *black triangles* show the previous incompletely malpositioned tunnel aperture. The tip of the femoral guide is placed within the anatomical femoral footprint through a far anteromedial portal. (**b**) Navigation view of the lateral wall and roof of the femoral intercondylar notch on the three-dimensional reconstructed image. The *white arrow* shows the previous incompletely malpositioned tunnel, and the *blue line* shows the tip of the femoral guide

Keeping the femoral guide tip at the target point, the knee is fully flexed. On the navigation display screen, the surgeon can then identify the whole image of the lateral wall of the femoral notch (Figs. 39.5 and 39.6). Additionally, the surgeon is able to monitor any apertures of previous tunnels on navigation screen (Figs. 39.5 and 39.6), even when the arthroscopic visualization of the lateral wall of the intercondylar notch is disturbed because of limited flow across the joint or an impeding fat pad in deep knee flexion. Next, the 3D image was rotated 90° on the navigation display screen, and the risk of a back wall blowout can be evaluated (Fig. 39.7a). Finally, the 3D image is rotated 180° to show the lateral aspect of the distal femur on the navigation monitor. Visualization of the virtual exit of the femoral tunnel on the monitor enables the surgeon to avoid communication between the primary and revision tunnel exits or collision between a new tunnel exit and a retained hardware on the lateral cortex (Fig. 39.7d, e). The total length of the femoral tunnel can be evaluated at the same time (Fig. 39.7a). During these procedures, the axial, coronal, and sagittal two-dimensional image of any point can also be viewed. These views are a powerful tool, allowing the surgeon to create a new femoral tunnel without any interference with the previous tunnel or the retained hardware [22] (Fig. 39.7b, c).

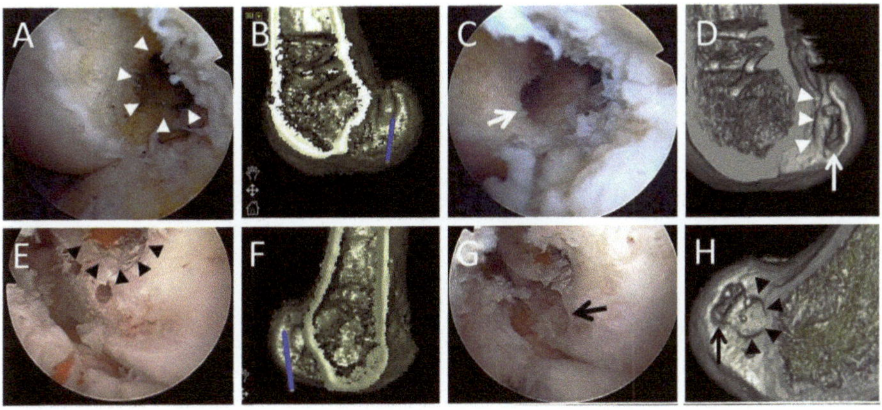

Fig. 39.6 (**a–d**) An illustrative case (*right knee*) with a bone defect after failed over-the-top route ACL reconstruction. (**a**) Arthroscopic view of the lateral wall of the femoral notch with a bone defect (*white triangles*) from the anteromedial portal. The knee was at 90° of flexion. (**b**) On the navigation computer screen, the surgeon can identify the whole image of the lateral wall of the femoral notch during surgery, whereas the natural morphology of the lateral wall of the intercondylar notch was destroyed by the previous reconstructive surgery.
Arthroscopic view (**c**) and medial view of a postoperative three-dimensional (3D) computed tomography (CT) reconstruction (**d**) of an anatomically created rectangular femoral tunnel (*white arrow*) for a bone-patellar tendon-bone (BPTB) graft overlapped with a proximal bone defect (*white triangles*).
(**e–h**) An illustrative case (*left knee*) with the previous incompletely malpositioned femoral tunnel. (**e**) Arthroscopic view of the lateral wall of the femoral notch with the previous incompletely malpositioned femoral tunnel (*black triangles*) from the anteromedial portal. The knee was at 90° of flexion. (**f**) The whole image of the lateral wall of the femoral notch and the previous incompletely malpositioned femoral tunnel are identified on the navigation computer screen.
Arthroscopic view (**g**) and medial view of a postoperative 3D CT reconstruction (**h**) of the anatomically created rectangular femoral tunnel (*black arrow*) for a BPTB graft without communication with the previous tunnel (*black triangles*)

39.6 Summary

Revision ACL surgery after failed primary ACL reconstruction requires careful preoperative planning using 3D CT. Although one-stage revision procedures should be performed whenever possible when proper or anatomical tunnel creation and secure graft fixation can be achieved, in cases with incompletely placed previous tunnel(s) or large bone defect, a staged procedure is sometimes required. A 3D fluoroscopy-based navigation system is a useful option in one-stage revision ACL reconstruction for technically demanding cases.

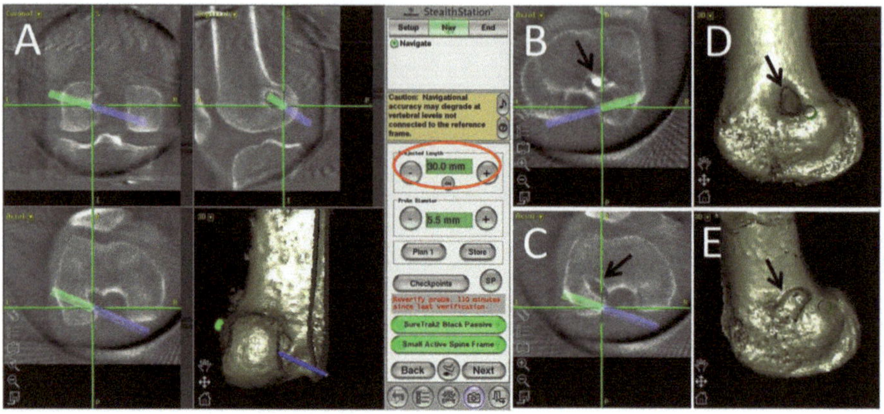

Fig. 39.7 Navigation view of the knee. Virtual tunnel routes are shown as *green columns* on the three- or two-dimensional (3D or 2D) model. (**a**) The 3D image is rotated 90° on the navigation screen in order to evaluate the risk of a back wall blowout. The total length of the femoral tunnel can be evaluated at the same time (*red circle*).
The retained metal hardware (**b**, *black arrow*) and the previous bone tunnel (**c**, *black arrow*) can be observed on the axial 2D image.
The image is rotated 180° to show the lateral aspect of the distal femur. Positional relation of the virtual exit of the femoral tunnel on the lateral cortex to the bone defect (**d**, *black arrow*) or the retained hardware (**e**, *black arrow*) can be observed

References

1. Niki Y, Matsumoto H, Enomoto H, Toyama Y, Suda Y (2010) Single-stage anterior cruciate ligament revision with bone-patellar tendon-bone: a case–control series of revision of failed synthetic anterior cruciate ligament reconstructions. Arthroscopy 26:1058–1065. doi:10.1016/j.arthro.2009.12.015
2. Safran MR, Harner CD (1996) Technical considerations of revision anterior cruciate ligament surgery. Clin Orthop Relat Res 325:50–64
3. Wong JW, Yip DK (2005) The peashooter device: an invaluable tool for bone grafting during revision anterior cruciate ligament surgery. Arthroscopy 21:1010. doi:10.1016/j.arthro.2005.04.096
4. Denti M, Lo Vetere D, Bait C, Schönhuber H, Melegati G, Volpi P (2008) Revision anterior cruciate ligament reconstruction: causes of failure, surgical technique, and clinical results. Am J Sports Med 36:1896–1902. doi:10.1177/0363546508318189
5. Magnussen RA, Debieux P, Benjamin B, Lustig S, Demey G, Servien E, Neyret P (2012) A CT-based classification of prior ACL femoral tunnel location for planning revision ACL surgery. Knee Surg Sports Traumatol Arthrosc 20:1298–1306. doi:10.1007/s00167-011-1814-4
6. Shino K, Nakata K, Nakamura N, Toritsuka Y, Nakagawa S, Horibe S (2005) Anatomically oriented anterior cruciate ligament reconstruction with a bone-patellar tendon-bone graft via rectangular socket and tunnel: a snug-fit and impingement-free grafting technique. Arthroscopy 21:1402
7. Shino K, Nakata K, Nakamura N, Toritsuka Y, Horibe S, Nakagawa S, Suzuki T (2008) Rectangular tunnel double-bundle anterior cruciate ligament reconstruction with bone-patellar tendon-bone graft to mimic natural fiber arrangement. Arthroscopy 24:1178–1183. doi: S0749-8063(08)00504-5 [pii]10.1016/j.arthro.2008.06.010

8. Shino K, Mae T, Nakamura N (2012) Surgical technique: revision ACL reconstruction with a rectangular tunnel technique. Clin Orthop Relat Res 470:843–852. doi:10.1007/s11999-011-1948-1
9. Shino K, Mae T, Take Y, Iuchi R, Nakagawa S (2015) One-stage revision anatomic anterior cruciate ligament reconstruction with rectangular tunnel technique. Asia-Pacific J Sports Med Arthroscopy, Rehabil Technol 2:43–48. doi:10.1016/j.asmart.2014.12.003
10. Hofbauer M, Murawski CD, Muller B, van Eck CF, Fu FH (2014) Revision surgery after primary double-bundle ACL reconstruction: AAOS exhibit selection. J Bone Joint Surg Am 96:e30. doi:10.2106/JBJS.M.01038
11. Groves C, Chandramohan M, Chew C, Subedi N (2013) Use of CT in the management of anterior cruciate ligament revision surgery. Clin Radiol 68:e552–e559. doi:10.1016/j.crad.2013.06.001
12. Ra HJ, Ha JK, Kim JG (2013) One-stage revision anterior cruciate ligament reconstruction with impacted bone graft after failed primary reconstruction. Orthopedics 36:860–863. doi:10.3928/01477447-20131021-07
13. Usman MA, Kamei G, Adachi N, Deie M, Nakamae A, Ochi M (2014) Revision single-bundle anterior cruciate ligament reconstruction with over-the-top route procedure. Orthop Traumatol Surg Res 101:71–75. doi:10.1016/j.otsr.2014.09.022
14. Said HG, Baloch K, Green M (2006) A new technique for femoral and tibial tunnel bone grafting using the OATS harvesters in revision anterior cruciate ligament reconstruction. Arthroscopy 22:796.e1–e3
15. Grote S, Helfen T, Mück F, Regauer M, Prall WC (2015) Femoral marrow cavity bone harvesting used for arthroscopic refilling of misplaced or enlarged bone tunnels in revision ACL surgery: an arthroscopically supported technique with antegrade intramedullary bone harvesting by a reamer-irrigator-aspirator (RIA) system. Knee Surg Sports Traumatol Arthrosc 23:808–815. doi:10.1007/s00167-013-2736-0
16. Franceschi F, Papalia R, Di Martino A, Rizzello G, Allaire R, Denaro V (2007) A new harvest site for bone graft in anterior cruciate ligament revision surgery. Arthroscopy 23:558.e1–e4. doi:10.1016/j.arthro.2006.07.054
17. Colombet P, Robinson J (2008) Computer-assisted, anatomic, double-bundle anterior cruciate ligament reconstruction. Arthroscopy 24:1152–1160. doi: S0749-8063(08)00423-4 [pii] 10.1016/j.arthro.2008.05.016
18. Tensho K, Kodaira H, Yasuda G, Yoshimura Y, Narita N, Morioka S, Kato H, Saito N (2011) Anatomic double-bundle anterior cruciate ligament reconstruction, using CT-based navigation and fiducial markers. Knee Surg Sports Traumatol Arthrosc 19:378–383. doi:10.1007/s00167-010-1217-y
19. Kawakami Y, Hiranaka T, Matsumoto T, Hida Y, Fukui T, Uemoto H, Doita M, Tsuji M, Kurosaka M, Kuroda R (2012) The accuracy of bone tunnel position using fluoroscopic-based navigation system in anterior cruciate ligament reconstruction. Knee Surg Sports Traumatol Arthrosc 20:1503–1510. doi:10.1007/s00167-011-1726-3
20. Nakagawa T, Takeda H, Nakajima K, Nakayama S, Fukai A, Kachi Y, Kawano H, Miura T, Nakamura K (2008) Intraoperative 3-dimensional imaging-based navigation-assisted anatomic double-bundle anterior cruciate ligament reconstruction. Arthroscopy 24:1161–1167
21. Taketomi S, Inui H, Nakamura K, Hirota J, Sanada T, Masuda H, Takeda H, Tanaka S, Nakagawa T (2014) Clinical outcome of anatomic double-bundle ACL reconstruction and 3D CT model-based validation of femoral socket aperture position. Knee Surg Sports Traumatol Arthrosc 22:2194–2201. doi:10.1007/s00167-013-2663-0
22. Taketomi S, Inui H, Nakamura K, Hirota J, Takei S, Takeda H, Tanaka S, Nakagawa T (2012) Three-dimensional fluoroscopic navigation guidance for femoral tunnel creation in revision anterior cruciate ligament reconstruction. Arthroscopy Tech 1:e95–e99
23. Shino K, Horibe S, Hamada M, Nakamura N, Nakata K, Toritsuka Y, Mae T (2002) Allograft anterior cruciate ligament reconstruction. Tech Knee Surg 1:78–85

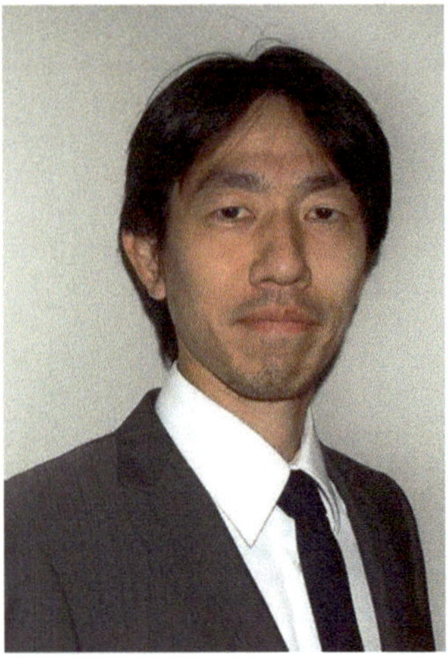

Shuji Taketomi, MD, PhD, Knee Surgery and Sports Medicine, Department of Orthopaedic Surgery, The University of Tokyo, Tokyo, Japan.

Part XI
Complications of ACL Reconstruction

Chapter 40
Complications of ACL Reconstruction

Satoshi Ochiai, Tetsuo Hagino, and Hirotaka Haro

Abstract Anterior cruciate ligament (ACL) reconstruction can be conducted endoscopically as a minimally invasive procedure. Moreover, since most of the patients who undergo ACL reconstruction are healthy young persons, the risk associated with ACL reconstruction is low. However, complications do occur at a considerable rate. Compared to other basic arthroscopic surgeries, the incidence of complications of ACL reconstruction is relatively high. A possible reason is that the procedures are complicated requiring bone preparation, tendon graft harvesting, and retention of internal fixation materials. The representative complications include anterior knee pain, limited range of motion in the knee, graft failure, infection, nerve injury, and deep vein thrombosis. In this chapter the status of occurrence of complications during and after ACL reconstruction, the risk factors, and treatments are discussed. Many of the complications can be prevented by performing the procedure cautiously and with scrupulous attention. It is important to perform ACL reconstruction fully aware of the potential intraoperative and postoperative complications and the prevention and management approaches.

Keywords Anterior cruciate ligament reconstruction • Operative complication • Arthroscopy

40.1 Introduction

The incidence of complications of arthroscopic knee surgeries in general is low; the rate was 0.27 % in our survey and ranged from 0.8 to 4.7 % in other previous studies [1]. Anterior cruciate ligament (ACL) reconstruction can also be conducted by arthroscopic surgery as a minimally invasive procedure. Moreover, since most of

S. Ochiai, M.D., PhD (✉) • T. Hagino, M.D., PhD
The Sports Medicine and Knee Center, National Hospital Organization, Kofu National Hospital, 11-35 Tenjin-cho, Kofu, Yamanashi 400-8533, Japan
e-mail: hxcmk230@ybb.ne.jp

H. Haro, M.D., PhD
Faculty of Medicine, Department of Orthopaedic Surgery, University of Yamanashi, Yamanashi, Japan

M. Ochi et al. (eds.), *ACL Injury and Its Treatment*,
DOI 10.1007/978-4-431-55858-3_40

Table 40.1 Incidence of complications associated with ACL reconstruction

Complication	Incidence (%)
Intraoperative	
Nerve injury (infrapatellar branch)	22–59 [7, 8]
Tunnel malposition	15 [18, 19]
Breakage (bioabsorbable interference screw)	3.4 [2]
Fracture (patellar) (blowout)	0.6–1.5 [2, 3] 1.2 [2]
Postoperative	
Anterior knee pain	11–56 [24, 25]
Limited knee range of motion	4–35 [32]
Graft failure	0.7–34.4 [42–45]
Infection	0.14–1.85 [52, 53]
Deep vein thrombosis	1.5–14 [60–62]

the patients who undergo ACL reconstruction are healthy young persons, the risk associated with ACL reconstruction is low. Nevertheless, complications do occur during and after reconstruction, and the rate is not necessarily low (Table 40.1). A possible reason is that although ACL reconstruction is an endoscopic surgery, the procedures are complicated requiring bone preparation, tendon graft harvesting, and retention of internal fixation materials. In this chapter the status of occurrence of complications associated with ACL reconstruction, the risk factors, and management approaches is discussed.

40.2 Intraoperative Complications

40.2.1 Bone and/or Cartilage Injury

When creating the femoral bone tunnel, drilling as well as placement and fixation of interference screws may cause blowout fracture in the posterior femoral cortex. The incidence of this type of fracture has been reported to be 1.2 % [2], and the causes include inappropriate size or position of the femoral bone tunnel and insufficient flexion of the knee joint during the surgical procedure.

When performing reconstruction using bone-patellar tendon-bone (BPTB) graft, patellar fracture may occur intraoperatively. The major causes are excessive bone cutting and aggressive levering. The reported incidence ranges from 0.6 to 1.5 % [2, 3].

Furthermore, manipulation of complicated surgical devices under the endoscope may cause damage to the articular cartilage. In recent years, the anteromedial portal technique, which has the merit of providing more anatomical placement of the bone tunnel, has grown in popularity. On the other hand, articular cartilage damage associated with this technique is becoming an issue. While creating the femoral bone tunnel using this method, the reamer head may injure the articular cartilage of the medial femoral condyle, and the risk increases as the portal is located far medial. In addition, drilling may also damage the articular cartilage of the lateral femoral condyle and the posterolateral knee structures. The risk increases during manipulation at a low knee flexion angle [4].

40.2.2 Nerve Injury

During ACL reconstruction, surgical manipulations may damage the nerves surrounding the knee joint. Caution has to be exercised.

The saphenous nerve may be injured during creation of the anteromedial portal for the endoscope or during harvest of the patellar tendon or the medial hamstring. Injury may occur during skin incision or manipulation of the tendon stripper when harvesting the medial hamstring [5, 6]. Although both the main trunk and the branches of the saphenous nerve may be injured, damage to the infrapatellar branch is particularly common (Fig. 40.1). The injury rates are as high as 22–59 % of all ACL reconstructions [7, 8]. Injury of the branch may lead to sensory disturbance from the anterior knee to the proximal leg and rarely causing painful neuroma or reflex sympathetic dystrophy [9, 10]. Recommendations to decrease the likelihood of nerve injury include making skin incisions for arthroscopy portals in a horizontal fashion parallel to the course of the nerve and in a flexed position to be directed

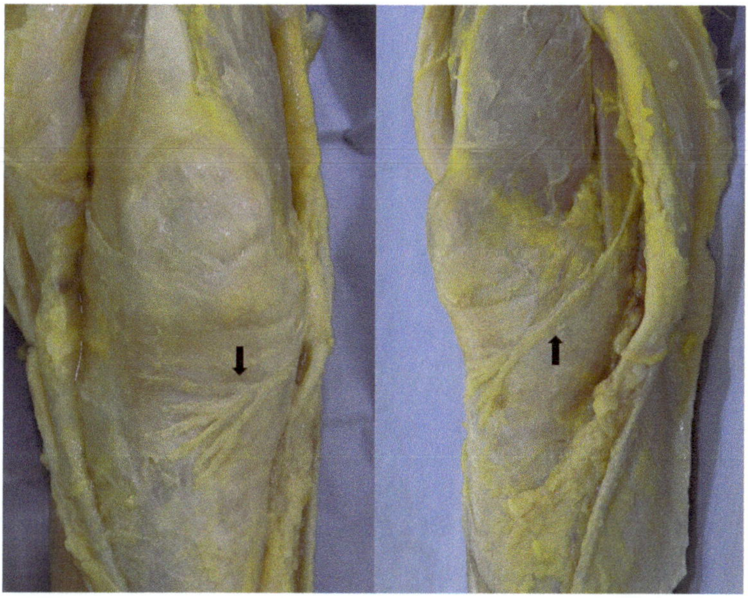

Fig. 40.1 Course of the infrapatellar branch of the saphenous nerve (*arrows*)
Standard skin incision has the risk of injuring the branch in ACL reconstructions both using hamstring graft and using bone-patellar tendon-bone graft

away from the course of the nerve [5]. In addition, attention has to be given to the direction of entry when using a tendon stripper.

The sciatic nerve may be injured when harvesting the medial hamstring using a tendon stripper. Injury to the sciatic nerve manifests drop foot and sciatic nerve numbness symptoms including extensive sensory disturbance. Attention has to be paid to the direction of entry of the tendon stripper. In patients with small physique, consideration has to be given to the fact that the hamstring runs near the sciatic nerve [11].

The peroneal nerve may be injured in ACL reconstruction using the anteromedial portal technique. By this technique, creating the bone tunnel toward the anatomical attachment site is considered to be easier compared to the conventional transtibial method. However, because the guide pin is inserted toward the posterior side of the lateral femoral condyle, the risk of peroneal nerve damage is increased. When performing ACL reconstruction using this method, it is recommended to drill the bone tunnel with the knee in hyperflexed position to be directed away from the course of the peroneal nerve [12, 13].

40.2.3 Vascular Injury

Although rare, injury of the blood vessels around the knee joint may occur during ACL reconstruction.

Popliteal artery and the adjacent arterial branch may be perforated by wire passing or drilling during placement of internal fixation materials on the tibial side or injured during dissection of the femoral ACL stump. The key to diagnosis is the development of signs of cyanosis and compartment syndrome due to the damaged blood vessels [14, 15].

Medial inferior genicular artery is the blood vessel coursing the medial side of the tibial condyle and may be injured during harvest of the hamstring or creation of the tibial bone tunnel. Pseudoaneurysm formation is often detected by swelling at the site of the injured artery several days after surgery [16, 17].

Arteriography is useful for definitive diagnosis of these vascular injuries. Depending on the site and severity of injury, treatment varies from embolization, surgical exploration, and repair or ligation, to artery bypass. Injury of the popliteal artery may require amputation, and urgent consultation with a vascular surgeon is essential. When performing surgery, it is important to have a good understanding of the vascular network including the abovementioned arteries and their branches.

40.2.4 Tunnel Malposition

Malposition of the bone tunnel through which the tendon graft passes may result in limited range of motion of the knee or rupture of the tendon graft. The incidence has been reported to be 15 % both on the tibial and femoral sides [18, 19]. Anteriorized positioning of the tibial tunnel causes impingement of the roof of the intercondylar notch, resulting in limited knee extension. Anteriorized positioning of the femoral tunnel causes excessive tension in the tendon graft, leading to limited knee flexion [20].

40.2.5 *Graft Fixation Error*

During ACL reconstruction, breakage of internal fixation material during fixation of the tendon graft and damage or laxity of the tendon graft accompanying poor reconstruction may occur. Bioabsorbable interference screws, which are increasingly popular because they do not require removal or hinder MRI examination, are more fragile than other internal fixation materials and therefore require attention during insertion. For these screws, intraoperative breakage rate of 3.4 % and intra-articular migration rate of 0.3 % have been reported [2, 21].

Endobutton is a representative internal fixation material used in ACL reconstruction. Endobutton malpositioning may be caused by inaccurate measurement of the bone tunnel length, insufficient overdrilling, and debris inside the bone tunnel. Intratunnel migration of the Endobutton occurs at an incidence of 1 % [2, 22, 23].

Occurrence of the above intraoperative complications is largely associated with surgical skill. While surgeons must have a good understanding of the anatomical relationship among nerves, blood vessels, and other structures before commencing surgery, many of the complications can be avoided by surgical manipulations at the optimal knee position, accurate insertion of the guide wire, confirmation using fluoroscopy, and furthermore combined use of notch plasty when the need arises.

40.3 Postoperative Complications

40.3.1 *Anterior Knee Pain*

Among the pains after ACL reconstruction, anterior knee pain (AKP) occurs at a relatively high frequency, ranging from 11 to 56 % [24, 25]. A preponderance in older population [26] and in females [27] has been reported, but the exact mechanism has not been identified. At one time, the occurrence of AKP caused by harvest of the bone-patellar tendon-bone (BPTB) graft was an issue. However, the pain is attenuated over time. Also, with the introduction of less invasive harvesting technique, the incidence of AKP associated with BPTB graft has shown to be similar to that for the hamstring tendon (HT) graft [28, 29]. AKP is often accompanied by restricted knee extension and lowered quadriceps strength, suggesting mutual relationship among the three [24].

Complex regional pain syndrome may occur after ACL reconstruction, albeit rarely, with an incidence of 4–7 % [30, 31]. In these cases, various symptoms manifest after surgery, including disproportionate continuing pain, sensory abnormality, edema, and articular contracture. Plain radiography may show a picture of local osteoporosis. On three-phase bone scintigraphy (Tc-99), uptake is often observed. After onset, remission may take several years.

Analgesic medication and systematic rehabilitation program are the mainstay for prevention and treatment. Preemptive analgesic technique of initiating continuous NSAIDs treatment from before surgery shows prophylactic effects for both AKP and complex regional pain syndrome [30].

40.3.2 Limited Range of Motion

The incidence of limited range of motion of the knee following ACL reconstruction ranges from 4 to 35 % [32]. Compared to loss of flexion, loss of extension significantly lowers knee performance, and extension loss exceeding 5° results in AKP and quadriceps weakness [32, 33]. The causes of loss of extension include nonanatomic placement of the graft, excessive graft tension, cyclops lesion, arthrofibrosis, and inappropriate rehabilitation [34].

Cyclops lesion refers to the nodular granulation tissue covering the fibrous tissue that forms after trauma or surgery to the ACL. The lesion arises anterior to the ACL. Loss of extension is caused by impingement of the ACL or the reconstructed ligament in the intercondylar notch upon knee extension [35] (Fig. 40.2a, b).

Arthrofibrosis caused by intra-articular or extra-articular metaplasia was shown to be induced by acute ACL reconstruction, leading to the recommendation of waiting for at least 3 weeks after injury before performing ACL reconstruction [36]. However, in recent years, early surgery during acute ACL injury has been considered to be safe in patients with little inflammatory reactions such as pain and swelling and in patients with little loss of motion [32].

The importance of proper surgical techniques and early aggressive rehabilitation for the prevention of limited range of motion has been advocated [32, 37]. Study has shown that aggressive rehabilitation mitigates weakening of muscle strength and AKP, while elongation and rupture of the tendon graft, which are concerns of this approach, are not observed [38]. However, for ACL reconstruction using the HT graft, increase of knee effusion and induction of tunnel enlargement as shown on CT have been reported. Therefore, it is necessary to monitor the patient's conditions during the rehabilitation program and modify if necessary [39, 40]. In patients with motion limitation unresponsive to rehabilitation therapy, arthrolysis or manipulation under anesthesia is required. Arthrolysis performed within 8 months after ACL reconstruction has been reported to achieve better outcome [41].

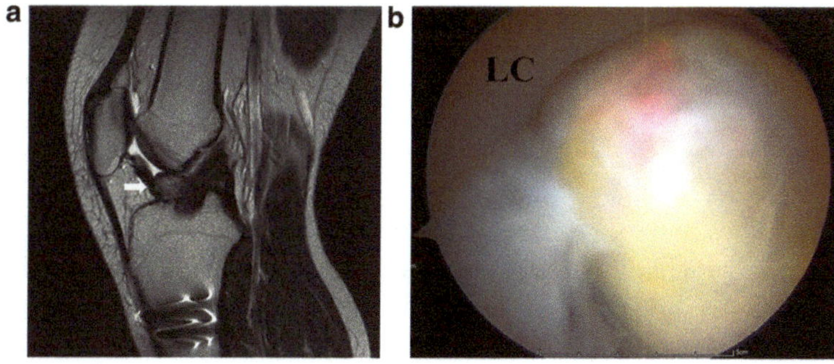

Fig. 40.2 Cyclops lesion formed after ACL reconstruction
(**a**) MRI shows a nodular lesion with clear margin in the intercondylar notch located anterior to the ACL graft (allow).
(**b**) Arthroscopic finding at the corresponding site shows a nodule attached to the tibial soft tissue, containing blood vessels on the surface.
LC lateral condyle of femur

40.3.3 Graft Failure

Although the incidence is relatively low, graft rupture may occur after ACL reconstruction. The reported rate of graft failure in BPTB grafts was 0.7–8.3 %; and among HT grafts, the rates were 1.6–16.7 % for the single-bundle method, 1.3–3.3 % for the double-bundle method, and 1.7–34.4 % for allografts [42–45]. For HT grafts, a prospective randomized study reported a significantly lower graft failure rate with the double-bundle method compared to the single-bundle method [44]. The rate of graft failure is significantly higher when using allografts than when using autografts, probably due to delayed remodeling [46]. On the other hand, another report found no significant difference in graft failure rate between reconstructions using allografts not chemically processed or irradiated and reconstructions using autografts [43].

The major causes of graft failure are trauma, inappropriate surgical technique, and problem with graft maturation. Trauma is the most common cause. The risk is especially high in the case of trauma occurring before graft maturation takes place and in the case of premature resumption of sports activities. Surgical technique issues include the location of bone tunnel, fixation method, and tension of the graft, while anterior placement of the femoral tunnel is considered to be the most common cause [47, 48].

The risk factors of graft failure after ACL reconstruction include young age, female, high activity level, and a contact mechanism of initial ACL injury [45, 49, 50]. For HT graft, a graft diameter of 8 mm or less has been proposed to be a risk factor [51]. Attention has to be paid to the fact that the graft tendon tends to have a smaller diameter in women. It is also necessary not to miss concurrent injuries in intra- and extra-articular structures and in the bones of patients who have a contact mechanism in the initial injury. In young persons with high activity level, it may be desirable to select the double-bundle method when HT graft is used or to use the BPTB graft that shows excellent graft fixation.

40.3.4 Infection

The rates of postoperative infection for the less invasive ACL reconstruction are low, ranging from 0.14 to 1.85 % [52, 53]. However, it should be noted that infection is a serious complication that occurs at a constant rate.

When infection occurs, the symptoms include pain, swelling, and reddening of the affected site; reduced range of motion due to pain; and persistent fever. However, even in noninfection cases, the same symptoms are also seen during the early postoperative period. Therefore, infection is difficult to diagnose and careful observation is necessary. For laboratory tests, hematological and biochemical tests include mainly C-reactive protein (CRP) and erythrocyte sedimentation rate (ESR) that are indicators of inflammatory reactions, white blood cell count in knee aspirate, and bacteriological culture to isolate the causative pathogen. Among the causative bacteria, *Staphylococcus aureus*, *Staphylococcus epidermidis*, and coagulase-negative staphylococci (CNS) are isolated at high rates [54, 55].

Various risk factors of infection have been reported, including a past history of knee surgery, meniscus suture during ACL reconstruction, and diabetes [56, 57]. In addition, the infection rate is higher when HT grafts are used compared to BPTB grafts and allografts. The difference in infection rate among different types of graft is probably due to the differences in graft preparation time and the difference in the amount of suture material placed inside the joint [57, 58].

Since postoperative infection may cause graft failure, loss of hyaline cartilage, and arthrofibrosis, prompt treatment is necessary [55, 58]. Treatment strategy involves arthroscopic irrigation and debridement, together with intravenous antibiotics [54, 56, 59]. Although there are many reports of good treatment outcome even with graft retention, removal of the graft or internal fixation material is necessary in cases not responding rapidly to treatment or in cases with poor graft condition [55].

40.3.5 Deep Vein Thrombosis

Deep vein thrombosis (DVT) is the formation of thrombus in the veins of the extremities or other sites caused by surgery, infection, prolonged immobility, and other factors. It is a serious complication because progression to pulmonary infraction is potentially life-threatening. Deep vein thrombosis that occurs after ACL reconstruction mainly involves the lower extremities. While symptoms of pain and swelling may be observed in some cases, many cases remain asymptomatic. Furthermore, it should be noted since symptoms resembling those of DVT are commonly seen in the early postoperative period

After ACL reconstruction, an accurate clinical diagnosis of DVT is often difficult. Various tests are being used to diagnose DVT, including venography, ultrasonography, and impedance plethysmography. Among them, venography has been reported to have the highest sensitivity [60, 61].

Lower extremity DVT after ACL reconstruction was thought to be a less frequently occurring complication, but studies using venography found an incidence of 14 % [60–62]. This rate is higher than that reported for general arthroscopic surgeries such as meniscus procedures. The possibility that bone debris generated during bone preparation procedures such as bone tunnel drilling may act as clotting factor precursors has been reported [60]. The incidence of DVT after ACL reconstruction is significantly higher in older patients and in females; hence old age and female gender are considered to be risk factors of DVT [61].

Some preventive measures against DVT after ACL reconstruction have been recommended, such as use of elastic stockings and prophylactic use of low molecular weight heparin, but no consensus has been reached [63, 64]. When DVT occurs, anticoagulant therapy, thrombolytic therapy, and vascular interventional radiology performed by specialists should be started promptly. In addition, lung contrast CT and other tests should be performed to detect pulmonary infarction.

40.3.6 Others

Other rare postoperative complications following ACL reconstruction include femoral, tibial, and patellar fractures [65–67], rupture of the patellar ligament [68], and migration or breakage of internal fixation materials [69]. Most of these complications occur during the early postoperative period. These complications should be borne in mind before repair of the surgically invaded bone and soft tissues and incorporation of the tendon graft are fully accomplished.

40.4 Conclusion

This chapter summarizes the representative complications associated with ACL reconstruction. Many of the complications can be prevented by performing the procedure cautiously and with scrupulous attention. It is important to perform ACL reconstruction fully aware of the potential intraoperative and postoperative complications and management approaches.

Acknowledgment The authors thank Professor Sen Takeda and Mr. Haruo Futamata of the Department of Anatomy and Cell Biology, University of Yamanashi Interdisciplinary Graduate School of Medicine and Engineering, for their support in the dissection of cadaver.

References

1. Hagino T, Ochiai S, Watanabe Y, Senga S, Wako M, Ando T, Sato E, Haro H (2014) Complications after arthroscopic knee surgery. Arch Orthop Trauma Surg 134 (11):1561–1564. doi:10.1007/s00402-014-2054-0
2. Almazán A, Miguel A, Odor A, Ibarra JC (2006) Intraoperative incidents and complications in primary arthroscopic anterior cruciate ligament reconstruction. Arthroscopy 22 (11):1211–1217
3. Berg EE (1996) Management of patella fractures associated with central third bone-patella tendon-bone autograft ACL reconstructions. Arthroscopy 12(6):756–759
4. Lubowitz JH (2009) Anteromedial portal technique for the anterior cruciate ligament femoral socket: pitfalls and solutions. Arthroscopy 25(1):95–101. doi:10.1016/j.arthro.2008.10.012. Review
5. Tifford CD, Spero L, Luke T, Plancher KD (2000) The relationship of the infrapatellar branches of the saphenous nerve to arthroscopy portals and incisions for anterior cruciate ligament surgery. An anatomic study. Am J Sports Med 28(4):562–567
6. Bertram C, Porsch M, Hackenbroch MH, Terhaag D (2000) Saphenous neuralgia after arthroscopically assisted anterior cruciate ligament reconstruction with a semitendinosus and gracilis tendon graft. Arthroscopy 16(7):763–766
7. Mochida H, Kikuchi S (1995) Injury to infrapatellar branch of saphenous nerve in arthroscopic knee surgery. Clin Orthop Relat Res 320:88–94
8. Portland GH, Martin D, Keene G, Menz T (2005) Injury to the infrapatellar branch of the saphenous nerve in anterior cruciate ligament reconstruction: comparison of horizontal versus vertical harvest site incisions. Arthroscopy 21(3):281–285
9. Pinar H, Ozkan M, Akseki D, Yörükoğlu K (1996) Traumatic prepatellar neuroma: an unusual cause of anterior knee pain. Knee Surg Sports Traumatol Arthrosc 4(3):154–156
10. Poehling GG, Pollock FE Jr, Koman LA (1988) Reflex sympathetic dystrophy of the knee after sensory nerve injury. Arthroscopy 4(1):31–35
11. Vardi G (2004) Sciatic nerve injury following hamstring harvest. Knee 11(1):37–39
12. Nakamura M, Deie M, Shibuya H, Nakamae A, Adachi N, Aoyama H, Ochi M (2009) Potential risks of femoral tunnel drilling through the far anteromedial portal: a cadaveric study. Arthroscopy 25(5):481–487. doi:10.1016/j.arthro.2008.11.010
13. Basdekis G, Abisafi C, Christel P (2008) Influence of knee flexion angle on femoral tunnel characteristics when drilled through the anteromedial portal during anterior cruciate ligament reconstruction. Arthroscopy 24(4):459–464. doi:10.1016/j.arthro.2007.10.012
14. Roth JH, Bray RC (1988) Popliteal artery injury during anterior cruciate ligament reconstruction: brief report. J Bone Joint Surg (Br) 70(5):840
15. Aldridge JM 3rd, Weaver JP, Mallon WJ (2002) Avulsion of the middle genicular artery: a previously unreported complication of anterior cruciate ligament repair. A case report. Am J Sports Med 30(5):748–750
16. Mello W, de Brito WE, Migon EZ, Borges A (2011) Pseudoaneurysm of the medial inferior genicular artery after anterior cruciate ligament reconstruction. Arthroscopy 27(3):442–445. doi:10.1016/j.arthro.2010.10.015
17. Milankov M, Miljkovic N, Stankovic M (2006) Pseudoaneurysm of the medial inferior genicular artery following anterior cruciate ligament reconstruction with hamstring tendon autograft. Knee 13(2):170–171
18. Hughes AW, Dwyer AJ, Govindaswamy R, Lankester B (2012) The use of intra-operative fluoroscopy for tibial tunnel placement in anterior cruciate ligament reconstruction. Bone Joint Res 1(10):234–237. doi:10.1302/2046-3758.110.2000086
19. Mehta VM, Paxton EW, Fithian DC (2009) Does the use of fluoroscopy and isometry during anterior cruciate ligament reconstruction affect surgical decision making? Clin J Sport Med 19 (1):46–48. doi:10.1097/JSM.0b013e3181915bd7

20. Fu FH, Bennett CH, Ma CB, Menetrey J, Lattermann C (2000) Current trends in anterior cruciate ligament reconstruction. Part II. Operative procedures and clinical correlations. Am J Sports Med 28(1):124–130. Review
21. Papalia R, Vasta S, D'Adamio S, Giacalone A, Maffulli N, Denaro V (2014) Metallic or bioabsorbable interference screw for graft fixation in anterior cruciate ligament (ACL) reconstruction? Br Med Bull 109:19–29. doi:10.1093/bmb/ldt038
22. Karaoglu S, Halici M, Baktir A (2002) An unidentified pitfall of Endobutton use: case report. Knee Surg Sports Traumatol Arthrosc 10(4):247–249
23. Vega R, Irribarra L, Filippi J (2005) Simple solution for failure of trailing sutures when using the EndoButton in anterior cruciate ligament reconstruction: the "Rescue Rein". Arthroscopy 21(8):1013
24. Niki Y, Hakozaki A, Iwamoto W, Kanagawa H, Matsumoto H, Toyama Y, Suda Y (2012) Factors affecting anterior knee pain following anatomic double-bundle anterior cruciate ligament reconstruction. Knee Surg Sports Traumatol Arthrosc 20(8):1543–1549. doi:10.1007/s00167-011-1746-z
25. Järvelä T, Kannus P, Järvinen M (2000) Anterior knee pain 7 years after an anterior cruciate ligament reconstruction with a bone-patellar tendon-bone autograft. Scand J Med Sci Sports 10 (4):221–227
26. Stapleton TR (1997) Complications in anterior cruciate ligament reconstructions with patellar tendon grafts. Sports Med Arthosc Rev 5:156–162
27. Aglietti P, Buzzi R, D'Andria S, Zaccherotti G (1993) Patellofemoral problems after intraarticular anterior cruciate ligament reconstruction. Clin Orthop Relat Res 288:195–204
28. Samuelsson K, Andersson D, Karlsson J (2009) Treatment of anterior cruciate ligament injuries with special reference to graft type and surgical technique: an assessment of randomized controlled trials. Arthroscopy 25(10):1139–1174. doi:10.1016/j.arthro.2009.07.021
29. Kartus J, Ejerhed L, Sernert N, Brandsson S, Karlsson J (2000) Comparison of traditional and subcutaneous patellar tendon harvest. A prospective study of donor site-related problems after anterior cruciate ligament reconstruction using different graft harvesting techniques. Am J Sports Med 28(3):328–335
30. Reuben SS, Ekman EF (2007) The effect of initiating a preventive multimodal analgesic regimen on long-term patient outcomes for outpatient anterior cruciate ligament reconstruction surgery. Anesth Analg 105(1):228–232
31. Reuben SS (2004) Preventing the development of complex regional pain syndrome after surgery. Anesthesiology 101(5):1215–1224. Review
32. DeHaven KE, Cosgarea AJ, Sebastianelli WJ (2003) Arthrofibrosis of the knee following ligament surgery. Instr Course Lect 52:369–381. Review
33. Sachs RA, Daniel DM, Stone ML, Garfein RF (1989) Patellofemoral problems after anterior cruciate ligament reconstruction. Am J Sports Med 17(6):760–765
34. Austin JC, Phornphutkul C, Wojtys EM (2007) Loss of knee extension after anterior cruciate ligament reconstruction: effects of knee position and graft tensioning. J Bone Joint Surg Am 89 (7):1565–1574
35. Jackson DW, Schaefer RK (1990) Cyclops syndrome: loss of extension following intra-articular anterior cruciate ligament reconstruction. Arthroscopy 6(3):171–178
36. Shelbourne KD, Wilckens JH, Mollabashy A, DeCarlo M (1991) Arthrofibrosis in acute anterior cruciate ligament reconstruction. The effect of timing of reconstruction and rehabilitation. Am J Sports Med 19(4):332–336
37. Cosgarea AJ, Sebastianelli WJ, DeHaven KE (1995) Prevention of arthrofibrosis after anterior cruciate ligament reconstruction using the central third patellar tendon autograft. Am J Sports Med 23(1):87–92
38. Kruse LM, Gray B, Wright RW (2012) Rehabilitation after anterior cruciate ligament reconstruction: a systematic review. J Bone Joint Surg Am 94(19):1737–1748. doi:10.2106/JBJS.K.01246. Review

39. Vadalà A, Iorio R, De Carli A, Argento G, Di Sanzo V, Conteduca F, Ferretti A (2007) The effect of accelerated, brace free, rehabilitation on bone tunnel enlargement after ACL reconstruction using hamstring tendons: a CT study. Knee Surg Sports Traumatol Arthrosc 15 (4):365–371
40. Majima T, Yasuda K, Tago H, Tanabe Y, Minami A (2002) Rehabilitation after hamstring anterior cruciate ligament reconstruction. Clin Orthop Relat Res 397:370–380
41. Aglietti P, Buzzi R, De Felice R, Paolini G, Zaccherotti G (1995) Results of surgical treatment of arthrofibrosis after ACL reconstruction. Knee Surg Sports Traumatol Arthrosc 3(2):8
42. Crawford SN, Waterman BR, Lubowitz JH (2013) Long-term failure of anterior cruciate ligament reconstruction. Arthroscopy 29(9):1566–1571. doi:10.1016/j.arthro.2013.04.014
43. Barber FA, Cowden CH 3rd, Sanders EJ (2014) Revision rates after anterior cruciate ligament reconstruction using bone-patellar tendon-bone allograft or autograft in a population 25 years old and younger. Arthroscopy 30(4):483–491. doi:10.1016/j.arthro.2013.12.022
44. Suomalainen P, Järvelä T, Paakkala A, Kannus P, Järvinen M (2012) Double-bundle versus single-bundle anterior cruciate ligament reconstruction: a prospective randomized study with 5-year results. Am J Sports Med 40(7):1511–1518. doi:10.1177/0363546512448177
45. Maletis GB, Inacio MC, Desmond JL, Funahashi TT (2013) Reconstruction of the anterior cruciate ligament: association of graft choice with increased risk of early revision. Bone Joint J 95-B(5):623–628. doi:10.1302/0301-620X.95B5.30872
46. Scheffler SU, Schmidt T, Gangéy I, Dustmann M, Unterhauser F, Weiler A (2008) Fresh-frozen free-tendon allografts versus autografts in anterior cruciate ligament reconstruction: delayed remodeling and inferior mechanical function during long-term healing in sheep. Arthroscopy 24(4):448–458. doi:10.1016/j.arthro.2007.10.011
47. George MS, Dunn WR, Spindler KP (2006) Current concepts review: revision anterior cruciate ligament reconstruction. Am J Sports Med 34(12):2026–2037
48. Carson EW, Simonian PT, Wickiewicz TL, Warren RF (1998) Revision anterior cruciate ligament reconstruction. Instr Course Lect 47:361–368. Review
49. Barrett AM, Craft JA, Replogle WH, Hydrick JM, Barrett GR (2011) Anterior cruciate ligament graft failure: a comparison of graft type based on age and Tegner activity level. Am J Sports Med 39(10):2194–2198. doi:10.1177/0363546511415655
50. Salmon L, Russell V, Musgrove T, Pinczewski L, Refshauge K (2005) Incidence and risk factors for graft rupture and contralateral rupture after anterior cruciate ligament reconstruction. Arthroscopy 21(8):948–957
51. Conte EJ, Hyatt AE, Gatt CJ Jr, Dhawan A (2014) Hamstring autograft size can be predicted and is a potential risk factor for anterior cruciate ligament reconstruction failure. Arthroscopy 30(7):882–890. doi:10.1016/j.arthro.2014.03.028
52. Indelli PF, Dillingham M, Fanton G, Schurman DJ (2002) Septic arthritis in postoperative anterior cruciate ligament reconstruction. Clin Orthop Relat Res 398:182–188
53. Torres-Claramunt R, Pelfort X, Erquicia J, Gil-González S, Gelber PE, Puig L, Monllau JC (2013) Knee joint infection after ACL reconstruction: prevalence, management and functional outcomes. Knee Surg Sports Traumatol Arthrosc 21(12):2844–2849. doi:10.1007/s00167-012-2264-3
54. Van Tongel A, Stuyck J, Bellemans J, Vandenneucker H (2007) Septic arthritis after arthroscopic anterior cruciate ligament reconstruction: a retrospective analysis of incidence, management and outcome. Am J Sports Med 35(7):1059–1063. doi:10.1177/0363546507299443
55. Kim SJ, Postigo R, Koo S, Kim JH (2014) Infection after arthroscopic anterior cruciate ligament reconstruction. Orthopedics 37(7):477–484. doi:10.3928/01477447-20140626-06. Review
56. McAllister DR, Parker RD, Cooper AE, Recht MP, Abate J (1999) Outcomes of postoperative septic arthritis after anterior cruciate ligament reconstruction. Am J Sports Med 27(5):562–570
57. Brophy RH, Wright RW, Huston LJ, Nwosu SK, MOON Knee Group, Spindler KP (2015) Factors associated with infection following anterior cruciate ligament reconstruction. J Bone Joint Surg Am 97(6):450–454. doi:10.2106/JBJS.N.00694

58. Binnet MS, Başarir K (2007) Risk and outcome of infection after different arthroscopic anterior cruciate ligament reconstruction techniques. Arthroscopy 23(8):862–868
59. Matava MJ, Evans TA, Wright RW, Shively RA (1998) Septic arthritis of the knee following anterior cruciate ligament reconstruction: results of a survey of sports medicine fellowship directors. Arthroscopy 14(7):717–725
60. Struijk-Mulder MC, Ettema HB, Verheyen CC, Büller HR (2013) Deep vein thrombosis after arthroscopic anterior cruciate ligament reconstruction: a prospective cohort study of 100 patients. Arthroscopy 29(7):1211–1216. doi:10.1016/j.arthro.2013.04.015
61. Ye S, Dongyang C, Zhihong X, Dongquan S, Jin D, Jianghui Q, Jizhen Q, Pu Y, Huacheng H, Wei S, Qing J (2013) The incidence of deep venous thrombosis after arthroscopically assisted anterior cruciate ligament reconstruction. Arthroscopy 29(4):742–747. doi:10.1016/j.arthro.2013.01.017
62. Cullison TR, Muldoon MP, Gorman JD, Goff WB (1996) The incidence of deep venous thrombosis in anterior cruciate ligament reconstruction. Arthroscopy 12(6):657–659
63. Marlovits S, Striessnig G, Schuster R, Stocker R, Luxl M, Trattnig S, Vécsei V (2007) Extended-duration thromboprophylaxis with enoxaparin after arthroscopic surgery of the anterior cruciate ligament: a prospective, randomized, placebo-controlled study. Arthroscopy 23(7):696–702
64. Camporese G, Bernardi E, Prandoni P, Noventa F, Verlato F, KANT (Knee Arthroscopy Nadroparin Thromboprophylaxis) Study Group et al (2008) Low-molecular-weight heparin versus compression stockings for thromboprophylaxis after knee arthroscopy: a randomized trial. Ann Intern Med 149(2):73–82
65. Berg EE (1994) Lateral femoral condyle fracture after endoscopic anterior cruciate ligament reconstruction. Arthroscopy 10(6):693–695
66. Delcogliano A, Chiossi S, Caporaso A, Franzese S, Menghi A (2001) Tibial plateau fracture after arthroscopic anterior cruciate ligament reconstruction. Arthroscopy 17(4):E16
67. Baums MH, Zelle BA, Schultz W, Ernstberger T, Klinger HM (2006) Intraarticular migration of a broken biodegradable interference screw after anterior cruciate ligament reconstruction. Knee Surg Sports Traumatol Arthrosc 14(9):865–868. Review
68. Christen B, Jakob RP (1992) Fractures associated with patellar ligament grafts in cruciate ligament surgery. J Bone Joint Surg (Br) 74(4):617–619
69. Bonamo JJ, Krinick RM, Sporn AA (1984) Rupture of the patellar ligament after use of its central third for anterior cruciate reconstruction. A report of two cases. J Bone Joint Surg Am 66(8):1294–1297

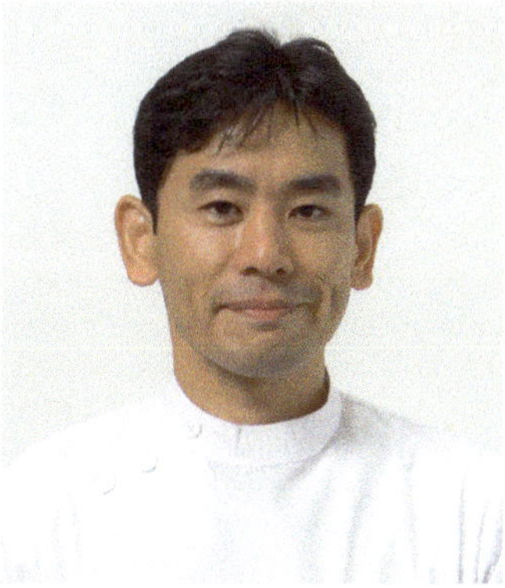

Satoshi Ochiai, M.D., PhD, The Sports Medicine and Knee Center, National Hospital Organization, Kofu National Hospital, Yamanashi, Japan.

Part XII
Future of ACL Reconstruction

Chapter 41
Future Challenges of Anterior Cruciate Ligament Reconstruction Biological Modulation Using a Growth Factor Application for Enhancement of Graft Healing

Mina Samukawa, Harukazu Tohyama, and Kazunori Yasuda

Abstract Although anterior cruciate ligament (ACL) reconstruction techniques using tendon autograft have improved markedly over the last couple of decades, the slow graft maturation may result in graft failure or elongation during the postoperative rehabilitation period. To improve the problems after ACL reconstruction in the near future, we should challenge to develop a new strategy to promote graft healing using biological modulation. Preclinical animal studies need scrutiny to see if further clinical trials are worthwhile. If a plurispecies approach is taken to confirm the findings, animal studies convey useful information for a better understanding on the effectiveness of biological modulation on ACL reconstruction. Our recent experimental findings using a plurispecies approach suggested that biological modulation by a TGF-beta1 application inhibits the deterioration of mechanical properties of the grafted tendon after ACL reconstruction. However, intraarticular administration of TGF-beta may be unsuitable for clinical application with an ACL reconstruction procedure, since recent studies reported that intraarticular administration of TGF-beta1 induced arthritic changes of the articular cartilage in the knee joint. The cell-based therapy with cellular activation by TGF-beta1 may be a potential solution against this problem. Translational research should be conducted to put biological modulation by a TGF-beta1 application into clinical use for the enhancement of graft healing after ACL reconstruction in the future.

Keywords ACL reconstruction • Biological modulation • Graft healing • Growth factor

---

M. Samukawa, PT, PhD (✉) • H. Tohyama
Faculty of Health Sciences, Hokkaido University, Kita 12, Nishi 5, Kita-ku, Sapporo, Hokkaido 060-0812, Japan
e-mail: mina@hs.hokudai.ac.jp

K. Yasuda
Hokkaido University School of Medicine, Sapporo, Hokkaido, Japan

M. Ochi et al. (eds.), *ACL Injury and Its Treatment*,
DOI 10.1007/978-4-431-55858-3_41

41.1 Introduction

Anterior cruciate ligament (ACL) reconstruction using tendon autograft has greatly improved over the last couple of decades [1]. While surgical techniques still need an adequate biological healing response to contribute satisfactory clinical outcomes, poor graft healing is considered as one of causes leading to nontraumatic ACL graft failure [2, 3]. Graft healing of ACL reconstruction is primarily attributed to the remodeling of intraarticular graft and intratunnel graft incorporation [4]. In ACL reconstruction, the strength of the grafted tendon is reduced at the early phase after surgery, and then it gradually increases [5–7]. The slow graft maturation may result in graft failure or elongation during the postoperative rehabilitation period. To solve these problems after ACL reconstruction, we should obtain scientific evidences of biological modulation for the graft remodeling after the surgery. There is a possibility that biological modulation could promote the graft healing after ACL reconstruction and enable more aggressive rehabilitation and an earlier return to sports activities for patients with ACL reconstruction.

Concerning the effects of biological modulation on clinical outcomes after ACL reconstruction, only several prospective studies were reported [8–14] (Table 41.1). Among methods for biological modulation, platelet-rich plasma (PRP) has received much attention in the field of sports medicine [15, 16]. PRP, which is a concentrated extract of platelets from autologous blood, contains growth factors in concentration 3–5 times of the normal plasma level [17–19]. Investigators conducted clinical studies about application of PRP to ACL reconstruction for acceleration of healing process and integration of the graft. However, prospective studies of biological modulation, e.g., PRP application, to ACL reconstruction showed mixed results. Ventura et al. [14] reported the effects of application of growth factors obtained by GPS Biomet-Merck technique on clinical outcomes at 6 months after ACL reconstruction using hamstring tendon graft and found no significant differences in clinical outcomes or knee laxity between the patients with and without application of growth factors. At this time, there is only one study showing that biological modulation improves anteroposterior knee stability after ACL reconstruction [10]. To develop a more effective method enabling to improve biomechanical function of the graft after ACL reconstruction, it is necessary to collect scientific evidences about the effects of biological modulation on knee biomechanics after ACL reconstruction.

Before clinical trials start, preclinical animal studies need scrutiny to see if further clinical trials are worthwhile. There is the evidence showing the homology of regenerative responses to biological stimulation in mammalian ligaments of the knee [20], although there are anatomical differences in ACLs between human and experimental animals [21]. If a plurispecies approach is taken to confirm the findings, animal studies of ACL reconstruction convey useful information for a better understanding on the effectiveness of biological modulation on graft healing after ACL reconstruction [22]. The authors has taken a plurispecies approach using several animal models in order to confirm the effects of the growth factor

Table 41.1 Summary of prospective studies about biological modulation on clinical outcomes after ACL reconstruction

Author (Year)	Study design	Biological modulation	Graft type	Follow-up (months)	Outcome measures	Finding
Silva et al. (2014) [8]	RCT	Bone marrow concentrate	Hamstring tendon	3	Imaging	No difference
Darabos et al. (2011) [9]	RCT	Autologous conditioned serum	Hamstring tendon or BTB	12	Imaging, questionnaire, biochemistry	Positive
Vogrin et al. (2010) [10]	RCT	Platelet-leukocyte gel	Hamstring tendon	6	Knee laxity	Positive
Silva et al. (2009) [11]	Comparative study without randomization	PRP	Hamstring tendon	3	Imaging	No difference
Orrego et al. (2008) [12]	RCT	Platelet concentrate plus bone plug	Hamstring tendon	6	Imaging	No difference
Huang et al. (2007) [13]	RCT	Hyaluronic acid	BTB	4	Clinical, questionnaire	Positive
Ventura et al. (2005) [14]	RCT	Growth factors (GPS Biomet-Merck technique)	Hamstring tendon	6	Clinical, knee laxity, imaging	No difference: (clinical/knee laxity) Positive (imaging)

application on graft healing after ACL reconstruction. In this chapter, the authors review scientific evidences of the effects of biological modulation with a growth factor application on graft healing after ACL reconstruction including recent findings of our studies using a plurispecies approach.

41.2 The Graft Remodeling After ACL Reconstruction

In ACL reconstruction, fibroblasts in the grafted tendon graft are necrotized immediately after its transplantation, and then numerous fibroblasts from extrinsic origins infiltrate the graft with revascularization [23, 24]. However, it is considered that the cell infiltration into a core portion of the graft occasionally occurs very slowly. For example, Delay et al. [25] reported a clinical case in which the core portion of the patellar tendon graft still remained necrotic even at the 18-month period after ACL reconstruction. Oaks et al. [26] examined biopsy samples of the grafted tendon in clinical ACL reconstruction cases and found that fibrils with a small diameter predominantly increase in the graft after its transplantation and still remain predominant at the 4-year period after surgery. The authors showed that fibroblast infiltration into the tendon after necrosis decreases the strength of the tendon with overexpression of type III collagen [27]. These structural changes in the grafted tendon after ACL reconstruction are considered to induce mechanical deterioration of autografts at the early phase after transplantation and then are very gradually restored over a long period [28].

In animal ACL reconstruction models, fibroblasts infiltrated into the grafted tendon overexpress vascular endothelial growth factor (VEGF), basic fibroblast growth factor (FGF), transforming growth factor (TGF)-beta, and platelet-derived growth factor (PDGF) in the grafted tendon after the implantation [29, 30]. Therefore, the fibroblasts infiltrated into the grafted tendon remodel the graft matrix via a complex growth factor network and implies that local application of these growth factors can moderate the healing graft after ACL reconstruction.

41.3 Promotion of Graft Healing with a Growth Factor Application

41.3.1 Vascular Endothelial Growth Factor (VEGF)

VEGF is well known as a potent mediator of angiogenesis [31]. The lack of vascularity within the graft after ACL reconstruction may induce degeneration or micro-ruptures of the grafted tendon during the postoperative period, since cell infiltration from the blood system is thought to be required for healing of the tissue with damage. Thus, there is a high possibility that an application of VEGF to the necrotized tendon graft enhances angiogenesis in the graft and accelerates remodeling of the graft after ACL reconstruction. To clarify the effects of local application of VEGF on graft healing after ACL reconstruction, the authors conducted animal experimental studies using a plurispecies approach. First, we histologically and mechanically examined the effects of a local application of VEGF to the in situ frozen-thawed rabbit ACL [32]. The in situ frozen-thawed rabbit ACL, which is anatomical but acellular, has been established as an ideal ACL graft rabbit model (Fig. 41.1) [33]. The local application of VEGF provided no significant effect on the mechanical properties of the ACL at 12 weeks after the in situ freeze-thaw procedure. On the other hand, the VEGF application significantly enhanced vascular endothelial cell infiltration and revascularization in the ACL at 3–12 weeks, respectively (Fig. 41.2). As a preclinical study model, we have recently established a sheep ACL reconstruction model using a doubled semitendinosus tendon autograft (Fig. 41.3) [34]. In response to the positive effects of VEGF application on cell infiltration and revascularization in the in situ frozen-thawed rabbit ACL, we conducted a preclinical animal study using a sheep model in order to examine the effect of local application on mechanical properties of the femur-graft-tibia complex after ACL reconstruction using a semitendinosus tendon graft [35]. As a result, we found that similar positive effects of VEGF application on cell infiltration and revascularization in the grafted tendon at 12 weeks after ACL reconstruction. However, the stiffness of the VEGF-treated femur-graft-tibia complex was significantly lower than that of the saline-treated graft at 12 weeks, while we failed to demonstrate a negative effect of VEGF application on ultimate failure load of the saline-treated graft. It is unclear exactly why our VEGF application

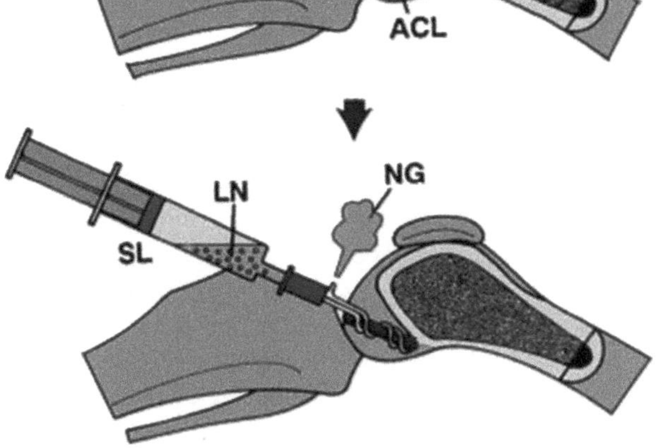

Fig. 41.1 The in situ frozen-thawed rabbit ACL model for a screening test of a growth factor application to the ACL graft. This procedure necrotizes the rabbit ACL without any damage of the anatomical ACL structure (From Ref. [33])

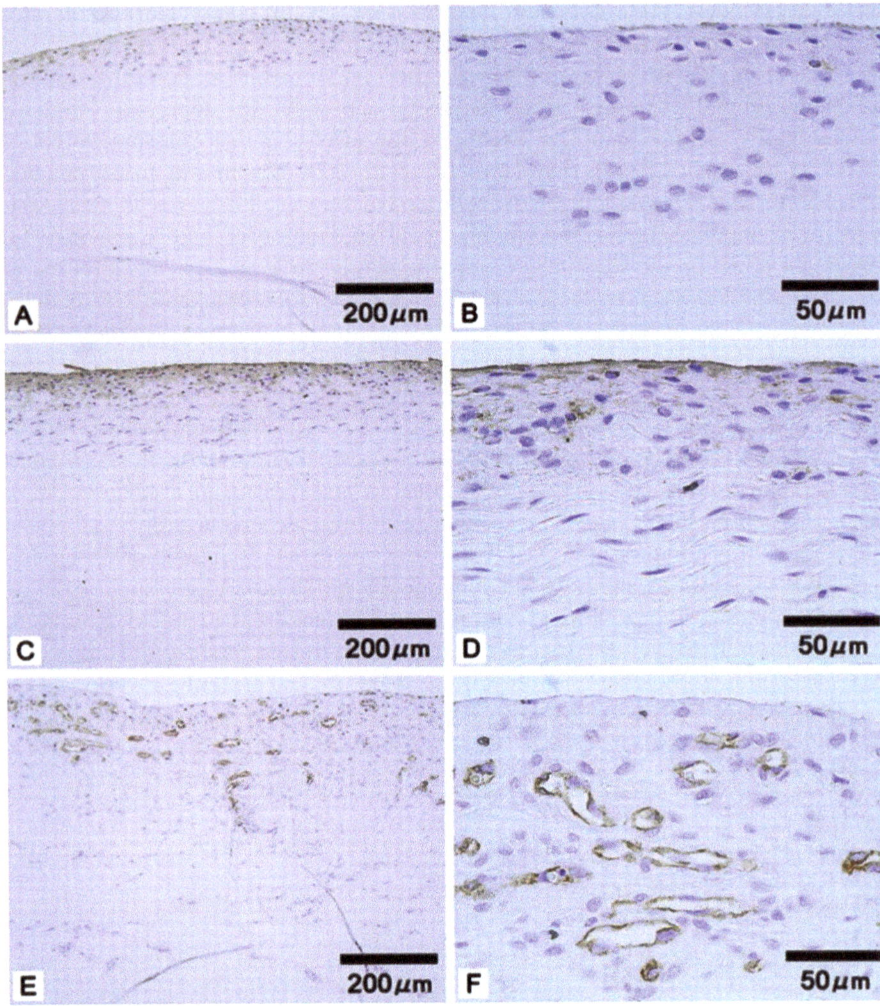

Fig. 41.2 Immunohistologies for vascular endothelial cells to evaluate the effects of local VEGF application on vessel formation in the ACL at 3 weeks after the in situ freeze-thaw treatment in the rabbit model (CD31 stain). The number of vessels with endothelial cells was significantly higher in the frozen-thawed ACLs with VEGF application (**e, f**) compared to those with the freeze-thaw treatment alone (**a, b**) and with phosphate-buffered saline application (**c, d**) (From Ref. [32])

reduced the stiffness of the grafted tendon after ACL reconstruction. Shrive et al. [36] and Tohyama et al. [37] reported that a number of newly formed vessels and infiltrative cells act as "flaws" resulting in the deterioration of the mechanical property of the tendon and ligament. Therefore, vascular invasion promoted by VEGF administration may cause graft weakening as soft tissue flaws. Therefore, we should take into account this adverse effect of VEGF application including PRP, which has a high content of VEGF, on the mechanical characteristics of the grafted tendon after ACL reconstruction surgery.

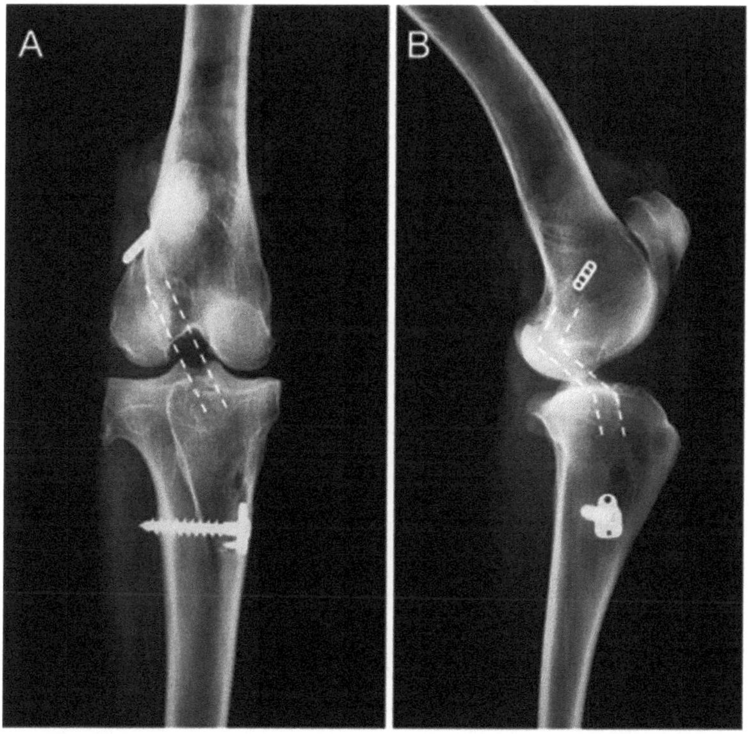

Fig. 41.3 The sheep ACL reconstruction model using a doubled semitendinosus tendon autograft for a preclinical test of a growth factor application to the ACL graft (From Ref. [49])

41.3.2 Transforming Growth Factor-Beta (TGF-Beta) and Epidermal Growth Factor (EGF)

Some of growth factors, such as TGF-beta, basic FGF, PDGF, and EGF, regulate the synthesis and degradation of collagen by the fibroblasts of tendons and ligaments. It is well known that TGF-beta enhances collagen synthesis in fibroblasts [38–40]. EGF significantly stimulates fibroblast proliferation in vitro [41]. A combined application of these two growth factors enhances these effects [42]. Therefore, we conducted following animal experimental studies using a plurispecies approach for the application of TGF-beta1 and EGF to ligament reconstruction. The authors examined in vivo effects of an application of TGF-beta1 and EGF on the in situ frozen-thawed ACL and found that a combined application of TGF-beta1 and EGF significantly inhibited the mechanical deterioration with significant reduction of the water content and significant changes of the collagen-fibril profile [33]. Based on these positive effects of local application of TGF-beta1 and EGF on a frozen-thawed rabbit ACL, the authors conducted a canine study that examined the effects of TGF-beta1 and EGF on a bone-patellar tendon-bone graft after ACL reconstruction as a preclinical study [43]. We then found that a combined application of

TGF-beta1 and EGF significantly improved mechanical strength of the femur-graft-tibia complex at 12 weeks after ACL reconstruction (Fig. 41.4). These findings suggest that a local application of TGF-beta1 and EGF is one of candidate biological modulations that can enhance graft healing after ACL reconstruction in the future. The authors also compared the effects of a local application among TGF-beta1, EGF, and PDGF-BB on mechanical properties of the in situ frozen-thawed rabbit ACL to clarify which growth factors dominantly affect the enhancement of graft healing after ACL reconstruction [44]. We found that an application of TGF-beta1 significantly inhibited the material deterioration that occurs in the in situ frozen-thawed ACL, while an application of EGF or PDGF-BB did not significantly affect the deterioration. The authors also found downregulation of MMP-13 mRNA and upregulation of type-1 collagen mRNA relative to type-3 collagen after TGF-beta1 stimulation in fibroblasts which had infiltrated the rat patellar tendon [45]. On the other hand, PDGF stimulation increased MMP-13 mRNA and decreased type-1 collagen mRNA relative to type-3 collagen. These findings suggest that TGF-beta1 is a key in the positive effects on graft healing after ACL reconstruction.

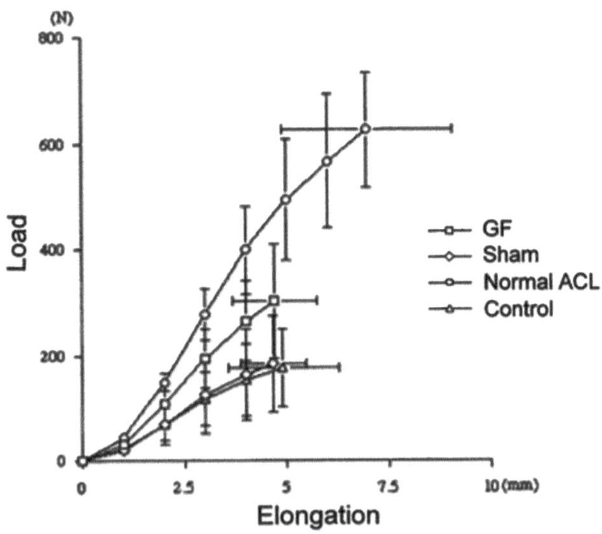

Fig. 41.4 The effects of a local application of TGF-beta and EGF on structural properties of the femur-graft-tibia complex after ACL reconstruction. The load-elongation curves of the femur-graft-tibia complexes in the knees with growth factor (*GF*) application, with fibrin sealant alone (sham), and without growth factor or fibrin sealant (control) groups and the normal femur-ACL-tibia complex (normal ACL). A combined application of TGF-beta1 and EGF significantly improved mechanical strength of the femur-graft-tibia complex at 12 weeks after ACL reconstruction (From Ref. [43]))

41.4 Promotion of Graft Healing with Cell-Based Therapy

As described above, TGF-beta1 has a positive effect on graft healing after ACL reconstruction. However, the intraarticular application of TGF-beta1 induces osteoarthritic changes in the knee joint [46, 47]. Therefore, the intraarticular administration of TGF-beta1 is considered unsuitable for clinical application during an ACL reconstruction. It is therefore necessary to develop a therapeutic method that can accelerate restoration of ACL graft strength without any detrimental effects to the knee joint. The authors conducted the rabbit study to clarify the effect of cell therapy with autologous synovial tissue-derived fibroblasts activated by TGF-beta1 on the in situ frozen-thawed ACL (Fig. 41.5) [48]. We wrapped the fibrin glue with autologous synovial tissue-derived fibroblasts after TGF-beta stimulation around the ACL following the freeze-thaw treatment. Histological observation found that

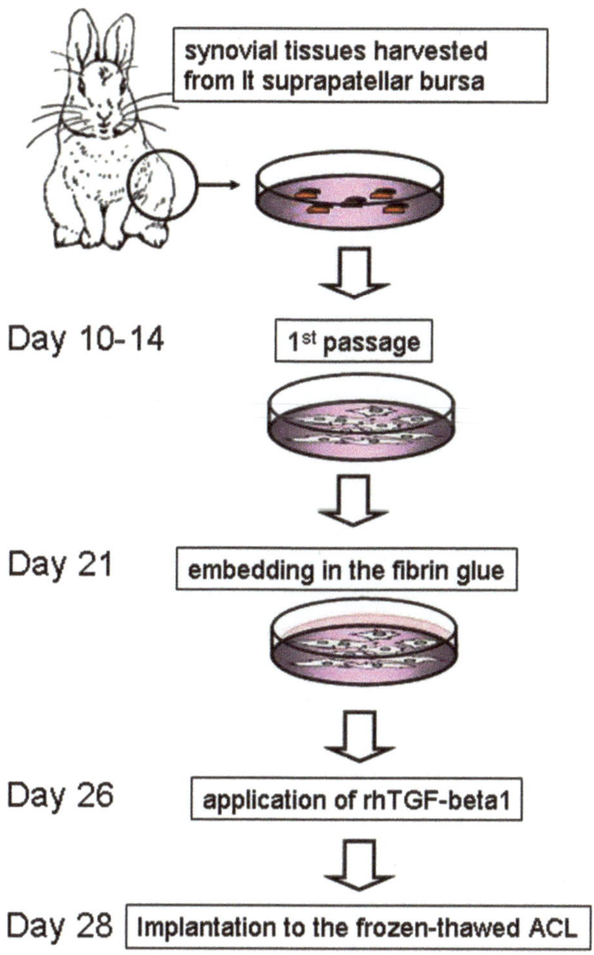

Fig. 41.5 The experimental protocol of the cell-based therapy with autologous synovial tissue-derived fibroblasts with TGF-beta1 application (From Ref. [48])

implantation of fibroblasts after TGF-beta stimulation accelerated cellular infiltration into the ACL following fibroblast necrosis. Biomechanically, the transplantation of synovial tissue-derived autologous fibroblasts activated by TGF-beta inhibited deterioration in the tangent modulus of the ACL after the freeze-thaw treatment. As a preclinical study, we examined the effect of cell therapy with autologous synovial tissue-derived fibroblasts activated by TGF-beta1 on the graft in a sheep ACL reconstruction model described above [49]. A fluorescence image with confocal microscope showed that the applied cells that were labeled before implantation infiltrated into the superficial portion of the graft at 1 week (Fig. 41.6). Biomechanically, the strength and the stiffness of the graft were significantly greater in the group with cell therapy using fibroblasts activated by TGF-beta1 than in the group without TGF-beta1 stimulation or without cell therapy. Histologically, no necrotic lesions were found in the midsubstance in the group with synovial tissue-derived fibroblasts activated by TGF-beta1, while necrotic lesions were observed in the core portion of the midsubstance in the group without cell therapy. Therefore, our cell-based therapy using fibroblasts activated by TGF-beta is a potential solution against the problem of graft deterioration after the transplantation.

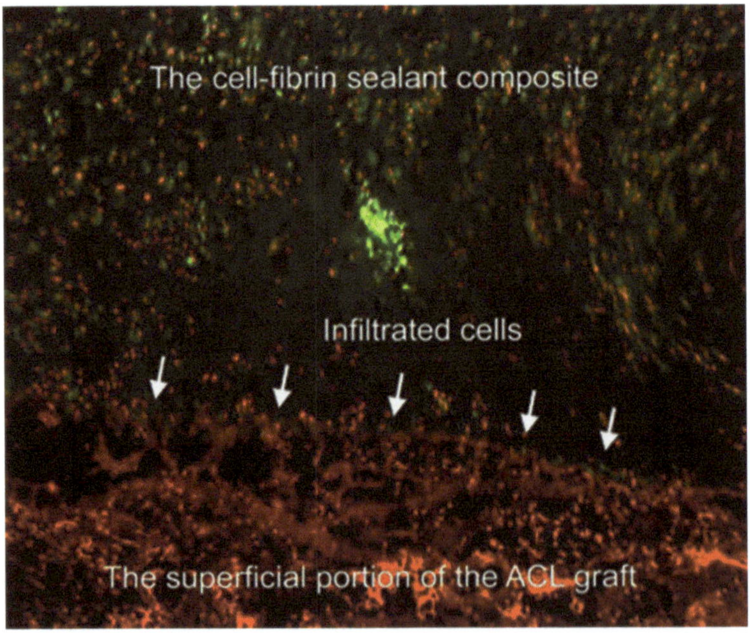

Fig. 41.6 A fluorescence image of the superficial portion of the ACL graft at 1 week after a sheep ACL reconstruction with the cell-based therapy with autologous synovial tissue-derived fibroblasts with TGF-beta1 application. Labeled fibroblasts (*arrows*) were observed in the superficial portion of the ACL graft (From Ref. [49])

41.5 Conclusions

Although tendon-bone healing at the tunnel interface is the weakest link of the graft complex at the early period after ACL reconstruction, the healing of the intraarticular midsubstance of the graft would be a key for the early return to sport activities and the prevention of nontraumatic ACL graft failure in the patients after ACL reconstruction. Scientific evidences in our animal studies with a plurispecies approach suggested that biological modulation by TGF-beta1 benefited healing of the intraarticular graft after ACL reconstruction. The authors previously reported that administration of TGF-beta1 significantly increased the bonding strength of the graft to the tunnel wall at 3 weeks in the canine ACL reconstruction model [50]. In addition, the systematic review suggested that TGF-beta may be beneficial to graft healing in ACL reconstruction through the promotion of healing at the tunnel-graft interface [51]. However, intraarticular administration of TGF-beta may be unsuitable for clinical application with an ACL reconstruction procedure, since recent studies reported that intraarticular administration of TGF-beta1 induced arthritic changes of the articular cartilage in the knee joint. The cell-based therapy with cellular activation by TGF-beta1 may be a potential solution against this problem. Translational research, which bridges the gap between basic and clinical research, should be conducted to put biological modulation by TGF-beta1 into clinical use for ACL reconstruction in the future.

References

1. Fu FH, Bennett CH, Ma CB, Menetrey J, Lattermann C (2000) Current trends in anterior cruciate ligament reconstruction. Part II. Operative procedures and clinical correlations. Am J Sports Med 28:124–130
2. Carson EW, Anisko EM, Restrepo C, Panariello RA, O'Brien SJ, Warren RF (2004) Revision anterior cruciate ligament reconstruction: etiology of failures and clinical results. J Knee Surg 17:127–132
3. Ekdahl M, Wang JH, Ronga M, Fu FH (2008) Graft healing in anterior cruciate ligament reconstruction. Knee Surg Sports Traumatol Arthrosc 16:935–947
4. Tohyama H, Yasuda K (2012) Basic science of ligament healing. In: Michel B, Annunziato A, Johan B, Steven MD, Jacques M (eds) The knee joint: surgical techniques and strategies. Springer, Paris, pp 43–50
5. Clancy WG Jr, Narechania RG, Rosenberg TD, Gmeiner JG, Wisnefske DD, Lange TA (1981) Anterior and posterior cruciate ligament reconstruction in rhesus monkeys. J Bone Joint Surg Am 63:1270–1284
6. Butler DL, Grood ES, Noyes FR, Olmstead ML, Hohn RB, Arnoczky SP, Siegel MG (1989) Mechanical properties of primate vascularized vs. nonvascularized patellar tendon grafts; changes over time. J Orthop Res 7:68–79
7. Ballock RT, Woo SL, Lyon RM, Hollis JM, Akeson WH (1989) Use of patellar tendon autograft for anterior cruciate ligament reconstruction in the rabbit: a long-term histologic and biomechanical study. J Orthop Res 7:474–485
8. Silva A, Sampaio R, Fernandes R, Pinto E (2014) Is there a role for adult noncultivated bone marrow stem cells in ACL reconstruction? Knee Surg Sports Traumatol Arthrosc 22:66–71

9. Darabos N, Haspl M, Moser C, Darabos A, Bartolek D, Groenemeyer D (2011) Intraarticular application of autologous conditioned serum (ACS) reduces bone tunnel widening after ACL reconstructive surgery in a randomized controlled trial. Knee Surg Sports Traumatol Arthrosc 19(suppl 1):S36–S46
10. Vogrin M, Rupreht M, Crnjac A, Dinevski D, Krajnc Z, Recnik G (2010) The effect of platelet-derived growth factors on knee stability after anterior cruciate ligament reconstruction: a prospective randomized clinical study. Wien Klin Wochenschr 122(suppl 2):91–95
11. Silva A, Sampaio R (2009) Anatomic ACL reconstruction: does the platelet-rich plasma accelerate tendon healing? Knee Surg Sports Traumatol Arthrosc 17:676–682
12. Orrego M, Larrain C, Rosales J (2008) Effects of platelet concentrate and a bone plug on the healing of hamstring tendons in a bone tunnel. Arthroscopy 24:1373–1380
13. Huang MH, Yang RC, Chou PH (2007) Preliminary effects of hyaluronic acid on early rehabilitation of patients with isolated anterior cruciate ligament reconstruction. Clin J Sport Med 17:242–250
14. Ventura A, Terzaghi C, Borgo E, Verdoia C, Gallazzi M, Failoni S (2005) Use of growth factors in ACL surgery: preliminary study. J Orthop Traumatol 6:76–79
15. Warth RJ, Dornan GJ, James EW, Horan MP, Millett PJ (2015) Clinical and structural outcomes after arthroscopic repair of full-thickness rotator cuff tears with and without platelet-rich product supplementation: a meta-analysis and meta-regression. Arthroscopy 31:306–320
16. Laver L, Carmont MR, McConkey MO, Palmanovich E, Yaacobi E, Mann G, Nyska M, Kots E, Mei-Dan O (2015) Plasma rich in growth factors (PRGF) as a treatment for high ankle sprain in elite athletes: a randomized control trial. Knee Surg Sports Traumatol Arthrosc 23:3383–3392
17. Foster TE, Puskas BL, Mandelbaum BR, Gerhardt MB, Rodeo SA (2009) Platelet-rich plasma from basic science to clinical applications. Am J Sports Med 37:2259–2272
18. de Vos RJ, Weir A, van Schie HT, Bierma-Zeinstra SM, Verhaar JA, Weinans H, Tol JL (2010) Platelet-rich plasma injection for chronic achilles tendinopathy: a randomized controlled trial. JAMA 303:144–149
19. Fallouh L, Nakagawa K, Sasho T, Arai M, Kitahara S, Wada Y, Moriya H, Takahashi K (2010) Effects of autologous platelet-rich plasma on cell viability and collagen synthesis in injured human anterior cruciate ligament. J Bone Joint Surg Am 92:2909–2916
20. McDougall JJ, Bray RC, Sharkey KA (1997) Morphological and immunohistochemical examination of nerves in normal and injured collateral ligaments of rat, rabbit, and human knee joints. Anat Rec 248:29–39
21. Proffen BL, McElfresh M, Fleming BC, Murray MM (2012) A comparative anatomical study of the human knee and six animal species. Knee 19:493–499
22. de Deyn PP, van Dam V (2010) General introduction to animal models of human conditions. In: de Deyn PP, van Dam V (eds) Animal models of dementia, Springer protocols (Series). Humana Press, New York, pp 3–13
23. Arnoczky SP, Tarvin GB, Marshall JL (1982) Anterior cruciate ligament replacement using patellar tendon. An evaluation of graft revascularization in the dog. J Bone Joint Surg 64A:217–224
24. Amiel D, Kleiner JB, Akeson WH (1986) The natural history of the anterior cruciate ligament autograft of patellar tendon origin. Am J Sports Med 14:449–462
25. Delay BS, McGrath BE, Mindell ER (2002) Observation on a retrieved patellar tendon autograft used to reconstruct the anterior cruciate ligament. A case report. J Bone Joint Surg 84A:1433–1438
26. Oakes BW (1993) Collagen ultrastructure in the normal ACL and in ACL graft. In: Jackson DW (ed) The anterior cruciate ligament. Current and future concepts. Raven Press, New York, pp 209–217
27. Tohyama H, Yasuda K, Uchida H (2006) Is the increase in type III collagen of the patellar tendon graft after ligament reconstruction really caused by "ligamentization" of the graft? Knee Surg Sports Traumatol Arthrosc 14:1270–1277

28. Tohyama H, Yasuda K (2015) Anterior cruciate ligament (ACL) healing: ACL graft biology. Sports Med Arthrosc Rev 13:156–160
29. Yoshikawa T, Tohyama H, Enomoto H (2006) Expression of vascular endothelial growth factor and angiogenesis in patellar tendon grafts in the early phase after anterior cruciate ligament reconstruction. Knee Surg Sports Traumatol Arthrosc 14:804–810
30. Kuroda R, Kurosaka M, Yoshiya S (2000) Localization of growth factors in the reconstructed anterior cruciate ligament: immunohistological study in dogs. Knee Surg Sports Traumatol Arthrosc 8:120–126
31. Ferrara N, Davis-Smyth T (1997) The biology of vascular endothelial growth factor. Endocr Rev 18:4–25
32. Ju YJ, Tohyama H, Kondo E, Yoshikawa T, Muneta T, Shinomiya K, Yasuda K (2006) Effects of local administration of vascular endothelial growth factor on properties of the in situ frozen-thawed anterior cruciate ligament in rabbits. Am J Sports Med 34:84–91
33. Sakai T, Yasuda K, Tohyama H, Azuma H, Nagumo A, Majima T, Frank CB (2002) Effects of combined administration of transforming growth factor-beta1 and epidermal growth factor on properties of the in situ frozen anterior cruciate ligament in rabbits. J Orthop Res 20:1345–1351
34. Kondo E, Yasuda K, Katsura T, Hayashi R, Kotani Y, Tohyama H (2012) Biomechanical and histological evaluations of the doubled semitendinosus tendon autograft after anterior cruciate ligament reconstruction in sheep. Am J Sports Med 40:315–324
35. Yoshikawa T, Tohyama H, Katsura T, Kondo E, Kotani Y, Matsumoto H, Toyama Y, Yasuda K (2006) Effects of local administration of vascular endothelial growth factor on mechanical characteristics of the semitendinosus tendon graft after anterior cruciate ligament reconstruction in sheep. Am J Sports Med 34:1918–1925
36. Shrive N, Chimich D, Marchuk L, Wilson J, Brant R, Frank C (1995) Soft-tissue "flaws" are associated with the material properties of the healing rabbit medial collateral ligament. J Orthop Res 13:923–929
37. Tohyama H, Yasuda K (2000) Extrinsic cell infiltration and revascularization accelerate mechanical deterioration of the patellar tendon after fibroblast necrosis. J Biomech Eng 122:594–599
38. DesRosiers EA, Yahia L, Rivard CH (1996) Proliferative and matrix synthesis response of canine anterior cruciate ligament fibroblasts submitted to combined growth factors. J Orthop Res 14:200–208
39. Deie M, Marui T, Allen CR (1997) The effects of age on rabbit MCL fibroblast matrix synthesis in response to TGF-beta 1 or EGF. Mech Aging Dev 97:121–130
40. Marui T, Niyibizi C, Georgescu HI (1997) Effect of growth factors on matrix synthesis by ligament fibroblasts. J Orthop Res 15:18–23
41. Scherping SC, Schmidt CC Jr, Georgescu HI (1997) Effect of growth factors on the proliferation of ligament fibroblasts from skeletally mature rabbits. Connect Tissue Res 36:1–8
42. Assoian RK, Frolik CA, Roberts AB (1984) Transforming growth factor-beta controls receptor levels for epidermal growth factor in NRK fibroblasts. Cell 36:35–41
43. Yasuda K, Tomita F, Yamazaki S, Minami A, Tohyama H (2004) The effect of growth factors on biomechanical properties of the bone-patellar tendon-bone graft after anterior cruciate ligament reconstruction: a canine model study. Am J Sports Med 32:870–880
44. Nagumo A, Yasuda K, Numazaki H, Azuma H, Tanabe Y, Kikuchi S, Harata S, Tohyama H (2005) Effects of separate application of three growth factors (TGF-beta1, EGF, and PDGF-BB) on mechanical properties of the in situ frozen-thawed anterior cruciate ligament. Clin Biomech 20:283–290
45. Tohyama H, Yasuda K (2011) Application of growth factors for enhancement of mechanical strength of grafted tendon following anterior cruciate ligament reconstruction. In: Klika V (ed) Biomechanics in applications. Intech, Croatia, pp 83–100

46. Hulth A, Johnell O, Miyazono K, Lindberg L, Heinegard D, Heldin CH (1996) Effect of transforming growth factor-beta and platelet-derived growth factor-BB on articular cartilage in rats. J Orthop Res 14:547–553
47. van Beuningen HM, van der Kraan PM, Arntz OJ, van den Berg WB (1994) Transforming growth factor-beta 1 stimulates chondrocyte proteoglycan synthesis and induces osteophyte formation in the murine knee joint. Lab Invest 71:279–290
48. Okuizumi T, Tohyama H, Kondo E, Yasuda K (2004) The effect of cell-based therapy with autologous synovial fibroblasts activated by exogenous TGF-beta1 on the in situ frozen-thawed anterior cruciate ligament. J Orthop Sci 9:488–494
49. Kondo E, Yasuda K, Katsura T, Hayashi R, Azuma C, Tohyama H (2011) Local administration of autologous synovium-derived cells improve the structural properties of anterior cruciate ligament autograft reconstruction in sheep. Am J Sports Med 39:999–1007
50. Yamazaki S, Yasuda K, Tomita F, Minami A, Tohyama H (2005) The effect of transforming growth factor-beta1 on intraosseous healing of flexor tendon autograft replacement of anterior cruciate ligament in dogs. Arthroscopy 21:1034–1041
51. Fu SC, Cheuk YC, Yung SH, Rolf CG, Chan KM (2014) Systematic review of biological modulation of healing in anterior cruciate ligament reconstruction. Orthop J Sports Med 2 (3):2325967114526687

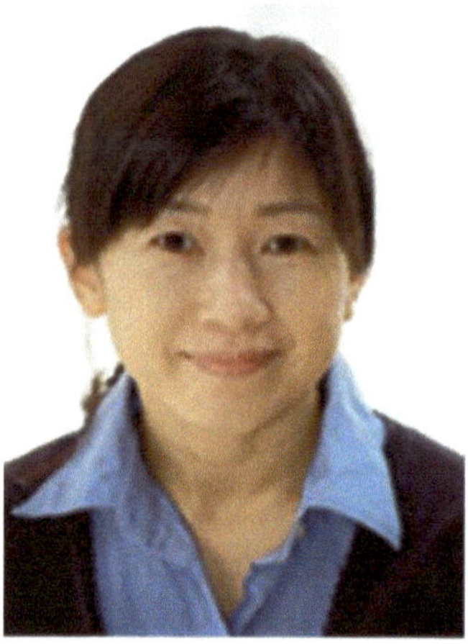

Mina Samukawa, PT, PhD, Faculty of Health Sciences, Graduate School of Health Sciences, Hokkaido University, Hokkaido, Japan.

Chapter 42
Strategies to Enhance Biological Tendon-Bone Healing in Anterior Cruciate Ligament Reconstruction

Tomoyuki Matsumoto and Ryosuke Kuroda

Abstract Tissue engineering techniques to enhance tendon-bone healing in anterior cruciate ligament (ACL) reconstruction, including stem cells and growth factors/cytokines, are gaining wide acceptance, and their clinical feasibility has also been recognized. Among them, vascular stem cells at the site of ruptured ACL, which have high proliferation and multi-differentiation potential, accelerate tendon-bone healing by enhancing angiogenesis and osteogenesis in human-rat xenotransplantation and canine autologous transplantation model of ACL reconstruction. A pilot clinical study, which used ruptured tissue for ACL reconstruction, indicated reduction of tunnel enlargement despite no improvement in clinical scores. However, for effective clinical application in future, detailed analysis is required regarding enrolled patient demographic parameters, such as age, sex, surgical timing, and type of ACL injury. This chapter highlights effectiveness of vascular stem cells application for early tendon-bone healing in ACL reconstruction, providing an insight for future strategies.

Keywords Tendon-bone healing • Stem cells • Ruptured tissue • Angiogenesis • Osteogenesis

42.1 Introduction

When an anterior cruciate ligament (ACL) is ruptured, the healing potential is considered to be extremely poor [1, 2]. Therefore, ACL reconstruction has become fairly standardized, with clinical success rates of 70–95 % [3–5]. Anatomical double-bundle (DB) reconstruction procedures using hamstring grafts have recently become widespread with promising results [6–9]. Whereas most surgical procedures in this area require healing and maturation of tendon grafts in a surgically

T. Matsumoto, M.D. (✉) • R. Kuroda
Department of Orthopaedic Surgery, Kobe University Graduate School of Medicine, 7-5-2 Kusunoki-cho, Chuo-ku, Kobe, Hyogo 650-0017, Japan
e-mail: matsun@m4.dion.ne.jp

M. Ochi et al. (eds.), *ACL Injury and Its Treatment*,
DOI 10.1007/978-4-431-55858-3_42

created bone tunnel, the attachment between the tendon and the bone is the weakest region in the early posttransplantation period [10, 11]. In fact, mechanical properties of the healing ligament did not return to normal 1 year after injury in both rabbit and canine models [12, 13]. Therefore, secure fixation of the tendon graft to the bone is a significant factor in allowing earlier and more aggressive rehabilitation and earlier return to sports and work.

Current treatment with hamstring grafts has achieved satisfactory anteroposterior and rotational stability but can cause significant tunnel enlargement [14, 15]. Tunnel widening is believed to be multifactorial in origin. Some mechanical causes are graft motion [15] and stress deviation inside the tunnel and inappropriate location of the graft and tunnel [16]. From a biological aspect, poor healing potential at the tendon-bone interface also results in tunnel enlargement. Large tunnels often require revision ACL surgery and necessitate staged procedures [17]. Therefore, enhancing tendon-bone healing and preventing bone tunnel enlargement are closely related and, therefore, vital in ACL reconstruction.

Tissue engineering techniques with stem cells or growth factors/cytokines have been explored to achieve early healing and better tendon-bone integration [18]. Several animal studies focused on enhancement of tendon-bone healing in ACL reconstruction used periosteum [19, 20], bone marrow stromal cells [21], bone marrow mesenchymal stem cells (MSCs) [20, 22], injectable tricalcium phosphate [23], and other growth factors [24–28]. Although these biological engineering strategies are currently experimental, they are expected to be used in clinical setting in the near future.

42.2 Blood Vessels as a Potential Target for Tendon-Bone Healing in ACL Reconstruction

Over the last decade, there have been considerable controversies regarding the ACL's intrinsic healing potential. Some surgeons are of the view that the ACL does not heal without reconstruction due to the lack of blood clot formation, insufficient vascular supply, deficits in intrinsic cell migration, impaired growth factor ability, and effects of synovial fluid on cell morphology [29, 30]. On the other hand, others have reported that the ACL spontaneously heals without surgery [31–33], or only with primary sutures [34–37]. In fact, during acute and subacute arthroscopic procedures for ACL reconstruction, a tibial stump is often visualized that can have connecting fibers to the femur and the tibia or between the posterior cruciate ligament and tibia, suggesting healing potential in ACL fibers. However, there is no scientific evidence till now.

Stem cells' qualities of high expansion, self-renewal, and multi-differentiation present a reasonable explanation for the healing potential of the ACL. Although some findings show the existence of MSC-like cells in human ACL tissues [38, 39], their origin and characteristics still remain unclear. Recently, blood vessels have been reported to be a richer supply of stem/progenitor cells with expression of CD34 and CD146 surface cell marker [40–43].

Matsumoto et al. demonstrated the presence in subacutely ruptured ACL tissues of CD34-expressing vascular cells with potential for multi-lineage differentiation that can be recruited to the ACL rupture site to support healing [44]. They confirmed the rich vascularity in the ruptured site and septum region when compared with mid-substance using H&E and immunohistochemical vascular staining. In addition, using immunohistochemistry and flow cytometry analysis, they confirmed recruitment of CD34+ and CD146+ cells with multi-lineage differentiation potential to the ruptured site when compared with the gathered cells as the mid-substance (Fig. 42.1a). These cells demonstrated multi-lineage differentiation potential including osteogenesis, adipogenesis, chondrogenesis, and endotheliogenesis (Fig. 42.1b). Covas et al. recently discovered that MSCs and pericytes are similar cells located in the vasculature wall, and they function as cell sources for repair and tissue maintenance [40, 45]. Findings reveal that CD34+ cells are committed not only to endothelial cells but also mural perivascular cells (i.e., pericytes and smooth muscle cells) [46, 47]. Similarly, vascular pericytes with CD146 expression may arise from CD34+ cells [41]. Furthermore, Zengin et al. reported the existence of endothelial progenitor cells and stem cells in a distinct zone between the smooth muscle and the adventitial layer of human adult vascular wall that are capable to differentiate among mature endothelial cells and hematopoietic and local immune cells, such as macrophages [43]. Based on these findings, CD34+ cells with high expansion and multi-differentiation potential in the ACL ruptured site, which were converted into cell population positive for CD146, CD44, CD90, and CD73 expression [44], may have similar characteristics of MSCs described over the last decade [48] and have a possibility to provide an attractive cell source for tissue repair and regeneration.

Among multi-lineage differentiation potentials, osteogenic and endothelial differentiations are especially important for ligament or tendon-bone healing. There are some reports concerning osteogenesis and angiogenesis/vasculogenesis for ligament or tendon-bone healing. To accelerate osteogenesis and/or angiogenesis for tendon-bone healing, vascular endothelial growth factor (VEGF), granulocyte colony-stimulating factor (G-CSF), transforming growth factor-β (TGF-β), bone morphogenetic protein 2 (BMP2), and BMP7 have recently received attention for their therapeutic potential [27, 28, 49–51]. However, Tei et al. reported that human G-CSF-mobilized peripheral blood CD34+ cells contribute to ligament healing via their endothelial differentiation (vasculogenesis) and enhanced intrinsic angiogenesis by VEGF secretion in a immunodeficient rat model [52]. In addition, Matsumoto et al. showed that peripheral blood CD34+ cells could be differentiated into osteoblasts and endothelial cells in a fracture model [53, 54]. Ratio of CD34+ cells is only 1 % in the peripheral blood cells [53] compared to 44 % [44] in ACL ruptured tissue cells, suggesting that isolation of CD34+ cells from the ACL tissue is less important than that from peripheral blood.

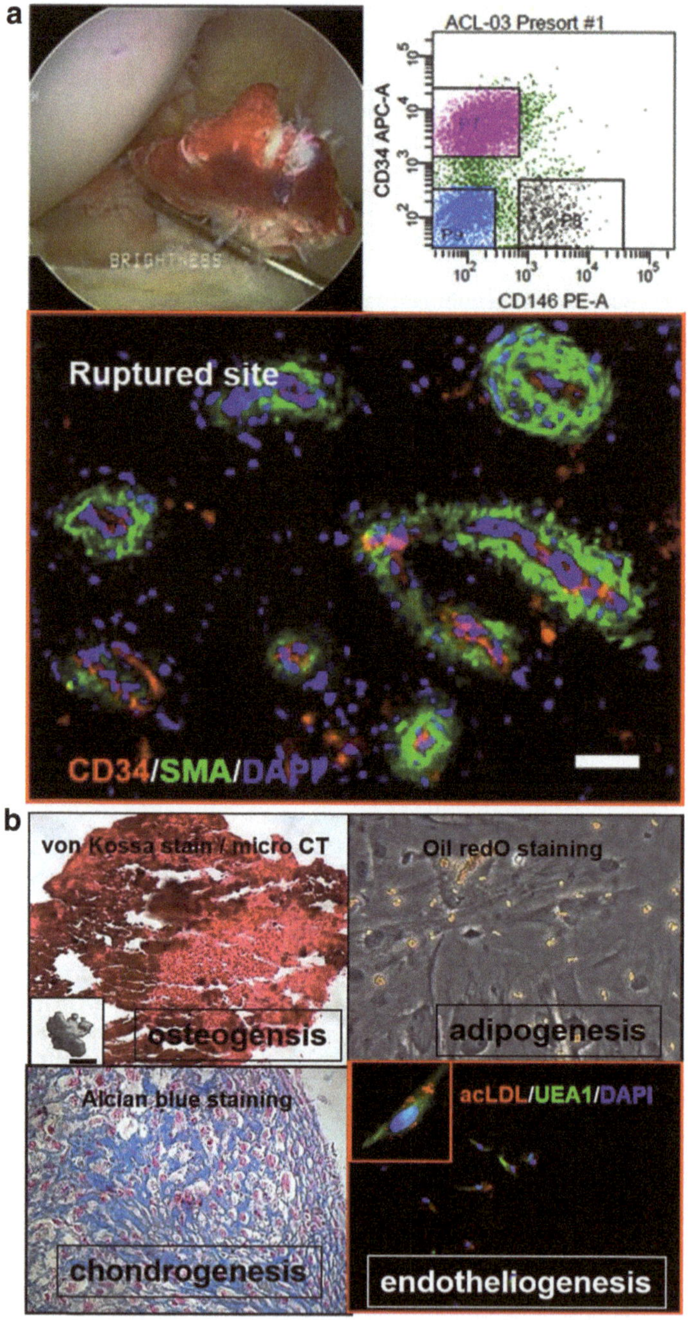

Fig. 42.1 In vitro experiments showing vascular stem cells in the ACL ruptured tissue
(**a**) Tissues showing more positive staining for CD34 in the ruptured site than in the mid-substance
(**b**) CD34-positive cells from ACL ruptured tissue showing multi-lineage differentiation potential including osteogenesis, adipogenesis, chondrogenesis, and endotheliogenesis

42.3 Therapeutic Potential of ACL-Derived Vascular Stem Cells or Ruptured Tissue for Tendon-Bone Healing in ACL Reconstruction

Based on the report showing the existence of CD34+ vascular stem cells in ACL ruptured tissue [44], Mifune Y et al. demonstrated that intracapsular transplantation of human ACL-derived CD34+ cells from the ruptured site contributed to tendon-bone healing via angiogenesis/vasculogenesis and osteogenesis in an immunodeficient rat model of ACL reconstruction [55]. Using a molecular approach, they confirmed enhanced intrinsic angiogenesis/osteogenesis and human-derived vasculogenesis/osteogenesis by intracapsular transplantation of human ACL-derived cells. Histological, radiological (CT), and biomechanical assessment exhibited early tendon-bone healing by cell transplantation. Nonselected as well as CD34+ cells contributed to tendon-bone healing and reduction of tunnel enlargement in a rat model of ACL reconstruction.

During cell therapy for ACL reconstruction, second-step arthroscopic surgery is unavoidable due to the necessity of cell isolation, cell culture, and cell expansion, thus affecting the clinical feasibility of CD34+ cell transplantation. Based on the rich supply of CD34+ cells in the ACL ruptured site [44] and effectiveness of nonselected cells in a rat ACL reconstruction model [55], Matsumoto et al. explored the effect of ACL ruptured tissue on tendon-bone healing in ACL reconstruction. To explore the feasibility of the use of ruptured tissue in the clinical setting, the study was designed as an autologous transplantation model with a large animal canine [56]. ACL ruptured tissue was harvested 2 days after ACL resection and was sutured to the grafts in the tibial tunnel in ACL reconstruction (Fig. 42.2a). The results in histological, CT, and biomechanical testing showed early tendon-bone healing and reduction of tunnel enlargement compared to control group (no tissue suture) (Fig. 42.2b). These findings may lead to the effectiveness of ruptured tissue in ACL reconstruction in the clinical application.

42.4 Clinical Application of ACL Ruptured Tissue in ACL Reconstruction

Based on previous findings, Matsumoto and Kuroda et al. compare 2-year clinical outcomes and tunnel enlargement of DB ACL reconstruction with and without suturing of the autologous ruptured tissue to the grafts in patients with subacute ACL injury (Fig. 42.3) [57]. In this study, 10 patients with subacute (within 3 months after injury) ACL rupture were randomly allocated to undergo DB ACL reconstruction with suturing of the ruptured tissue to hamstring grafts or conventional DB ACL reconstruction in two equal control groups ($n = 5$ each). The results showed significant reduction in tunnel enlargement as assessed with 3D-MDCT in the tissue group, especially at the femoral side. However, the postoperative Lysholm score, anterior

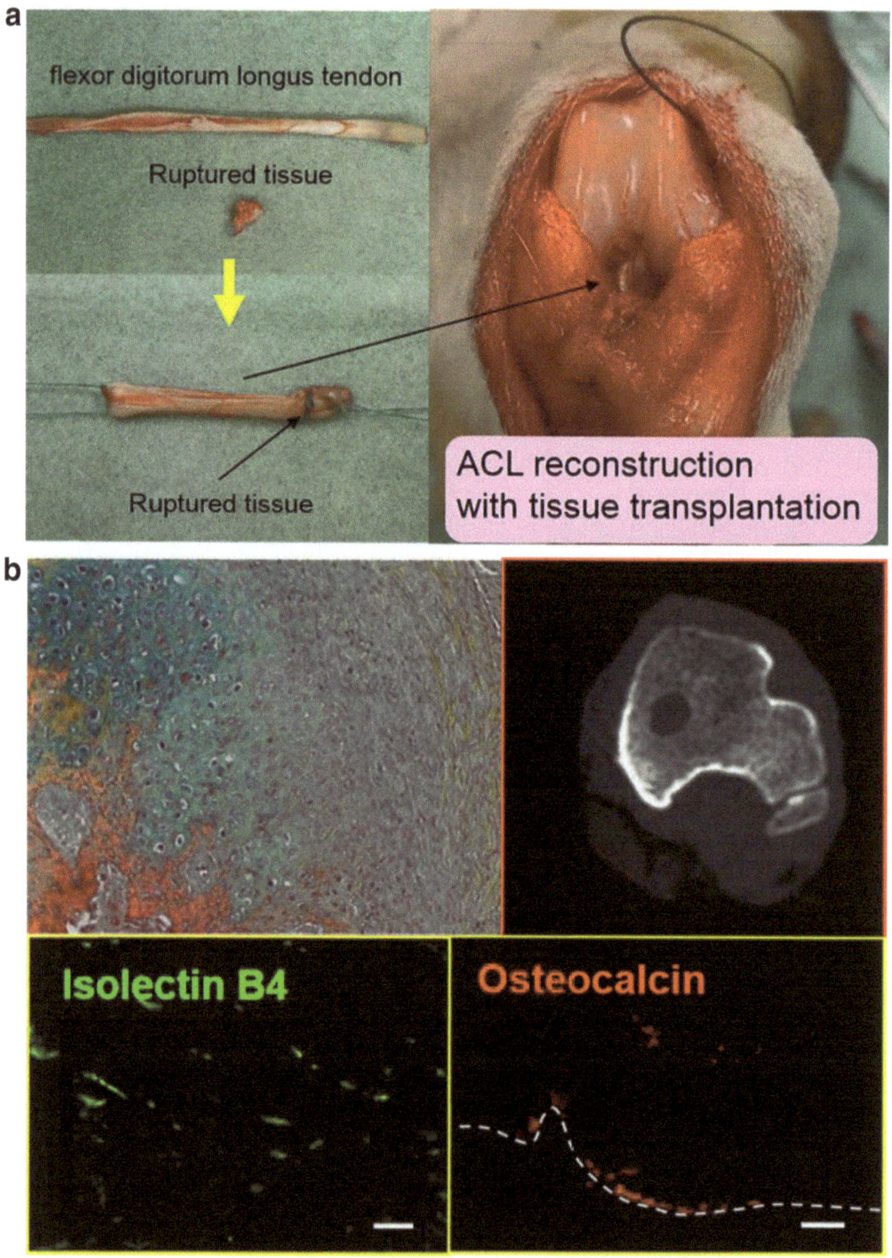

Fig. 42.2 Preclinical study using canine ACL reconstruction model
(**a**) ACL reconstruction was performed using tendon graft with ruptured tissue
(**b**) Autologous tissue transplantation exhibited early tendon-bone healing and bone tunnel reduction via enhanced angiogenesis and osteogenesis

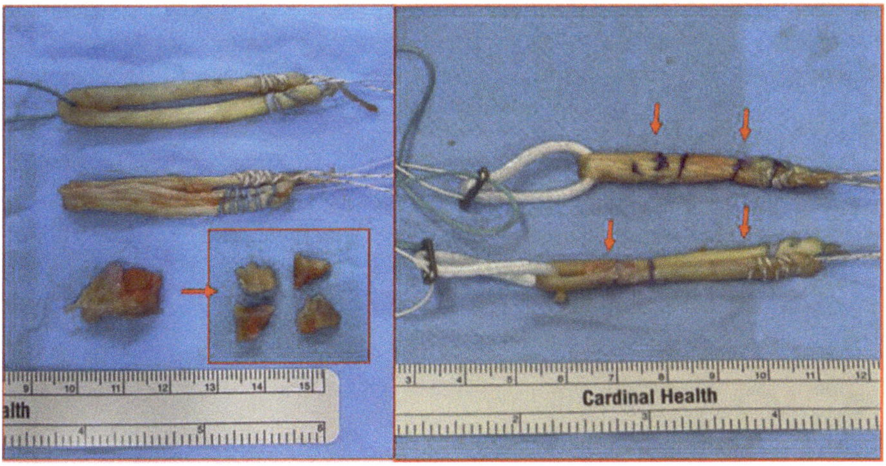

Fig. 42.3 A pilot clinical study using ruptured tissue in ACL reconstruction surgery
ACL reconstruction was performed with the use of ruptured tissues which were sutured to the grafts located in the tunnels

stability of the knee measured with the KT-1000 arthrometer, and rate of negative manual pivot shift test did not differ significantly between the two groups. In several animal studies, the use of periosteum [19, 20], bone marrow mesenchymal stem cells [20, 22], injectable tricalcium phosphate [23], and growth factor [26–28] was reported to enhance tendon-bone healing in ACL reconstruction. Among those, application for human ACL reconstruction was only limited to periosteum with promising results [58–60]. Chen CH et al. reported after their 2–7-year clinical follow-up in 312 patients that satisfactory results could be achieved with the periosteum-enveloping hamstring tendon graft in single-bundle ACL reconstruction with minimal tunnel widening (more than 1 mm tunnel widening: 5.4 % of femoral and 6.1 % of tibial side). Considering this comparison, concept for the treatment is similar and successful tunnel reduction was found on radiographs [58]. If the strategy using ruptured tissue has advantages over previous strategies for enhancement of tendon-bone healing, the ruptured ACL tissue can be used with easy clinical settings without any additional incision, procedure, and cell isolation and expansion.

Preservation of the remnant ACL reconstruction has recently received attention focused on the existence of mechanoreceptors in the ACL remnant that contribute to the proprioceptive function of the ACL [61–65]. However, the intrinsic healing potential of ACL remnants after ACL reconstruction has not been fully investigated. In the pilot study based on a previous series [44, 55, 56], the rupture site of the ACL remnant was harvested and transplanted to the grafts to augment healing, especially at the tendon-bone integration site. This technique is reliable, simple, surgeon-friendly, and inexpensive, and thus clinically feasible.

To predict outcomes of ACL reconstruction surgery, the characteristics of patients should be considered. Uefuji et al. recently reported that ruptured ACL remnants have a healing potential with multi-lineage differentiation, including osteogenesis and endotheliogenesis; however, this potential is age dependent and decreases with age, as CD34+ cells were more prevalent in the ACL remnants in younger patients [66]. ACL remnants in younger patients exhibited high proliferation and great multi-lineage differentiation potential, especially in osteogenic and endothelial differentiation. Furthermore, with the use of in vivo rat ACL reconstruction model, Nakano et al. reported that the healing potential of human ACL-derived cells on the maturation of tendon-bone healing is dependent on the patient's age [67]. Considering these evidences, patient age can be one of the factors that influence postoperative outcomes in healing potential for ACL-derived cells or remnant. In the near future, other demographic factors such as interval between injury and surgery, sex, type of injury, and patient activity level should be assessed to explore other factors that impact ACL remnant-derived cells in the healing potential of reconstructed ACL.

References

1. Beynnon BD, Johnson RJ, Abate JA, Fleming BC, Nichols CE (2005) Treatment of anterior cruciate ligament injuries, part I. Am J Sports Med 33(10):1579–1602. doi:10.1177/0363546505279913
2. Sundar S, Pendegrass CJ, Blunn GW (2009) Tendon bone healing can be enhanced by demineralized bone matrix: a functional and histological study. J Biomed Mater Res B Appl Biomater 88(1):115–122. doi:10.1002/jbm.b.31157
3. Aglietti P, Giron F, Buzzi R, Biddau F, Sasso F (2004) Anterior cruciate ligament reconstruction: bone-patellar tendon-bone compared with double semitendinosus and gracilis tendon grafts. A prospective, randomized clinical trial. J Bone Joint Surg Am 86-A(10):2143–2155. doi:86/10/2143 [pii]
4. Bach BR Jr, Tradonsky S, Bojchuk J, Levy ME, Bush-Joseph CA, Khan NH (1998) Arthroscopically assisted anterior cruciate ligament reconstruction using patellar tendon autograft. Five- to nine-year follow-up evaluation. Am J Sports Med 26(1):20–29
5. Beynnon BD, Johnson RJ, Fleming BC, Kannus P, Kaplan M, Samani J, Renstrom P (2002) Anterior cruciate ligament replacement: comparison of bone-patellar tendon-bone grafts with two-strand hamstring grafts. A prospective, randomized study. J Bone Joint Surg Am 84-A (9):1503–1513
6. Fu FH, Shen W, Starman JS, Okeke N, Irrgang JJ (2008) Primary anatomic double-bundle anterior cruciate ligament reconstruction: a preliminary 2-year prospective study. Am J Sports Med 36(7):1263–1274. doi:10.1177/0363546508314428
7. Fujita N, Kuroda R, Matsumoto T, Yamaguchi M, Yagi M, Matsumoto A, Kubo S, Matsushita T, Hoshino Y, Nishimoto K, Araki D, Kurosaka M (2011) Comparison of the clinical outcome of double-bundle, anteromedial single-bundle, and posterolateral single-bundle anterior cruciate ligament reconstruction using hamstring tendon graft with minimum 2-year follow-up. Arthroscopy 27(7):906–913. doi:10.1016/j.arthro.2011.02.015
8. Muneta T, Koga H, Mochizuki T, Ju YJ, Hara K, Nimura A, Yagishita K, Sekiya I (2007) A prospective randomized study of 4-strand semitendinosus tendon anterior cruciate ligament reconstruction comparing single-bundle and double-bundle techniques. Arthroscopy 23 (6):618–628. doi:10.1016/j.arthro.2007.04.010
9. Yasuda K, Kondo E, Ichiyama H, Kitamura N, Tanabe Y, Tohyama H, Minami A (2004) Anatomic reconstruction of the anteromedial and posterolateral bundles of the anterior cruciate

ligament using hamstring tendon grafts. Arthroscopy 20(10):1015–1025. doi:10.1016/j.arthro.2004.08.010
10. Ballock RT, Woo SL, Lyon RM, Hollis JM, Akeson WH (1989) Use of patellar tendon autograft for anterior cruciate ligament reconstruction in the rabbit: a long-term histologic and biomechanical study. J Orthop Res 7(4):474–485. doi:10.1002/jor.1100070404
11. Grana WA, Egle DM, Mahnken R, Goodhart CW (1994) An analysis of autograft fixation after anterior cruciate ligament reconstruction in a rabbit model. Am J Sports Med 22(3):344–351
12. Weiss JA, Woo SL, Ohland KJ, Horibe S, Newton PO (1991) Evaluation of a new injury model to study medial collateral ligament healing: primary repair versus nonoperative treatment. J Orthop Res 9(4):516–528
13. Woo SL, Inoue M, McGurk-Burleson E, Gomez MA (1987) Treatment of the medial collateral ligament injury. II: structure and function of canine knees in response to differing treatment regimens. Am J Sports Med 15(1):22–29
14. Fauno P, Kaalund S (2005) Tunnel widening after hamstring anterior cruciate ligament reconstruction is influenced by the type of graft fixation used: a prospective randomized study. Arthroscopy 21(11):1337–1341. doi:S0749-8063(05)01186-2 [pii] 10.1016/j.arthro.2005.08.023
15. L'Insalata JC, Klatt B, Fu FH, Harner CD (1997) Tunnel expansion following anterior cruciate ligament reconstruction: a comparison of hamstring and patellar tendon autografts. Knee Surg Sports Traumatol Arthrosc 5(4):234–238
16. Ekdahl M, Nozaki M, Ferretti M, Tsai A, Smolinski P, Fu FH (2009) The effect of tunnel placement on bone-tendon healing in anterior cruciate ligament reconstruction in a goat model. Am J Sports Med 37(8):1522–1530. doi:0363546509332503 [pii] 10.1177/0363546509332503
17. Getelman MH, Friedman MJ (1999) Revision anterior cruciate ligament reconstruction surgery. J Am Acad Orthop Surg 7(3):189–198
18. Petrigliano FA, McAllister DR, Wu BM (2006) Tissue engineering for anterior cruciate ligament reconstruction: a review of current strategies. Arthroscopy 22(4):441–451. doi:S0749-8063(06)00109-5 [pii] 10.1016/j.arthro.2006.01.017
19. Chen CH, Chen WJ, Shih CH, Yang CY, Liu SJ, Lin PY (2003) Enveloping the tendon graft with periosteum to enhance tendon-bone healing in a bone tunnel: a biomechanical and histologic study in rabbits. Arthroscopy 19(3):290–296. doi:10.1053/jars.2003.50014
20. Karaoglu S, Celik C, Korkusuz P (2009) The effects of bone marrow or periosteum on tendon-to-bone tunnel healing in a rabbit model. Knee Surg Sports Traumatol Arthrosc 17(2):170–178. doi:10.1007/s00167-008-0646-3
21. Ouyang HW, Goh JC, Lee EH (2004) Use of bone marrow stromal cells for tendon graft-to-bone healing: histological and immunohistochemical studies in a rabbit model. Am J Sports Med 32(2):321–327
22. Lim JK, Hui J, Li L, Thambyah A, Goh J, Lee EH (2004) Enhancement of tendon graft osteointegration using mesenchymal stem cells in a rabbit model of anterior cruciate ligament reconstruction. Arthroscopy 20(9):899–910. doi:10.1016/j.arthro.2004.06.035
23. Huangfu X, Zhao J (2007) Tendon-bone healing enhancement using injectable tricalcium phosphate in a dog anterior cruciate ligament reconstruction model. Arthroscopy 23(5):455–462. doi:10.1016/j.arthro.2006.12.031
24. Anderson K, Seneviratne AM, Izawa K, Atkinson BL, Potter HG, Rodeo SA (2001) Augmentation of tendon healing in an intraarticular bone tunnel with use of a bone growth factor. Am J Sports Med 29(6):689–698
25. Nakase J, Kitaoka K, Matsumoto K, Tomita K (2010) Facilitated tendon-bone healing by local delivery of recombinant hepatocyte growth factor in rabbits. Arthroscopy 26(1):84–90. doi:10.1016/j.arthro.2009.06.029
26. Rodeo SA, Suzuki K, Deng XH, Wozney J, Warren RF (1999) Use of recombinant human bone morphogenetic protein-2 to enhance tendon healing in a bone tunnel. Am J Sports Med 27(4):476–488

27. Sasaki K, Kuroda R, Ishida K, Kubo S, Matsumoto T, Mifune Y, Kinoshita K, Tei K, Akisue T, Tabata Y, Kurosaka M (2008) Enhancement of tendon-bone osteointegration of anterior cruciate ligament graft using granulocyte colony-stimulating factor. Am J Sports Med 36 (8):1519–1527. doi:10.1177/0363546508316282
28. Yoshikawa T, Tohyama H, Katsura T, Kondo E, Kotani Y, Matsumoto H, Toyama Y, Yasuda K (2006) Effects of local administration of vascular endothelial growth factor on mechanical characteristics of the semitendinosus tendon graft after anterior cruciate ligament reconstruction in sheep. Am J Sports Med 34(12):1918–1925
29. Frank CB, Jackson DW (1997) The science of reconstruction of the anterior cruciate ligament. J Bone Joint Surg Am 79(10):1556–1576
30. Murray MM, Martin SD, Martin TL, Spector M (2000) Histological changes in the human anterior cruciate ligament after rupture. J Bone Joint Surg Am 82-A(10):1387–1397
31. Fujimoto E, Sumen Y, Ochi M, Ikuta Y (2002) Spontaneous healing of acute anterior cruciate ligament (ACL) injuries – conservative treatment using an extension block soft brace without anterior stabilization. Arch Orthop Trauma Surg 122(4):212–216
32. Kurosaka M, Yoshiya S, Mizuno T, Mizuno K (1998) Spontaneous healing of a tear of the anterior cruciate ligament. A report of two cases. J Bone Joint Surg Am 80(8):1200–1203
33. Sandberg R, Balkfors B, Nilsson B, Westlin N (1987) Operative versus non-operative treatment of recent injuries to the ligaments of the knee. A prospective randomized study. J Bone Joint Surg Am 69(8):1120–1126
34. Drogset JO, Grontvedt T, Robak OR, Molster A, Viset AT, Engebretsen L (2006) A sixteen-year follow-up of three operative techniques for the treatment of acute ruptures of the anterior cruciate ligament. J Bone Joint Surg Am 88(5):944–952. doi:88/5/944 [pii] 10.2106/JBJS.D. 02876
35. Marshall JL, Warren RF, Wickiewicz TL (1982) Primary surgical treatment of anterior cruciate ligament lesions. Am J Sports Med 10(2):103–107
36. Marshall JL, Warren RF, Wickiewicz TL, Reider B (1979) The anterior cruciate ligament: a technique of repair and reconstruction. Clin Orthop Relat Res 143:97–106
37. Strand T, Molster A, Hordvik M, Krukhaug Y (2005) Long-term follow-up after primary repair of the anterior cruciate ligament: clinical and radiological evaluation 15–23 years postoperatively. Arch Orthop Trauma Surg 125(4):217–221. doi:10.1007/s00402-004-0766-2
38. Lee IC, Wang JH, Lee YT, Young TH (2007) Development of a useful technique to discriminate anterior cruciate ligament cells and mesenchymal stem cells-the application of cell electrophoresis. J Biomed Mater Res A 82(1):230–237. doi:10.1002/jbm.a.31163
39. Lee SY, Miwa M, Sakai Y, Kuroda R, Matsumoto T, Iwakura T, Fujioka H, Doita M, Kurosaka M (2007) In vitro multipotentiality and characterization of human unfractured traumatic hemarthrosis-derived progenitor cells: a potential cell source for tissue repair. J Cell Physiol 210(3):561–566. doi:10.1002/jcp.20890
40. Crisan M, Yap S, Casteilla L, Chen CW, Corselli M, Park TS, Andriolo G, Sun B, Zheng B, Zhang L, Norotte C, Teng PN, Traas J, Schugar R, Deasy BM, Badylak S, Buhring HJ, Giacobino JP, Lazzari L, Huard J, Peault B (2008) A perivascular origin for mesenchymal stem cells in multiple human organs. Cell Stem Cell 3(3):301–313. doi:S1934-5909(08)00337-8 [pii] 10.1016/j.stem.2008.07.003
41. Howson KM, Aplin AC, Gelati M, Alessandri G, Parati EA, Nicosia RF (2005) The postnatal rat aorta contains pericyte progenitor cells that form spheroidal colonies in suspension culture. Am J Physiol Cell Physiol 289(6):C1396–C1407. doi:00168.2005 [pii] 10.1152/ajpcell.00168. 2005
42. Tavian M, Zheng B, Oberlin E, Crisan M, Sun B, Huard J, Peault B (2005) The vascular wall as a source of stem cells. Ann N Y Acad Sci 1044:41–50
43. Zengin E, Chalajour F, Gehling UM, Ito WD, Treede H, Lauke H, Weil J, Reichenspurner H, Kilic N, Ergun S (2006) Vascular wall resident progenitor cells: a source for postnatal vasculogenesis. Development 133(8):1543–1551. doi:dev.02315 [pii] 10.1242/dev.02315

44. Matsumoto T, Ingham SM, Mifune Y, Osawa A, Logar A, Usas A, Kuroda R, Kurosaka M, Fu FH, Huard J (2012) Isolation and characterization of human anterior cruciate ligament-derived vascular stem cells. Stem Cells Dev 21(6):859–872. doi:10.1089/scd.2010.0528
45. Covas DT, Panepucci RA, Fontes AM, Silva WA Jr, Orellana MD, Freitas MC, Neder L, Santos AR, Peres LC, Jamur MC, Zago MA (2008) Multipotent mesenchymal stromal cells obtained from diverse human tissues share functional properties and gene-expression profile with CD146+ perivascular cells and fibroblasts. Exp Hematol 36(5):642–654. doi:S0301-472X (08)00005-2 [pii] 10.1016/j.exphem.2007.12.015
46. Iwasaki H, Kawamoto A, Ishikawa M, Oyamada A, Nakamori S, Nishimura H, Sadamoto K, Horii M, Matsumoto T, Murasawa S, Shibata T, Suehiro S, Asahara T (2006) Dose-dependent contribution of CD34-positive cell transplantation to concurrent vasculogenesis and cardiomyogenesis for functional regenerative recovery after myocardial infarction. Circulation 113(10):1311–1325
47. Yeh ET, Zhang S, Wu HD, Korbling M, Willerson JT, Estrov Z (2003) Transdifferentiation of human peripheral blood CD34 + −enriched cell population into cardiomyocytes, endothelial cells, and smooth muscle cells in vivo. Circulation 108(17):2070–2073. doi:10.1161/01.CIR. 0000099501.52718.70 01.CIR.0000099501.52718.70 [pii]
48. Pittenger MF, Mackay AM, Beck SC, Jaiswal RK, Douglas R, Mosca JD, Moorman MA, Simonetti DW, Craig S, Marshak DR (1999) Multilineage potential of adult human mesenchymal stem cells. Science 284(5411):143–147
49. Martinek V, Latterman C, Usas A, Abramowitch S, Woo SL, Fu FH, Huard J (2002) Enhancement of tendon-bone integration of anterior cruciate ligament grafts with bone morphogenetic protein-2 gene transfer: a histological and biomechanical study. J Bone Joint Surg Am 84-A(7):1123–1131
50. Mihelic R, Pecina M, Jelic M, Zoricic S, Kusec V, Simic P, Bobinac D, Lah B, Legovic D, Vukicevic S (2004) Bone morphogenetic protein-7 (osteogenic protein-1) promotes tendon graft integration in anterior cruciate ligament reconstruction in sheep. Am J Sports Med 32 (7):1619–1625
51. Yasuda K, Tomita F, Yamazaki S, Minami A, Tohyama H (2004) The effect of growth factors on biomechanical properties of the bone-patellar tendon-bone graft after anterior cruciate ligament reconstruction: a canine model study. Am J Sports Med 32(4):870–880
52. Tei K, Matsumoto T, Mifune Y, Ishida K, Sasaki K, Shoji T, Kubo S, Kawamoto A, Asahara T, Kurosaka M, Kuroda R (2008) Administrations of peripheral blood CD34-positive cells contribute to medial collateral ligament healing via vasculogenesis. Stem Cells 26(3):819–830. doi:10. 1634/stemcells.2007-0671
53. Matsumoto T, Kawamoto A, Kuroda R, Ishikawa M, Mifune Y, Iwasaki H, Miwa M, Horii M, Hayashi S, Oyamada A, Nishimura H, Murasawa S, Doita M, Kurosaka M, Asahara T (2006) Therapeutic potential of vasculogenesis and osteogenesis promoted by peripheral blood CD34-positive cells for functional bone healing. Am J Pathol 169(4):1440–1457. doi:10.2353/ajpath. 2006.060064
54. Mifune Y, Matsumoto T, Kawamoto A, Kuroda R, Shoji T, Iwasaki H, Kwon SM, Miwa M, Kurosaka M, Asahara T (2008) Local delivery of granulocyte colony stimulating factor-mobilized CD34-positive progenitor cells using bioscaffold for modality of unhealing bone fracture. Stem Cells 26(6):1395–1405. doi:10.1634/stemcells.2007-0820
55. Mifune Y, Matsumoto T, Ota S, Nishimori M, Usas A, Kopf S, Kuroda R, Kurosaka M, Fu FH, Huard J (2012) Therapeutic potential of anterior cruciate ligament-derived stem cells for anterior cruciate ligament reconstruction. Cell Transplant 21(8):1651–1665. doi:10.3727/ 096368912X647234
56. Matsumoto T, Kubo S, Sasaki K, Kawakami Y, Oka S, Sasaki H, Takayama K, Tei K, Matsushita T, Mifune Y, Kurosaka M, Kuroda R (2012) Acceleration of tendon-bone healing of anterior cruciate ligament graft using autologous ruptured tissue. Am J Sports Med 40 (6):1296–1302. doi:10.1177/0363546512439026
57. Matsumoto T, Kuroda R, Matsushita T, Araki D, Hoshino Y, Nagamune K, Kurosaka M (2014) Reduction of tunnel enlargement with use of autologous ruptured tissue in anterior

cruciate ligament reconstruction: a pilot clinical trial. Arthroscopy 30(4):468–474. doi:10.1016/j.arthro.2013.12.014
58. Chen CH, Chang CH, Su CI, Wang KC, Liu HT, Yu CM, Wong CB, Wang IC (2010) Arthroscopic single-bundle anterior cruciate ligament reconstruction with periosteum-enveloping hamstring tendon graft: clinical outcome at 2 to 7 years. Arthroscopy 26 (7):907–917. doi:10.1016/j.arthro.2009.11.011
59. Li H, Jiang J, Wu Y, Chen S (2012) Potential mechanisms of a periosteum patch as an effective and favourable approach to enhance tendon-bone healing in the human body. Int Orthop 36 (3):665–669. doi:10.1007/s00264-011-1346-z
60. Robert H, Es-Sayeh J (2004) The role of periosteal flap in the prevention of femoral widening in anterior cruciate ligament reconstruction using hamstring tendons. Knee Surg Sports Traumatol Arthrosc 12(1):30–35. doi:10.1007/s00167-003-0380-9
61. Adachi N, Ochi M, Uchio Y, Iwasa J, Ryoke K, Kuriwaka M (2002) Mechanoreceptors in the anterior cruciate ligament contribute to the joint position sense. Acta Orthop Scand 73 (3):330–334. doi:10.1080/000164702320155356
62. Ochi M, Abouheif MM, Kongcharoensombat W, Nakamae A, Adachi N, Deie M (2011) Double bundle arthroscopic anterior cruciate ligament reconstruction with remnant preserving technique using a hamstring autograft. Sports Med Arthrosc Rehabil Ther Technol 3:30. doi:10.1186/1758-2555-3-30
63. Ochi M, Adachi N, Deie M, Kanaya A (2006) Anterior cruciate ligament augmentation procedure with a 1-incision technique: anteromedial bundle or posterolateral bundle reconstruction. Arthroscopy 22(4):463 e461–463 e465. doi:10.1016/j.arthro.2005.06.034
64. Ochi M, Adachi N, Uchio Y, Deie M, Kumahashi N, Ishikawa M, Sera S (2009) A minimum 2-year follow-up after selective anteromedial or posterolateral bundle anterior cruciate ligament reconstruction. Arthroscopy 25(2):117–122. doi:10.1016/j.arthro.2008.10.011
65. Yasuda K, Kondo E, Kitamura N, Kawaguchi Y, Kai S, Tanabe Y (2012) A pilot study of anatomic double-bundle anterior cruciate ligament reconstruction with ligament remnant tissue preservation. Arthroscopy 28(3):343–353. doi:10.1016/j.arthro.2011.08.305
66. Uefuji A, Matsumoto T, Matsushita T, Ueha T, Zhang S, Kurosaka M, Kuroda R (2014) Age-related differences in anterior cruciate ligament remnant vascular-derived cells. Am J Sports Med 42(6):1478–1486. doi:10.1177/0363546514529092
67. Nakano N, Matsumoto T, Takayama K, Matsushita T, Araki D, Uefuji A, Nagai K, Zhang S, Inokuchi T, Nishida K, Kuroda R, Kurosaka M (2015) Age-dependent healing potential of anterior cruciate ligament remnant-derived cells. Am J Sports Med 43(3):700–708. doi:10.1177/0363546514561436

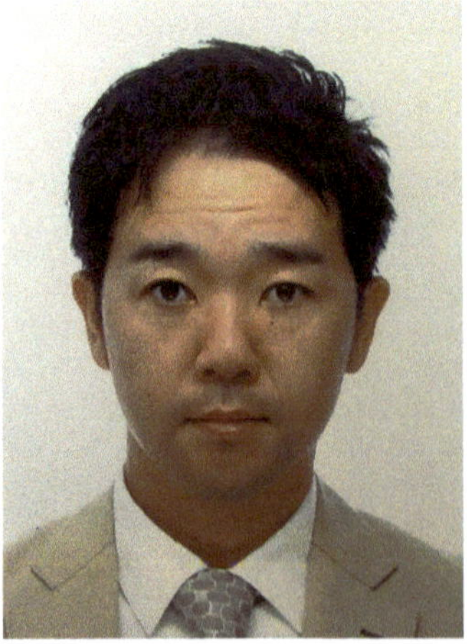

Tomoyuki Matsumoto, M.D., Department of Orthopaedic Surgery, Kobe University Graduate School of Medicine, Hyogo, Japan.

Chapter 43
Tissue Engineering Approach for ACL Healing

Takeshi Shoji, Tomoyuki Nakasa, and Mitsuo Ochi

Abstract Anterior cruciate ligament (ACL) injuries have become increasingly prevalent and account for a large proportion of knee ligament injuries among young, active individuals. The management of ACL injuries is technically demanding because of their poor healing potential. At present, ACL reconstruction with intra-articular grafts is still gold standard; however, these approaches sometimes lead to several problems such as secondary osteoarthritis and inadequate restoration of functional knee stability. Progress in science and technology has enabled the development of tissue engineering techniques, with basic research being applied clinically. The improved knowledge of healing, along with recent progress in regenerative medicine, has resulted in the discovery of novel biologically augmented ACL repair techniques that have satisfactory outcomes in preclinical studies. In the past decade, we have investigated tissue regeneration in animal models of musculoskeletal disorders by using tissue engineering approach, such as cells, scaffold, microRNA, and delivery systems, which has been relatively easy to apply and develop in clinical settings. In this section, we specifically discuss the available tissue engineering options for managing ACL injuries and introduce our challenges to achieve better outcomes for ACL reconstruction and for the overall healing of native ACL.

Keywords Anterior cruciate ligament • Tissue engineering • MicroRNA • Stem cells • Scaffold

43.1 Introduction

The anterior cruciate ligament (ACL) is the major stabilizer of the knee, and it functions to limit rotation and anterior translation of the tibia. Injuries to ACL have become increasingly prevalent and account for a large proportion of knee ligament

---

T. Shoji, M.D., Ph.D. (✉) • T. Nakasa, M.D., Ph.D.
Department of Orthopaedic Surgery, Graduate School of Biomedical Sciences, Hiroshima University, 1-2-3 Kasumi, Minami-ku, Hiroshima 734-8551, Japan
e-mail: readymade_jpn@yahoo.co.jp

M. Ochi, M.D., Ph.D.
President of Hiroshima University, 1-3-2 Kagamiyama, Higashi-Hiroshima 739-8511, Japan

M. Ochi et al. (eds.), *ACL Injury and Its Treatment*,
DOI 10.1007/978-4-431-55858-3_43

injuries among young, active individuals [1]. A completely torn ACL rarely heals spontaneously, and most partial ACL tears eventually progress to complete rupture [2]. Hefti et al. have reported no regeneration after complete ACL transection in rabbits, and very slow and incomplete regeneration after partial rupture. Similar results have been shown in other species [3]. Several factors have been reported to be responsible for this limited healing capacity, including the surrounding tissues, blood supply, nutrient delivery, biomechanical forces, and synovial fluid, as well as the supply of growth factors. Failure healing of ACL causes instability of the knee, which usually leads to early osteoarthritis (OA) of the affected knee [4]. Although the repair or reconstruction of ACL after rupture is important for the stability of the knee and for prevention of future OA, the management of ACL injuries is technically demanding, and the acceptable options are limited [5]. At present, ACL reconstruction with intra-articular grafts is the most broadly accepted procedure for young and active patients [6]. ACL reconstruction has been demonstrated to improve clinical instability of the knee joint, to reduce knee laxity, and to decrease the risk of late meniscus tear [4, 7, 8]. However, previous reports mentioned that ACL reconstruction does not fully restore the functional dynamic stability of the knee, and the rates of return to pre-injury activity level vary from 37 to 75 % [8–11]. Furthermore, patients remain at higher risk for early onset OA even after ACL reconstruction [12, 13]. Over the last decade, substantial efforts have been made to understand ligament healing and to improve surgical reconstruction.

Ligaments comprise two different areas including the ligament itself and its bony attachments, and the healing and regeneration processes of which are complicated. After ligament injury, the vessels are disrupted and a blood clot forms in the wound area. The blood clot acts as a scaffold for the inflammatory and mesenchymal cells, thus creating a tridimensional environment which enables the cells to migrate, attach, and proliferate in the healing process [14]. The platelets in the blood clot and the injured cells release their growth factors and pro-inflammatory mediators consisting of mainly platelet-derived growth factor (PDGF), basic fibroblast growth factor (bFGF), insulin-like growth factor (IGF), epidermal growth factor (EGF), and vascular endothelial growth factor (VEGF). Neutrophils and macrophages are the first-line inflammatory cells which also release several growth factors and cytokines into the wound area, which accelerate the inflammation and cause the absorption of more inflammatory cells in the wound area [15]. Thereafter, FGF and VEGF play essential roles in the collagen production of fibroblasts, regulation of inflammation, proliferation of endothelial cells, and acceleration of angiogenesis [16]. When the mesenchymal cells infiltrate the injured area, some cells differentiate to fibroblasts when exposed to bFGF, and others which are mainly exposed to VEGF differentiate to endothelial cells [17]. Fibroblasts are the main cell types responsible in collagen production, while the endothelial cells are responsible for angiogenesis and vessel production [5, 17]. Then, collagen and immature blood vessels are produced in the wound area, and at the same time fibroplasia occurs [14]. Thus, angiogenesis, the formation of new blood vessels from a preexisting vessel, is an essential step in the process of ligament healing. However, angiogenesis and regeneration in the injured ACL occur at a very slow rate, and their magnitude increase does not reach a sufficient level for appropriate healing to occur, leading to insufficient healing [18].

Numerous studies have attempted to determine the effects of various growth factors and genes on the ligament engineering system with regard to cell proliferation, ECM synthesis, neovascularization, and mechanical properties [19–23]. Recent advancements in functional biological/tissue engineering techniques, including growth factors, stem cells, and bioscaffolds, have helped researchers to introduce novel biologic ACL repair approaches, and they might help the ligament healing in surgical reconstruction and/or the native structure. Basically, tissue engineering can be divided into four major categories: tissue scaffolds, growth factors, stem cells, and gene therapy.

43.1.1 Biomaterial Scaffolds in Ligament Tissue Engineering

Scaffolds play an important role in tissue engineering because an application of growth factors and stem cells has low clinical value without them. Tissue scaffolds have several duties, but their major role is to provide a suitable environment for cell attachment, migration, proliferation, matrix remodeling and regeneration [14]. The synthetic scaffolds are firstly produced by polymerization of the synthetic materials [12, 28, 29]. The Leeds-Keio (LK) open-weave polyester ligament, which is a synthetic ligament substitute and was thought to encourage ingrowth of collagen fibers and the generation of a new ligament, was widely used in the 1980s and early 1990s for ACL replacement [28]. Thereafter, the Ligament Advanced Reinforcement System (LARS; Surgical Implants and Devices, Arc-sur-Tille, France) and radio frequency-generated glow discharge (RFGGD)-treated LK ligament (LKII) were introduced [29]. However, incidences of postoperative complications related with chronic inflammatory reactions have been noted. Thus these failures indicated these synthetic artificial ligament graft had poor "ligamentization" in the knee joint after implantation [30]. The newer ones are those constructed by the biologic-based molecules such as collagen, elastin, chitosan, hyaluronic acid, demineralized bone matrix, fibrin, gelatin, etc. [24–27]. Although many scaffolds combined with cell type and growth factors have been examined for ACL tissue engineering, relatively few have been translated to in vivo performance, and more advancements in this arena are needed.

43.1.2 Growth Factors in Ligament Tissue Engineering

The use of growth factors has gained a lot of attention in the treatment of soft tissue injuries since the late 1990s. A wide range of growth factors, including IGF, TGF-β,

PDGF, VEGF, and FGF, have been used previously to improve ligamentous tissue repair [19, 20, 31–34]. They have been shown to have positive effects on various biological processes needed to improve ACL healing. Yoshikawa T. et al. reported that an exogenous VEGF application for ACL reconstruction can induce an increase in knee laxity, and others have reported TGF-b, FGF, EGF, and PDGF significantly affect biomechanical properties of ACL [31–34]. However, there are some concerns regarding the use of growth factors. Yoshikawa T. et al also reported that an exogenous VEGF application decreases the stiffness of the grafted tendon after ACL reconstruction [34]. Furthermore, the understanding of the signaling events of these growth factors and the way of stimulating or repressing the immunologic and vascularization responses are not well established. Thus, further experiments regarding the optimized use of growth factors, such as the short life span of these factors, delivery and maintenance, are needed for significant advances in the application of these growth factors.

Platelet-rich plasma (PRP), which contains a wide range of growth factors, garnered much attention as a novel, noninvasive treatment. Through in vitro and animal studies, several investigators have studied the positive influence of PRP on the proliferation of osteoblasts and tenocytes in tendon–bone interface healing [35, 36]. However, PRP augmentation when used in ACL reconstruction has shown no statistically significant difference regarding clinical outcomes, tunnel widening, and graft integration, thus the further experiments are also needed for significant advances in the application of PRP [37].

43.1.3 Stem Cells in Ligament Tissue Engineering

Due to their demonstrable multipotency, mesenchymal progenitor cells (MPCs), marrow-derived mesenchymal stem cells (MSCs), and adipose-derived stromal or stem cells (ADSC) have been the subject of extensive research in vitro and in preclinical studies in tissue engineering research. They are attractive cell sources for regenerative medicine because of their ability to differentiate into osteogenic, adipogenic, and chondrogenic lineages. We previously reported improved histology and biomechanics in rat torn ACL-injured models using intra-articular injection of MSCs [38], and others also have shown improved biomechanics in other models of ACL injury [39–41]. These findings are encouraging considering the therapeutic potential of MSCs in the healing of ligaments, although there are several limitations in optimizing the MSC applications in ACL repair. One limitation is the need to employ the proper methods of effective differentiation of these multi-pluripotent cells into specific cell types. Another is the delivery and maintenance of these cells into the wound site.

43.1.4 Gene Therapy in Ligament Tissue Engineering

Gene therapy might be a recent promising strategy to transfer the genetic information to target cells and to apply various therapeutic factors essential to the healing of injured tissues [42, 43]. Gene therapy can be used for the delivery of growth factors, and it may have the potential to modulate biochemical changes following a ligament injury such as variations in collagen expression. Hildebrand et al. reported the application of gene transfer to normal and ACL-injured knees in a rabbit model [44]. They concluded that adenoviral vectors are able to express more efficiently than retroviral vectors in ACL cells and can lead to a long period of gene expression in vivo. Madry H et al. demonstrated that the stable FGF-2 expression via direct recombinant adeno-associated virus vector-mediated gene transfer enhances the healing of experimental human ACL lesions by activating key cellular and metabolic processes [42]. Others reported the ability of vector-laden hydrogels in in situ gene delivery to the injury site for potential biological repair of the ACL [45]. However, unresolved challenges exist in this therapy, including trans-infection of the target cells with foreign genes, targeting the right gene at the right location in the right cells and expressing sufficiently at the right time while minimizing adverse reactions [46, 47].

43.2 Our Challenges in Tissue Engineering Approaches for ACL Injury

In the past decade, we have investigated tissue regeneration in animal models of musculoskeletal disorders by using cells, scaffold, and delivery systems which has been relatively easy to apply and develop in clinical settings. Moreover, microRNA (miRNA), which is important in biological processes and in the pathogenesis of human diseases, has been used in research on regenerative medicine.

43.2.1 Tendon to Bone Healing

Successful ACL reconstruction with a tendon graft requires solid healing of the tendon graft in the bone tunnels [48]. A complete bone tunnel healing of a ligament graft may occur as late as 6–12 months after surgery, and the weakest part during early healing is the attachment between tendon and bone [49]. Thus tendon to bone incorporation of tendon grafts within the bone tunnel is a major concern when using a tendon graft for ligament reconstruction. Furthermore, hamstring grafts have been associated with a higher incidence of bony tunnel widening, and the strength of this attachment is crucial for the success of the ACL reconstruction [50]. We applied commercially available enamel matrix derivative (EMD) (EMDOGAIN; Biora,

Malmö, Sweden) for better healing of the tendon graft in the bone tunnels. EMD is extracted from the tooth germs of the immature porcine mandible and is composed of many proteins, such as amelogenin, enamelin, seathlin, and proteases, with amelogenin as the main component (>90 %) [51]. It induces ligament fibroblast proliferation and migration, total protein synthesis, alkaline phosphatase activity, and mineralization, and it stimulates MSCs [52]. These proteins have been used clinically in regenerative periodontal procedures. In experimental models and clinical studies, EMD has been shown to promote the regrowth and regeneration of natural supporting structures, including cementum, periodontal ligament, and alveolar bone. In experimental rat ACL reconstruction models, we filled 40 μl of EMD with propylene glycol alginate as a carrier protein in the space around the tendon–bone interface on the tibial side. We demonstrated that EMD, when filled in around the tendon–bone interface, accelerates tendon–bone healing at 8 weeks in histological analysis and at 8 and 12 weeks in biomechanical analysis (Fig. 43.1). EMD has not previously been used clinically in the knee joint, and to date, we have applied it in clinical study.

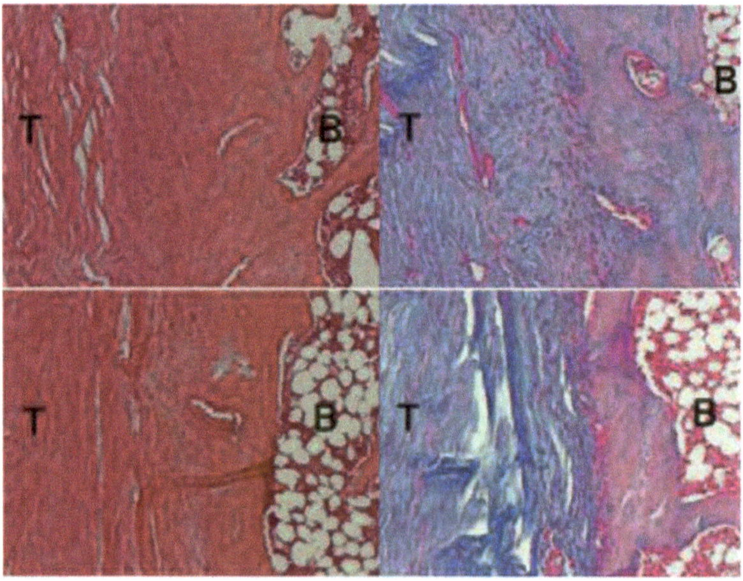

Fig. 43.1 Histological images showing evaluation of the tendon–bone interface of a specimen at 8 weeks after surgery, for the enamel matrix derivative group (EMD+) (*top row*) and the control group (EMD–) (*bottom row*). Abundant perpendicular collagen fibers connecting to the bone and Sharpey's fibers were observed in the EMD+ group (*top*); they were not seen in the control group (*bottom*) (*left panels*, hematoxylin and eosin staining; *right panels*, azan staining. *T* tendon, *B* bone; original magnification × 100)

43.2.2 Application of Stem Cells

For the cell source, we focused on MSC and endothelial progenitor cell (EPC). With MSCs, we evaluated biomechanically and histologically whether intra-articularly injected MSCs can accelerate the healing of a partially torn ACL using a rat model. We created an ACL partially transected model in rats and injected 1×10^6 MSCs into the knee joint [38]. We demonstrated that the transected area was covered with healing tissues at 2 and 4 weeks after MSC injection, and we found that the ultimate failure load of the femur–ACL–tibia complex was significantly improved by intra-articular MSC injection (Fig. 43.2).

EPCs have been reported to play an important role for pathophysiological neovascularization in various ischemic tissues, and they also have the therapeutic potential to facilitate tissue repair/regeneration and modulate the regenerating environment. We confirmed that bone marrow-derived EPCs may contribute to the tissue repair by augmenting neovascularization following spinal cord injury, thus we think that these cells can be applied to the ligament tissue engineering in the future [53].

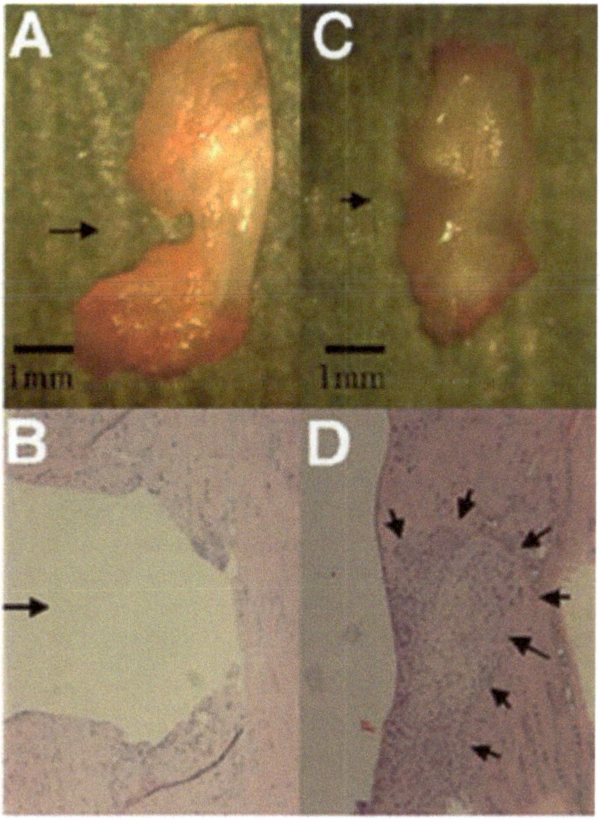

Fig. 43.2 Specimen at 4 weeks: macroscopic observations in (**a**) MSC(−) group and (**c**) MSC(−) group and histological appearance in (**b**) MSC(−) group and (**d**) MSC(−) group (H&E staining, original magnification × 100) (*arrows*, transected area)

43.2.3 Application of miRNAs

In addition to cell therapy, we examined the potential of tissue regeneration by miRNA which are important in biological processes and human diseases. MiRNAs are a class of noncoding RNA that regulate gene expression posttranscriptionally and are recognized as one of the major regulators of a variety of biological processes, for example, the cell cycle, immune function, and metabolism [54, 55]. MiRNAs regulate gene expression by binding 30 UTR of their target mRNAs before translational repression or mRNA degradation. Many miRNAs are evolutionarily conserved across phyla, identified from nematodes to humans. Because miRNAs are of crucial importance in the pathogenesis of human diseases, including in the orthopedic field, miRNAs have attracted attention for developing a novel therapeutic strategy. To date, hundreds of human miRNAs have been identified, and they are known to regulate several mRNAs with distinct effects on individual genes in a single cell. Several therapeutic trials examining the regulation of endogenous miRNAs that are related to disease pathogenesis through *in vivo* administration of specific antisense oligoribonucleotides or double-stranded miRNAs have been reported [56–58].

MiRNA-210 (miR-210) is known to be extremely important in angiogenesis and is upregulated in response to hypoxia, subsequently affecting endothelial cell survival, migration, and differentiation. Overexpression of miR-210 in endothelial cells can stimulate the formation of a capillary structure [59]. We hypothesized that miR-210 administration by intra-articular injection would accelerate ACL healing via enhancement of angiogenesis [60]. We created an ACL partially transected model in rats and injected intra-articular double-stranded (ds) miR-210 with atelocollagen soon after injury. Histological analysis confirmed that the transected area was covered with healing tissue by miR-210 injection at 4 weeks after injury (Fig. 43.3). We confirmed that an intra-articular injection of miR-210 mimic could improve the biomechanical properties of partially transected ACL, achieving good coverage of healing tissue with abandoned vessels on the injured site by upregulation of VEGF, FGF2, and collagen type 1, suggesting the possibility of miRNA therapy for ACL injury.

Interestingly, several miRNA candidates for fibrosis or tendon fibroblast proliferation and osteogenesis have been reported. For example, miR-21, miR-29b, miR-133b, miR-155 and let-7 were reported to have relationships with fibrosis or tendon fibroblast proliferation, and miR-26a and miR-222 were reported to have an osteogenic potential [61–63]. Thus, it is likely that the combination of miRNA injection with or without surgical procedures may be more useful and have much ability for the ligament itself and for tendon to bone healing.

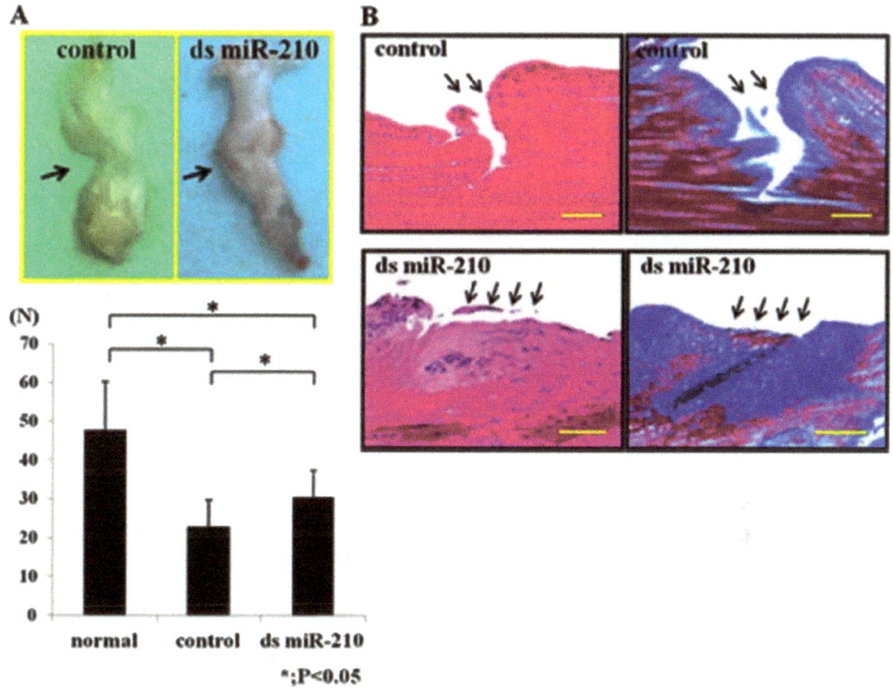

Fig. 43.3 (**a**) Macroscopic findings of the ACL at 4 weeks after intra-articular injection of ds RNA. (**b**) Histological findings of ACL at 4 weeks. *Left panels* indicate H&E staining and *right panels* indicate Masson trichrome staining. *Arrows* indicate the site of resection of ACL. (**c**) The ultimate failure load after partial resection of rat anterior cruciate ligament (n = 5). The ultimate failure load of the ds miR-210 group was significantly higher than that of the control group at 4 weeks after surgery (Data were calculated as means ± SD. *;p < 0.05)

43.2.4 Cell Delivery System

For tissue regeneration, it is essential to accumulate cells effectively at the injured site. Therefore, a cell delivery system or method to accumulate cells in the desired area is required. In our experimental model, MSCs were labeled with ferumoxides, dextran-coated superparamagnetic iron oxide nanoparticles approved by the US Food and Drug Administration as a magnetic resonance contrast agent for hepatic imaging of humans. Our cell delivery system uses a minimally invasive external magnetic force device (Fig. 43.4). We originally made an external magnetic device that generated a high magnetic force, and we succeeded in accumulating magnetically labeled MSCs (m-MSCs) in the desired area [64]. Our study also confirmed that the proliferation and chondrogenic, osteogenic, and adipogenic differentiation of m-MSCs were not affected by magnetic labeling and exposure to a magnetic force. To date, clinical trials are on set in the knee joint [65].

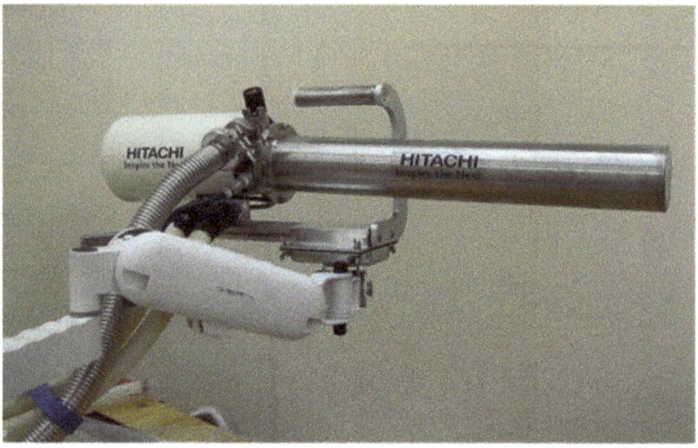

Fig. 43.4 External magnetic device

43.3 Future Perspectives

In our studies, the use of stem cells and miRNA has led to the effective regeneration of musculoskeletal tissues including ACL. The current and future objective is more effective and less invasive cell-based therapy with spatial control of transplanted cells by means of an external magnetic force.

Although the tissue engineering approach has led to the emergence of novel biologically augmented ACL repair techniques, unresolved challenges exist in optimizing these applications for ACL repair. Analysis of efficiency, safety, delivery, and maintenance methods, as well as the mechanism of tissue regeneration by cells, scaffolds, and miRNAs, is needed. This will lead to a more promising regenerative medicine, involving the development of a new generation of therapy. As for the cell therapy in tissue regeneration, its mechanism is yet to be fully elucidated. Analysis of miRNA/exosome, which circulates microvesicle packaging miRNAs in cell therapy, has the potential to clarify this mechanism, thus leading to a novel alternative cell therapy for tissue regeneration. Several reports have revealed that therapeutic trials by administration of synthetic miRNA or modified antisense in vivo have been conducted in many fields; hence, miRNA therapy in clinical orthopedics will be introduced in the near future. It is likely that the combination of miRNAs and an external magnetic device will be more useful and safe, so any accompanying challenges should be examined to discover the most effective and least invasive methods. As for the cell therapy, mobilization from bone marrow (in vivo expansion) with G-CSF (granulocyte colony-stimulating factor) and subsequent apheresis will be required in order to obtain plenty of "EPCs," because of their low frequency. Therefore, as a future option, ex vivo cell expansion by the use of optimized medium containing growth factor/cytokine cocktails has been tried, to establish a less invasive and less costly approach for EPC-assisted tissue regeneration. Furthermore, well-controlled human trials are needed to assure the ultimate efficacy of these novel approaches.

In conclusion, recent advances in the area of tissue engineering and regenerative medicine coupled with an improved understanding of the requirements for ACL healing offer great potential for new insights which would result in significant imminent achievements. The present study suggested therapeutic potential of our strategy in the treatment of ACL injury, and they will be a promising future candidate for ACL injury treatment. Future work should focus on further refinement of these techniques, in an effort to improve the clinical outcomes followed by their translation into effective human application.

References

1. Hewett TE, Di Stasi SL, Myer GD (2013) Current concepts for injury prevention in athletes after anterior cruciate ligament reconstruction. Am J Sports Med 41:216–224
2. Taylor DC, Posner M, Curl WW, Feagin JA (2009) Isolated tears of the anterior cruciate ligament: over 30-year follow-up of patients treated with arthrotomy and primary repair. Am J Sports Med 37:65
3. Hefti FL, Kress A, Fasel J, Morscher EW (1991) Healing of the transected anterior cruciate ligament in the rabbit. J Bone Joint Surg 73A:373–383
4. Ochi M, Adachi N, Uchio Y, Deie M, Kumahashi N, Ishikawa M, Sera S (2009) A minimum 2-year follow-up after selective anteromedial or posterolateral bundle anterior cruciate ligament reconstruction. Arthroscopy 25(2):117–122
5. Oryan A, Moshiri A, Meimandi-Parizi AH (2013) Graft selection in ACL reconstructive surgery: past, present and future. Curr Orthop Pract 24:321–333
6. Fithian DC, Paxton EW, Stone ML et al (2005) Prospective trial of a treatment algorithm for the management of the anterior cruciate ligament-injured knee. Am J Sports Med 33 (3):335–346
7. Fu FH, Karlsson J (2010) A long journey to be anatomic. Knee Surg Sports Traumatol Arthrosc 18:1151–1153
8. Kanaya A, Ochi M, Deie M, Adachi N, Nishimori M, Nakamae A (2009) Intraoperative evaluation of anteroposterior and rotational stabilities in anterior cruciate ligament reconstruction: lower femoral tunnel placed single-bundle versus double-bundle reconstruction. Knee Surg Sports Traumatol Arthrosc 17(8):907–913
9. Ristanis S, Giakas G, Papageorgiou CD, Moraiti T, Stergiou N, Georgoulis AD (2003) The effects of anterior cruciate ligament reconstruction on tibial rotation during pivoting after descending stairs. Knee Surg Sports Traumatol Arthrosc 11:360–365
10. Gobbi A, Diara A, Mahajan S, Zanazzo M, Tuy B (2002) Patellar tendon anterior cruciate ligament reconstruction with conical press-fit femoral fixation: 5-year results in athletes population. Knee Surg Sports Traumatol Arthrosc 10:73–79
11. Ardern CL, Webster KE, Taylor NF, Feller JA (2011) Return to the preinjury level of competitive sport after anterior cruciate ligament reconstruction surgery: two-thirds of patients have not returned by 12 months after surgery. Am J Sports Med 39:538–543
12. Chu CR, Beynnon BD, Buckwalter JA et al (2011) Closing the gap between bench and bedside research for early arthritis therapies (EARTH): report from the AOSSM/NIH U-13 Post-Joint Injury Osteoarthritis Conference II. Am J Sports Med 39:1569–1578
13. Murray JR, Lindh AM, Hogan NA et al (2012) Does anterior cruciate ligament reconstruction lead to degenerative disease?: thirteen-year results after bone-patellar tendon-bone autograft. Am J Sports Med 40:404–413

14. Moshiri A, Oryan A (2012) Role of tissue engineering in tendon reconstructive surgery and regenerative medicine: current concepts, approaches and concerns. Hard Tissue 1:11
15. James R, Kesturu G, Balian G, Chhabra AB (2008) Tendon: biology, biomechanics, repair, growth factors, and evolving treatment options. J Hand Surg [Am] 33:102–112
16. Peng H, Wright V, Usas A, Gearhart B, Shen HC et al (2002) Synergistic enhancement of bone formation and healing by stem cell-expressed VEGF and bone morphogenetic protein-4. J Clin Invest 110:751–759
17. Hankemeier S, Keus M, Zeichen J (2005) Modulation of proliferation and differentiation of human bone marrow stromal cells by fibroblast growth factor 2: Potential implications for tissue engineering of tendons and ligaments. Tissue Eng 11:41–49
18. Bray RC, Leonard CA, Saio PT (2003) Correlation of healing capacity with vascular response in the anterior cruciate and medial collateral ligaments of the rabbit. J Orthop Res 21:1118–1123
19. Petrigliano FA, McAllister DR, Wu BM (2006) Tissue engineering for anterior cruciate ligament reconstruction: a review of current strategies. Arthroscopy 22(4):441–451
20. Kobayashi D, Kurosaka M, Yoshiya S, Mizuno K (1997) Effect of basic fibroblast growth factor on the healing of defects in the canine anterior cruciate ligament. Knee Surg Sports Traumatol Arthrosc 5:189–194
21. Meike H, Patrik P, Manuela K, Lothar S, Franz J (2010) BMP12 and BMP13 gene transfer induce ligamentogenic differentiation in mesenchymal progenitor and anterior cruciate ligament cells. Cytotherapy 12:505–513
22. Miyaki S, Ushida T, Nemoto K, Shimojo H, Itabashi A, Ochiai N, Miyanaga Y, Tateishi T (2001) Mechanical stretch in anterior cruciate ligament derived cells regulates type I collagen and decorin expression through extracellular signal-regulated kinase ½ pathway. Mater Sci Eng C17:91–94
23. Wang Y, Tang Z, Xue R, Singh GK, Lv Y, Shi K, Cai K, Deng L, Yang L (2011) TGF-b1 promoted MMP-2 mediated wound healing of anterior cruciate ligament fibroblasts through NF-kB. Connect Tissue Res 52(3):218–225
24. Drury JL, Mooney DJ (2003) Hydrogels for tissue engineering: scaffold design variables and applications. Biomaterials 24:4337–4351
25. Kim BS, Putnam AJ, Kulik TJ, Mooney DJ (1998) Optimizing seeding and culture methods to engineer smooth muscle tissue on biodegradable polymer matrices. Biotechnol Bioeng 57:46–54
26. Chen J, Xu J, Wang A, Zheng M (2009) Scaffolds for tendon and ligament repair: review of the efficacy of commercial products. Expert Rev Med Devices 6:61–73
27. Natalie L et al (2015) Evaluation of polycaprolactone scaffold with basic fibroblast growth factor and fibroblasts in an athymic rat model for anterior cruciate ligament reconstruction. Tissue Eng Part A Volume 21, Numbers 11 and 12
28. Fujikawa K, Iseki F, Seedhom BB (1989) Arthroscopy after anterior cruciate reconstruction with the Leeds-Keio ligament. J Bone Joint Surg (Br) 71(4):566–570
29. Li H, Chen C, Zhang S et al (2012) The use of layer by layer self-assembled coatings of hyaluronic acid and cationized gelatin to improve the biocompatibility of polyethylene terephthalate artificial ligaments for reconstruction of the anterior cruciate ligament. Acta Biomater 8:4007–4019
30. MaCalus VH, Kawakami Y, Christopher D, Murawski BS, Fu FH (2015) Tissue engineering of ligaments for reconstructive surgery. Arthroscopy 31(5):971–979
31. Azuma H, Yasuda K, Tohyama H et al (2003) Timing of administration of transforming growth factor-beta and epidermal growth factor influences the effect on material properties of the in situ frozen-thawed anterior cruciate ligament. J Biomech 36:373–381
32. Kondo E, Yasuda K, Yamanaka M, Minami A, Tohyama H (2005) Effects of administration of exogenous growth factors on biomechanical properties of the elongation-type anterior cruciate ligament injury with partial laceration. Am J Sports Med 33:188–196

33. Nagumo A, Yasuda K, Numazaki H et al (2005) Effects of separate application of three growth factors (TGF-beta1, EGF, and PDGF-BB) on mechanical properties of the in situ frozen-thawed anterior cruciate ligament. Clin Biomech 20:283–290
34. Yoshikawa T, Tohyama H, Katsura T, Kondo E, Kotani Y, Matsumoto H, Toyama Y, Yasuda K (2006) Effects of local administration of vascular endothelial growth factor on mechanical characteristics of the semitendinosus tendon graft after anterior cruciate ligament reconstruction in sheep. Am J Sports Med 34:1918–1925
35. Pietrzak WS, Eppley BL (2005) Platelet rich plasma: biology and new technology. J Craniofac Surg 16:1043–1054
36. Vavken P, Sadoghi P, Murray MM (2011) The effect of platelet concentrates on graft maturation and graft-bone interface healing in anterior cruciate ligament reconstruction in human patients: a systematic review of controlled trials. Arthroscopy 27:1573–1583
37. Cervellin M, de Girolamo L, Bait C, Denti M, Volpi P (2012) Autologous platelet-rich plasma gel to reduce donor-site morbidity after patellar tendon graft harvesting for anterior cruciate ligament reconstruction: a randomized, controlled clinical study. Knee Surg Sports Traumatol Arthrosc 20:114–120
38. Kanaya A, Deie M, Adachi N, Nishimori M, Yanada S, Ochi M (2007) Intra-articular injection of mesenchymal stromal cells in partially torn santerior cruciate ligaments in a rat model. Arthroscopy 23(6):610–617
39. Awad HA, Boivin GP, Dressler MR, Smith FN, Young RG, Butler DL (2003) Repair of patellar tendon injuries using a cell-collagen composite. J Orthop Res 420–431
40. Ouyang HW, Cao T, Zou XH, Heng BC, Wang LL, Song XH, Huang HF (2006) Mesenchymal stem cell sheets revitalize nonviable dense grafts: implications for repair of large-bone and tendon defects. Transplantation 82:170–174
41. Pittenger MF (2008) Mesenchymal stem cells from adult bone marrow. Methods Mol Biol 449:27–44
42. Madry H, Kohn D, Cucchiarini M (2013) Direct FGF-2 gene transfer via recombinant adeno-associated virus vectors stimulates cell proliferation, collagen production, and the repair of experimental lesions in the human ACL. Am J Sports Med 41:194–202
43. Attia E, Brown H, Henshaw R, George S, Hannafin JA (2010) Patterns of gene expression in a rabbit partial anterior cruciate ligament transection model: the potential role of mechanical forces. Am J Sports Med 38:348–356
44. Hildebrand KA, Deie M, Allen CR et al (1999) Early expression of marker genes in the rabbit medial collateral and anterior cruciate ligaments: the use of different viral vectors and the effects of injury. J Orthop Res 17:37–42
45. Pascher A, Steinert AF, Palmer GD et al (2004) Enhanced repair of the anterior cruciate ligament by in situ gene transfer: evaluation in an in vitro model. Mol Ther 10:327–336
46. Schwabe P, Greiner S, Ganzert R, Eberhart J, Dahn K et al (2012) Effect of a novel nonviral gene delivery of BMP-2 on bone healing. ScientificWorldJournal 560142
47. Heyde M, Partridge KA, Oreffo RO, Howdle SM, Shakesheff KM et al (2007) Gene therapy used for tissue engineering applications. J Pharm Pharmacol 59:329–350
48. Goradia VK, Rochat MC, Grana WA, Rohrer MD, Prasad HS (2000) Tendon-to-bone healing of a semitendinosus tendon autograft used for ACL reconstruction in a sheep model. Am J Knee Surg 13:143–151
49. Rodeo SA, Arnoczky SP, Torzilli PA, Hidaka C, Warren RF (1993) Tendon-healing in a bone tunnel: a biomechanical and histological study in the dog. J Bone Joint Surg Am 75-A:1795–1803
50. L'Insalata JC, Klatt B, Fu FH, Harner CD (1997) Tunnel expansion following anterior cruciate ligament reconstruction: a comparison of hamstring and patellar tendon autografts. Knee Surg Sports Traumatol Arthrosc 5:234–238
51. Kadonishi Y, Deie M, Takata T, Ochi M (2012) Acceleration of tendon–bone healing in anterior cruciate ligament reconstruction using an enamel matrix derivative in a rat model. J Bone Joint Surg (Br) 94-B:205–209

52. Rodrigues TL, Marchesan JT, Coletta RD et al (2007) Effects of enamel matrix derivative and transforming growth factor-beta1 on human periodontal ligament fibroblasts. J Clin Periodontal 34:514–522
53. Kamei N, Kwon SM, Kawamoto A, Ii M, Ishikawa M, Ochi M, Asahara T (2012) Contribution of bone marrow-derived endothelial progenitor cells to neovascularization and astrogliosis following spinal cord injury. J Neurosci Res 90(12):2281–2292
54. Ambros V (2004) The functions of animal microRNA. Nature 431(7006):350–355
55. Bartel DP, Chen CZ (2004) MicroRNA: genomics, biogenesis, mechanism, and function. Cell 116(2):281–297
56. Elmen J, Lindow M, Schutz S, Lawrence M, Petri A, Obad S et al (2008) LNA-mediated microRNA silencing in non-human primates. Nature 452:896–899
57. Krutzfeldt J, Rajewsky N, Braich R, Rajeev KG, Tuschl T, Manoharan M et al (2005) Silencing of microRNAs in vivo with 'antagomirs'. Nature 438:685–689
58. Tazawa H, Tsuchiya N, Izumiya M, Nakagama H (2007) Tumor-suppressive miR-34a induces senescence like growth arrest through modulation of the E2F pathway in human colon cancer cells. Proc Natl Acad Sci U S A 104:15472–15477
59. Fasanaro P, D'Alessandra Y, Di Stefano V, Melchionna R, Romani S, Pompilio G, Capogrossi MC, Martelli F (2008) MicroRNA-210 modulates endothelial cell response to hypoxia and inhibits the receptor tyrosine kinase ligand ephrin-A3. J Biol Chem 283(23):15878–15883
60. Shoji T, Nakasa T, Yamasaki K, Kodama A, Miyaki S, Niimoto T, Ohuhara A, Kamei N, Adachi N, Ochi M (2012) The effect of intraarticular injection of microRNA-210 on ligament healing in a rat model. Am J Sports Med 40(11):2470–2478
61. Mendias CL, Gumucio JP, Lynch EB (2012) Mechanical loading and TGF-beta change the expression of multiple miRNAs in tendon fibroblasts. J Appl Physiol 113:56–62
62. Martin MM, Lee EJ, Buckenberger JA, Schmittgen TD, Elton TS (2006) MicroRNA-155 regulates human angiotensin II type 1 receptor expression in fibroblasts. J Biol Chem 281:18277–18284
63. Luzi E, Marini F, Sala SC, Tognarini I, Galli G, Brandi ML (2008) Osteogenic differentiation of human adipose tissue-derived stem cells is modulated by the miR-26a targeting of the SMAD1 transcription factor. J Bone Miner Res 23:287–295
64. Kobayashi T, Ochi M, Yanada S, Ishikawa M, Adachi N, Deie M, Arihiro K (2008) A novel cell delivery system using magnetically labeled mesenchymal stem cells and an external magnetic device for clinical cartilage repair. Arthroscopy 24(1):69–76
65. Kamei G, Kobayashi T, Ohkawa S, Kongcharoensombat W, Adachi N, Takazawa K, Shibuya H, Deie M, Hattori K, Goldberg JL, Ochi M (2013) Articular cartilage repair with magnetic mesenchymal stem cells. Am J Sports Med 41(6):1255–1264

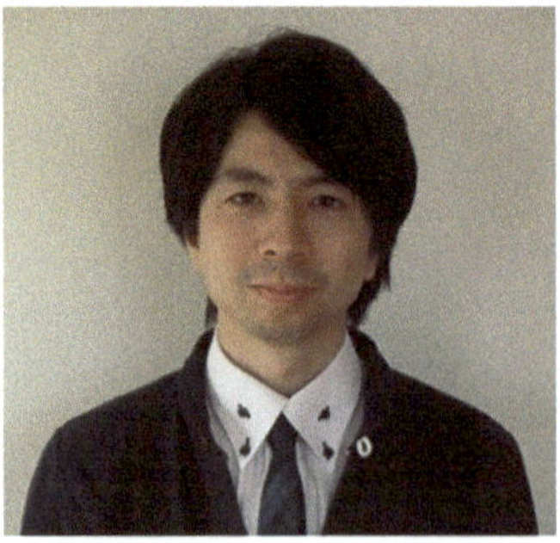

Takeshi Shoji, M.D., Ph.D. Department of Orthopaedic Surgery, Graduate School of Biomedical Sciences, Hiroshima University, Hiroshima, Japan.

Kolibri 360 GmbH
Ferdinand-Jühlke-Straße 7
99095 Erfurt, Deutschland
produktsicherheit@kolibri360.de